Recent Management in Otorhinolaryngology
(Diagnosis & Treatment)

Recent Management in Otorhinolaryngology

(Diagnosis & Treatment)

S.P.S. Yadav MS, MNAMS, FAMS
Senior Professor, Deptt. of Otorhinolaryngology, Head & Neck Surgery,
PGIMS, Pt. B.D. Sharma University of Health Sciences, Rohtak (Haryana)

R.K. Ranga MS (ENT)
Director, Bharat ENT & Endoscopy, Head and Neck Surgery Hospital,
Bhiwani (Haryana)

CBS

CBS PUBLISHERS & DISTRIBUTORS PVT. LTD.
NEW DELHI • BENGALURU • PUNE • KOCHI • CHENNAI

ISBN: 978-81-239-2049-8

First Edition : 2012

Published by Satish Kumar Jain and produced by V.K. Jain for
CBS Publishers & Distributors Pvt. Ltd.,
CBS Plaza, 4819/XI, Prahlad Street, 24 Ansari Road, Daryaganj,
New Delhi - 110 002, India
Ph.: 23289259, 23266861, 23266867 • Fax: 011-23243014
E-mail: delhi@cbspd.com, cbspubs@airtelmail.in
Website: www.cbspd.com

Branches:

- ***Bengaluru:*** 2975, 17th Cross, K.R. Road,
  Bansankari 2nd Stage, Bengaluru - 560 070
  Ph.: +91-80-26771678/79 Fax: +91-80-26771680
  E-mail: cbsbng@gmail.com, bangalore@cbspd.com
- ***Pune:*** Bhuruk Prestige, Sr. No. 52/12/2+1+3/2,
  Narhe, Haveli (Near Katraj-Dehu Road By-pass), Pune - 411051
  Ph.: +91-20-64704058/59, 32342277 • E-mail: pune@cbspd.com
- ***Kochi:*** 36/14, Kalluvilakam, Lissie Hospital Road,
  Kochi - 682018, Kerala
  Ph.: +91-484-4059061-65 • Fax: +91-484-4059065
  E-mail: cochin@cbspd.com
- ***Chennai:*** 20, West Park Road, Shenoy Nagar, Chennai - 600030
  Ph.: +91-44-26260666, 26208620 • Fax: +91-44-42032115
  E-mail: chennai@cbspd.com

Printed at:
Aegean Offset Printers, Greater Noida (UP)

Dedicated to

Our Parents,

Teachers

and

Beloved Students

Foreword

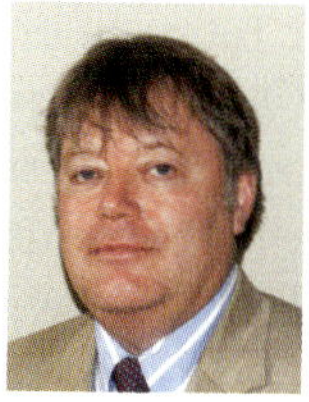

Otolaryngology is a speciality which attracts surgeons who pioneer and embrace new technology, as well as adapt and improve tried and tested treatment methods; all with the one aim of achieving optimum patient care. It is not a specialty which stands still, but one which is at the forefront of progress. It remains essential to relate modern concepts and treatment methods, to the underlying scientific basis, and principles which underpin our practice.

It is an honour for me to write the forward to this new textbook which achieves just such a balance. The anatomic and scientific basis of ENT disease is used throughout the textbook as the foundation stones on which thorough, concise and practical descriptions of current treatment and practice is built, to deliver a comprehensive précis of contemporary management.

Whether the reader is an advanced undergraduate student, a surgeon in training, or a trained specialist wanting to update their knowledge; this book 'Recent Management in Otorhinolaryngology: Diagnosis and Management' will be an invaluable aid and guide.

The layout is clear, the full breadth of the specialty included and the emphasis on cutting edge techniques is to be welcomed in this compact and comprehensive tome. The contributors to this textbook from India and abroad are recognised experts in their fields, and their knowledge distilled to provide key learning points for the reader. The editors Dr. SPS Yadav and Dr. Rupender K Ranga are to be applauded, the contributors lauded; as the readers will be rewarded with a greater understanding and knowledge, in a specialty renowned for endeavour.

Graham J. Cox BDS FRCS
Consultant ENT Surgeon
Macmillan Head and Neck Surgical Oncologist
Honorary Senior Clinical Lecturer
Oxford University Hospitals, UK

Foreword

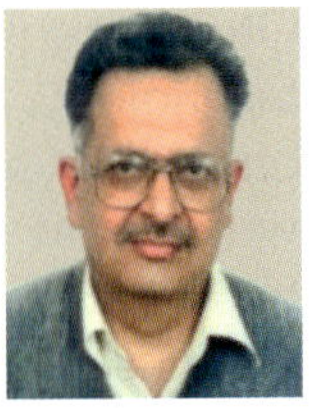

I have been privileged to write the foreword to this book 'Recent Management in Otorhinolaryngology: Diagnosis and Management'. I congratulate Prof. (Dr.) S.P.S. Yadav and Dr. Rupender K. Ranga for publishing such a wonderful and informative book.

This multi-author book under the editorship of Prof. (Dr.) S.P.S. Yadav and Dr. Rupender K. Ranga will definitely be a milestone for residents and ENT practitioners in our country and abroad. I know both the editors since they were postgraduate students, who have extensive training and experience in this field and are certainly well qualified to complete this dynamic work. The editors and chapter authors are pioneers in their respective fields of otorhinolaryngology and head & neck surgery. This book covers 47 chapters with broad spectrum of recent advances in the field of otorhinolaryngology and head & neck surgery in the form of anatomy, pathology, investigations, medical and surgical treatment.

Overall, the book is easy to read, very well illustrated, not only with microscopic, endoscopic and cadaveric photographs, but also with a lot of illustrative drawings which complement and add to the quality of chapters.

I believe that this book will be an excellent academic contribution, valuable tool and boon to all MS, DLO, DNB students as well as otorhinolaryngologists across the world in the field of recent advances: diagnosis and management. The book is definitely very promising for the future.

Prof. (Dr.) S.K. Kacker
M.S., F.R.C.S. (London), F.A.M.S.
Otorhinolaryngologist and Head & Neck Surgeon,
Former Director & Prof., AIIMS, New Delhi

Preface

The concepts in otorhinolaryngology have dramatically changed over the last few decades. The impetus for this book 'Recent Management in Otorhinolaryngology: Diagnosis and Treatment' was to highlight the major paradigm shifts and bring them together in one volume. The book was written to provide comprehensive review, concise, complete and accessible clinical information with recent advances in the diagnosis and management. In almost every chapter one can find important insights or pearls that, until now, have only been taught verbally by mentors to students.

As otorhinolaryngologists it is our privilege and duty to continually expand the scope of knowledge about recent advances in diagnosis and management and to develop new and better treatment modalities. Authors believe that "A picture is worth a thousand words and seeing believes".

All the chapters have been designed to understand surgical anatomy, pathophysiology as well as basic clinical, radiological evolution and treatment either by medical or surgical means. In the last few decades there has been dramatic developments in medical technology like high definition microscopes, wide-angle telescopes and cameras with image-guided sinoscopy, high power microdebrider, laser, radiofrequency, gamma knife, CT, MRI, PET, cochlear implant and robotic surgery. All these have contributed to make it be possible in the present which was impossible in the past.

After 19th century these were the evidence-based advances with comprehensive knowledge about pathophysiology and treatment of ear, nose, throat, head & neck ailments. The cosmetic surgery is also not lagging behind. It is the desire of everyone to have a graceful look of head & neck region, so rhinoplasty, laser surgery, augmentation plasty and hair transplant procedures have assumed much significance now-a-days.

We are highly indebted to all the contributing authors from India and abroad who have shared their time and experience to help us in bringing out this edition of the book. Among these authors are oto-rhinolaryngologists, head & neck surgeons and other specialists who are pioneers in their fields.

In this edition, we have selected topics in the fields of ear, nose, throat, head & neck region that will help to solve the challenging clinical situations in day-to-day practice when confronted with ear, nose, throat, head & neck and cosmetic ailments after primary medical care. We hope that these articles in the book will help and guide the otorhinolaryngologists and head & neck surgeons.

We wish that readers enjoy reading this text and feel enlightened by the recent advances within field of otorhinolaryngology and head & neck surgery. It will up quest the knowledge, best possible patient care and keeping otorhinolaryngology as the most vibrant of medical specialities.

Utmost care has been taken to minimize the mistakes but as you all know it is never perfect. Readers are requested to write back/email to point out any errors which will be corrected in the next edition. Suggestions and criticism are welcome with open arms.

Prof. (Dr.) S.P.S. Yadav
Sr. Prof., Deptt. of Otorhinolaryngolgy,
Head & Neck Surgery, PGIMS,
Pt. B.D. Sharma University of Health Sciences,
Rohtak (Haryana)
Email: bharatentbwn@sify.com

Dr. Rupender K. Ranga
Director, Bharat ENT & Endoscopy,
Head & Neck Surgery Hospital,
Rohtak Gate, Bhiwani (Haryana)
Email: rupenderent@yahoo.co.in

Acknowledgement

Praise to the Almighty God, who made us able to complete this book successfully.

Today, otorhinolaryngology, head & neck surgery is developing at an incredibly rapid pace. In this era, it is essential to update our knowledge on recent advances in diagnosis and management. Efficient and appropriate management of ear, nose, throat, head & neck ailments will improve our name and fame in the society.

We are highly indebted to all the contributing authors from India and abroad who have shared their time and experience to help us in bringing out this edition of the book. Among these authors are otorhinolaryngologists, head & neck surgeons and other specialists who are pioneers in their fields.

We would like to express our sincere thanks to all the contributors from our country and abroad who supported us in all respects to make this endeavour successful.

We are thankful to Surender Sabharwal, Anil Bhayana and Chand Ram Brar. We are also thankful to Brij Mohan Singh, Dharmvir and Anurag Trivedi of CBS Publishers & Distributors Pvt. Ltd. who constantly supported us to complete the format of the book.

We are sure this book will prove a milestone in the recent diagnosis and management in ear, nose, throat, head & neck ailments.

Prof. (Dr.) S.P.S. Yadav
Sr. Prof., Deptt. of Otorhinolaryngolgy,
Head & Neck Surgery, PGIMS,
Pt. B.D. Sharma University of Health Sciences,
Rohtak (Haryana)
Email: bharatentbwn@sify.com

Dr. Rupender K. Ranga
Director, Bharat ENT & Endoscopy,
Head & Neck Surgery Hospital,
Rohtak Gate, Bhiwani (Haryana)
Email: rupenderent@yahoo.co.in

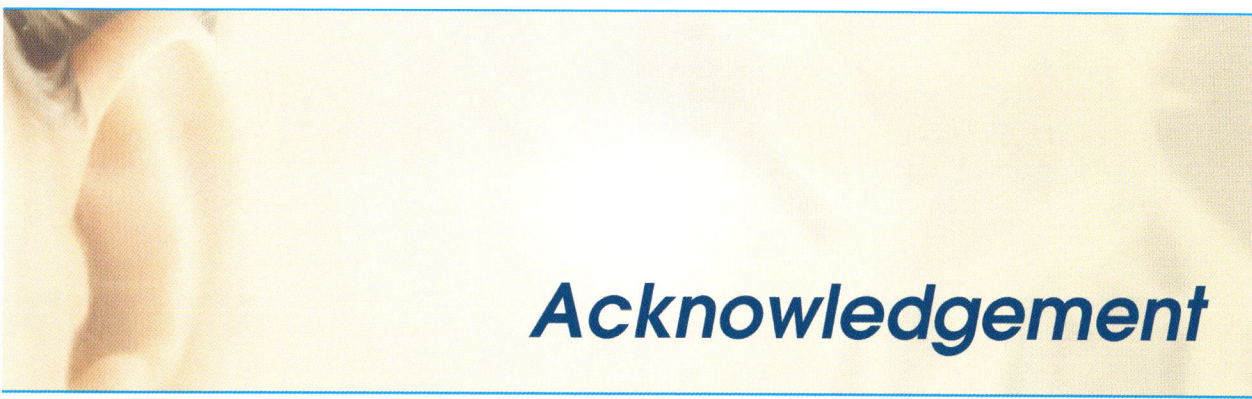

I sincerely acknowledge my esteemed teachers Prof. S.K. Kacker, Prof. P. Ghosh, Dr. B.M. Abrol and Dr. V.P. Sood who imparted the knowledge to me in the subject of otolaryngology during my training as postgraduate student in AIIMS. I also acknowledge all my postgraduate students who are responsible more or less for whatever I have achieved as a teacher.

Prof. (Dr.) S.P.S. Yadav

This book was made possible because of my close academic association with my eminent teacher Dr. (Prof.) S.P.S. Yadav. I am indebted to him for being a dynamic, wonderful teacher, mentor and for unlimited patience, generously sharing his profound knowledge and wisdom with me. His consummate skill to guide, interpretation, continuous constructive criticism with newer ideas has been an inspiration to me. He is always accessible, helpful and without his guidance this book would not have seen the light of the day.

Gratitude to my father late Sh. Jage Ram Ranga and my mother Smt. Murti Devi who inspired and blessed me to make the format of the book lucid, illustrative and comprehensive.

I am grateful to my wife Dr. Saroj Bala for her unconditional love and support and sacrifices to take care of my children Bharat and Himanshi for their studies and healthy environments.

I am also grateful to Mr. Brij Mohan Singh of CBS Publishers & Distributors Pvt. Ltd. for encouraging me to publish this book.

Dr. Rupender K. Ranga

List of Contributors

Dr. Arpit Agrawal
Resident, Deptt. of Otorhinolaryngolgy,
Head & Neck Surgery, PGIMS,
Pt. B.D. Sharma University of Health Sciences,
Rohtak (Haryana)
Email: arpitcalling@yahoo.co.in

Dr. Rahul Agrawal
Agrawal ENT Hospital & Research Institute,
H-15, Chetakpuri, Gwalior (M.P.)
Email: agrawalrahul77@rediffmail.com.

Dr. R.G. Aiyer
Prof. & Head, Dept. of ENT, Head & Neck Surgery,
SSG Hospital & Medical College, Vadodara
(Gujarat)
Email: drrgaiyer@hotmail.com

Dr. P.K. Anand
Director, Anand Nursing Home, Rohtak Gate,
Bhiwani (Haryana)
Email: drpkanand@yahoo.co.in

Dr. Vipin Arora
Assistt. Prof., Deptt. of ENT, UCMS & GTB Hospital,
Delhi
Email: vipinar@yahoo.com

Dr. Saroj Bala
Medical Officer, In-charge ESI Dispensary,
Bhiwani (Haryana)
Email: sarojranga17@gmail.com

Dr. Gaurav Bambha
Resident, Deptt. of ENT, Govt. Medical College,
Chandigarh (U.T.)
Email: gauravbambha@yahoo.co.in

Dr. S.K. Bansal
Anesthesiologist, Bansal Villa, Jhankar Road,
Bhiwani (Haryana)
Email: skbansal55@gmail.com

Prof. (Dr.) Brajendra Baser
Director, Akash Hospital, Prof. & HOD, Deptt. of
Otorhinolaryngology, SAIMS Medical College,
Indore (MP)
Email: baserbv@gmail.com

Dr. P.S. Bhandari
Prof., Deptt. of Burns and Plastic Surgery,
G.B. Pant Hospital, New Delhi - 2
Email: drpsbhanddari@yahoo.com

Dr. Patrick J. Bradley
Prof. of Head & Neck, Oncologic Surgery, Deptt. of
Otorhinolaryngology, Head & Neck Surgery,
University Hospitals, Nottingham NG7 2UH,
England
Email: pjbradley@zoo.co.uk

Dr. Grace Budhiraja
Sr. Resident, Deptt. of Otolaryngology & Head &
Neck Surgery, PGI MER, Chandigarh (U.T.)
Email: dr.gracebudhiraja148@yahoo.co.in

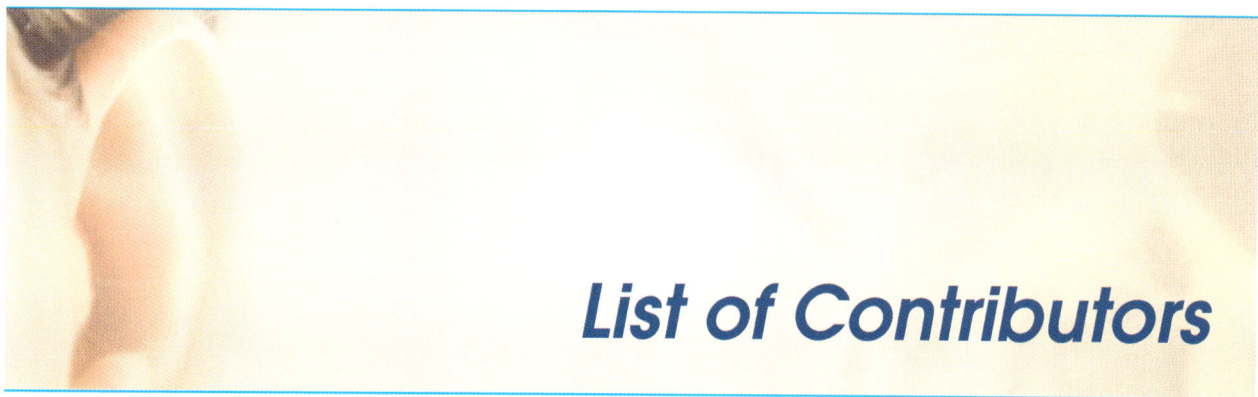

Dr. Arjun Dass
Prof. & Head, Deptt. of ENT, Govt. Medical College, Chandigarh (U.T.)
Email: adkusum@yahoo.com

Dr. Anuj Goel
Assistant Prof. Deptt. of Otorhinolaryngology, Saraswathi Institute of Medical Sciences, Hapur (U.P.)
Email: dranujgoel@rediffmail.com

Dr. Joginder Singh Gulia
Prof., Deptt. of Otorhinolaryngolgy, Head & Neck Surgery, PGIMS, Pt. B.D. Sharma University of Health Sciences, Rohtak (Haryana)
Email: jsgulia@hotmail.com

Dr. A.K. Gupta
Prof. & Head, Deptt. of Otolaryngology & Head & Neck Surgery, Unit-II, PGI MER, Chandigarh (U.T.)
Email: akpgi@yahoo.com

Dr. Nishi Gupta
Associate Director & Head, Deptt. of ENT, Dr. Shroff's Charity Eye Hospital, New Delhi
Email: gupta_nishi@hotmail.com

Dr. Rajeev Gupta
ENT Consultant, Sir Ganga Ram Hospital, New Delhi
Email: rgentclinic2@yahoo.co.in

Dr. K.K. Handa
Director, Deptt. of Otorhinnolaryngology, Head & Neck Surgery, Medanta Medicity, Gurgaon (Haryana)
Email: handak@hotmail.com

Dr. Bachi T. Hathiram
Prof. & Head, Deptt. of Otolaryngology & Head & Neck Surgery, TN Medical College & BYL Nair Charitable Hospital, Mumbai - 8
Email: bachi.hathiram@rediffmail.com

Dr. Abdulla Ibrahim
Associate Prof., Deptt. of ORLHNS, MOH, Dubai, UAE
Email: draibrahim@gmail.com

Dr. Narayan Jayashankar
Deptt. of Otorhinolaryngology, Head & Neck Surgery, Dr. Balabhai Nanavati Hospital, Mumbai
Email: drnaryanj@gmail.com

Prof. (Dr.) Mohan Kameshwaran
Consultant, Deptt. of Implant Otology, Madras ENT Research Foundation, Chennai (T.N.)
Email: merfmk30@yahoo.com

Dr. Vicky S. Khattar
Assistant Professor, Deptt. of Otolaryngology & Head & Neck Surgery, TN Medical College & BYL Nair Charitable Hospital, Mumbai - 8
Email: vickykhattar@rediffmail.com

Dr. Shenal Kothari
Associate Professor, Deptt. of Otorhinolaryngology, SAIMS Medical College, Indore (MP)
Email: drshenal@gmail.com

Dr. Agadurappa Mahadevaiah
Consultant, Basavanagudi ENT Care Centre and Sagar Apollo Hospital, Bengaluru
Email: bent@bgl.vsnl.net.in

Dr. Ravi Mehar
Associate Prof., Dept. of ENT, Head & Neck Surgery, MAMC, New Delhi
Email: ravimehar@gmail.com

Dr. Madhuri Mehta
Director, Deptt. of ENT, Jindal Institute of Medical Sciences, Hissar (Haryana)
Email: madhurimehta@gmail.com

Dr. Firdous Quader Minu
Consultant, ENT, Head & Neck and Cosmetic Surgery, Cosmetic Surgery Centre Ltd., 72, Satmasjid Road, Dhaka - 1209, Bangladesh
Email: fqm_ent@yahoo.com

Dr. Sonal Modi
Director, Laddha ENT Institute, Akola (Maharashtra)
Email: sonalrmodi2003@yahoo.co.in

Dr. Anil K. Monga
Sr. Consultant, Sir Ganga Ram Hospital, New Delhi
Email: dramonga@yahoo.com

Dr. K.P. Morwani
Chief, Deptt. of Otorhinolaryngology, Head & Neck Surgery, Dr. Balabhai Nanavati Hospital, Mumbai
Email: drmorwani@gmail.com

Dr. Ashutosh Nangia
Sr. Resident, Deptt. of Otorhinolaryngology, Head & Neck Surgery, Safdarjang Hospital, New Delhi
Email: anangia@hotmail.com

Dr. Deepti Jain Nangia
DNB (Std), Deptt. of Otorhinolaryngology, Head & Neck Surgery, Safdarjang Hospital, New Delhi
Email: docdips11@yahoo.co.in

Dr. Inder Pal Nangia
Director, Nangia ENT Hospital, 118 Model Town, Gurgaon (Haryana)
Email: ipnangia@yahoo.com

Dr. Dipak Ranjan Nayak
Prof. & Head, Deptt. of ENT - Head & Neck Surgery, Kasturba Medical College, Manipal (Karnataka)
Email: drnent@rediffmail.com

Dr. C. Preetam
Sr. Resident, Deptt. of Otorhinolaryngology, Head & Neck Surgery, AIIMS, New Delhi

Dr. N. Prepageran
Prof., Department of Otorhinolaryngology, University of Malaya Medical Center, Kuala Lumpur - 50603, Malaysia
Email: prepageran@yahoo.com

Dr. S. Raghunandhan
Consultant, Deptt. of Implant Otology, Madras ENT Research Foundation, Chennai (T.N.)
Email: drraghunandhan@sify.com,

Dr. Rajesh Rajput
Sr. Professor & Head, Deptt. of Endocrinology, PGIMS, Pt. B.D. Sharma University of Health Sciences, Rohtak (Haryana)
Email: drrajeshrajput@live.in

Prof. (Dr.) Balakrishnan Ramaswamy
Prof. & Head of ENT, Head & Neck Surgery Deptt., Kasturba Medical College, Manipal - 576104 (Karnataka)
Email: baluent@yahoo.com

Dr. Rupender Kumar Ranga
Director, Bharat ENT & Endoscopy, Head & Neck Surgery Hospital, Rohtak Gate, Bhiwani (Haryana)
Email: rupenderent@yahoo.co.in

Dr. Rijuneeta
Associate Professor, Deptt. of Otolaryngology & Head & Neck Surgery, PGI MER, Chandigarh (U.T.)
Email: rijuneeta@yahoo.com

Dr. Sanjay Sachdeva
Director, ENT Head & Neck Surgery, Fortis Healthcare, New Delhi
Email: sachi25@gmail.com

Dr Ravi Sehrawat
Resident, Deptt. of CTVS, PGIMS, Pt. B.D. Sharma University of Health Sciences, Rohtak (Haryana)

Dr. Rohtas Singh Sehrawat
Reader, Deptt. of Anesthesiology, JCD Dental College, Sirsa (Haryana)

Dr. J.B. Sharma
Sr. Consultant, Deptt. of Medical Oncology, Action Cancer Hospital, Paschim Vihar, New Delhi - 110063
Email: dr_sharmajb@rediffmail.com

Dr. Shruti
Sr. Resident, Deptt. of Otolaryngology and Head & Neck Surgery, PGIMER, Chandigarh (U.T.)

Dr. Sayeed Ahmed Siddiky
Consultant, ENT, Head & Neck and Cosmetic Surgery, Cosmetic Surgery Centre Ltd., 72, Stamasjid Road, Dhaka - 1209, Bangladesh
Email: surgeon.siddiky_2004@yahoo.com

Dr. G.B. Singh
Associate Professor, Deptt. of Otolaryngology, Head & Neck Surgery, Lady Hardinge Medical College & Associated Hospital, New Delhi - 110001.
Email: gbsnit@yahoo.co.in

Dr. Ishwar Singh
Director Prof., Deptt. of ENT & Head & Neck Surgery, MAMC, Associated Lok Nayak Hospital, New Delhi - 110002
Email: drishwarsinghmamc@yahoo.co.in

Dr. Jagat Singh
Professor, Deptt. of Otorhinolaryngolgy, Head & Neck Surgery, PGIMS, Pt. B.D. Sharma University of Health Sciences, Rohtak (Haryana)
Email: drjagatsingh@gmail.com

Dr. Jagdeepak Singh
Associate Professor & Incharge, ENT-II, Govt. Medical College, Amritsar (Punjab)
Email: singhjagdeepak@yahoo.co.in

Prof. (Dr.) P.P. Singh
Director-Professor & Head, Deptt. Of ENT, UCMS & GTB Hospital, Delhi
Email: drppsingh@hotmail.com

Rahul Jeet Singh
Rahul Computers, Bhiwani (Haryana)
Email: rahul0105@yahoo.co.in

Dr. Surinder K. Singhal
Associate Professor, Deptt. of ENT, Head & Neck Surgery, Govt. Medical College Hospital, Chandigarh (U.T.)
Email: singhalsks@gmail.com

Dr. Sanjay Singla
Director, Singla Hospital, Opp. Court, Bhiwani (Haryana)
Email: sanjay5050@rediffmail.com

Dr. Shubhrica
9J/30 Medical Enclave, PGIMS, Pt. B.D. Sharma University of Health Sciences, Rohtak (Haryana)

Dr. Susheela Taxak
Prof. Deptt. of Anesthesiology, PGIMS, Pt. B.D. Sharma University of Health Sciences, Rohtak (Haryana)
Email: susheela_taxak@hotmail.com

Dr. Alok Thakkar
Additional Professor, Deptt. of Otorhinolaryngology & Head & Neck Surgery, AIIMS, New Delhi
Email: drathakar@gmail.com

Dr. Anshul Vijay
Resident, Deptt. of Otorhinolaryngology, SAIMS Medical College, Indore (MP)

Dr. Vicknes Waran
Professor, Division of Neurosurgery, University Malaya Medical Centre

Dr. Jyoti Yadav
Prof. Deptt. of Physiology, PGIMS, Pt. B.D. Sharma University of Health Sciences, Rohtak (Haryana)

Neha Yadav
Speech Therapist and Audiologist, Bharat ENT Endoscopy Hospital, Rohtak Gate, Bhiwani
Email: nehayaduvanshi.aslp@gmail.com

Prof. (Dr.) S.P.S. Yadav
Sr. Prof. Deptt. of Otorhinolaryngolgy, Head & Neck Surgery, PGIMS, Pt. B.D. Sharma University of Health Sciences, Rohtak (Haryana)
Email: bharatentbwn@sify.com

Contents

SECTION 4

SECTION 5

SECTION 6

SECTION 7

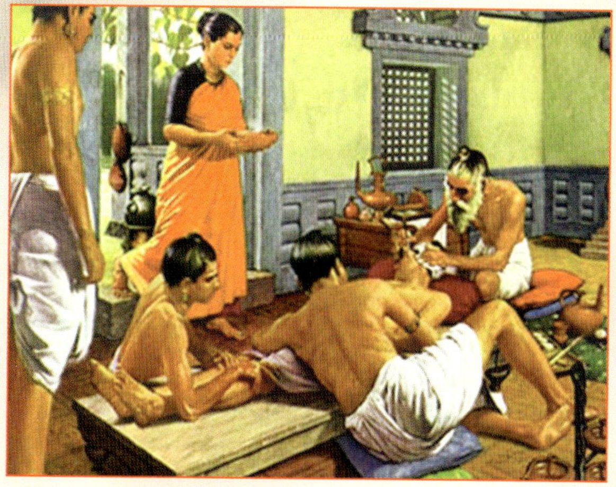

SECTION 1

History of Otorhinolaryngology

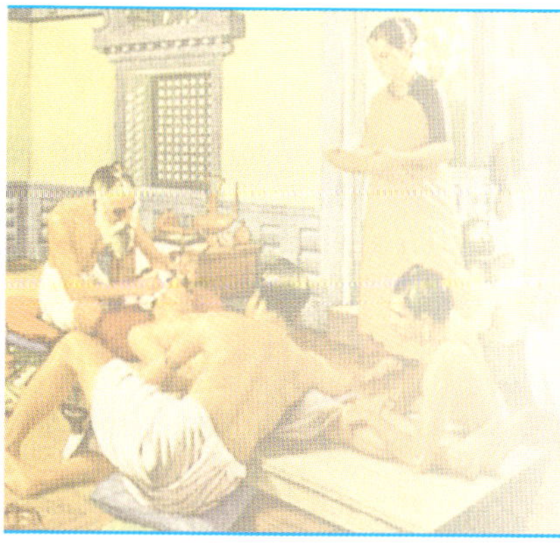

CHAPTER 1

Otorhinolaryngology: Past, Present and Future

S.P.S. Yadav, Jagat Singh, R.K. Ranga

The ears, nose and throat have intrigued mankind since the earliest time. The early attention towards them was due to their relations to breathing, eating, smell, taste, hearing and the cosmetic reasons. The folklore remedies are being used since the prehistoric time, like wearing of rings in the ear to cure wean ears, black lamb's wool to ward off deafness, juice of snail, a wild goat's gall, urine of bull, the blood of moles and juice of plants, vegetables and fruit as ear drops. For nose bleeds, the patient's own blood, hemlock, moss and many other plant remedies; cold water and vinegar or salt poured over the forehead. For the affection of the throat – liniment derived from centipedes, juice of crab, and owl's brain; plant remedies as bishop wart and garlic; local applications such as the dung of lamb, the juice of a snail, gargles of sheep's or goat's milk, etc.

Ancient history

The first medical evidence found in the Egyptian tomb at Thebes of Pharaoh Sahura dating back to the 5th dynasty (c. 3500 BC) a tablet is dedicated to a physician who made his nostril well. Oldest surgical treatise, the Edwin Smith Papyrus (17th century BC), describes treatment of fractured nose.

Atharva Veda (Ca 700 BC) contains much medical information including the diseases of ears, nose and throat regarding quinsy, uvulotomy and possibly tonsillectomy. Fractured nose was treated by raising the depressed bone by special instrument and maintained with a hollow tube in the nostril. The most noteworthy achievement was creating of new noses by flaps from cheek or forehead to replace the lost tissue of noses as a punishment of adultery.

Hippocrates (400 BC) no longer considered medicine as magic. He is remembered for his noble ethical code, "the Hippocratic oath". He was also the first to examine the tympanic membrane. Hippocrates removed the nasal polyps and observed associated high palate with irregular teeth. One of his most interesting observations is otitis and meningitis after head injury. He advocated fracture setting of nose within 36 hours of injury. He wrote that ulcers on tonsils with formation of spider web membrane was not good sign as they bring breathing difficulty (probably diphtheria).

Aristotle (384–322 BC) the philosopher physician laid the foundations of comparative anatomy and embryology. Celsius a first century Roman nobleman wrote a medical encyclopedia "De Medicina" in 8 volumes. He stated that otitis might lead to death or insanity. He advised killing of the insect with vinegar before removal from ear. An incision into the palate above uvula was recommended for quinsy and gave earliest description of dissection method of tonsillectomy with finger nails and bistoury.

Aretaeus of Cappadocia (about 80–160 AD) described the tracheostomy for relief of suffocation.

Galen (131 AD) first applied the term labyrinth to the inner ear. He described that the auditory nerve connected the ear with the brain. He noted that otitis media was a sequel of infectious diseases and can cause intracranial complication. He advocated removal of carious bone by an incision behind the ear. He described the anatomy and physiology of the upper airway. He observed that the air follows a curve before entering trachea which has two advantages – (1) the deflection allows cold air to warm, and (2) pollutants do not land directly in trachea. He thought the larynx was the instrument of voice. He was first to describe the laryngeal ventricle and the vocal cords. Galen recognized six pairs of intralaryngeal muscles and divided them as openers and closures of larynx. He interrupted the recurrent nerves to produce aphonia.

Middle ages and the renaissance

After the fall of Western Roman Empire in 476 AD, there were centuries of stagnation in the management of the ear, nose and throat diseases. In the east, Byzantine compilers wrote synopsis of medicine and surgery of early years of Christian era. The one achievement of Byzantine was to preserve the culture and manuscripts of ancient Greece, and with the fall of Constantinople in 1453, the priceless manuscripts and art treasures disseminated throughout the Mediterranean countries, particularly in Italy.

The work of Aetius (500–550 AD) described tonsillectomy. It also described that the visible foreign body in the throat should be removed with forceps; otherwise, the patient is given a piece of raw meat on a string, which was pulled up after swallowing. Alexander (525–605) forbid opium in otitis as it disguised the symptoms.

Paul (Paulus Aegineta, 690), the last Byzantine compiler wrote earache may be cured by oil in which onion has been boiled. The nasal polyps should be removed with polypus scalpel and for inaccessible polyp a knotted cord is introduced into nose and pulled out through mouth. He described the laryngotomy in cases of inflammation of mouth and palate (possibly diphtheria).

1

Renaissance – 17th century

With the Renaissance, experimental investigation, like dissection and examining bodies, came in vogue. The first anatomical textbook was the "Anathomia" written by Mundinus (1316) as a result of the practice of dissection and postmortems. Guy de Chauliac (1300–1367 AD), described the importance of anatomy as the basis of surgery. He first used the ear speculum to facilitate sunlight into meatus for removing foreign body from the ear.

Leonardo da Vinci (1452–1519), the great artist, first accurately depicted the maxillary and frontal sinuses. Andreas Vesalius (1514–1564), a Belgian physician described choana, malleus, incus, oval and round windows, fenestra anterior and posterior; maxillary, frontal and sphenoid sinuses and declared these contain air. He described the cartilages of larynx except the epiglottis. The stapes was described by Ingrassia few years later.

Bartolomeus Eustachius (1520–1574), worked exclusively on the ear. He described accurately the structure, course and relations of eustachian tube. Grabriel Pallopios (1523–1562), a surgeon and anatomist coined the terms cochlea, labyrinth, Fallopian canal, velum palate tympanum, chorda tympani, trigeminal, auditory and glossopharyngeal nerves. Fallopius invented the wire snare for the removal of nasal polypi. Volcher Coiter (1534–1600) of Holland described the tympanum, the ossicles, eustachian tube, the cochlea, auditory nerve and physiology of hearing.

Hieronmus Mercurialis (1530–1605 AD) gave the first clinical manual of otology in 1584. Antonio Musa Brasavola (1490–1554) first accurately performed laryngotomy in 1546. The trocar and cannula were used by Sanctorius (1561–1636).

Fabricius (1537–1619), a pupil of Fallopius, described structure of ear. He removed foreign body ear with small hook and warned about the injury to tympanic membrane. He gave the best description of tracheotomy. He first used vertical, instead of transverse, incision at 3rd and 4th tracheal rings and recommended two-winged cannula for tracheostomy. The word "tracheostomy" was first described by Thomas Fienus (1567–1631).

17th and 18th centuries

Highmore (1613–1685) reported a case in 1651 of dentogenic abscess of the maxillary antrum, treated by extracting canine tooth. Schneider (1614–1680), described the origin of nasal secretion from the anterior and posterior inflamed nasal mucosa rather than from the cranial cavity.

Joseph Duverney (1648–1730) described that the eustachian tube ventilated the middle ear and explained the mechanism of the bone conduction.

Antonio Scarpa (1747–1832) discovered the membranous labyrinth was a replica of the bony labyrinth. He also described the saccule, utricle, the perilymph and endolymph as the contents of bony and membranous labyrinth. Antonio Valsalva (1665–1723) divided the ear in three parts – outer, middle, and inner ear. He used the term "labyrinth" for entire inner ear and scala vestibuli and scala tympani were parts of the cochlea. He used the name "Eustachian" for the pharyngotympanic tube in honour of Eustachius and suggested "Valsalva manoeuvre" in cases of eustachian tube blockage.

Jean Louis Petit (1674–1750) removed pus from mastoid by exploring the air cells.

Giovanni Battista Morgagni (1682–1771) described the ventricles of the larynx; and nasal spurs and deviations were due to relative overside of the bones of the upper jaw. Quelmaltz (1750) published a treatise on the deviations of the nasal septum as a result of pressure in difficult labour, fall in infancy, pushing of finger in the nose in childhood as well as inflammatory conditions. George Martine (1702–1743) did the first tracheostomy in Britain and suggested the use of double tracheostomy tubes.

Benjamin Guy Babington (1794–1865) invented laryngoscope. He used a hand-mirror to reflect the light. Jonathan Wathen (1755) described the eustachian tube catheterization. Ferrein first (1742) used the term "vocal cords". Haller (1761) wrote about the role of the nose, throat and sinuses to produce the resonance.

Physick (1828) modified the uvulotome of Benjamin Bell into a tonsillotome, the predecessor of tonsil guillotine.

Flourens (1794–1867) described that the acoustic nerve has two parts – the cochlear for hearing, and the vestibular part for equilibrium. Prosper Meniere (1799–1862) suggested that the vertigo could be due to inner ear instead of intracranial disease. Today we use the term "Meniere's Disease" in his honour.

EH Weber, with the help of his brother Wilhelm, described the first tuning-fork test (1834) bearing his name "Weber's test". Adolf Rinne and D. Scwabeback of Berlin in 1885 published additional information on the tuning-fork tests.

19th century

The invention of the otoscope by Jean Pierre Bonnafont in 1834 and the laryngoscope by Turck and Czermak in the late 1850s, accelerated clinical understanding of the anatomy and pathology.

Bacteria and microorganisms were first observed with a microscope by Antonie van Leuwenhoek (1676). British surgeon Joseph Lister (1865) proved the principles of antisepsis in the treatment of wounds.

In the middle of the century, Helmholtz propounded piano theory of hearing. Thomas Buchanan published "Physiological Illustrations of the Organ of Hearing" in 1828. He recommended the use of artificial light to inspect the tympanic membrane.

James Yearsley (1805–1869) founded the Metropolitan Ear Institute in London in 1838, which later developed to the Metropolitan Ear, Nose, and Throat Hospital, the first hospital of its kind in the world. He was the first to practice as an ear, nose, and throat specialist. He performed many tonsillectomies. He introduced the "artificial ear drum", a small pellet of moistened cotton-wool placed on perforation. He suggested that "almost all diseases of the ear originate in morbid mucous membrane of the throat and nose".

Joseph Toynbee (1815–1866) dissected more than 2000 temporal bones, known as the Toynbee Collection in the Museum of the Royal College of Surgeons. He published "Disease of the Ear" in 1860. He noted that the eustachian tube was not permanently open, but lightly closed. He first described otosclerosis.

James Hinton (1822–1874) was a close and lifelong friend of Toynbee. Hinton edited the second edition of Toynbee's "Disease of the Ear". He made a supplement to the book including a number of his own observations. He noted that aural polyp arose in middle ear. He showed that the cholesteatoma might cause death by eroding the bone and spread of infection to the brain. William Wilde (1815–1876) described the method of treating acute mastoiditis, known as the "Wilde's incision".

J.F.L. Deschamps (1804) wrote the first paper on the nose and nasal sinuses and stated that the sinuses had nothing to do with olfaction. He divided nasal polypi into fungous and vascular, mucous and lymphatic, scirrhous, and sarcomatous. He recognized the symptoms of acute frontal sinusitis.

Francois Magendie (1813) described the role of epiglottis in laryngeal physiology. John Reid (1838) showed that the superior laryngeal nerve was sensory and the recurrent nerve supplies muscles, except the cricothyroid muscle.

Frederick Ryland (1837) published diseases of the larynx. Horace Green (1850) removed a laryngeal tumour before the invention of the laryngoscope. Patrick Heron Watson (1832–1907) performed the first laryngectomy in 1866 on syphilitic larynx. The patient died of pneumonia. Christian Billroth (1829–94) was the first to remove the larynx in cancer in 1873.

Gurdon Buck (1807–1877), a general surgeon in New York, was the first to perform a successful thyrotomy for the removal of a laryngeal cancer. J. Solis Cohen (1838–1927), of Philadelphia, was the first in America to perform a laryngectomy.

Hippolyte Cloquet (1821) described deviations of nasal septum, fracture of the nose and rhinoplasty. Grunwald published "Nasal Suppuration" in 1893. Adams (1875) recommended surgery on a deviated nasal septum. G. Caldwell of America (1893) and Henery Luc of France (1894) independently suggested Caldwell-Luc method. Ogston (1884) performed a frontal sinus operation. Luc of France also designed a similar operation. This method became known as the Ogston-Luc operation. Killian (1895) described an operation on the frontal sinus designed to avoid deformity. Jansen described around the same time the principles and technique of the modern frontal sinus operation.

Carl Koller (1884) used the topical cocaine for anaesthesia in eye surgery which was copied by rhinologists.

Hans Wilhelm Meyer of Copenhagen (1868) described clinical features of adenoids. Morell Mackenzie (1837–1892) is regarded as the true founder of the modern tonsil operation. His guillotine was a modification of the one devised by Physick.

Joseph P O'Dwyer (1885) intubated cases of diphtheria, however, introduction of diphtheria antitoxin by Behring in 1890–1893 reduced the number of cases requiring intubation or tracheostomy.

Manoel Garcia (1840) was the first laryngoscopist and is known as the "Father of Laryngology". John Avery (1844) invented the laryngoscope. Ludwig Turck (1857) described the clinical appearance of laryngeal disease using laryngoscope. Johann Czermak (1857) developed the first practical, precision, laryngoscope. The removal of the first laryngeal polyp with the aid of the laryngoscope was completed by G.R. Lewin on July 20th, 1860. In 1866, Mackenzie established the Throat Hospital in Golden Square, London. He published his first book, "Use of the Laryngoscope", which reviewed the history of the laryngoscope and included a description of the new instruments and methods of examination. Mackenzie's textbook, "Disease of the Throat and Nose", which had been called the "laryngologist's bible" included one volume published in 1880 that dealt with the pharynx, larynx, and trachea and a second volume published in 1884 that dealt with the nose and esophagus. In 1887, Mackenzie, with the help of Norris Wolfenden, founded the monthly "Journal of Laryngology", which added "otology", making it concerned exclusively with the speciality of otolaryngology.

On April 23, 1895, Kirstein of Berlin used a flat spatula and a Caspar's prismatic incandescent lamp to see the interior of the larynx.

19th century and 20th century

John Cunningham Saunders (1805) founded Moorfields, the first speciality hospital in London for diseases of the eye and ear. In 1816, John Harrison Curtis founded the ear dispensary and in 1845 it became the Royal Ear Hospital. In 1838, James Yearsley founded the Metropolitan Ear, Nose, and Throat Hospital. The Throat Hospital, Golden Square, was founded by Morell Mackenzie in 1863 and joined with the London Throat Hospital in 1914. In 1939, it joined with the Central London Throat and Ear Hospital which was founded by Lennox Browne in 1874 and became known as the Royal National Throat, Nose, and Ear Hospital.

In Scotland, the Edinburgh Royal Infirmary opened its ear and throat department in 1883. The Aberdeen Royal Infirmary instituted a department for diseases of the ear, nose, and throat under Henry Peterkin in 1909. In Dublin, Ireland, the St. Mark's Eye and Ear Infirmary was founded by Wilde in 1844. In Belfast, Ireland, the Eye and Ear Dispensary began in 1844.

The British journal, "Journal of Laryngology and Otology", was founded by Morell Mackenzie and Norris Wolfenden in 1887. In 1896, Gustav Killian of Freiburg, "Father of Bronchoscopy" adapted the oesophagoscope for the direct examination of the trachea.

THE DEVELOPMENT OF OTOLARYNGOLOGY

Otorhinolaryngology was founded through the amalgamation of otology and laryngology specialities with distinct, separate backgrounds. Otology existed within the realm of general surgeons, who had developed the myringoplasty (Sir Astley Cooper, 1802) and the artificial tympanic membrane (Joseph Toynbee, 1853).

Otology

The American Otological Society was founded in 1868. Most believe that otology became a separate speciality in 1861, when Dr. Adam Politzer was appointed the first lecturer in diseases of the auditory organ at the Vienna Medical School. In 1873, Dr. Politzer and his rival, Dr. Joseph Gruber, the 2 forefathers of Viennese otology, established the first department of otology at the school.

Otorhinolaryngology

In his 1907 work, "Gescichte der Ohrenheilkunde", Dr. Adam Politzer wrote that the study of otology and rhinology had been fused. In the USA the fusion of the practice of otology, rhinology, and laryngology accelerated with the 1895 founding of the American Laryngological, Rhinological, and Otological Society, "The Triological Society". American Board of Otolaryngology was created in 1924.

Julius Lempert (1938) wrote a paper on creating a new oval window. Lampert also introduced the motor-driven drill in mastoid surgery.

The American Academy of Ophthalmology and Otolaryngology (AAOO) was founded in 1903. In 1979, the academy split into the American Academy of Ophthalmology and the American Academy of Otolaryngology. In 1980 the American Academy of Otolaryngology changed its name to the American Academy of Otolaryngology – Head and Neck Surgery (AAO-HNS).

By the end of the Civil War in 1865, both the Miami Medical College and the Medical College of Ohio had established professorship in otology. In 1875, the first professorship of laryngology was established at the Medical College of Ohio. Ophthalmology and otolaryngology became separate units at the Miami Medical College in 1894. The college appointed a dynamic young surgeon, Christian Holmes, as clinical professor of otology. Holmes was instrumental in separating the study and treatment of the eye from the ear, nose and throat.

In the early years of the 20th century, otolaryngologists mostly treated ear and sinus infections. Mastoidectomies, radical maxillary sinus surgery, ethmoidectomies and sphenoidectomies were the most frequently performed procedures. Tonsillectomies and adenoidectomies were mainly performed by general practitioners. Antibiotics brought an end to acute mastoiditis and the major complications of otitis media, as well as a decline in the number of tonsillectomies and adenoidectomies.

By the 1950s, the combinations of antibiotics, asepsis, reliable anaesthesia and the operating microscope heralded a new era in the treatment for diseases of the ear, nose and throat like surgery of the labyrinth, decompression of the facial nerve, treatment of suppuration of the petrous apex of the temporal bone.

The pioneering use of the endoscope in ENT by Jackson and the implementation of the fibre optic light by Hopkins in 1953, shaped the modern ENT diagnostics and treatment.

The field of otolaryngology continued to expand in the 1970s and 1980s, incorporating head and neck oncologic surgery, neurotology and pediatric head and neck disorders, upper airway allergy, laser surgery and sinus surgery.

Aran and Lê Bel, (1968) in Bordeaux, France, established the basis for electrocochleography. Jewet et al. (1970) recorded brain stem potentials. Linear tomography was introduced in 1932. Computed tomography in 1972 and magnetic resonance imaging in 1982 improved diagnostic capabilities. Optic fibre endoscopes developed by Hopkins (1954) revolutionized endoscopy. In the last 30 years, laryngology has gradually evolved. The concept of phonosurgery by Von Leden was initially restricted to laryngeal microsurgery to remove lesions on vocal folds. Thyroplasty was published by Isshiki in 1976. In 1998, the first larynx transplant was carried out in Cleveland.

Messerklinger brought back the use of endoscopes, using it for diagnostic and surgical procedures in the nose. David Kennedy, Heinz Stammberger, Wolfgang Draf and, in Brazil, Aldo Stamm were major participants in the popularization of the use of modern endoscopy in sinonasal surgeries. CT scan also helped much in the development of functional endoscopic sinus surgery. Gerard Guiot (1970) was the first to use endoscopy for a trans-sphenoidal approach in neurosurgery.

OTOLARYNGOLOGY IN THE MILLENNIUM

Diseases of the ear, nose, throat, head and neck have a profound effect on the health and quality of life of millions of patients around the globe. New millennium brought many exciting advances like solving the puzzle of cancer.

Work is being done to develop an implantable hearing aid for "nerve" deafness. Image guidance system can make sinus surgery more precise and lead to better surgical results.

In the not-too-distant future, a new type of injectable treatment for allergic rhinitis will become available.

Current preclinical research into a tissue-engineered trachea and tissue-engineered cartilage for ear and nasal reconstruction has shown promising results and so has the brain stem implants.

Principles of Laser in otorhinolaryngology and head and neck surgery

Laser means light amplification by stimulated emission of radiation. Lasers work on the theory of stimulated emission given by Albert Einstein in 1917. Ali Javan built the first helium-neon gas laser in 1961. C. Kumar and N. Patel introduced the CO_2 laser in 1962 which was first used in head and neck surgery in 1972 by Jako and Strong.

Depending on the medium used, lasers can be classified as solid state (Ruby, Nd-YAG, KTP), semiconductor (Gallium arsenide laser), liquid, gaseous (CO_2) and free electron. The reaction of the laser energy with tissue can be photoablative, photochemical, photomechanical or photothermal. The laser light strikes tissues and scatters till all light is absorbed or reflected. The light absorbed heats up the tissues which produces a series of changes. These changes are of denaturation, coagulation, vaporization, carbonization and incandescence. Cutting using laser produces haemostasis by causing coagulation.

1

In otolaryngology lasers are used in:

- Stapedectomy/stapedotomy and tympanomastoid surgery: CO_2, KTP, Argon.
- Endonasal dacryocystorhinostomy: Holmium YAG, KTP.
- Nasal and sinus surgery, telangiectasia destruction, antrostomy and turbinate reduction: Holmium YAG, KTP, Nd YAG, Argon.
- Nasal polyposis: CO_2.

Photodynamic therapy

Photodynamic therapy is a type of photochemotherapy where, in addition to light and the drug, oxygen is administered to complete the process. The drug known as a photosensitizer accumulates within the cell and interacts with light and oxygen to produce 'singlet' oxygen which damages cell membranes leading to cell death.

This therapy has been put to use in squamous cell carcinomas of the oral cavity, nasopharynx; oesophageal carcinoma and metastatic squamous carcinoma in neck and inverted papilloma.

Contact endoscopy

Contact endoscopy was first described by Desormeaux in 1865. He had managed to obtain a direct view of the bladder mucosa. It has now been used in otorhinolaryngology to assess vocal cord pathology, nasal mucosa, nasopharynx, oropharynx, oral cavity and the trachea.

It is possible to detect microvascular changes and/or alterations in surface epithelium which are suggestive of subclinical stages of disease.

Contact endoscopy provides us with a global perspective of the disease process with the facility of cellular and vascular mapping. It can be undertaken under local anaesthesia on an outpatient basis.

The mucosal surface to be examined is gently cleaned with a saline moistened swab or gentle suction. It is then stained with 1% methylene blue applied on a piece of gelfoam. The endoscope tip is then gently placed against the mucosa for examining. This procedure needs to be carried out fast as the staining lasts for about 4–5 minutes before gradually disappearing.

Optical coherence tomography

Optical coherence tomography (OCT), a relatively new optical imaging modality, allows high-resolution, cross-sectional imaging of tissue microstructure. OCT can image with an axial resolution of 1–5 μm and has an imaging depth of 2–3 mm in non-transparent tissue.

OCT is of particular benefit in areas where non-keratinised epithelium is separated from underlying stroma by a smooth basement membrane zone. The advantages of this technique are that it can be performed in situ and nondestructively; the images are high resolution, 10–100 times that of a conventional MRI or ultrasound; the imaging is performed in real time, OCT is fibreoptically based and is therefore compatible with a wide variety of instruments. Further, OCT instruments are compact, portable and have relatively low cost.

OCT may prove helpful in the diagnosis of hyperplasia, early-stage keratosis and papillomas, and carcinoma in-situ.

Polarization-sensitive OCT is an adjunct to conventional OCT that provides information about tissue microstructure by exploiting information contained in the polarization state of the light that is backscattered or backreflected.

Image-guided surgery

This is also known as computer-aided surgery, navigational surgery and computer-guided surgery. In this MRI, CT or combined image data sets are used to create three-dimensional (3D) reconstructions of the operative volume. These 3D reconstructions can be used to plan, practice or navigate during a surgical procedure.

Preoperative imaging alerts the surgeon to anatomical variations that are inherent or caused due to the disease or previous surgery.

Two fundamental processes: registration and tracking are required for intraoperative image guidance. Registration is the process that relates the patient in the operation theatre to preoperatively taken image data sets. Tracking is the mechanism of following the position of the patient or an instrument within the operative field. There are several tracking methods, the earliest being mechanical arms fitted with potentiometers based on magnetic field distribution which are effective and cheap. However, infrared light sensors are most commonly used today. They are active or passive devices. The active ones sense infrared light from LEDs attached to the patient or location probe. The passive devices detect infrared light from metallic balls attached to the patient or probe, with the light source located on the sensing device itself.

This surgery has a good scope in areas of the skull base and endoscopic sinus surgery especially in difficult revision cases such as Draf types 2 and 3 procedures and trans-sphenoidal, trans-nasal endoscopic hypophysectomy. In otology it has helped in locating the facial nerve, identifying lesions of the petrous apex and internal acoustic meatus like meningiomas and vestibular schwannomas.

Positron emission tomography and integrated PET

Positron emission tomography provides a means of identifying pathology based on altered tissue metabolism. This functional imaging technique relies on a radioactive molecule (radiotracer) that decays with positron emission. The tracer is given intravenously and is taken into cells. This tracer is trapped in the cells more so by malignant cells which can be measured in vivo as they decay by positron emission. Positrons collide with electrons producing photons which are detected and reassembled into images that represent tracer uptake in the body part scanned. The majority of studies use 2-[18 F] fluoro-2-deoxy-D-glucose which reflects glucose metabolism. Cancer cells have a greater avidity for glucose than normal cells. It helps in detecting occult metastatic nodal disease, distant metastasis and recurrent/residual tumour. It has limited value in differentiation of benign and malignant tumours, however, it can be helpful in post-treatment evaluation. In practice, FDG-PET is routinely considered eight weeks or more following RT in head and neck malignancies. FDG-PET is also helpful in assessment of cochlear implant and their pattern on stimulation of the central nervous system.

Integrated PET/CT

The advantages of integrated PET/CT include superior localization of lesions and better distinction between physiological uptake and pathology. With PET/CT, CT is acquired followed by PET. This accurately localizes occult primary, recurrence and pulmonary metastasis not identified on FDG.

Robotic surgery

Over the past several years, major innovations have been made in the area of robotic surgical procedures. Used in a variety of different surgical settings, robotic applications have significantly simplified many complex procedures. For patients, the benefits include less blood loss, less pain, and quicker recovery times. In otolaryngology, robotic surgical techniques can be used in head and neck cancer cases, facial plastic surgery, and airway procedures.

CONCLUSION

Otorhinolaryngology is very advancing branch since time immemorial. Many eminent workers in this field contributed to light up this field. In the beginning of the 19th century they used clinical anatomical approach to make the diagnosis by matching findings on post mortem with clinical signs found in life. In 20th century lots of advances in the field of otology, rhinology, larnygology, head and neck surgery due to improvement in technology like microscope, endoscopes, laser, photodynamic therapy, image-guided endoscopy, CT, MRI and PET. Robotic surgery has simplified many complex procedures with many benefits like less blood loss, less pain and quicker recovery time.

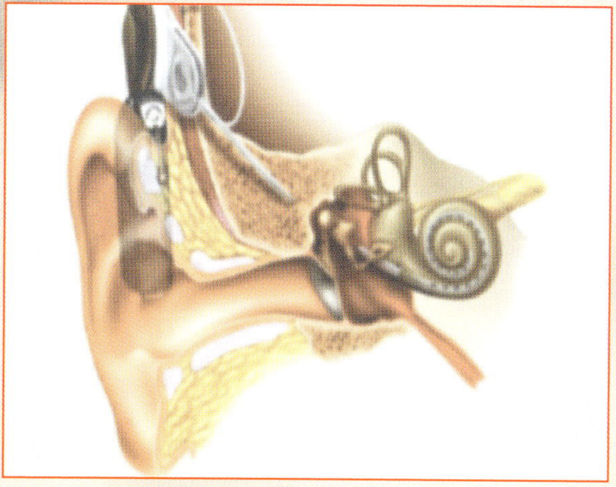

SECTION 2

Otology

CHAPTER 2

Surgical Anatomy of Temporal Bone

K.P. Morwani, Rahul Agrawal, Narayan Jayashankar

Surgical anatomy of temporal bone can be understood only by dissection. It is the most complicated bone of human body which can be mastered by regular dissection only. In this chapter we will be showing few labelled photographs of temporal bone at different stages of dissection. It will guide the readers during their dissection and will help understand the relevant surgical anatomy.

To start with dissection the reader should be well versed with the microscope, drill machine and dissection instruments.

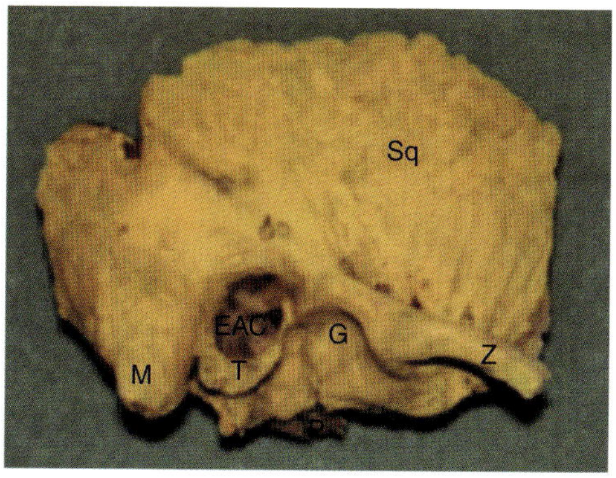

Fig. 2.1. Surface anatomy of right temporal bone. Sq – squamous part of temporal bone, Z – root of zygoma, G – glenoid fossa, T – tympanic bone, Mt – mastoid tip, P – petrous part of temporal bone, EAC – external auditory canal.

Few basic points of dissection which need to be remembered are:

1. Use of largest size of burr for any particular area.
2. Check the direction of drill bit i.e. clockwise or anticlockwise.
3. Regular suction irrigation.
4. Drilling should always be parallel to any important structure and should be medial to lateral.
5. Appreciate the colour difference in bone.
6. Use diamond burr whenever close to any important structure. How close is a matter of experience?
7. Cavity should be widened and saucerised simultaneously, so that we get adequate exposure inside.

CONCLUSION

Learning anatomy of temporal bone is first step for any otologist. For mastering otology and giving good surgical results thorough knowledge of temporal bone is essential, which can be gained only by regular dissection. This chapter is only a guide for dissection.

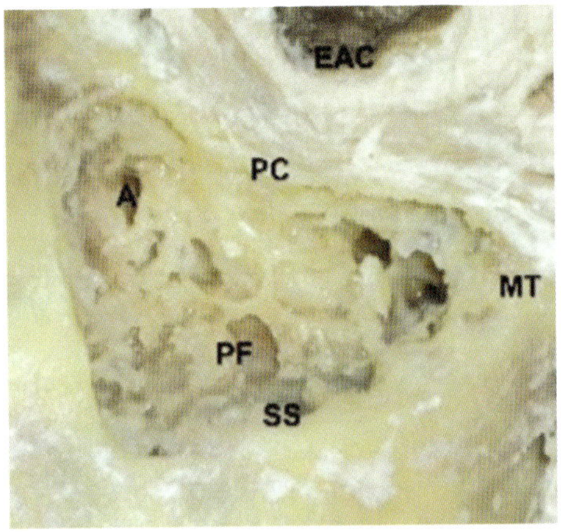

Fig. 2.2. Right temporal bone as seen when starting for cortical mastoidectomy. Antrum (A) is the first landmark to be identified, which is just coming in view. Inferior to antrum will be bulge of lateral semicircular canal. Appreciate the colour difference between the cells lateral to posterior fossa dura (PF) and that lateral to sigmoid sinus (SS). Note that cavity is widened enough to get adequate exposure of antrum. Once antrum is identified dissection is continued to delineate tegmen plate and followed posteriorly to sinodural angle, sigmoid sinus and posterior fossa dura. Once these landmarks are clear further dissection is carried out anteriorly by thinning the posterior canal wall and inferiorly by following sigmoid sinus into jugular bulb. MT – mastoid tip, PC – posterior canal wall, EAC – external auditory canal.

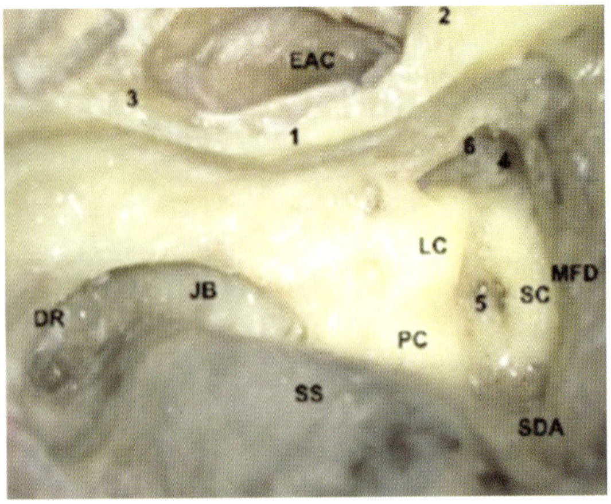

Fig. 2.4. Right temporal bone after canal wall down mastoidectomy. Note the amount of bone between posterior annulus and vertical segment of facial nerve. Removal of this bone is termed by author as thinning of facial ridge, which is required to expose the sinus tympani. Also note that anterior attic wall is in line with anterior canal wall, and inferior canal wall is in line with floor of mastoid cavity. If floor of mastoid cavity is inferior to the floor of external auditory canal then either the mastoid tip cavity should be obliterated with bone pate or muscle, or mastoid tip should be excised. MFD – middle fossa dura, SDA – sinodural angle, SS – sigmoid sinus, F (2G) – facial nerve (2nd genu), F (V) – facial nerve (vertical segment), R – round window niche, St – Stapedial tendon, P – promotory, M – malleus, I – incus, LC – lateral semi-circular canal.

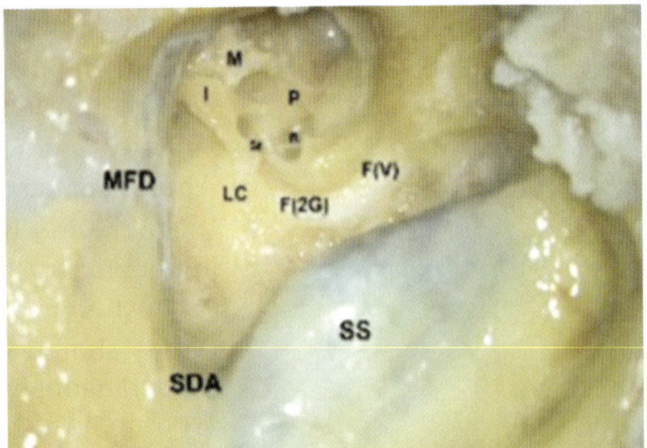

2

Fig. 2.3. Left temporal bone after cortical mastoidectomy. For identification of fallopian canal, landmarks are – anterior end of digastrics ridge (landmark for inferior end of vertical segment of facial nerve) and bulge of lateral semi-circular canal (landmark for 2nd genu). Drilling is done with a large diamond burr from above downwards with regular suction irrigation. Change in colour of bone and appearance of perifacial vessels (bleeds in surgery) indicates that fallopian canal is near. After every few strokes of drill, area should be visualized in high magnification. EAC – external auditory canal, LC – lateral semi-circular canal, SC – superior semi-circular canal, PC – posterior semi-circular canal, MFD – middle fossa dura, SDA – sinodural angle, SS – sigmoid sinus, DR – digastrics ridge, JB – jugular bulb, 1 – posterior external auditory canal wall, 2 – superior external auditory canal wall, 3 – inferior external auditory canal wall, 4 – antrum, 5 – area for sub-arcuate artery, 6 - incus.

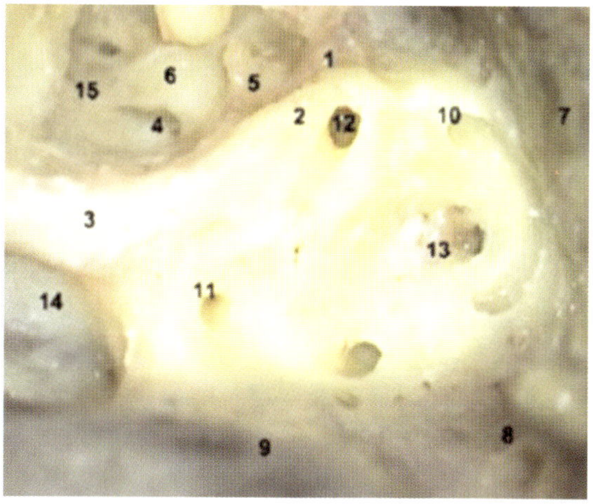

Fig. 2.5. Left temporal bone after canal wall down mastoidectomy and labyrinthectomy. Appreciate the landmarks for facial nerve. Ampullary end of superior semicircular canal is landmark for labyrinthine segment of facial nerve. Anterior wall of lateral semicircular canal is landmark for 2nd genu of facial nerve. Ampullary end of inferior semicircular canal is landmark for vertical segment of facial nerve. Once these three landmarks are identified the entire bone posterior to them can be removed up to internal auditory canal. Superior limit is middle fossa dura and inferior limit is cochlear aqueduct (landmark for lower cranial nerves). Non-ampullary end of superior and inferior canal are followed into crus commune which leads to the vestibule. 1 – facial nerve (transverse segment), 2 – facial nerve (2nd genu), 3 – facial nerve (vertical segment), 4 – round window niche, 5 – stapes, 6 – promotory, 7 – middle fossa dura, 8 – sinodural angle, 9 – posterior fossa dura, 10 – ampullary end of superior semicircular canal, 11 – ampullary end of posterior semicircular canal, 12 – ampullary end of lateral semicircular canal, 13 – area for sub-arcuate artery, 14 – jugular bulb, 15 – hypotympanum.

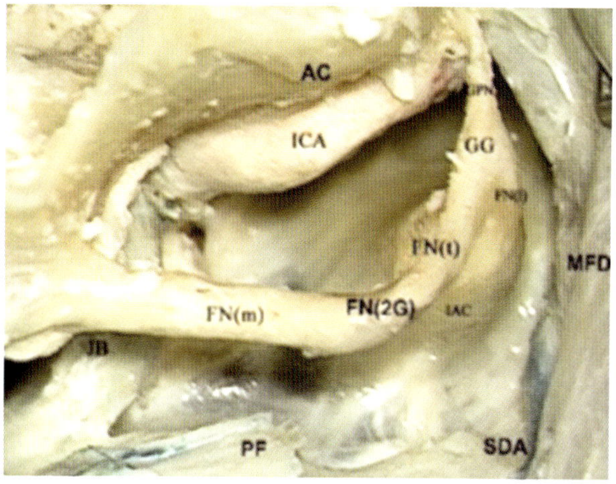

Fig. 2.6. Left temporal bone after complete temporal bone dissection leaving behind facial nerve intact. AC – anterior canal wall, ICA – internal carotid artery, GPN – greater superficial petrosal nerve, GG – geniculate ganglion, FN (t) – facial nerve (transverse segment), FN (2G) – facial nerve (2nd genu), FN (m) – facial nerve (vertical segment), IAC – internal auditory canal, MFD – middle fossa dura, SDA – sinodural angle, PF – posterior fossa dura, JB – jugular bulb.

SUGGESTED READING

1. May M. Anatomy of the facial nerve (spatial orientation of fibers in the temporal bone). *Laryngoscope*, 1973; 83 : 1311–29.
2. Gulya AJ, Schukenecht HF. Anatomy of the temporal bone with surgical implications. Parthenon Pub Group, New York, 1995.
3. Swartz JD, Harns Berger HR. Imaging of the temporal bone 3rd edition. Thieme, New York, 1998.
4. Nadal JB, Mckenna MJ. Surgery of the ear and temporal bone. Lippincott Williams & Wilkins, 2005.
5. Brackmann DE, Shelton C, Arriaga MA. Otologic Surgery, 3rd edition. Elsevier Health Science, Philadelphia, 2010.
6. Tos M. Manual of middle ear surgery: Mastoid surgery and reconstructive procedure. Thieme, New York, 1995.
7. Wiet RJ. Ear and Temporal Bone Surgery: Minimizing risks and complications. Thieme, New York, 2006.
8. Richard RG. Ear Surgery. Springer Verlag, Berlin, Heidelberg, 2008.
9. Sanna M, Khraist T, Falconim, Russo A. The temporal bone – A manual for dissection and surgical approaches. Thieme, New York, 2005.

CHAPTER 3

Otitis Media: An Overview and Recent Advances

D.R. Nayak, B. Ramaswamy

Otitis media is a major health problem around the world and is responsible for significant morbidity and financial burden for patients and lot of work for healthcare providers. Though the mortality due to complications following acute otitis media has significantly reduced in this antibiotic era, the incidence of complications due to cholesteatoma is still high especially in rural areas of developing/ underdeveloped countries. Deafness due to otitis media is often correctable with appropriate intervention. Advances in technology like CT imaging, audiology and surgical techniques have revolutionized its management but are not available to all.

Definition of otitis media

Inflammation of the mucoperiosteal lining of the middle ear cleft which may be acute or chronic.

Classification of otitis media

Acute otitis media

- Non-suppurative
    - Acute viral (non-suppurative) otitis media
    - Barotraumatic otitis media
- Suppurative
    - Acute suppurative otitis media
    - Acute necrotizing otitis media
- Reccurent acute otitis media.

Chronic otitis media

- Nonspecific
    - Chronic suppurative otitis media
        - ◊ Tubotympanic type
            - Inactive (mucosal) chronic otitis media (COM): Permanent perforation without discharge
            - Active (mucosal) COM: Permanent perforation with intermittent muco-purulent often profuse non-foul-smelling ear discharge
            - Healed COM: Tympanosclerosis; healed perforation
        - ◊ Atticoantral type
            - Inactive (squamous) COM: Retraction of pars flacida/pars tensa (usually posterior superior quadrant) with no cholesteatoma
            - Active (squamous) COM: Usually associated with foul-smelling scanty purulent ear discharge
                - Retraction pocket with cholesteatoma
                - Secondary acquired cholesteatoma
    - Chronic non-suppurative otitis media
        - ◊ Otitis media with effusion
        - ◊ Otitis media without effusion
            - Retracted TM
            - Chronic adhesive otitis media
            - Tympanosclerosis
            - Cholesterol granuloma
- Specific
    - Tuberculous otitis media
    - Syphilitic otomastoiditis

ACUTE OTITIS MEDIA

Acute otitis media refers to acute inflammation of the mucoperiosteal lining of the middle ear cleft characterized by acute pain in the ear, deafness, mucopurulent ear discharge and may be associated with complications depending on the stage of the disease.

Reccurent acute otitis media (AOM) may occur on coexisting otitis media with effusion (OME) and are interrelated. AOM is characterized by constitutional symptoms unlike OME where pain and fever etc. are absent.

Incidence

In developed countries, acute otitis media (AOM) is the most common reason for antibiotic prescription, with possible links to rising rates of antibiotic-resistant bacteria. The incidence of AOM from longitudinal birth cohort studies in developed countries range from 0.125 to 1.2 episodes per child-year. Otitis media is the cause of nearly 20% of all hearing loss (Jacob, 1998).

- ASOM is more common in children than adults. Peak incidence is at the age of 6–18 months.
- 60% of children below 1 year of age and 80% of children below 3 years of age develop at least one episode of variable severity.
- Incidence is more in boys than girls but exact reason for this relation is not known.
- It is more common in Native Americans than African Americans.
- Prevalent in rural than in urban population. This reflects on the socioeconomic factor in its causation. There is a need to improve living conditions and health services in rural areas (Minja and Machemba, 1996).

Etiopathology

ASOM is a common complication of influenza and a major complication of measles. This condition is more commonly seen in children than adults. The pathophysiology of the disease is multifactorial. The eustachian tube dysfunction following viral URTI, secondary bacterial infection, compromised immunological status, and other social and environmental factors including poor economy, overcrowding, can all contribute to the persistent and recurrent disease. Child's immune system develops with more and more immunological challenge. Hence they are immunologically more susceptible to recurrent respiratory tract infections. Moreover, the eustachian tube in a child is short, wide and horizontal compared to an adult. Feeding habits in an infant in lying down position causes nasopharyngeal reflux which can be an additional factor for developing ASOM. **Patulous eustachian tube as a result of 1st/2nd branchial arch anomalies or a hypotonic eustachian tube due to neuromuscular incoordination is often prone for bacterial infection.** Persistent nasal discharge is also responsible for its causation. **Flask model with long neck explains the role of eustachian tube in middle ear that prevents infection.** Short and wide eustachian tube as in children is prone to infection.

Risk factors include environmental tobacco smoke, season, lack of breast-feeding, younger age, respiratory viral infection, exposure to other children, immature immune system and possibly genetic factors. Children with cleft palate and Down's syndrome are prone to ear infections. First episode of ASOM before 6 months of age may be related to anatomical abnormalities or minor immunologic deficiency. Children with formula feeding are at a risk. Breast-feeding allows for passive transmission of antibodies, typically with breast-feeding for more than 3 months. Breast milk contains anti-infective agent like immunoglobulin A & G, leukocytes, complement components, interferon, glycoprotein, glycolipids, glycosaminoglycan, oligosaccharides, and lactadherin.

Milk may protect against otitis media in a child by blocking the attachment of bacterial pathogens to respiratory mucosa. Anti-inflammatory factors in the breast milk like antioxidants, lactoferrin, tumour necrosis factor, etc. limit the infection. Altered immune system like HIV, immune suppression secondary to drugs, IgA deficiency, Kartagener's syndrome are at great risk to suffer from otitis media. Immunoglobulin G2 and G4 are responsible for immunity against polysaccharide antigens and deficiency of these antibodies leads to otitis media as in Down's syndrome. Previous exposure or immunization may have a preventive role by suppressing colonization of nasopharynx by pathogens. High incidence of otitis media in twins indicate a strong genetic component being involved (Casselbrant et al., 1999).

Smoking and environmental pollutants especially passive smoking which is commonly seen among children of smokers is responsible for structural and physiological changes in respiratory mucosa and can result in goblet cell hyperplasia and hypersecretion. Heavy maternal smoking is a serious risk factor that can be associated with recurrent acute otitis media.

The innate immune system is a critical first response to infection, particularly as passive maternal antibodies decline and during the maturation of the infant adaptive immune response. Deficiency of strain-specific antibodies increases the susceptibility to recurrent infections. Swimming pools are common source of infection where pre-pool prevalence of infections is high. School/day-care going children are more prone for ASOM due to contact/droplet infection of the respiratory tract.

The factors contributing to ASOM can be summarized as follows:

Contributing factors

- Rhinitis and sinusitis
- Tonsillitis and nasopharyngitis
- Influenza and exanthemas
- Trauma of tympanic membrane
- Nasopharyngeal tumours
- Pulmonary infection
- Patulous eustachian tube
- Faulty feeding habits in infants
- Immunodeficiency syndromes
- Overcrowding
- Tobacco and pollutant exposure
- Barotrauma
- Climate change
- Chronic systemic disorders (leukemia, anemia)

Precipitating factors

- Pre-existing middle ear effusion
- Barotrauma
- Acoustic trauma
- Nasal/nasopharyngeal surgery
- Nasal/nasopharyngeal pack
- Swimming and diving

Pathogenesis

Route of spread of infection to middle ear

- Eustachian tube
- Perforation of tympanic membrane including traumatic perforation.
- Iatrogenic
  - Myringotomy/ventilation tube
  - Tympanotomy
- Haematogenous
- Peritubal lymphatics

Factors affecting the severity of infection

1. Virulence of infecting organism: More virulent organism like β-haemolytic streptococcus causing acute necrotizing otitis media.
2. Resistance and age of the patient: Affect the susceptible individual.
3. Inadequate and improper treatment: Can lead to chronic stage and can also be associated with complication. Can also cause non-suppurative middle ear effusion – persists for over 30 days in 40% of children
4. Prior infection: Makes the individual more susceptible.
5. Degree of pneumatization of the mastoid: More the pneumatization more is the mucosal surface area that is involved and causes more severe inflammation.

Microbiology

Viral

The disease usually starts as a viral infection (Rhinovirus 24%, Respiratory Syncitial Virus 13% are the most common types followed by Cytomegalovirus, Measles virus, Ebstein-Barr Virus) followed by secondary bacterial infection. Some studies have shown viruses as the main causative factor in AOM. In one of the studies up to 50% of isolates had grown viruses (Jacob et al., 1997). Respiratory syncitial virus and adenovirus are responsible for persistent purulent otitis media.

Bacterial

Positive bacterial culture is seen in 65–70% of cases (Ludman, 1998). The main pathogens associated with otitis media are *Streptococcus pneumoniae* (30–50%), *Haemophilus influenzae* (20–30%) and *Moraxella catarrhalis* (10–20%). Haugsten and Lorentzen (1980) found the organism isolated in a series of 297 patients with otitis media as *Streptococcus pneumoniae* (33%), *Haemophilus influenzae* (17%), *Streptococcus pyogenes* group A (7%), *Staphylococcus aureus* (10% apathogenic bacteria including *Staphylococcus epidermidis* (30%). Gram-negative bacilli such as *Pseudomonas aeruginosa*, various *Proteus* species, *Klebsiella pneumoniae* and *E. coli* have been reported.

Desmukh (1998) in his study in India found that *Streptococcus pneumoniae* (30–40%), *Haemophilus influenzae* (> 20%) and *Moraxella catarrhalis* (7–20%) account for 80% of all cases of AOM. *Staphylococcus aureus* are seen in some children. *Streptococcus pyogenes* are commonly seen in older children, *Chlamydia pneumoniae* in smaller children and gram-negative bacteria like *E. coli* and *Pseudomonas* are responsible for 20% of cases and are commonly seen in newborns.

Clinicopathological stages

The authors have divided the acute suppurative otitis media into the following stages as the treatment planning and methods of evaluation are different for each of these stages. The stage of exudation and suppuration before perforation has a different management protocol than after perforation. The stages can be divided as follows:

1. Stage of hyperemia
2. Stage of exudation and suppuration
3. Stage of perforation and discharge
4. Stage of resolution
5. Stage of acute coalescent mastoiditis
6. Stage of complications

1. Stage of hyperemia (congestion)

Pathology

- Edema and congestion of the mucoperiosteal lining of the middle ear cleft along with dilatation of the radial vessels of the drum (Fig. 3.1).
- Occlusion of eustachian tube.
- Absorption of air from the middle ear cleft.
- Negative pressure in middle ear leading to retraction of tympanic membrane.

Clinical features

Symptoms

- Blocked feeling in the ear following URTI.
- Mild ache/discomfort.
- +/– Fever and other associated symptoms.

Signs

- Tympanic membrane is retracted.
- Hyperemia and congestion of tympanic membrane with distorted landmarks.
- Dilatation of radial blood vessels of TM gives cartwheel appearance (Fig. 3.2).

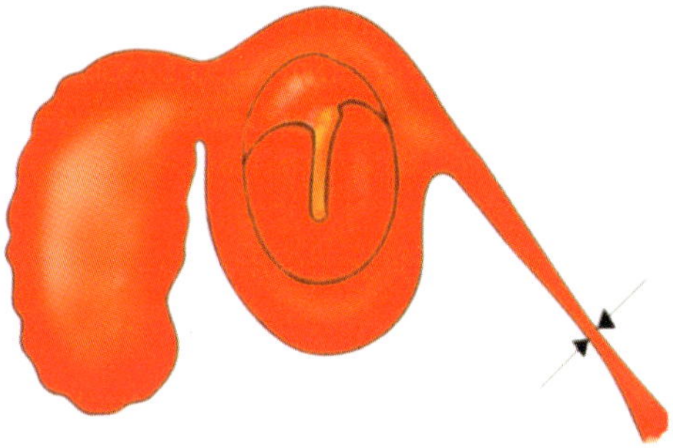

Fig. 3.1. Hyperemia of the entire mucoperiosteal line of the middle ear cleft associated with eustachian tube blockage following mucosal edema in ASOM. Arrow shows site of tubal blockage.

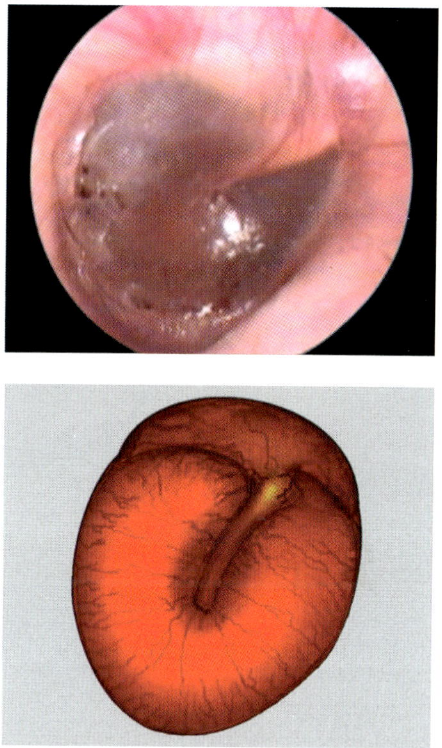

Fig. 3.2 A & B. Hyperemic tympanic membrane associated with retraction. Dilated radial blood vessels may be noted (cartwheel appearance).

3

2. Stage of exudation and suppuration

Pathology

Stage of exudation

- Increased permeability leads to accumulation of inflammatory exudates in the middle ear cleft and increased secretion by the goblet cells and mucous glands. There is also decreased drainage of the middle ear cleft due to eustachian tube occlusion.

- Non-purulent fluid in middle ear initially (serum-containing fibrin, red blood cells, and polymorphonuclear leukocytes) from the dilated, permeable capillaries of the mucoperiosteum.
- Polymorphonuclear infiltration.

Stage of suppuration

- The mucoperiosteum of the tympanomastoid compartment becomes thickened with the formation of new capillaries and fibrous tissue, infiltrated with lymphocytes, plasma cells, and polymorphonuclear leukocytes to form a very thick mucosal lining resembling granulation tissue.
- Accumulation of pus in the tympanomastoid compartment under tension (Fig. 3.3).
- The bony septae of the mastoid air cells system are not affected.

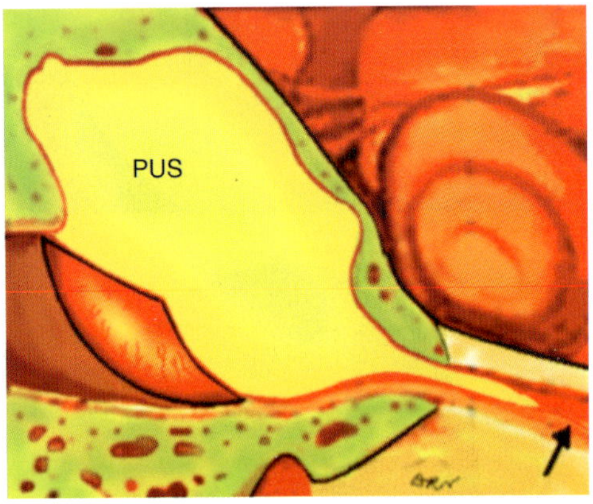

Fig. 3.3. Accumulation of mucopurulent inflammatory exudates in the middle ear causing bulging of the drum. Black arrow shows occlusion of the Eustachian tube.

Clinical features in stage of exudation

Symptoms

- Irritable child.
- Unexplained cause of crying in a child.
- Otalgia and deafness.
- Autophony is present due to accumulation of exudates in the middle ear.
- Fever.
- Toxic symptoms are usually absent.

Signs (Fig. 3.4)

- Thick, congested and bulging drum.
- Tuning fork test: Shows features of conductive deafness.
- Grossly congested and edematous TM.

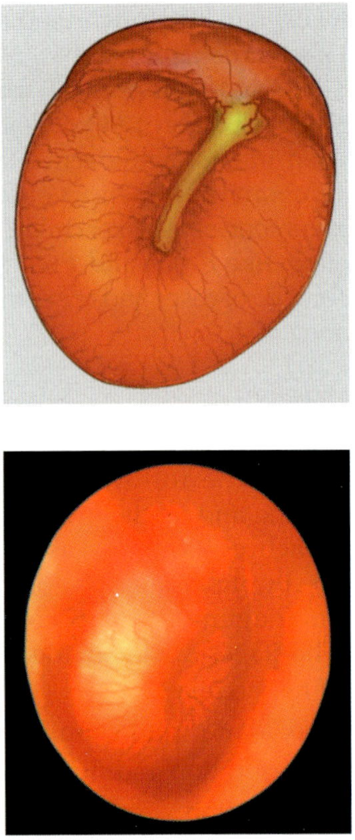

Fig. 3.4 A & B. Congested and bulging drum with prominent radial blood vessels.

Clinical features in stage of suppuration

Symptoms

- Increasing earache and deafness as the secretions gets accumulated further in the middle ear.
- Autophony.
- Fever, toxic symptoms are often present.
- Severe otalgia at its peak which is throbbing in nature.

Signs (Fig. 3.5)

- Bulging and congested tympanic membrane can be seen on otoscopy.
- Pus pointing is often present.

3. Stage of perforation and discharge

Pathology

- Pus in the middle ear is under intense tension causing pressure necrosis of the tympanic membrane at the site of maximum pressure. The fibrous layer is first to be involved causing protrusion of skin and mucosa (pus pointing).

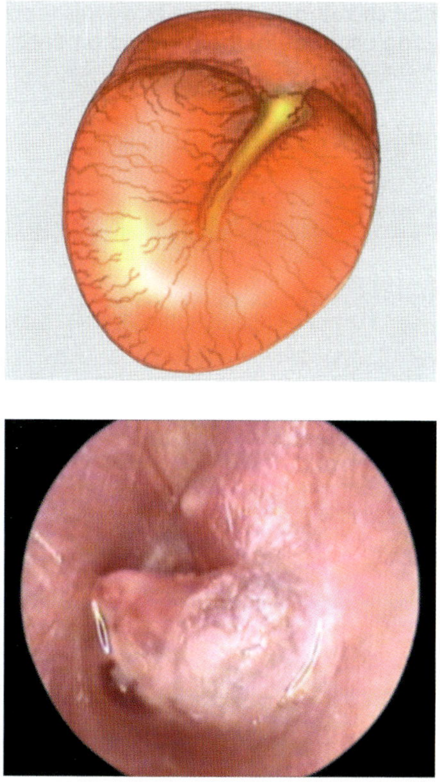

Fig. 3.5 A & B. Congested and bulging drum with process pressure necrosis (A) and pus pointing (black arrow) in the anteroinferior quadrant (B) of the tympanic membrane.

- Pus pointing which eventually gives way and the discharge comes out through a small perforation.
- Commonest site of rupture is anteroinferior quadrant.
- Middle ear mucosa is congested and swollen due to inflammatory edema.

Clinical features

Symptoms

- Otalgia at its peak before rupture of tympanic membrane.
- Mucopurulent, blood stained ear discharge.
- Otalgia subsides with onset of discharge.

Signs

Rupture of the drum occurs and is associated with initial blood stained mucopurulent discharge which later becomes mucopurulent. Pulsatile ear discharge with classical 'Lighthouse sign' is seen through a pin-hole or small perforation. Pain subsides with the onset of ear discharge (Fig. 3.6).

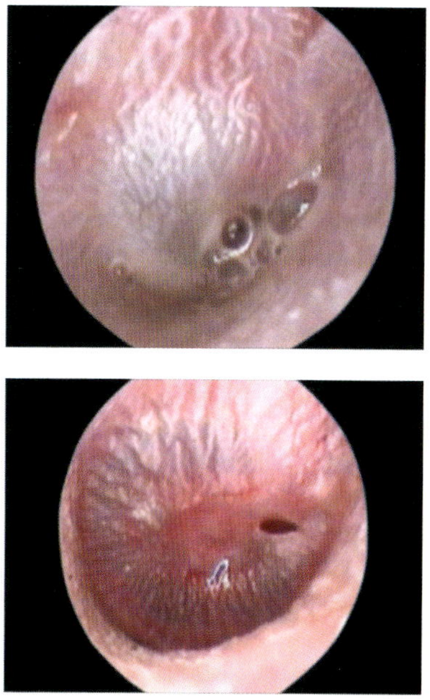

Fig. 3.6 A & B. A small perforation in the tympanic membrane with pulsatile mucopurulent ear discharge. Drum is also congested.

4. Stage of healing and resolution

Pathology

Middle ear cleft inflammatory changes resolve and ear becomes dry. Perforation eventually heals and hearing is restored.

Clinical features

Symptoms

- Acute symptoms subside with blocked feeling in the ear and mild hearing loss initially.
- Ear becomes dry.
- Eventually hearing is restored after perforation heals.

Signs

- Perforation is seen usually in the antero-inferior quadrant of the tympanic membrane with granulation at the perforation margin. Discharge may be negligible or completely stopped (Fig. 3.7).
- Later perforation heals with a scar (thin drum) (Fig. 3.8).

5. Stage of acute coalescent mastoiditis (surgical mastoiditis)

It was common in pre-antibiotic era and is rarely seen today. It starts as a natural extension of ASOM into the mastoid compartment.

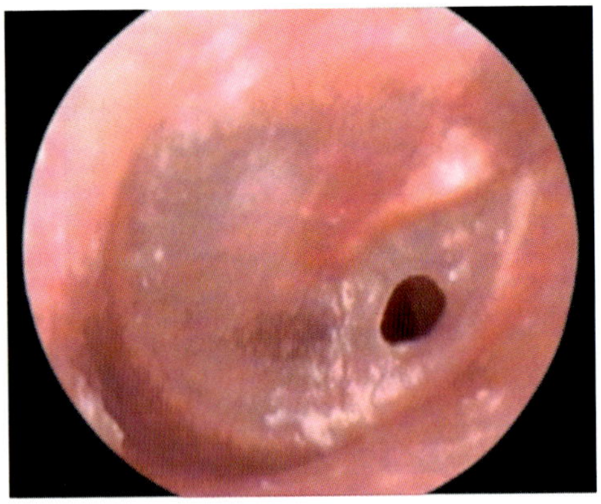

Fig. 3.7. Reduced inflammatory changes and a dry small perforation in the anteroinferior quadrant of the pars tensa.

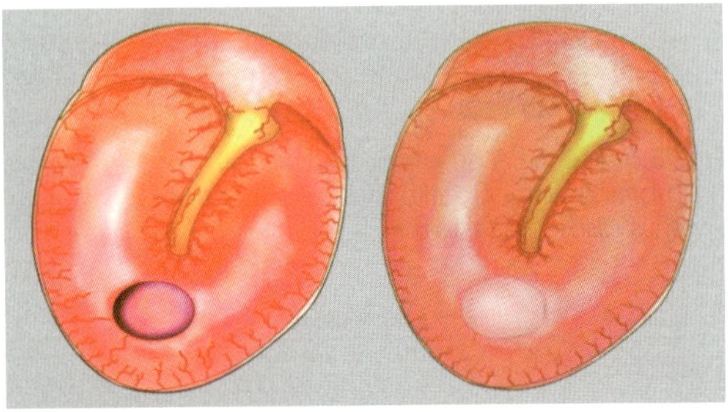

Fig. 3.8 A & B. A small dry perforation in the anteroinferior quadrant of the pars tensa (A) which eventually heals (B).

Pathology

- Progressive thickening of the mucoperiosteum obstructs drainage of the mucopurulent secretions through the aditus.
- Accumulation of pus under pressure, along with persistent noticeable hyperemia, results in venous stasis, localized acidosis.
- Inadequate drainage and demineralization leads to the absorption of calcium from the adjacent bony walls.
- Continued new blood vessel formation in bone, along with the activity of numerous osteoclasts, acts to soften and destroy the decalcifying septae resulting in the coalescence of the mastoid air cells (Fig. 3.10) and is called as the stage of coalescence mastoiditis or **surgical mastoiditis (empyema of the mastoid)**.
- Further progress can lead to bony erosion of the adjacent walls and spread of infections to related structure causing complications.

Flowchart showing sequence of events leading to coalescence of the mastoid air cells

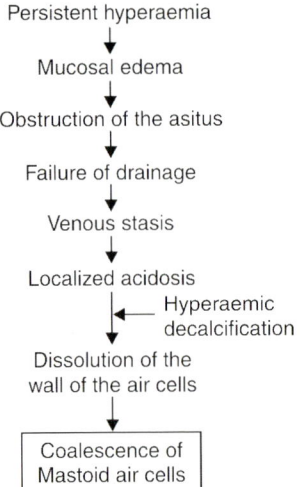

Persistent hyperaemia
↓
Mucosal edema
↓
Obstruction of the asitus
↓
Failure of drainage
↓
Venous stasis
↓
Localized acidosis
↓ ← Hyperaemic decalcification
Dissolution of the wall of the air cells
↓
Coalescence of Mastoid air cells

Clinical features

Symptoms

- Ear pain reappears which is severe and throbbing in nature and may localize to the postauricular region.
- Fever, malaise are often present.
- Painful postauricular swelling may be present.
- Ear discharge is profuse thick and mucopurulent.
- Deafness increases.
- Constitutional symptoms may be present.

Signs

- Thickening of periosteum of mastoid.
- Erythema, edema and increase in local temperature over the mastoid area.
- Mastoid tenderness can be elicited.
- Discharge is copious and profuse and reappears immediately after cleaning (+ve reservoir sign).
- Central perforation with swollen middle ear mucosa.
- Sagging of posterior-superior meatal wall due to erosion of posterior superior bony meatal wall.
- Deepening of postauricular sulcus may be noted associated with a fluctuant swelling in the postauricular area.
- Protrusion of the auricle.

Urgent surgical intervention is required to prevent impending complications and hence called surgical mastoiditis.

6. Stage of complications

- Close relations of middle ear to important structures within the temporal bone, extra-temporal region and the intracranial compartments make it susceptible to various complications following middle ear infection, especially following coalescent mastoiditis.
- This was a leading cause of death in the pre-antibiotic era.
- Advanced diagnostic and therapeutic techniques have reduced the mortality and morbidity.
- Complications can be classified broadly into
  - Extracranial
  - Intracranial

Extracranial complications

- Mastoid abscess: Depending on its site where it presents, this may be further classified as:
  - Postauricular subperiosteal/subcutaneous abscess. This is the most common type of mastoid abscess. It may rupture to form a discharging mastoid fistula.
  - Bezold's abscess: Situated in relation to the upper end of sternocliedomastoid muscle. Pus tracks down from the tip of the mastoid.
  - Citelli's abscess: It is situated in the sub-mandibular region with pus tracking along the posterior belly of the digastrics muscle.
  - Zygomatic abscess.
  - Luc's abscess: Deep meatal (subtemporal) abscess or abscess in the infratemporal fossa. It is usually an inferior extension of the zygomatic abscess.
  - Parapharyngeal abscess: Originates from the peritubal cells.
- Labyrinthitis: This is due to destruction of the labyrinth especially in the region of the lateral semicircular canal. Depending on its severity is can be:
  - Circumscribed labyrinthitis
  - Serous labyrinthitis
  - Suppurative labyrinthitis
  - Dead labyrinth
- Facial paralysis (LMN)
- Petrositis with Gradinigo's syndrome (discharge in the ear, diplopia due to abducent nerve palsy and deep temporal pain due to involvement of the trigeminal nerve).
- Otogenic tetanus: This is rarely seen today.
- Persistent perforation and chronic otitis media.

Intracranial complications (Fig. 3.9)

- Meningitis: Presence of headache, altered sensorium.
- Extradural abscess.
- Subdural abscess.
- Lateral sinus thrombophlebitis.
- Brain abscess (cerebellar or temporal lobe).
- Superior sagittal sinus thrombophlebitis.
- Otitic hydrocephalus.
- Cortical venous thrombophlebitis.

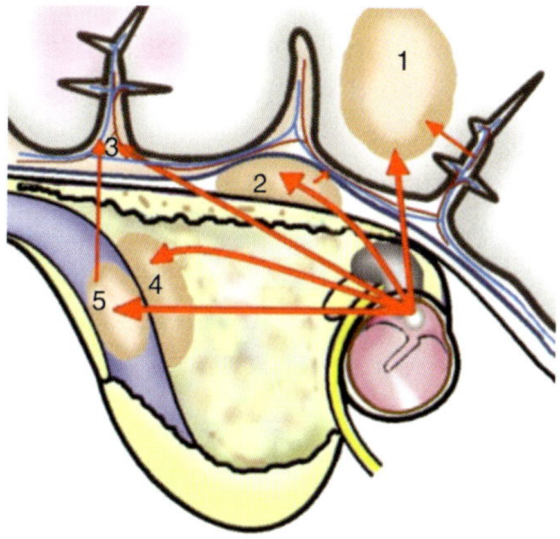

Fig. 3.9. Intracranial complications of otitis media. 1. Brain abscess, 2. Extradural abscess, 3. Subdural abscess, 4. Perisinus abscess, 5. Lateral sinus thrombophlebitis.

Diagnosis of impending intracranial complication

- Elevation of temperature with toxic features (brain abscess, meningitis) and hectic rise of temperature (lateral sinus thrombophlebitis).
- Signs of neck stiffness, meningismus and papillaedema should be looked for.
- Greisinger's sign (edema over mastoid cortex) in lateral sinus thrombophlebitis.
- Headache (parietal or occipital) indicates intracranial complication.
- Drowsiness, nausea, vomiting, irritability, altered mental status, lethargy.
- Focal neurologic signs (e.g., ataxia, occulo-motor deficits, seizure, etc. can be seen in cerebellar or temporal lobe abscess).
- X-ray mastoids: Evidence of bony erosion.
- CT scan with intra- or extra-cranial extension.

3

Investigations

1. **Complete blood picture:** It includes hemoglobin, total and differential count and ESR.
2. **Examination under microscope:** To confirm the clinical findings and the ear discharge can be cleared to visualize better.
3. **Audiological investigations:** An audiometric evaluation may be obtained. Pure tone audiometry and Impedance audiometry are commonly done.
   - **Pure tone audiometry (PTA):** Shows conductive hearing loss of varied AB gap depending on the stage of the disease.
   - **Tympanometry:** It is a useful investigation in infants and young children to know if there is fluid in the ear or eustachian tube dysfunction.
4. **Radiological investigations:**
   - X-ray mastoids:
     - Cloudiness (haziness) of the air cells.
     - Destruction of the intercellular septae in coalescent mastoiditis (Fig. 3.10).

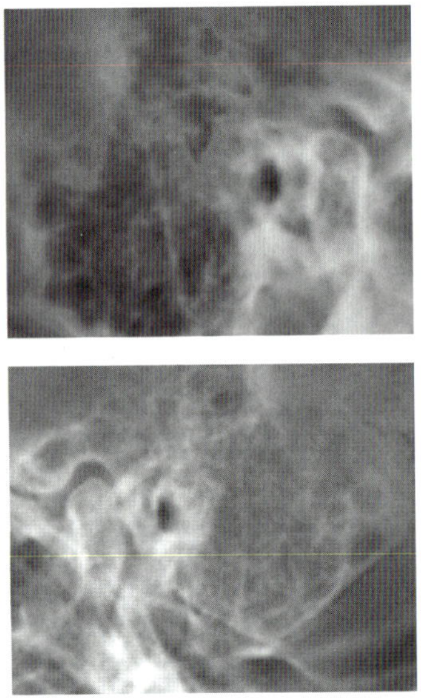

Fig. 3.10 A & B. Hazy mastoid air cells on the left side compared to right.

   - CT scan (Fig. 3.11):
     - Haziness with loss of intercellular septae due to coalescence.
     - Opacification of the mastoid air cells and middle ear by inflammatory swelling of mucosa and by collection of fluid.

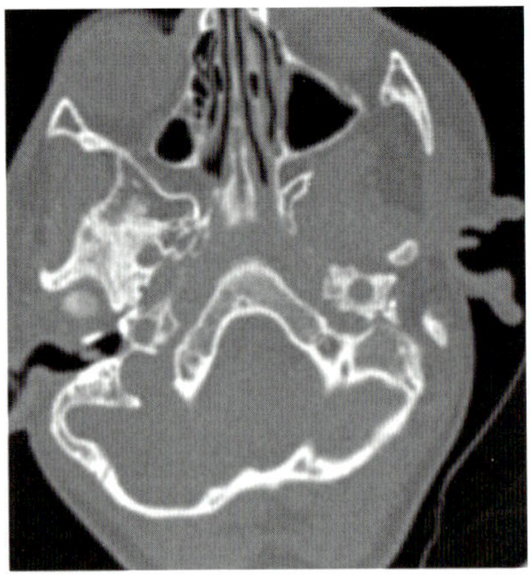

Fig. 3.11. CT scan of temporal bone with left coalescent mastoiditis with subperiosteal mastoid abscess.

     - Loss of sharpness or visibility of mastoid cell walls due to demineralization, atrophy, or necrosis of bony septa.
     - Haziness or distortion of the mastoid outline, possibly with visible defects of the tegmen or mastoid cortex.
     - Enhancement of areas of abscess formation.
     - Elevation of periosteum of mastoid process or posterior cranial fossa.
   - MRI: Helpful in showing inflammatory processes and differentiating certain tumours.
5. **Culture and sensitivity:** Ear swab is taken for culture and sensitivity if the ear is discharging or following myringotomy.

Treatment

Medical

Patient with acute suppurative otitis media are best managed medically before the stage of exudation or after the stage of perforation to facilitate early healing. The most common form of treatment given is as follows:

- **Antibiotics:** Co amoxyclav is the most preferred antibiotic as it is effective against β-lactamase resistant organism and is given at a dose of 80–90 mg/kg/d of amoxicillin component, 6.4 mg/kg/d of clavulanate component in divided dosage of 8–12 hourly. In case of allergy to penicillin, oral cefuroxime axetil (suspension: 30 mg/kg/d; tablet 250 mg bid) can be given. Alternatively Clarithromycin or Azithromycin can be given in similar dosage.

- Intramuscular (IM) ceftriaxone (administered as a single IM injection of 50 mg/kg on 3 consecutive days) can be given in severe case with potential complications.
- **Analgesics and antipyretcs:** Paracetamol with or without aceclofenac/ibuprofen can be given for fever and pain.
- **Local decongestants:** Xylometazoline/oxymetazoline nasal drops are useful to maintain eustachian tube patency and should be given for a short duration.
- **Systemic decongestants:** Phenylephrine/pseudoephedrine is useful to facilitate faster recovery and helps in reducing ear discharge.

Surgical

Myringotomy: This is indicated in stage of exudation and suppuration to let out the pus collecting under tension. This prevents formation of a perforation and helps in relieving pain immediately. The pus thus released can be collected for culture and sensitivity. This helps in selection of antibiotics in refractory cases.

Indications for myringotomy include the following:

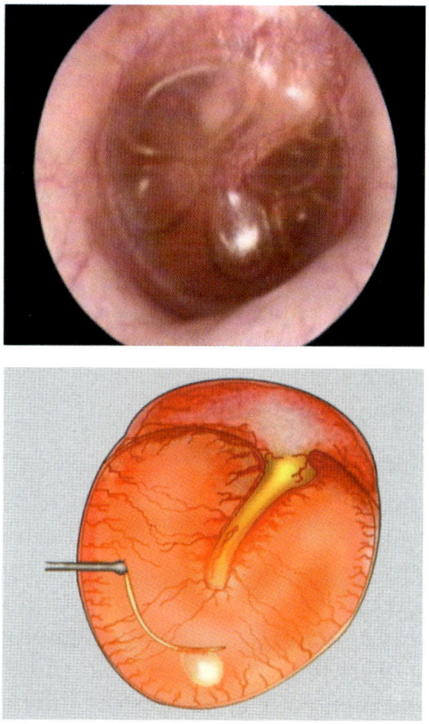

Fig. 3.12. Fluid in middle ear and myringotomy being done in the posteroinferior quadrant to drain the fluid from the middle ear.

- Toxic child with severe otalgia.
- Recurrent AOM with persistent exudates in middle ear with intact tympanic membrane following inadequate antibiotic therapy.
- Potential to develop complication/has developed complication.
- Poor response to antibiotic therapy.
- ASOM in new born child.
- ASOM in immune deficiency patients.

Technique: Under general anesthesia, curvilinear incision is made in the postero-inferior quadrant of the tympanic membrane where there is maximum bulge using a myringotomy knife as shown in Fig. 3.12. Posterosuperior quadrant is avoided to prevent injury to the incudostapedial joint.

Cortical mastoidectomy: This is the treatment of choice for acute coalescent mastoiditis/masked mastoiditis and is done as an emergency to exenterate the diseased air cells and to prevent intra-/extracranial complications.

Surgical treatment of predisposing conditions like deviated nasal septum, adenoid hypertrophy, sinusitis, etc should be considered whenever indicated.

Prevention

1. Treatment of underlying predisposing conditions of nose, sinuses, nasopharynx and throat such as sinusitis, chronic tonsillitis, and adenoid hyperplasia can prevent recurrent ASOM.
2. Improvement of living conditions like proper ventilation, hygiene, overcrowding, etc. are important factor that needs to be addressed.
3. Blowing the nose during acute URTI should be avoided.
4. Administration of trivalent influenza-A vaccine has shown to decrease frequency of ASOM during influenza epidemic. HiB conjugated vaccine when administered in early life reduces the risk of AOM. Heptavalent vaccine to *S. pneumoniae* is now in widespread use and has made an impact in the number of cases of invasive pneumococcal disease confined to only seven strains.

SPECIAL FORMS OF OTITIS MEDIA

1. **Acute necrotizing otitis media:** It is a special form of acute otitis media seen mostly in infants and children following Influenza, scarlet fever,

measles, mumps etc. and other systemic illness. Virulent strain bacteria like beta hemolytic streptococcus is the main causative agent. The patient develops spontaneous large perforation of tympanic membrane with fowl smelling mucopurulent ear discharge. The perforation is often very large (subtotal) involving the entire pars tensa with an intact annulus and can be associated with ossicular discontinuity. These patients often develop permanent perforation and go to chronic stage. Patient may require tympanoplasty in addition to medical treatment if the perforation doesn't heal.

2. **Acute epitympanitis:** It is a rare form of acute otitis media where the inflammatory changes are confined to epitympanum and posterior and superior mesotympanum (Fig. 3.13). It is usually associated with an acellular type of mastoid. The resultant perforation is seen in pars flacida and is a true perforation and should be differentiated from attic retraction pocket. Treatment is same as ASOM.

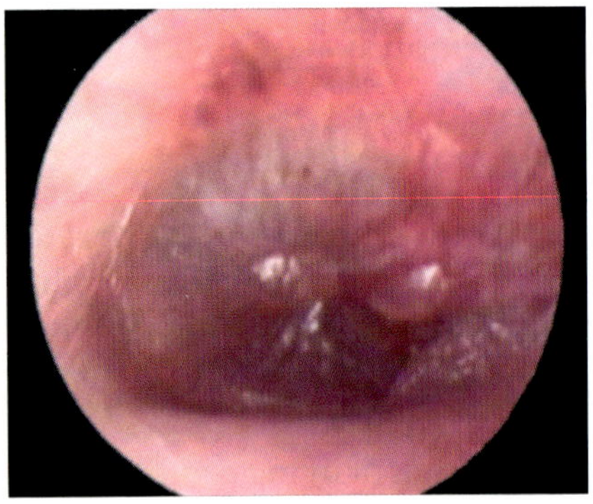

Fig. 3.13. Congestion predominantly in the pars flaccida in acute epitympanitis.

ACUTE VIRAL OTITIS MEDIA

It occurs usually as an extension of viral infection of nasal passages into the middle ear. The pathological changes that can be noted include degeneration of ciliated columnar cells leaving the basal layer of non ciliated cuboidal cells that recovers in a period of two weeks (Hilding, 1944). The virus can induce release of cytokines and other inflammatory mediators like histamine, bradykinin, interleukins etc that provokes eustachian dysfunction. Loss of cilliary activity, inflammatory edema, negative middle pressure following tubal obstruction and increased mucus production leads to temporary collection of transudate in the middle ear. The classical features of acute suppurative otitis media are usually absent as they are often subclinical.

3

BAROTRAUMATIC OTITIS MEDIA

It is an acute traumatic inflammatory condition associated with sudden change of atmospheric pressure in comparison to middle ear pressure leading to soft tissue damage of the ear and collection of non-serous fluid in the middle ear cleft.

Etiology

Predisiposing factors

- Eustachian tube dysfunction.
- Respiratory tract infection.
- Infants and young children who have difficulty in dilating the eustachian tube (by swallowing) due to adenoid hypertrophy, submucous cleft palate, etc.
- Any obstructive nasal and nasopharyngeal pathology.
- Obstructive pathology like exostosis can predispose to external ear barotraumas (reverse ear squeeze).

Precipitating factors

- Airplane flight.
- Scuba diving.
- Sky diving.
- High-altitude mountain climbers.
- High-impact sports.
- Deep sea divers

Causes

- Damage caused by sudden, increased pressure in the surrounding air, such as occurs in the rapid descent of an airplane.
- Deep sea diving during ascent.

Mechanism

A pressure difference of 90 mm of Hg or more between atmospheric and middle ear can result in eustachian tube locking due to elastic lips of the eustachian tubal orifice in the nasopharynx, which cannot be opened by Valsalva maneuver. The presence of predisposing factor can cause locking of the tube even with lesser pressure difference. On air travel during ascent, the atmospheric pressure is reduced and there is passive exit of the air from the middle ear through the eustachian tube. During rapid descent the middle ear pressure is low and the atmospheric pressure is high at the sea level. This Sudden negative pressure leads to locking of the eustachian tube that causes middle/inner ear injuries.

A sudden descent in water (as seen in deep sea diving) leads to sudden increase in ambient water pressure in the external ear. This causes a relative negative middle ear pressure. The damage caused by sudden descent in air by 6000 metres is equivalent to the damage caused by sudden descent in salt water by only 5 metres.

Pathology of barotraumas

External ear (reverse ear squeeze)

- Hemorrhage into the skin of the ear canal forming blebs.
- Rupture of them may cause tympanic membrane perforation.

Middle ear (middle ear squeeze)

- Retraction of the pars tensa and pars flacida.
- Transudation.
- Hemorrhagic effusion.
- Rupture of tympanic membrane.
- Rupture of round window membrane.
- Ossicular discontinuity.
- Divers using oxygen can develop delayed barotrauma as a result of absorption of oxygen present in the middle ear.

Clinical features

- Fullness/block sensation in the ear.
- Otalgia.
- Deafness.
- Vertigo/alternobaric vertigo (vertigo without hearing loss and tinnitus).
- Tinnitus.
- Tympanic membrane may be hemorrhagic, congested and retracted.
- Tuning fork test may show features of conductive/mixed hearing loss.
- Nystagmus is present if inner ear is involved.
- Severe neurologic or respiratory symptoms may occur due to associated cerebral/pulmonary edema.

Investigations

- Pure tone audiogram to assess hearing.
- Impendance audiometry if tympanic membrane is intact and the effusion is suspected.
- Examination under microscope to assess the tympanic membrane and middle ear pathology.

Treatment

- The effusion usually clears over a period of few days to few weeks.
- Nasal decongestants and systemic decongestants.
- Antihistamines.
- Antibiotics may help prevent infection.
- Auto-insufflation by valsalva may be helpful but should be carefully done and force should be avoided to prevent pneumoencephalus.
- Labyrinthine sedative if the patient is having vertigo.
- Systemic steroids may help in resolution of eustachian tube edema and effusion.
- Myringotomy and grommet insertion in case of severe otalgia or persistent effusion.
- In case of round window rupture, emergency exploration and closure of leak by fat/fascia may be done to prevent permanent sensorineural hearing loss.
- Tympanoplasty may be required to treat ruptured tympanic membrane/ossicular discontinuity.

CHRONIC NON-SUPPURATIVE OTITIS MEDIA

A chronic inflammatory condition of the mucoperiosteal lining of the middle ear cleft without suppuration and with an intact tympanic membrane.

Types

- Eustachian tube (ET) dysfunction.
- Otitis media with effusion.
- Atelectasis.
- Adhesive otitis media.
- Tympanosclerosis.

ET dysfunction

It is a localized condition termed as salpingitis (acute/chronic) which is prelude to most of the middle ear pathology.

Characteristics

- Cause of all forms of otitis media.

- Common in children.
- Can be congenital/acquired.
- Anatomical ET obstruction (mechanical).
- Functional ET obstruction (dysfunction of muscles opening the tube).

Causes of eustachian dysfunction

Mechanical

- Mucosal edema due to infection/allergy.
- Adenoid hypertrophy.
- Polyp or tumour in nasopharynx.
- Stricture.
- Trauma.

Functional

- Cleft palate.
- Craniobasal anomalies.
- Velopharyngeal insufficiency.
- Patulous ET.

Risk factors

- Smoking/passive smoking.
- Allergy.

Clinical features

Symptoms

- Blocked sensation/discomfort in the ears.
- Clicking sounds more on swallowing.
- Tinnitus.
- Mild deafness.

Signs

- Retracted tympanic membrane.
- Cone of light – absent/distorted/displaced.
- Apparent fore-shortening of the handle of malleus which appears more horizontal (Fig. 3.14).
- Prominent lateral process.
- Prominent malleolar folds.

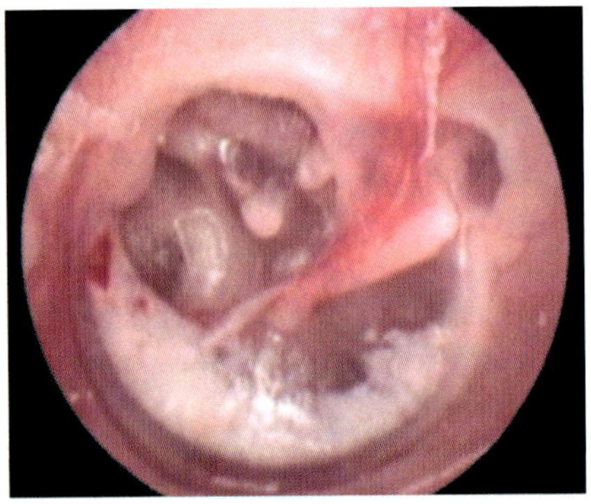

Fig. 3.14. Retracted, adhesive and tympanosclerotic TM.

3

- Restricted mobility of the drum on Valsalva/Toynbee/Segalisation.

Investigations

- Pure tone audiometry.
- Impedence audiometry (tympanogram).

Treatment

- Treat the cause.
- Valsalva manoeuvre.
- Auto-inflation methods in children:
  - Balloon blowing.
  - Toy trumpet blowing.
- Myringotomy and grommet insertion if symptoms do not improve.
- Endoscopic eustachian balloon tuboplasty:

It is found to be a feasible and safe procedure to inflate the ET by a balloon to dilate the cartilaginous and bony segment of eustachian tube (Ockermann, 2010).

Otitis media with effusion (OME)

OME can be acute, subacute or chronic. The effusion is said to be acute up to 3 weeks duration, subacute if of 3–12 weeks duration and after that as chronic. Acute OME has been discussed under AOM. The chronic type has been described below.

Synonyms

- Serous otitis media.
- Secretory otitis media.
- Glue ear.
- Mucinous otitis media.
- Seromucinous otitis media.

Definition

Chronic inflammation of the middle ear cleft characterized by accumulation of serous or mucoid non-purulent fluid, in the middle ear behind an intact tympanic membrane.

Chronic OME is middle ear effusion without signs and symptoms of infection. Commonly they are asymptomatic but may have hearing loss or balance disturbances.

Etiology

Multi-factorial

- E tube dysfunction (as described earlier).
- URTI/allergy.

- Miscellaneous.
- Mucociliary dysfunction.
- Feeding habits.
- Socioeconomic.
- Living conditions.
- Smoking.

More common in children because:

- Upper respiratory tract infections are more common.
- Eustachian tube is short, wide and horizontal in children compared to adults.
- Adenoid tends to hypertrophy and obstruct the ET orifice in the nasopharynx.
- Feeding habits in an infant- nasopaharyngeal reflux more common.

Risk factors in children

- Passive smoking.
- Allergy.
- Play school.
- Deprived of breast-feeding.
- Overcrowding at home.
- GERD.

Pathogenesis

- ET dysfunction: It is the important predisposing factor.
- Immunological mechanisms are probably involved in the pathogenesis that is known to be multifactorial in origin, and this mechanism is an important factor in secretory otitis media. Immunological changes involves IgG and its subclasses. IgE may be involved in allergy associated OME.
- IgA is a late defense mechanism which may prevent bacteriolysis by IgG and its compliments acting as a blocking antibody.
- No suppuration – more mechanical than infective although microorganisms are detected in the fluid.
- Chronic negative pressure in middle ear leads to transudation – 'Hydrops ex-vacuo theory'.
- Low grade inflammatory response is seen as evidenced by presence of inflammatory mediators such as interleukins, cytokines, etc. in the middle ear effusion. T cell lymphocytes activation has been noted in the middle car fluid and in the blood of these patients.
- Role of surfactant is under evaluation.
- Increased mucous secretion due to glandular hypertrophy (secretory).
- Decreased drainage leading to accumulation of fluid.
- Accumulation of non-purulent fluid
- Microhemorrhage – organization of haem pigment – bluish colour (blue drum in glue ear).

Micobiology

The bacterial spectrum of OME closely resemble that of AOM. Common micro organism isolated are *Streptococcus pneumoniae, H. influenzae, M. catarrhalis* and *S. pyogenes*. About 50% of viral infections are caused by respiratory syncitial virus. Adenovirus and influenza virus have been isolated in certain cases.

Pathology

- Initally acute and later chronic inflammatory change in the mucosa.
- Incresed goblet cells and mucus production.
- Normal increase in the size of the middle ear cleft with age is affected in children following OME.
- Functional effects on cilia, producing alteration in the mucociliary clearance mechanism.

Clinical features

Symptoms

- This condition is commonly seen in children who are often asymptomatic.
- High index of suspicion should be present among parents, teachers and family physician, if the child is inattentive to call, or is not doing well in school.
- Behavioral changes.
- Delayed speech and language development.
- Reccurent earache.
- A grown up child may complain of hearing loss/block sensation in the ear.
- Autophony.
- Tinnitus.
- Features of underlying nasal/nasopharyngeal pathology.

Signs

- The tympanic membrane may be dull and lusterless with amber hue and may be bluish as a result of microhemorrhage.

- Retracted/bulging drum with restricted mobility on siegelization,
- Air fluid level or air bubbles may be seen that moves with when the child cries.
- Should look for signs of underlying nasal or nasopharyngeal pathology.
- Craniofacial anomalies including cleft palate, bifid uvula etc should be ruled out.
- In adolescents and adults, nasopharyngeal neoplasm should be ruled out.

Sequelae of OME

- Thinning of the TM due to histological degeneration of lamina propria and decrease in thickness of fibrous layer.
- Atelectatic changes and adhesive otitis media (Fig. 3.14).
- Erosion of long process of incus.
- Predisposition to breakdown and perforation.
- Tympanosclerosis/myringosclerosis, ossicular fixation.
- Cholesterol granuloma.
- Retraction pocket and cholesteatoma formation.
- Ultrahigh frequency hearing loss and abnormality of balance probably due to inflammatory mediators and neurotoxins.

Investigations

- Tympanometry: Shows a B type or a C2 curve. It is an easy to perform and useful screening procedure for school children.
- PTA – If it can be done will show features of conductive hearing loss.
- Diagnostic endoscopy if patient cooperates.
- Radiological:
  - Plain radiographs – PNS and X-ray soft tissue nasopharynx lateral view.
  - CT imaging of PNS.
- Allergy tests if nasal allergy is suspected.
- Tympanocentesis confirms the diagnosis.

3

Management

Medical

- Treat underlying nasal/nasopharyngeal pathology.
- Antihistaminic and decongestants have been tried however clinical evidence is lacking.
- Mucolytic like ambroxol, bromohexine, carbo-cysteine, etc.
- Antibiotics though of limited use like Co amoxyclav, macrolides, and cephalosporin can be used if indicated in cases like reccurent otitis media or if the patient is receiving systemic steroid as a prophylaxis.
- 3–4 weeks of antibiotic therapy is helpful according to some studies. Same antibiotic as used in ASOM is recommended.
- Steroids – Topical/systemic have proved beneficial in clearing middle ear effusion. It helps in controlling inflammatory mediators and relieves the tubal/ peritubal edema.
- Immunodeficiency state should be treated.
- AUTOINFLATION
  - Valsalva.
  - Autovent device.
- Hearing aid: In those patients who are not willing or are not fit for surgery.

Wait and watch with medical treatment and follow up with serial tympanogram

Surgical

- Myringotomy and grommet insertion: Myringotomy is done in the anterior quadrants (Fig. 3.16) of pars tensa with a myringotomy knife and a suitable ventilating tube (grommet) is inserted. Various types of commonly used grommets are as follows (Fig. 3.15):
  - Tita prosthesis bent tube
  - Armstrong
  - Armstrong with tail
  - Donaldson
  - Shah
  - Shah with tail
  - Shepard
  - Shepard with tail
  - T tube straight tube
- Laser-assisted myringotomy.
- Cortical mastoidectomy in selected cases like persistent otorrhoea after grommet insertion or not cured after repeated grommet insertion including double grommet.

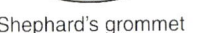

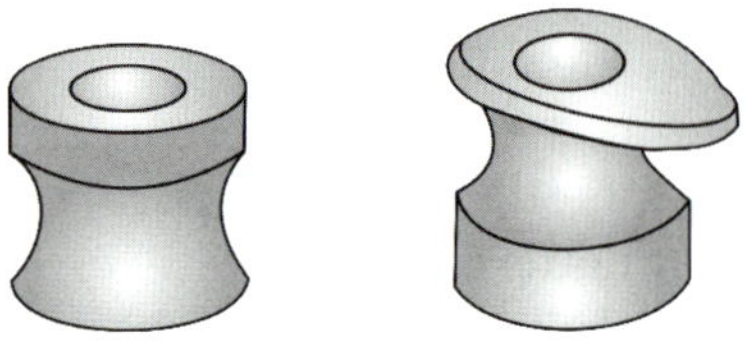

Fig. 3.15. Types of gromet.

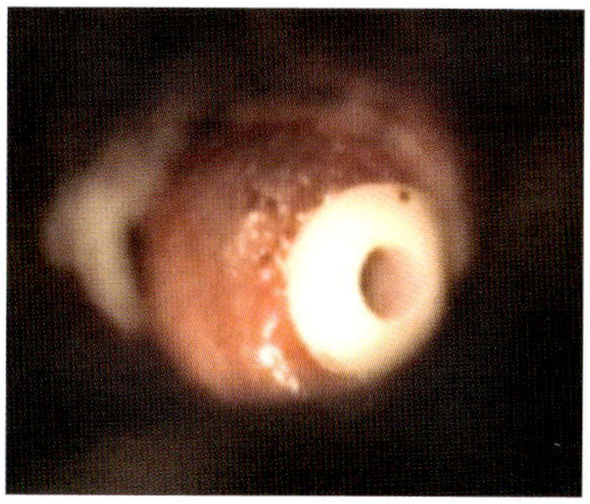

Fig. 3.16. Intraoperative picture showing grommet after insertion.

- Endoscopic balloon assisted eustachian tuboplasty (BET) has been found to be a feasible and safe alternative procedure to inflate the ET. It significantly helps to improve ET function.
- Surgical treatment of underlying cause like endoscopic adenoidectomy, turbinoplasty, endoscopc sinus surgery, etc.

CHRONIC SUPPURATIVE OTITIS MEDIA

A chronic inflammatory condition of the muco-periosteal lining of the middle ear cleft with suppuration associated with a perforation in the tympanic membrane.

Tubotympanic disease (TTD)

Chronic inflammation of the muco-periosteal lining of the middle ear cleft characterized by intermittent copious non-foul smelling mucoid/mucopurulent ear discharge associated with a central perforation of the tympanic membrane (pars tensa).

Etiology

- Unresolved ASOM – more than 3 months.
- Non-healing traumatic perforation.
- Perforation caused by above fails to heal because of presence of septic focus.
- Thin drum as a sequelae of OME can get perforated by trivial trauma.
- Following long stay ventilation tube such as Goode 'T' tube can be associated with residual perforation.

Route of spread

- Through eustachian tube:
  - Rhinitis, sinusitis, adenoiditis, etc.
- Through the external auditory canal via pre-existing perforation.
- Mastoid reservoir of infection.

Risk factors

- Smoking.
- Passive smoking.
- Overcrowding at home.
- Deprived breast feeding during infancy.
- Play school.
- ASOM.
- Low immune status.
- Respiratory allergy.
- GERD.
- Leukaemia.

Microbiology

Usually mixed flora of gram +ve, gram –ve, anaerobic.

- *S. pneumoniae*
- *H. influenzae*
- *M. catarrhalis*
- *P. aeruginosa*
- *Proteus*
- *E. coli*
- *Klebsiella*
- Bacteroides
- Fungal infection may be coexisting.

Pathology

- Occurs as a consequence of unresolved acute suppurative otitis media/trauma for more than 3 months duration.
- Mucosal disease is predominantly in the eustachian tube, anterior and inferior mesotympanum hence called tubotympanic. Histopathologically the mucosa is hyperplastic and edematous with increased glandular activity. In late stages the mucosa can undergo subepithelial fibrosis and collagen deposition, hyalinization of collagen and calcium deposition (tympanosclerosis).
- As this usually do not produce complications even if untreated, hence called safe type.
- Rarely due to ingrowing squamous epithelium/squamous metaplasia can cause secondary acquired cholesteatoma.
- Inflammatory granulation following focal osteitis can lead to aural polyp formation.
- Ossicular erosion can occur due to osteoclastic activity/avascular necrosis/hyperemic decalcification. Common sites are long process of incus and crura of the stapes.
- Often associated with poor pneumatization.

- The mastoid air cell system undergoes secondary sclerosis with new bone formation.
- Subepithelial micro-hemorrhage can lead to foreign body granulomatous response to cholesterol crystals (cholesterol granuloma) which appear as yellow – brown semisolid material that may fill the middle ear or mastoid cavity.

Types

- Inactive (mucosal) chronic suppurative otitis media (CSOM): Permanent perforation without discharge.
- Active (mucosal) CSOM: Permanent perforation with intermittent mucopurulent often profuse non foul smelling ear discharge.
- Healed CSOM: Healed perforation which may be associated with tympanosclerosis.

Clinical features

Ear discharge

- Onset as ASOM/traumatic perforation
- Intermittent, mucoid or mucopurulent, usually non-foul smelling and non-blood stained.
- Increases with URTI/entry of water into the ear.
- Decreases with resolution of URTI/medications.

Hearing impairment

- **Usually mild to moderate.**
- Non-progressive.
- Paradoxical effect may be present with hearing improvement at the time of ear discharge.

Tinnitus

May be present during acute exacerbation.

Vertigo

- Occasional and mild.
- Sometimes due to 'caloric' effect/ototoxic ear drops.

Otalgia

- Due to acute exacerbations.
- Co-existent secondary otitis externa.

On examination

- **Characteristic ear discharge** in the middle ear and external auditory canal may be present as described under symptoms. Depending on the presence of discharge the disease may be classified clinically into the following stages:
  - **Active:** Discharge is present at the time of examination
  - **Quiescent:** Discharge is absent at the time of examination and is dry on history for less than 6 months duration.
  - **Inactive:** Discharge is absent at the time of examination and is dry on history for more than 6 months duration.
  - **Healed:** Perforation has healed spontaneously with a scar/thin drum (monomeric TM) or after surgery.
- **Central perforation** – perforation in the pars tensa with an intact margins/annulus all around. The size of the perforation can vary from pin hole to a large or sub-total defect (Fig. 3.17).

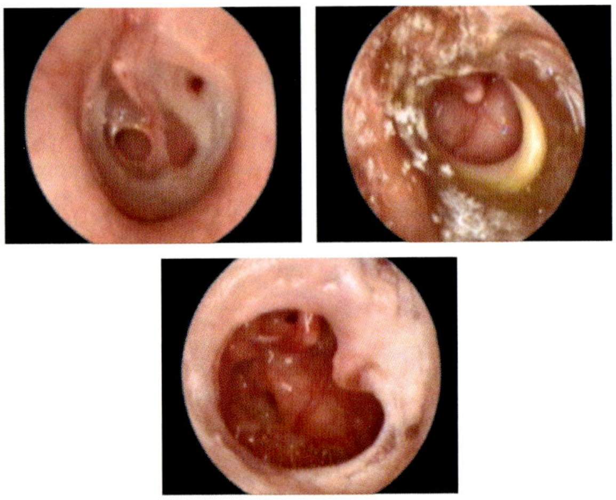

Fig. 3.17. Various sizes of central perforation.

- **Middle ear mucosa** – May be pale/congested/edematous/polypoidal and can be associated occasionally with aural polyp. Ingrowing epithelium and squamous metaplasia should be looked for to rule out secondary acquired cholesteatoma.
- **Handle of malleus** may appear foreshortened due to retraction and incudo-stapedial joint may be discontinuous. Tympanosclerosis may involve the ossicles causing fixation.
- **Tuning fork tests:** Show features of conductive deafness.
- **Foci of sepsis** in nose/sinus/nasopharynx/external ear, etc. may be present.
- Mastoid reservoir sign may be seen in the active stage where in discharge reappears after mopping.

Investigations

1. **Examination under microscope (EUM)** is used to confirm the findings seen on otoscopic examination. Meticulous suction cleaning can be done under magnification before examination to look for the status of ossicular chain, mucosal pathology and hidden cholesteatoma.
2. **Otoendoscopy:** Straight and angled endoscope can detect pathology in inaccessible recesses which may not be detected by microscope. It also helps in photographic documentation.
3. **An audiometric evaluation must be obtained.**
   - Pure tone audiogram (PTA): Is done to confirm and graphically document the type and the severity of hearing loss. If the cochlear reserve is poor, the ossiculoplasty is deferred.
   - Patch test: A cigarette foil can be used to close the perforation and PTA is repeated to know if a simple myringoplasty is sufficient or ossiculoplasty is indicated.
   - Anatomical patency of the eustachian tube can be assessed by tympanometry which will show a flat curve and increased external canal volume if the tube is completely blocked.
4. **Ear swab for culture and sensitivity in active stage.**
5. **Radiology:**
   - X-ray mastoid:
     - Haziness with intact intercellular septae may be present (mastoid reservoir of infection).
     - Secondary sclerosis of mastoid air cells.
   - X-ray of PNS/CT OMC: To rule out sinusitis.
   - X-ray lateral view nasopharynx: To rule out adenoid hypertrophy.
   - CT scan:
     - Cloudiness of the mastoid air cells and middle ear by inflammatory swelling of mucosa and by collection of fluid.
     - Secondary sclerosis of mastoid air cells.
6. **Diagnostic nasal endoscopy:** Is done to rule out nasal and nasopharyngeal pathology.

Treatment

- Depends on the stage
- Objective of treatment
  - Active stage: Make the ear dry
  - Quiescent stage: Maintain the ear dry
  - Inactive stage: Reconstruct the middle ear
  - Healed stage: Observe/reconstruct ossicles
- Medical treatment
- Surgical treatment

Active stage

Objective of the treatment in this stage is to eliminate infection including septic foci so that the ear can be dry.

- Aural toilet:
  - Dry mopping: It can be done under vision by an otologist using a sterile ear bud. The patient can be trained to use an ear bud to clean the discharge from the outer part of the canal with aseptic precaution. He should take care not to injure the canal/drum.
  - Suction clearance: It is an extremely effective method of aural toilet that can be performed meticulously by using a fine suction tip under microscope.
  - Syringing should not be advised as it can promote infection.
- Antibiotics
  - Systemic:
    - ◊ Broad-spectrum or based on culture sensitivity antibiotic should be given in active infection.
    - ◊ Ototoxic drugs like aminoglycosides should be avoided although in case of pseudomonas infection it may be given under proper monitoring to prevent cochlear damage.
  - Topical: Antibiotic, antifungal, antiseptic with or without steroid ear drops should be used for not more than a month by displacement method.
    - ◊ Ciprofloxacin/ofloxacin, acetic acid with or without steroid are preferred over neomycin or gentamycin.
- Nasal decongestants/antihistamines/steroid nasal spray if indicated.
- Aural hygiene should be maintained:
  - Prevention of entry of water.
  - Should use clean ear buds along with antiseptics for aural cleaning.

- Treat the septic focus – rhinitis/sinusitis/adenoiditis, etc. surgically whenever indicated.
- If ear discharge persists suspect mastoid reservoir of infection and a cortical mastoidectomy may be done if no other septic foci can be detected.

Quiescent stage

- Aural hygiene should be maintained.
- Prompt treatment of URT infection is necessary to prevent reactivation of mucosal disease.
- Focus of infection should be treated if any.
- Some surgeons avoid middle ear reconstruction in this stage as spontaneous closure can occur following removal of septic focus or otherwise. If no septic focus is found a tympanoplasty can be performed.

Inactive stage

Surgical intervention is the mainstay of treatment.

- EUM and cauterization of the margin of the perforation with 10% $AgNO_3$/3% trichloroacetic acid (small/medium-sized perforation) may be tried to promote healing.
- 1% sodium hyaluronate application to the margins of the perforation may be tried to promote closure.
- Myringoplasty: Repair of the perforated drum by a suitable graft material like temporalis fascia, tragal perichondrium, vein graft, fat, etc.
- Tympanoplasty: Reconstrucion of the middle ear pathology (ossiculoplasty has been discussed separately).
- A BAHA can be considered to improve hearing in cases of bilateral tympanosclerosis involving the footplate.

Pre-requisites for myringoplasty/tympanoplasty

- NO SEPTIC FOCUS.
- Good eustachian tube function.
- Good COCHLEAR RESERVE (for tympanoplasty there should be no SN loss).
- Avoid in children.

3

Myringoplasty (Fig. 3.18)

This refers to reconstruction of the perforated tympanic membrane. The aim of the surgery is to achieve permanent closure of the perforation with dry ear and improved hearing. Graft is placed on

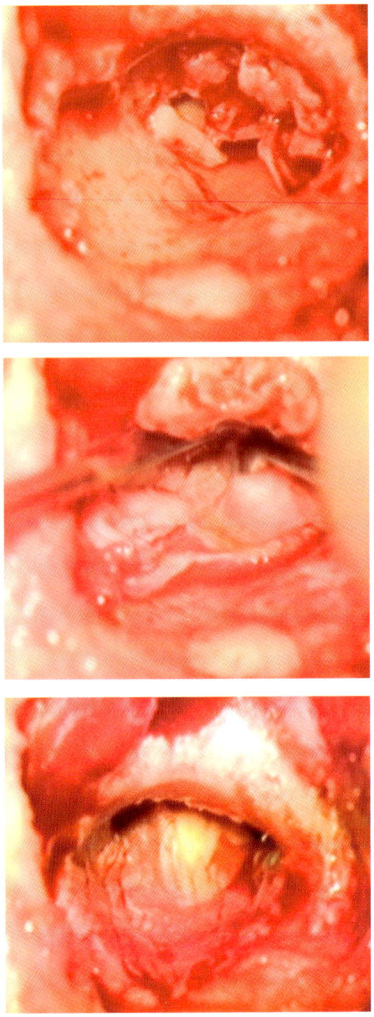

Fig. 3.18. Various stages og myringoplasty. (a) Elevation of tympanomeatal flap. (b) Placement of temporalis fascia with underlay technique. (c) Tympanomeatal flap in place.

the fibrous layer/annulus in overlay (onlay) technique and under the fibrous annulus in the underlay technique. Approaches to the middle ear may be transmeatal (endomeatal), end-aural or post-auricular. The post-auricular approach gives better exposure. Graft materials commonly used include the temporalis fascia, tragal perichondrium, conchal perichondrium etc. The advantages of the onlay technique include better visualization of the anterior recess, addressing the anterior canal overhang and higher graft take-up rate without reducing the depth of the middle ear space. Underlay technique is simple and easy to perform and is more suitable for small/ medium perforations. This technique has the advantage of preventing anterior blunting and early healing.

Tympanoplasty

This refers to the surgical procedure involving the reconstruction of the tympanic membrane and the ossicular chain. Banzer (1640) first attempted repair of a TM perforation using pigs bladder as a lateral graft. Berthold coined the term myringoplasty and placed cork plaster against TM to remove epithelium and then applied a full thickness skin graft. This procedure was popuarized by Zollner and Wullstein in 1956. Storrs (1961) introduced the use of temporalis fascia grafting by underlay technique which was originally described by Shea in 1957 by using a vein graft. House (1961), Glasscock and Sheehy 1967 developed and refined techniques for lateral grafting (Overlay).

Wullstein (1956) described tympanoplasty into five types:

- Type I tympanoplasty
  - TM is grafted to an intact ossicular chain.
- Type II tympanoplasty
  - Malleus is partially eroded. Graft is placed over eroded malleus or incus.
- Type III tympanoplasty
  - Malleus and incus are eroded.
  - Graft is placed over the stapes suprastructure.
- Type IV tympanoplasty
  - Stapes suprastructure is eroded but footplate is mobile.
  - Graft is placed over a mobile foot plate and round window is protected by the graft.
  - In type IV tympanoplasty mobile foot plate is exposed while round window is shielded with a fascia.
- Type V tympanoplasty
  - Graft is placed on a fenestration in the horizontal semicircular canal.
- Type VI: Round window is left exposed to direct impact of soud waves. Mobile foot plate is protected. (Sono inversion) This technique was added later by Garcia-Ibanez.

Type three has been modified further with the use of sculpture cartilage/bone and partial ossicular replacement prosthesis by various authors. Merchant et al. have classified type three into the following types:

I. Type three minor columella (graft/prosthesis placed between stapes head and tympanic membrane/handle of malleus).

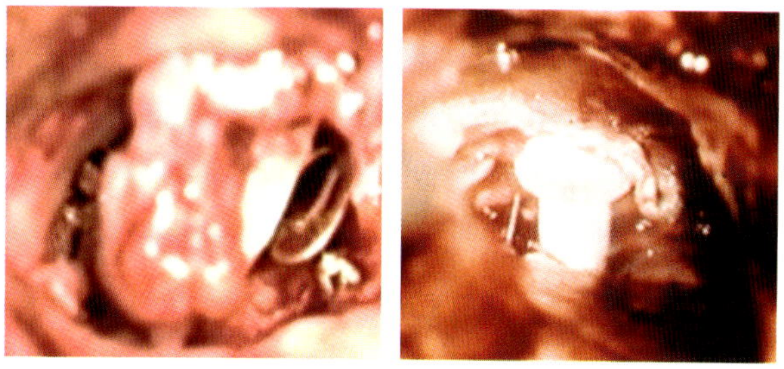

Fig. 3.19. Ossciculoplasty using (a) titanum PORP and (b) Plastipore PORP.

II. Type three major columella (graft/prosthesis placed between the stapes footplate and tympanic membrane/handle of malleus) (Fig. 3.19).

III. Type three stapes columella (facial graft placed on the head of stapes).

Atticoantral disease (cholesteatoma)

Chronic inflammation of the middle ear cleft usually confined to posterior superior mesotympanum, attic, aditus and mastoid antrum associated with a bone eroding condition called cholesteatoma.

- Cholesteatoma is defined as a three dimensional epidermal sac and connective tissue in the middle ear cleft, lined by keratinizing stratified squamous epithelium which has lost its self-cleansing property causing accumulation of keratin and desquamated cells inside the sac.
- Expansion of the cholesteatoma sac at the expense of surrounding structures including bone can give rise to various intra-/extracranial complications
- Called dangerous type of CSOM because of the associated life threatening complications.

Etiopathogenesis

- Impaired tubular function and infantile otitis media.
- Inadequate ventilation of the middle ear cleft.
- Middle ear effusion/atelectasis.
- Retraction pocket.
- Cholesteatoma (presence of skin in the middle ear cleft).
- Entrapment of squamous epithelium within the temporal bone.
- Congenital.
- Traumatic/iatrogenic: Implantation of squamous epithelium in the middle ear cleft.
- Secondary acquired cholesteatoma.

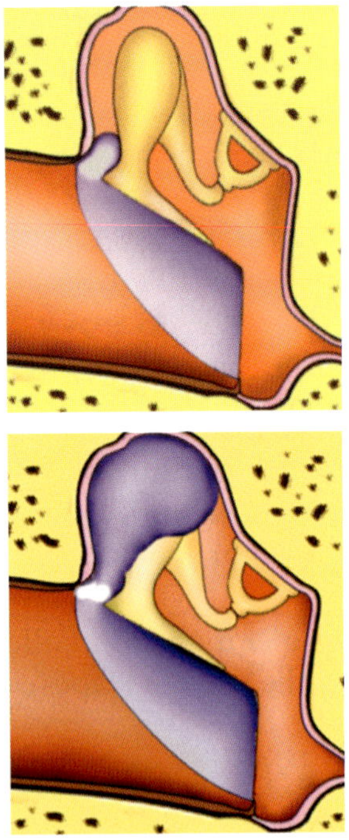

Fig. 3.20. Pathogenesis of attic cholesteatoma by invagination.

Pathology

A cholesteatoma is a benign growth of skin in an abnormal location such as the middle ear or petrous apex and is a destructive and expanding disease.

Congenital

- Developmentally epidermoid cell rests present in the temporal bone.
- Forms skin in the middle ear cleft/temporal bone/CP angle.

Acquired (acquired later in life)

- Primary
- Secondary

Primary acquired: Occurs in a previously non-discharging ear associated with retraction pocket due to ventilator defect in the middle ear leading to:

- **Invagination of the tympanic membrane** commonly seen in the pars flacid/postero-superior quadrant of pars tensa. Reasons for retraction are eustachian tube dysfunction, chronic inflammation, tympanic membrane atrophy and poor mastoid pneumatization. Retraction pocket should be considered precursor to cholesteatoma (Fig. 3.20).
- **Immigration** of cone like extensions of skin into the middle ear due to **basal cell hyperplasia** of the external ear canal skin/tympanic membrane at the tympanic sulcus as a papillary ingrowth of epithelium as described by Ruedi (1978).

Secondary acquired: Occurs in a previously discharging/diseased middle ear with perforation or due to implantation of squamous epithelium into the middle ear.

- Irritation: Chronic inflammation causes cuboidal epithelium to undergo transformation to keratinized squamous epithelium (squamous metaplasia).
- Implantation: Mastoid and middle ear surgery and penetrating trauma can be associated with implantation of squamous epithelium in the middle ear especially grommet insertion, overlay myringoplasty, injury to the tympanic membrane.
- Migration through the tympanic membrane perforation and is commonly seen in the marginal perforation.

Bony erosion and expansion

- Mechanical theory: Long-standing pressure on the surrounding bone by the expansion of cholesteatoma sac due to continuous deposition of desquamated debris.
- Enzyme/chemical theory: Osteoclast mediated release of certain lysosomal enzymes like collagenase, hyoluronidase, elastase, etc. by cholesteatoma causes bony resorption. The osteoclast activation is probably due to release of inflammatory mediators such as cytokine interleukin-1α from macrophases and epidermal keratinocytes. Other factors suggested as prostaglandins, cathepsin-d and parathyroid hormone like protein.

Common sites of erosion of significance

- Long process of incus.
- Stapes suprastructure.
- Lateral attic wall.
- Lateral semicircular canal.
- Fallopian canal.
- Dural plate.
- Sinus plate.

Clinical features

Atticoantral disease can remain silent for several years. Moreover the initial symptoms are mild due to scanty ear discharge and minimal hearing loss causing delay in seeking medical attention. However, as it is an unsafe disease the patient may present directly with complication.

Symptoms (uncomplicated)

- **Ear discharge:** Purulent/thick mucopurulent/blood stained, scanty, foul smelling and persistent discharge with no obvious precipitating factors like URTI.
- **Impaired hearing:** Extent of hearing loss is not proportional to the pathology in the middle ear unlike tubotympanic type of disease. Cholesteatoma may bridge the gap between the eroded ossicles.
- **Tinnitus** may be present occasionally following associated sensorineural hearing loss.

Symptoms (complicated)

- **Earache:** Due to external otitis/extradural abscess/trigeminal nerve involvement in petrositis.
- **Vertigo:** Due to erosion of lateral semicircular canal.
- **Headache, blurring of vision, projectile vomiting, etc.** can be present due to petrositis, meningitis and other impending intracranial complications.
- **Facial paralysis** due to the involvement of fallopian canal.

Signs

- Characteristic discharge as mentioned in the symptoms. Discharge has a fishy odor and is usually scanty.
- Perforation is either attic, marginal or total.
- Attic crust.
- Cholesteatoma seen as:
  - Pearly white sac through translucent TM.
  - Pearly white flakes of epithelium through mouth of the sac.
  - Ingrowing skin though perforation.
- Presence of granulation/polyp at the margin of the perforation or attic.
- Evidence of bone erosion in the form of scutum erosion or natural cavity may be seen (Fig. 3.21).
- Signs of complication: For example, facial palsy/lateral rectus palsy, nystagmus/fistula test positive. Signs of complications as described under acute otits media may be present.

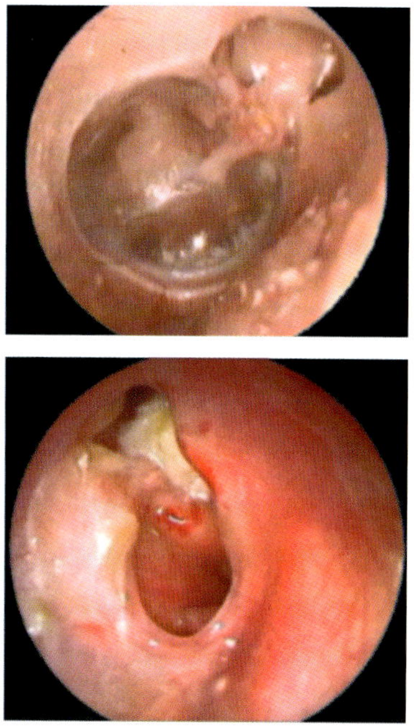

Fig. 3.21. Attic retraction and cholesteatoma with perforation.

Investigations

- **EUM (examination under microscope):** It is one of the most important investigations in otological examination. It gives magnification, better illumination and allows the surgeon to use both hands for instrumentation. Discharge and crusts can be removed meticulously by using the suction apparatus for better assessment of the ear pathology.
- **Otoendoscopy:** The angled endoscope helps in the visualization of the hidden areas including facial recess, sinus tympani and the fundus of the retraction pocket, etc.
- **Pure tone audiometry:** Is done to confirm and graphically document the type and the severity of hearing loss including the AB gap. The noted hearing loss may not be proportional to the pathology.
- **X-ray mastoids – lateral oblique view (Schuller's view):** Evidence for bony erosion and cavity should be looked for. It also gives the information about the position and the status of the dural and the sinus plates. The cholesteatoma cavity is usually smooth lined with a zone of sclerosis around it and a cotton wool appearance inside the cavity.
- **CT scan of the temporal bone/brain:** HR CT temporal bone helps in accurate assessment of

3

the extent of lesion in the middle ear cleft, status of the ossicles, labyrinth, facial canal, dural plate, sinus plate, sigmoid sinus etc. MRI is useful in the assessment of intracranial complications.

- **Ear swab for C/S:** May help in choosing the antibiotic for perioperative period and for the treatment of complications of the otitis media.

Treatment

Objectives

- Primary objective: "To make the ear SAFE"
- Secondary objective:
  - Make the ear dry
  - Preserve the hearing
  - Restore the hearing loss

Surgery: This is the mainstay of treatment for cholesteatoma. Conservative treatment may be considered in elderly and immune-compromised patients who are at surgical risk and in them regular suction clearing of retraction pocket/cholesteatoma under microscope may help in slowing the progression of the disease. Surgical procedure on the only hearing ear may be considered only when progressive enlargement of cholesteatoma is present or there are threatened complications.

The choice of the surgical procedure depends on the extent and the type of disease and the cochlear reserve.

In early lesions:

- **Atticotomy:** Early attic cholesteatoma may be managed by inside-out atticotomy followed by planned reconstruction of the scutum by cartilage and fascia graft.
- **Canal up procedures like combined approach tympanoplasty (CAT):** This has the advantage of preserving the posterior canal wall and its function and thus avoiding the open mastoid cavity problems. The essential steps of this surgery includes:
  - Cortical mastoidectomy.
  - Anterior tympanotomy: Middle ear approached by raising the tympanomeatal flap.
  - Posterior tympanotomy: Posterior tympanum is approached through the facial recess by drilling in the chordofacial angle.
  - Tympanoplasty.
- CAT is suitable for retraction pocket or early primary acquired cholesteatoma/posterior superior marginal perforation with granulation tissue without cholesteatoma. This approach is contraindicated in extensive cholesteatoma and if the patient is not willing for a 'second look' operation which may be necessary after 6–12 months.

In extensive cholesteatoma, a canal wall down procedure should be considered like modified radical mastoidectomy with or without tympanoplasty and a radical mastoidectomy.

Modified radical mastoidectomy (MRM) (Figs. 3.22 & 3.23)

This surgery can be done by both inside out and outside in technique. The purpose of this surgery is to exenterate the entire tympano-mastoid segment of the middle ear cleft, excise all the middle ear disease with preservation of parts of un-involved tympanic membrane and ossicles and to exteriorize the mastoid cavity by canal wall down procedure and a meatoplasty. This facilitates a large enough meatus for easy examination of the external auditory canal and mastoid cavity as well providing ventilation of this area. It is crucial to remove and exenterate all possible air cells as the mucosa within these cells can trap cholesteatoma matrix and cause recurrence. Also, the remnant mucosa can cause a discharging ear.

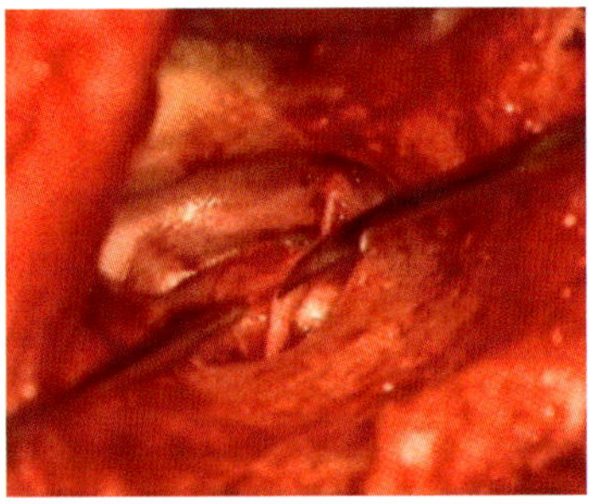

Fig. 3.22. Intraopertive photo showing retraction pocket with cholesteatoma sac.

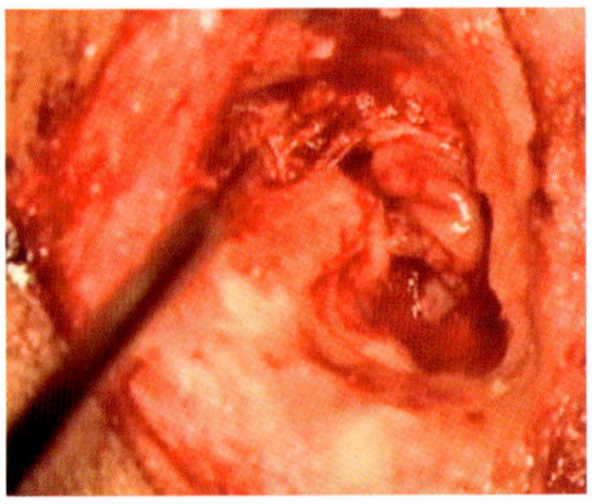

Fig. 3.23. Complete exposure of the cholesteatoma sac by inside out technique.

3

Modified radical mastoidectomy with tympanoplasty (Figs. 3.25 & 3.26)

If the surgeon is sure of the clearance of the disease a tympanoplasty may be combined. This includes reconstruction of ossicular defect as discussed under tubotympanic disease. Grafting of the drum also prevents mucosal growth into the cavity. This also facilitates early healing of the cavity. Attempts should be made to reduce the size of the cavity by suitable obliteration techniques thereby avoiding possible cavity problems.

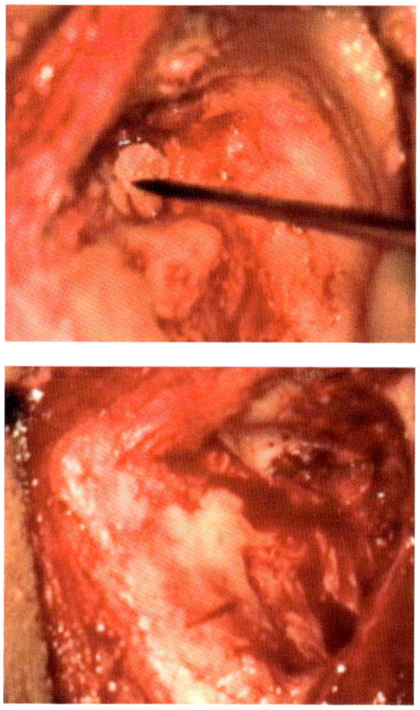

Fig. 3.25. Post MRM tympanoplasty using (a) cartilage graft as TORP; (b) placement of temporalis fascial graft.

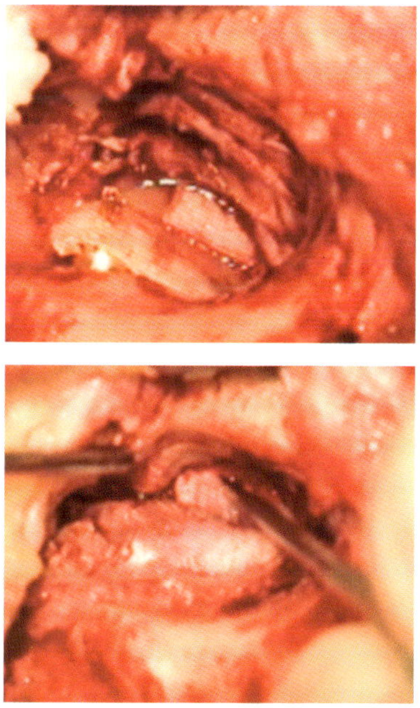

Fig. 3.26. Post MRM tympanoplasty using (a) gold implant mounted on choncal cartilage (b) placement of temporalis fascial graft.

'Inside-out' attico-antrostomy

It helps in reducing the size of the open mastoid cavity and thus in avoiding post-mastoidectomy cavity problems. This procedure is also known as Bondy's mastoidectomy.

Radical mastoidectomy

Radical mastoidectomy involves the removal of the mastoid air cells, the tympanic membrane, the involved malleus, incus, chordatympani, and mucoperiosteal lining which converts the middle ear and the mastoid into one cavity. This procedure is not commonly performed these days. May be considered in patients who already have developed complications or in whom there is no cochlear reserve.

Mastoid obliteration (Fig. 3.27)

Various methods have been described to obliterate the mastoid cavity partially or completely to reduce post-mastoidectomy cavity and its problems. Necessity of regular follow up following mastoid surgery and discharge from the mastoid cavity is

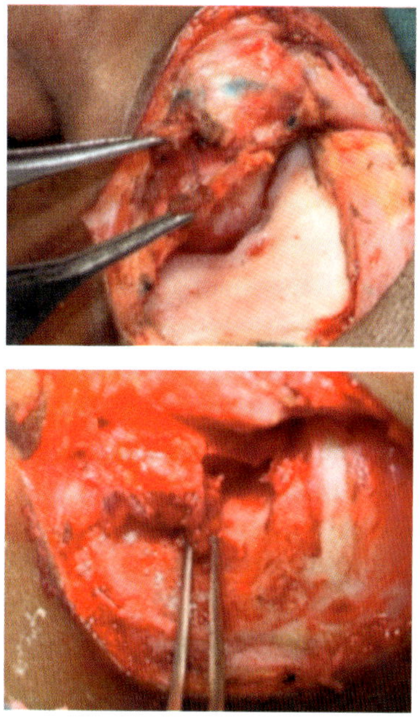

Fig. 3.27. A. Musculoperiosteal flap being raised, B. Flap being used for inferior recess after MRM.

3

the main problem associated with canal wall down procedure. The presence of a potential space in the tip region of the mastoid bowl has been implicated as a cause for collection of debris and subsequent discharge (Balakrishna et al., 2005). Palva et al., 1968 described anteriorly based musculoperiosteal flap for mastoid obliteration. Hongkong flap (pedicled vascularized superficial temporopareital flap) based on the posterior branch of superficial temporal artery (Van Hassaelt et al., 1995). According to Ugo Fisch, temporalis muscle flap is best avoided as it would prevent superior exteriorization. Weiss et al. (1992) described mastoid tip amputation and turning the mastoid periosteum into the cavity.

Posterior canal wall reconstruction

This may be done to deepen the middle ear space which gives favorable results if ossiculoplasty is being considered. It can be staged or can be done in the same sitting. Reconstruction can be done using otologus material like bone dust and chips, cortical bone graft, tragal or scaphoid cartilage. Synthetic material like hydroxylapatite may be used however extrusion can be a problem.

CONCLUSION

Otitis media is a major health problem around the world and is responsible for significant morbidity. It is an important cause of preventable hearing loss, particularly in the developing world. The WHO definition requires only 2 weeks of otorrhoea, but otolaryngologists tend to adopt a longer duration, e.g., more than 3 months of active disease.

Mortality due to complications following acute otitis media has been reduced significantly following timely treatment with antibiotics by the general practitioners and pediatrician but masked mastoiditis following inadequately treated acute otitis media needs special attention. Availability of polyvalent influenza and pneumococcal vaccine has shown promising results in reducing the incidence. Complications following chronic otitis media are sometimes seen following cholesteatoma due to late diagnosis and delayed surgical intervention. High index of suspicion about chronic otitis media by parents, teachers, family physician, pediatrician etc and early referral to otorhinolaryngologist will help in preventing/restoring the hearing loss and other sequelae of otitis media.

3

SUGGESTED READING

1. Goycoolea MV, Hueb MM, Ruah C. Definitions and terminology. *Otolaryngol Clin North Am*, 1991, 24 (4): 757–61.
2. Smith AW, Hatcher J, Mackenzie, IJ, Thompson S, Bal J, Mac P, Okoth-Olende C, Oburra H, Wanjohi Z. Randomised control of chronic suppurative otitis media in Kenyan school children. *Lancet*, 1996, 348: 1128–33.
3. Textbook of diseases of the ear; Ludman & Wright, 6th edition, Arnold Publishers, 1998.
4. Ballenger's Otolaryngology and Head & Neck Surgery; Snow & Wackym, Centenial edition, 2009.
5. Glasscock-Shambaugh's Surgery of the Ear, 7th edition, A. J. Gulya, Lloyd B. Minor, Glasscock, Zina Juliana Gulya, Dennis Poe, People Medical Publications House, USA. 2010.
6. Chronic otitis media – Burden of Illness and Management Options, World Health Organization, Geneva, Switzerland, 2004
7. Textbook of Ear Nose Throat-Head & Neck surgery, 2nd revised edition, Hazarika, Nayak, Balakrishna, CBS Publishers New Delhi, 2011.
8. Scott-Brown's Otorhinolaryngology: Head and Neck Surgery, 7th edition, Vol-3, George G Browning and Linda M Luxon, 2007
9. Bluestone CD, Klein JO. Otitis Media in infants and children. 3rd ed. Philadelphia:W.B. Saunders, 2001.
10. Jacob A, Rupa V, Job A and Joseph A. Hearing loss and otitis media in a rural primaryschool in South India. *Int J Ped Otorhinolaryngol*, 1997, 39: 133–38.
11. Rupa V, Jacob A, Joseph A. Chronic suppurative otitis media: prevalence and practices among rural South Indian children.
12. Minja BM and Machemba A. Prevalence of Otitis media hearing impairment and cerumen impaction among school children in in rural and urban Dar-es-Salam, Tanzania. *Int J Pediatr Otorhinolaryngol*, 1996, 37: 29–34.
13. Bluestone CD, Klein JO. Otitis media and eustachian tube dysfunction. *In:* Bluestone CD, Stool SE, Alper CM, Arjmand EM, Casselbrant ML, Dohar JE, Yellon RF. eds. Pediatric Otolaryngology. Philadelphia, PA: Saunders; 2003: 474–687.
14. Casselbrant M, Mandel EM, Kurs-Lasky M, et al. The heritability of otitis media: a twin and triplet study. *JAMA*, 1999; 282: 2125–30.
15. Casselbrant ML, Mandel EM, Rockette HE, Kurs-Lasky M, et al. The genetic component of middle ear disease in the first 5 years of life. *Arch Otolaryngol Head Neck Surg*, 2004; 130(3): 273–8.
16. Desmukh CT: Acute otitis media in children – treatment options, *J Postgrad Med*, 1998, 44(3): 81–4.
17. Ockermann T, Reineke U, Upile T, Ebmeyer J, Sudhoff HH. Balloon dilation eustachian tuboplasty: A feasibility study. *Otol Neurotol*, 2010; 31(7): 1100–3.

18. Wullstein H. Theory and practice of tympanoplasty. *Laryngoscope*, 1956, 66: 1076–1093.
19. Storrs LA; Myringoplasty with use of fascia graft. *Arch Otolarygol*, 1961; 74: 45–9.
20. Shea JJ Jr: Vein graft closure of ear perforation. *J Laryngol Otol*, 1960; 74: 358–62.
21. Austin and Shea; A new system of tympanoplasty using vein graft. *Laryngoscope*, 1961; 71: 596–602.
22. Derald E Brackmann et al. Otologic Surgery, Elsevier Health Science, 2001.
23. Hilding, AC.; Middle-ear pressure under basal conditions. *Otolaryngol*, 1944; 113, 829–32.
24. Sheehy JL, Glasscock ME. Tympanic membrane grafting with temporalis fascia. *Arch Otolaryngol*, 1967; 86: 391–402.
25. Sheehy JL. Surgery of chronic otitis media, Otolaryngology Vol 1, Revised edition, Philadelphia: Harper & Row, 1985.
26. Balakrishnan R, Kailesh P, Parul P, Nayak D. Inferior Recess Obliteration in an Open Cavity Mastoidectomy. *Indian J Otol*, 2005; 11: 5–9.
27. Nayak D R, Balakrishnan R, Hazarika P & Mathew PT. Role of cortical mastoidectomy in the results of myringoplasty for dry tubotympanic disease. *Indian J Otol*, 2003; 9: 11–15.
28. Palva, T et al.: Radical mastoidectomy with cavity obliteration. *Arch Otolaryngol*, 1968; 88: 119–123.
29. Van Hassaelt et al.; The Hongkong vascularized temporalis fascial flap for optimal reconstruction of mastoid cavity. *Laryngoscope*, 1992; 102: 289–99.
30. Weiss MH, Simon CP, Jin CH, David RE; Surgery for recurrent and residual cholesteatoma. *Laryngoscope*, 1992; 102: 145–51.

CHAPTER 4

Management of Cholesteatoma With Inside-Out Technique

Madhuri Mehta, K.P. Morwani

Cholesteatoma as we all know always starts in the attic in Prussack's space (except in congenital cholesteatoma, fortunately a very rare condition). This space is between pars flaccida, neck of the malleus and lateral malleolar fold. Further on it may extend towards middle ear, leading to erosion of lenticular process/long process of incus and suprastructure of stapes. On the way it may erode fallopian canal and may further extend to meso- and hypotympanum. The second route of spread which is more frequently seen is via the aditus to the antrum and from here to sinodural angle and mastoid tip. On the route it may erode lateral semicircular canal with formation of a fistula. At times it goes beyond the boundaries of temporal bone and then it can spread:

1. **Extracranially:** Disease can erode mastoid bone and cause abscess around or anywhere in the vicinity of mastoid bone. If it erodes tip of mastoid, it can form abscess around SCM muscle (Bezold's abscess), it can cause zygomatic abscess and Luc's abscess.

2. **Intracranially:** Which can be in the following manner:
   - (a) Along the infracochlear cells up to petrous apex leading to Gradenigo's syndrome.
   - (b) Supralabyrinthine cells eroding the tegmen leading to spread to the temporoparietal area.
   - (c) Erosion of sinus plate leading to thrombosis of sigmoid sinus or perisinus abscess.
   - (d) Via solid angle and retrolabyrinthine cells into cerebellar area
   - (e) After spreading into intracranial space manifesting as meningitis, encephalitis, hydrocephalus, extradural, subdural and brain abscess.

Philosophy of outside-in approach

Many decades back outside-in technique seemed to be the sound approach as patient would reach the surgeon with extensive disease and cholesteatoma having already spread to mastoid cortex or beyond the confines of mastoid bone. By approaching from outside-in, the surgeon was directly on disease by minimum gouging of mastoid cortex (by hammer and gouge in pre-drill era). Anyway the aim of surgery in those days was to decompress the mastoid cortex and remove as much cholesteatoma as possible.

However, competent the surgeon might have been, there was no chance of performing finer steps like surgery over fallopian canal or labyrinthine block because of lack of fine instruments and proper illumination and magnification. Outside-in technique was performed with the crude instruments surgeon had in those days.

The myth that cholesteatoma could not be eradicated completely was true for that era, because of limited training and the inadequate equipments available at that time. They did not indulge in ossiculoplasty and tympanoplasty for the same reasons.

Philosophy of inside-out technique

With present level of understanding of cholesteatoma disease, tremendous scope of practising dissection on the temporal bones, advances in technology like microscopes, microdrills, fine burr points (cutting and diamond), various other very fine instruments to handle each anatomical location and finally with improved anaesthesia techniques, our target should be to achieve perfect results and bring the incidence of residual cholesteatoma disease to < 1%.

We all know that the disease (cholesteatoma) starts in attic. One wonders why the surgeon should approach the attic by drilling through all the healthy bone of mastoid cortex. In inside-out mastoidectomy, the philosophy is to follow the cholesteatoma from where it starts i.e. attic. Keeping this in mind, starting from attic, we keep on drilling around the cholesteatoma in all dimensions. However, in cases of mastoid fistula, disease is followed from outside-in technique thus sticking to the principle of following the disease.

Today, the priority and aim of the surgeon is to make ear safe, dry, maintain or improve the hearing level, avoid dizziness postoperatively, avoid cavity formation or create small-sized cavity thus avoiding the possibility of performing disfiguring meatoplasty. In short patient's ear should be non-doctor dependent for rest of his life after cholesteatoma surgery.

Due to increasing awareness and better health care system in urban scenario the disease is often restricted to attic or antrum (in almost 40–60% of the cases). These cases require either atticotomy or atticoantrostomy for clearance of cholesteatoma, followed by repair of outer attic or atticoantral wall. In case disease extends beyond the antrum or involves the complete mastoid air cell system, we perform canal wall down technique. Fortunately fair number of cases have sclerosed mastoid thus reducing the workload of surgeon and size of cavity is restricted. In cases mastoid is partially cellular and cavity is big, we do partial obliteration of the cavity and if mastoid cavity is very big, then we go for complete obliteration of the cavity with various techniques. Cases with sclerosed mastoid, with either low lying dura or forward sigmoid sinus, prove hazardous for surgeon, if approached by outside-in technique.

In cholesteatoma surgery, it is mandatory to remove the cholesteatoma matrix completely along with all the cells and mucosa under it. Incomplete mastoidectomy leaves some air cells containing mucosa which leads to discharging cavity as the mucosa produces mucus in the cavity.

The present article describes the surgical technique and benefits of inside-out mastoidectomy as also discuss the potential pitfalls and causes of failure in cholesteatoma surgery.

METHOD

The surgery can be performed either by endaural or postaural route. However, these days postaural route is practised by most of the surgeons. The procedure is performed under general anesthesia and in cooperative adults in local anaesthesia.

Postaural route

Skin incision is given 2 mm behind the postaural groove. The superior extent of the incision is from a point above the helix, the anterior limit being along a vertical line drawn from tragus superiorly. The inferior limit is at the mastoid tip or up to a horizontal plane just below the floor of the external canal (Fig. 4.1).

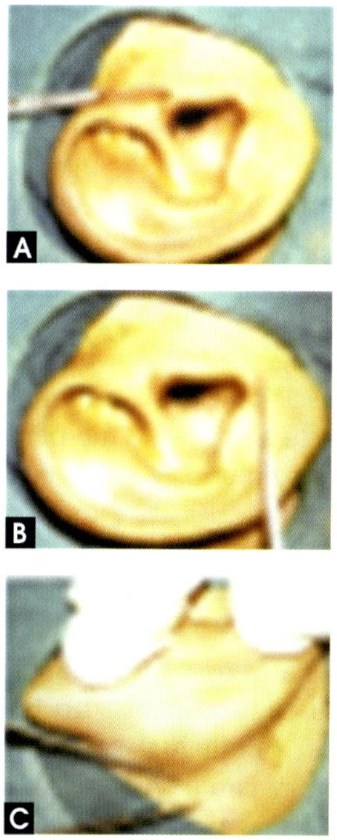

Fig. 4.1A, B, C. Skin incision. (A) Anterosuperiorly upto anterior canal wall. (B) Inferiorly upto mastoid tip. (C) 2–3 mm away from the groove.

4

Cross hatches incision is important as improper alignment of suturing can lead to displacement of pinna inferiorly or superiorly. The posterior margin of skin is mobilized for a few millimetres which helps in retaining the mastoid retractor as well as closing both layers of incision in single layer.

Harvesting temporalis fascia graft

A large fascia graft of rough dimension 3 cm × 3 cm is harvested without damaging temporalis muscle under it (Fig. 4.2).

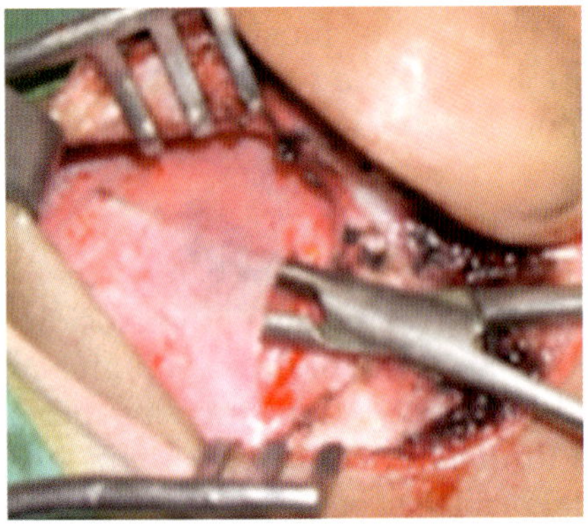

Fig. 4.2. Thin temporalis fascia graft being harvested without damaging any muscle fibres under it.

Musculoperiosteal flap incision

First incision is C-shaped given in 3/4th circumference along the bony margins of external auditory canal (EAC). It starts anteriosuperiorly from base of zygoma going along superior margin of bony EAC, further curving along the posterior canal wall and ends at the floor of canal (Fig. 4.3A).

Second incision is placed horizontally from base of zygoma going posteriorly between superficial temporalis muscle and postaural muscle (Fig. 4.3A). Postaural muscle along with the periostium is then mobilized posteroinferiorly to expose mastoid bone adequately (Fig. 4.3B). The main advantage of mobilizing the muscle periosteum posteriorly is that it can be utilized if required as a pedicle flap to partially reduce the size of cavity in posteroinferior part.

4

The external auditory canal skin is then elevated in 3/4th of its circumference up to annulus thus exposing roof, posterior wall and floor of the external auditory canal. All the skin is advanced upwards and forwards towards the pinna and retracted (Fig. 4.4A). This prevents the damage to the skin with the burr while performing the inside-out technique.

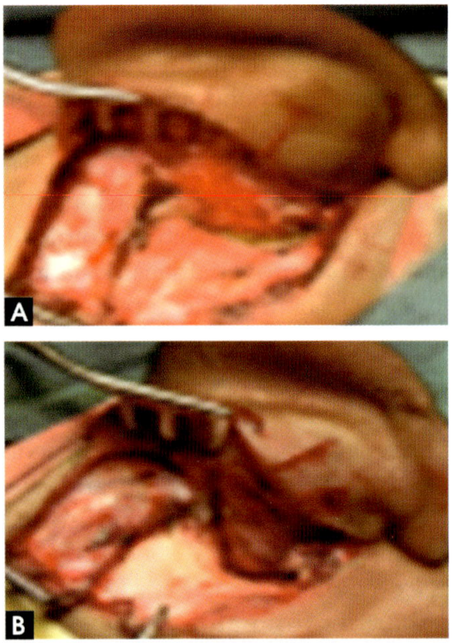

Fig. 4.3A & B. (A) Musculoperiosteum incision along 3/4th circumference of the canal and between superficial temporal and post aural muscle. (B) Mobilization of 3/4th circumference of canal upto annulus.

The floor cartilage is then exposed and excised (Fig. 4.4B) either at this stage or later on. This helps in widening the canal at floor level and also lengthens the released skin to reach the floor of cavity during meatoplasty. The other uses of floor cartilage are for reconstruction outer attic or attico-

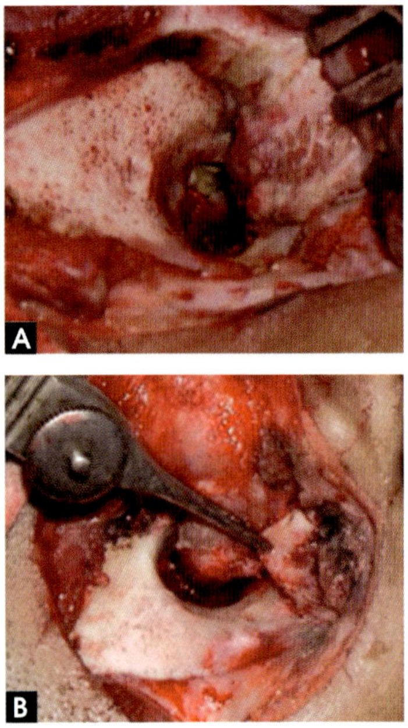

Fig. 4.4A & B. (A) Mobilization of 3/4th circumference of canal skin laterally. (B) Floor cartilage being removed.

antral wall. Piece of cartilage can also be used to obliterate sinodural angle and mastoid tip or depth of cavity and ossiculoplasty by cutting it into various sizes and shapes.

Bone work in limited cholesteatoma

1. *Widening the canal and collecting the bone dust*

Bone drilling is started with a large-sized cutting burr. While drilling the healthy outer bony canal wall, a few drops of saline are used for irrigation and the resultant bone dust is collected (Fig. 4.5A). This is kept in a small container along the edge (Fig. 4.5B) so that the saline drains into the container and the bone dust is relatively dry for later use, if required, to obliterate bony sockets or to reduce size of cavity in depth and width.

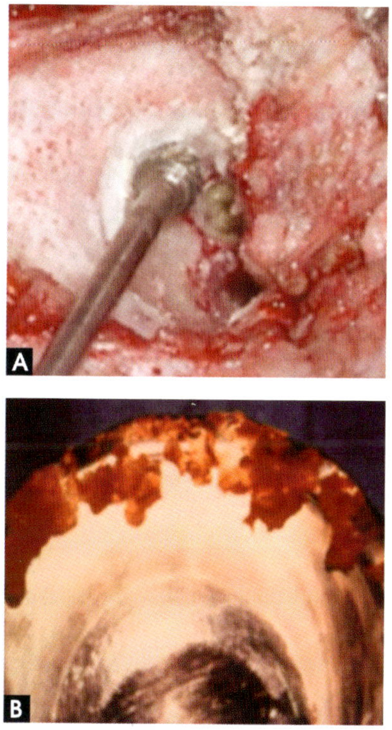

Fig. 4.5A & B. (A) Widening of the external auditory canal in 3/4th of the circumference starting from lateral to medial and collection of bone dust.

The bony external canal is then gradually widened in 3/4th of its circumference starting laterally and proceeding medially towards the annulus (Fig. 4.9B). In case of anterior canal wall bulge skin flap is mobilized in complete circumference laterally to expose the canal totally and canaloplasty is performed.

2. *Drilling of bone to expose cholesteatoma sac completely*

(a) Cholesteatoma may involve partial or complete attic.

(b) Cholesteatoma may extend into the antrum.

(c) Cholesteatoma may extend marginally beyond antrum.

In above situations drilling stops here and necessary reconstruction is performed.

(d) If cholesteatoma extends further up to sinodural angle or mastoid tip than we perform canal wall down procedure.

Important step

If the mucosa on the floor of attic or antrum is too oedematous then one can perform simple mastoidectomy as conventionally performed in cases of oedematous mucosa of promontory, to achieve adequate ventilation, for residual air cells in mastoid. Simple mastoidectomy should also be performed in cases of adhesive pathology. Fortunately this is not required very often.

The drilling is carried on in the attic to expose the sac. The cholesteatoma sac is then followed into attic removing the outer attic wall. If the incudostapedial joint is intact, it is dislocated to prevent transmission of the burr vibrations to the stapes. In case the sac is limited to the attic or the antrum, the sac is removed completely in continuity under higher magnification, and the outer attic wall or atticoantral wall defect is reinforced with cartilage having perichondrium intact. Either floor, tragal or conchal cartilage may be used for ossiculoplasty.

(a) Disease involving partial attic

This is a case of plastered drum posteroinferiorly and retracted posterosuperiorly. After widening canal in 3/4th circumference, the end of epithelium is visible in posterosuperior compartment, which is elevated with the plastered drum to expose posterosuperior compartment of middle ear (Fig. 4.6 – 1, 2). The granulation tissue may be found over and around the long process of incus and stapes suprastructure (Fig. 4.6 – 3, 4). The mucosa in this area may be edematous and drum is plastered, a simple mastoidectomy by exposure of antrum is performed to clear the ventilation pathway. The minimal attic defect is repaired with cartilage along with necessary ossiculoplasty (Fig. 4.6).

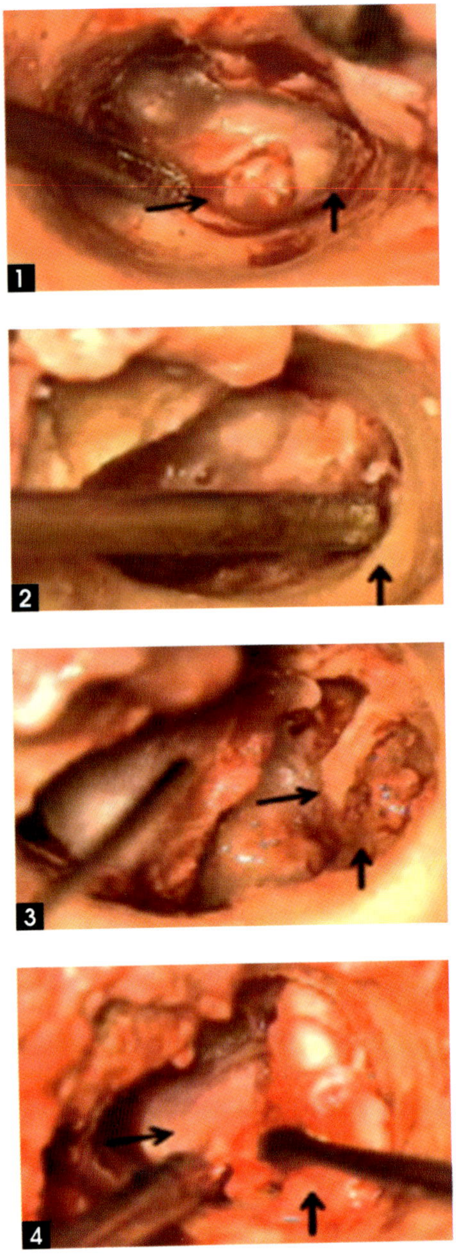

Fig. 4.6. Surgical steps when the disease is limited to attic and/or antrum (left ear). (1) Plastered drum posterosuperiorly. (2) Partial atticotomy – end of false epithelium. (3, 4) Granulations around long process of incus and suprastructure stapes.

(b) Cholesteatoma involving attic and antrum

The drilling is started in the attic. We expose the sac completely and once we see the end of sac in all dimensions, we mobilize the sac completely and in continuity up to middle ear. The next two sets of photo will be showing the various steps of surgery in which disease is limited to attic (Fig. 4.7) or antrum (Fig. 4.8). The posterior-superior defect is reinforced with cartilage having perichondrium intact. Ossiculoplasty is performed if required and drum repaired with fascia graft using underlay technique. If the mucosa on the floor of attic or antrum is too edematous then one can perform simple mastoidectomy to achieve adequate ventilation for residual air cells in mastoid.

Cholesteatoma extending beyond antrum into mastoid, requiring canal wall down technique

The steps of surgery are:

- Bone work before removal of cholesteatoma
- Bone work after removal of cholesteatoma
- Ossiculoplasty
- Obliteration of the cavity
- Tympanic membrane reconstruction
- Meatoplasty

Bone work before removal of cholesteatoma

- Widening of canal and collecting bone dust (Figs. 4.5A & B and 4.9B).
- Drilling is started in inside-out manner from attic towards mastoid (Figs. 4.9C & D).
- Steps till antrum same as described earlier.
- From here on drilling is carried further to expose the cholesteatoma sac towards the sinodural angle and mastoid tip (Figs. 4.9E & F).
- Drilling is done lateral and around the cholesteatoma sac in a circular manner and continued, till we reach the end of cholesteatoma sac in all dimensions, which is then removed in continuity towards attic and middle ear under higher magnification (Figs. 4.9G, H, I & J). Lowering and thinning of facial ridge is carried out simultaneously, to exteriorize the cholesteatoma sac completely (Fig. 4.9J).

Important steps

Lowering facial ridge bone to open facial recess

It is an important step and is done simultaneously with inside-out technique, rather facial ridge is never created. Drilling of the anterior aspect of the posterior canal wall at the level of annulus, from region of attic to the floor, going along the vertical course of fallopian canal is termed lowering of facial ridge. This step opens up facial recess and also

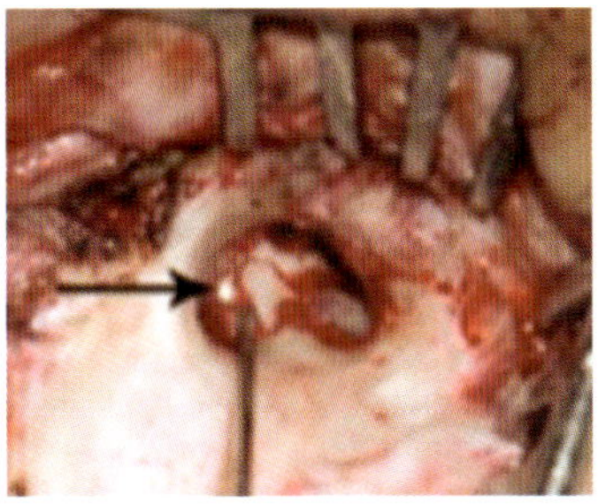

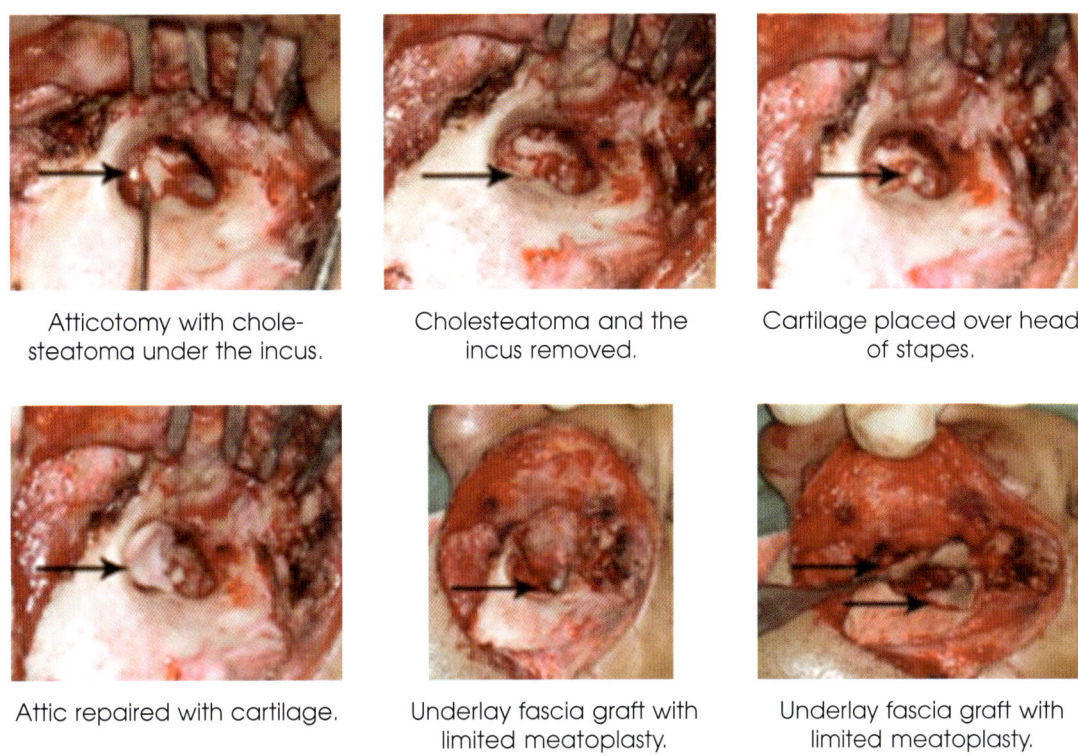

Atticotomy with cholesteatoma under the incus.

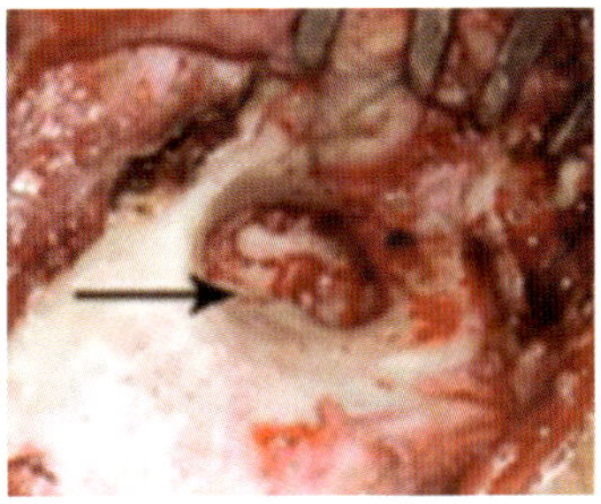

Cholesteatoma and the incus removed.

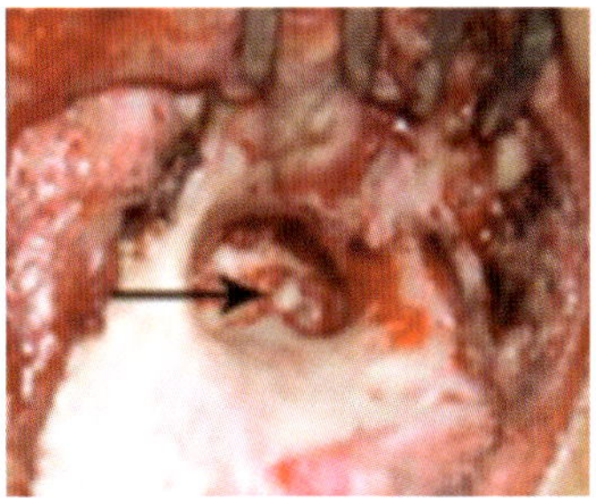

Cartilage placed over head of stapes.

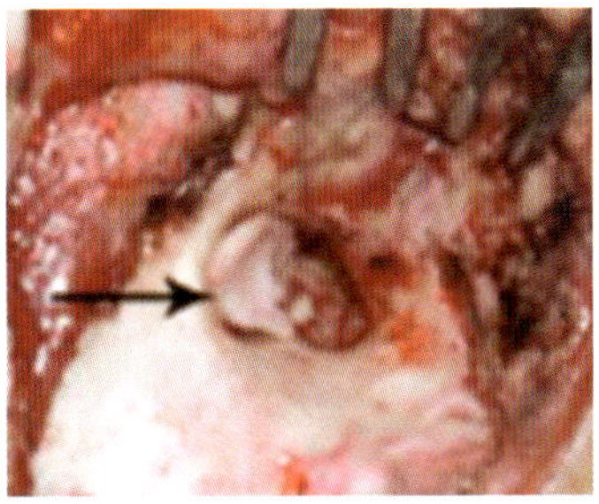

Attic repaired with cartilage.

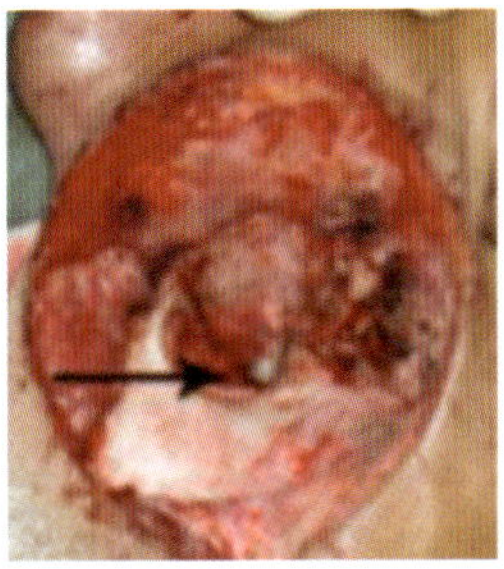

Underlay fascia graft with limited meatoplasty.

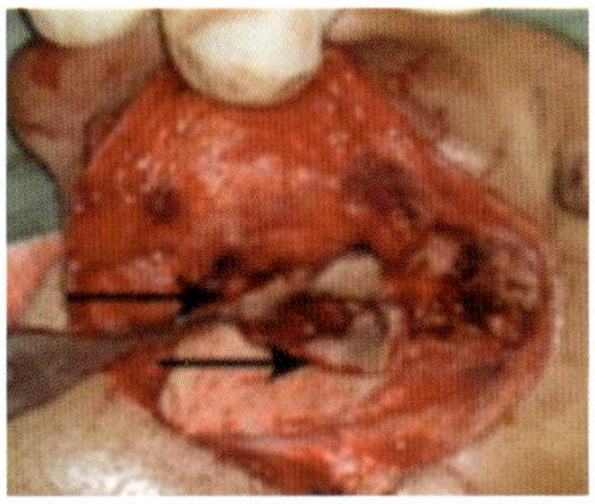

Underlay fascia graft with limited meatoplasty.

Fig. 4.7. Right ear. Various surgical steps of attic cholesteatoma excision and reconstruction (canal wall up technique).

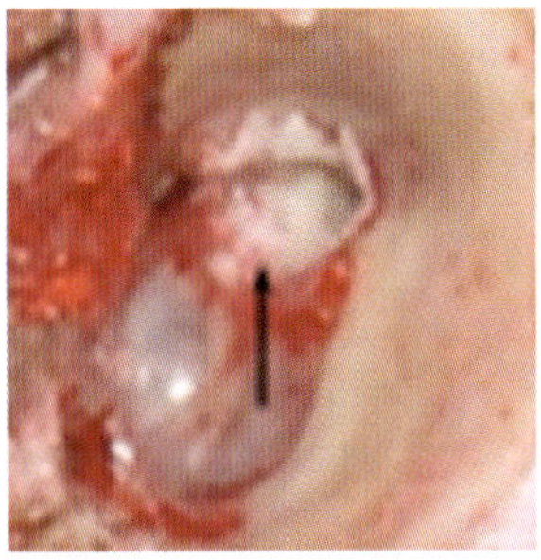

Attic cholesteatoma.

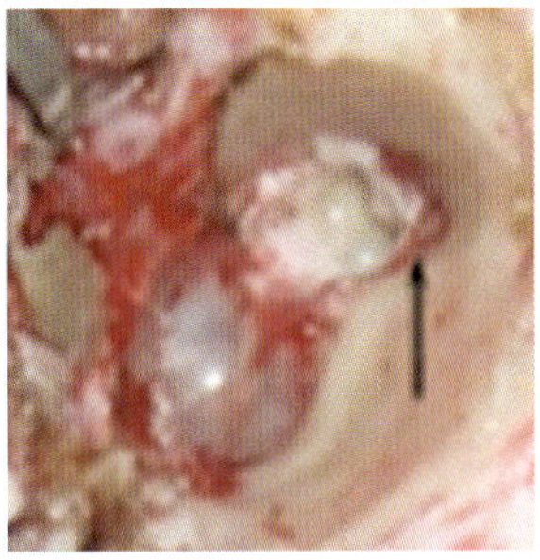

End of cholesteatoma in antrum.

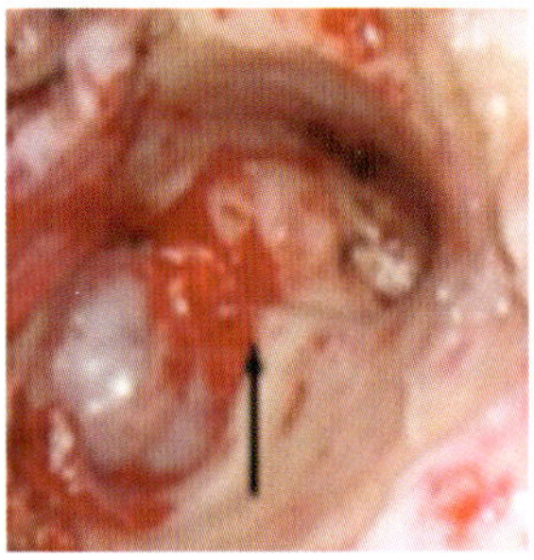

Clearance of matrix.

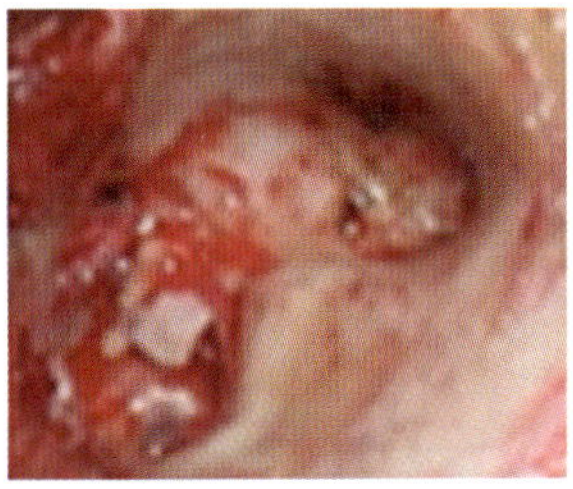

Ossiculoplasty.

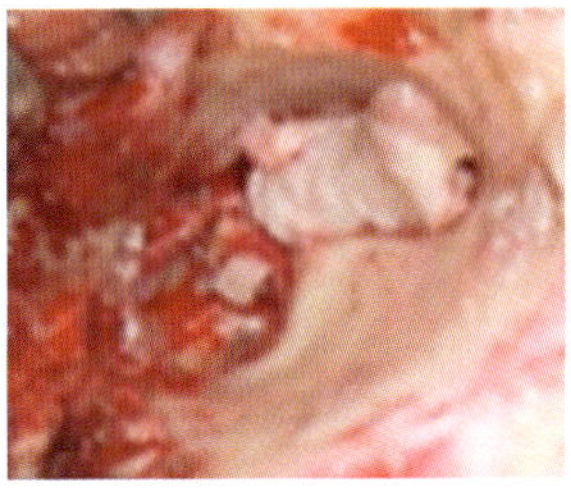

Reconstruction of attic.

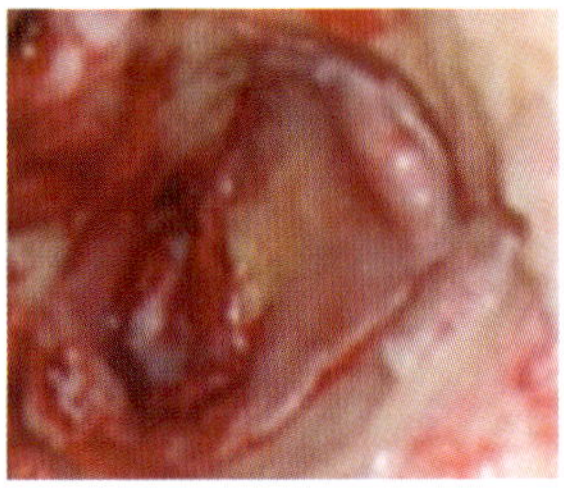

Placement of fascia and replacement of TM flap.

Fig. 4.8. Left ear. Various surgical steps of atticoantral cholesteatoma excision and reconstruction (canal wall up technique).

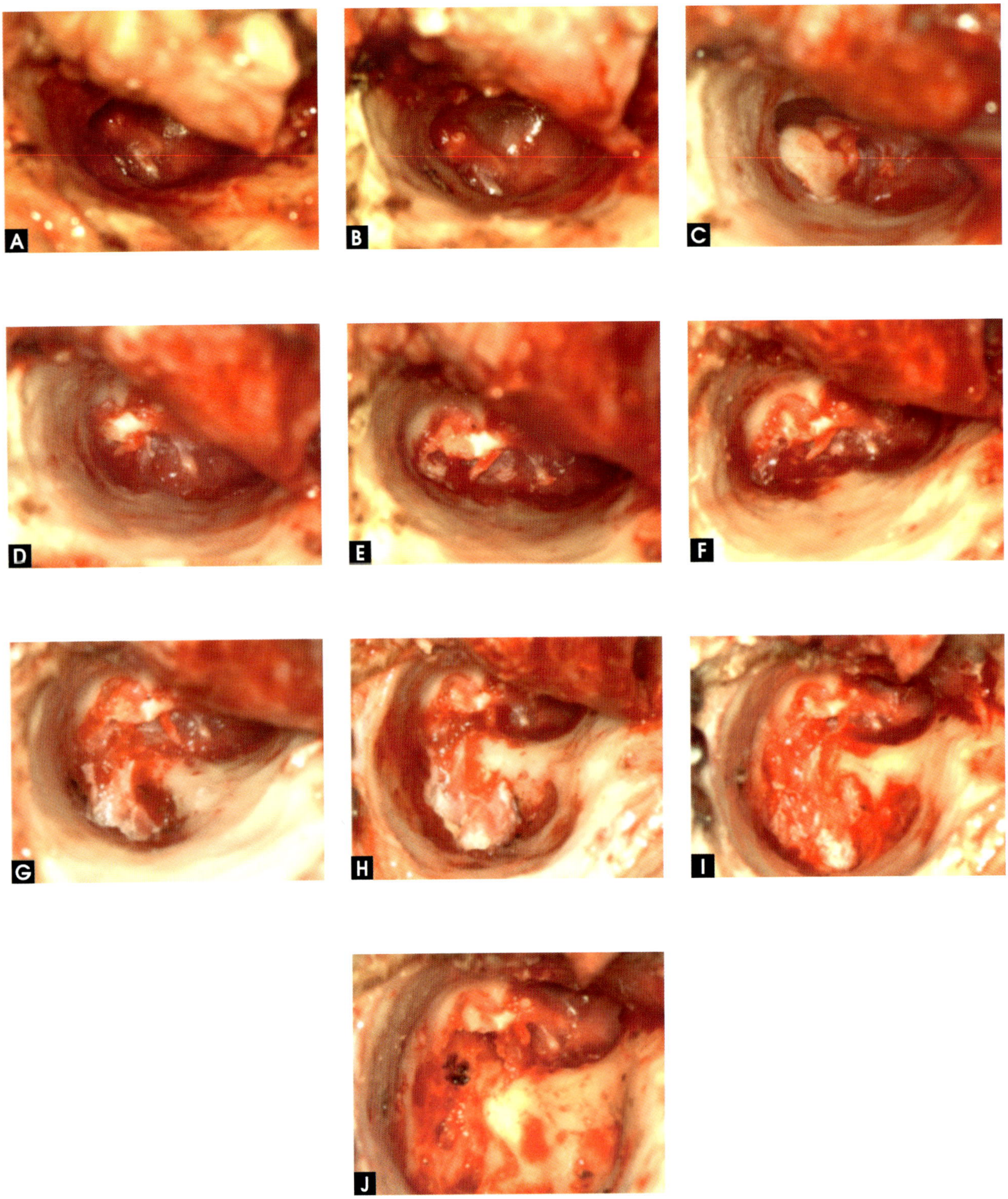

Fig. 4.9A to J. Various surgical steps for cholesteatoma extending beyond antrum into mastoid (canal wall down technique). (A) Post. canal wall skin elevated and retracted. (B) Widening the canal in 3/4th of its circumference, from lateral to medial direction. (C, D) Drilling started in attic, in inside-out manner. (E, F) Drilling around the cholesteatoma, towards mastoid. (G, H, I) Lowering the facial ridge along with end of cholesteatoma reached in all directions. (J) Cholesteatoma matrix removed in continuity toward attic and middle ear.

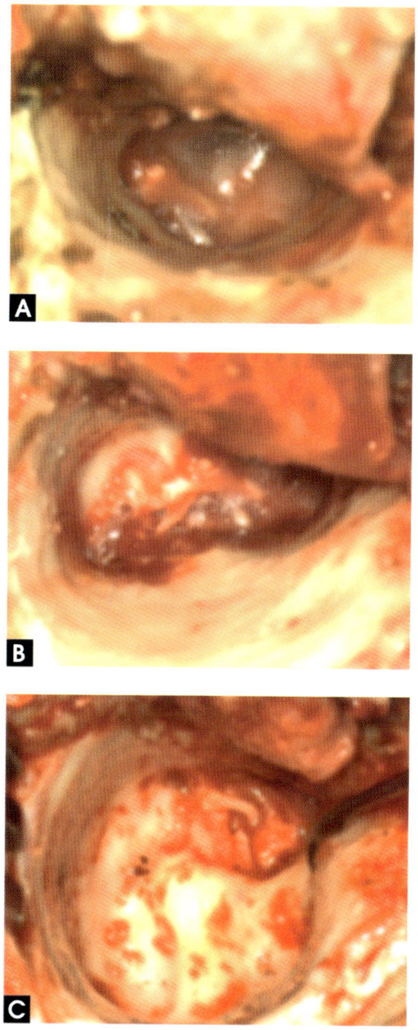

Fig. 4.10A, B & C. Right ear. Lowering of facial ridge.

makes one cavity out of two i.e. EAC and mastoid cavity (Fig. 4.10).

Thinning of the facial ridge to open sinus tympani

If cholesteatoma is reaching under the tympanic recess or pyramid, the anterior border of fallopian canal in its vertical course is drilled with diamond burr (of diameter wider than the fallopian canal width) to expose the cholesteatoma matrix completely in sinus tympani. Pyramid can also be drilled if cholesteatoma is lying under it (Figs. 4.11 & 4.12A, B) showing the exposed complete course of facial nerve and bone anterior to it.

In the middle ear, if the incus is surrounded by cholesteatoma or if there is necrosis of the long process, the incus is removed along with cholesteatoma. Similarly, head of malleus is amputated

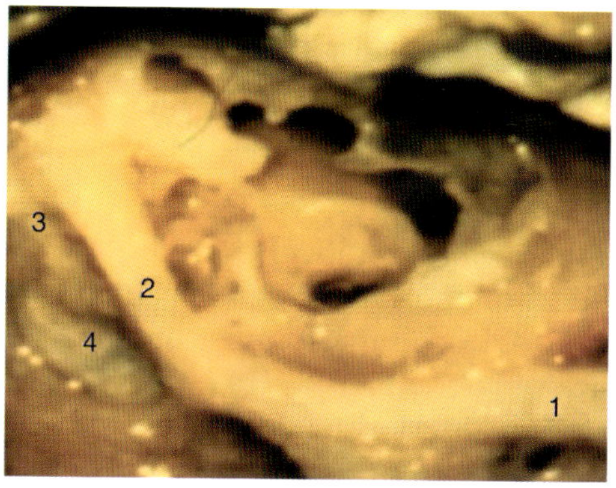

Fig. 4.11. Right ear. Relation of exposed facial nerve with the pyramid (*Courtesy:* Dr. M.V. Kirtane).

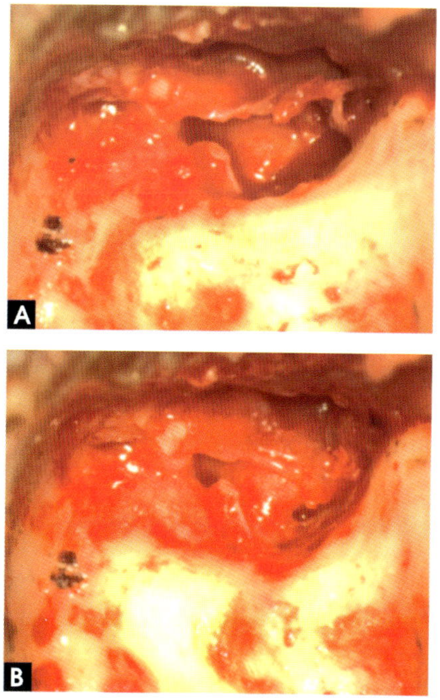

Fig. 4.12 A & B. Right ear. (A) Removal of bone anterior to vertical course of Fallopian canal. (B) Thinning of fascial ridge to expose sinus tympani.

to clear disease around and under it. Great care is taken to remove cholesteatoma from dura, sigmoid sinus, exposed facial nerve and fistulas of semicircular canal or footplate. In these cases, it is necessary to expose healthy dura, sigmoid sinus or facial nerve around the cholesteatoma or granulation tissue and a plane is found between the healthy area and the sac or granulation tissue.

Important steps

In extensive disease with dizziness or paresis of facial nerve, one has to be very cautious while peeling off cholesteatoma sac from vital structures.

Look for LSCC fistula under higher magnification and do not use big suction canula/sharp instruments whenever on LSCC fistula or exposed horizontal portion of facial nerve (mostly both conditions coexist). Lysis of the horizontal portion of facial nerve and rarely of chorda along with the big fistula of the lateral semicircular canal are diagnostic of Koch's mastoiditis in absence of frank cholesteatoma.

As far as labyrinthine fistula is concerned we believe in removing cholesteatoma matrix completely from fistula and repairing it at the end of procedure. Trick is to perform hydro-dissection that is excessive washing of the area. Have smallest suction canula tip to elevate the matrix and dissect out with fine pick and needle under high magnification.

Repair of fistula

To prevent dizziness postoperatively we have to repair labyrinthine fistula and defect in footplate of stapes adequately. Labyrinthine fistula is repaired in three layers – soft tissue, bone dust which is held in position with bone wax and further covered with fascia graft. Footplate defect is repaired with perichondrium, periostium or vein graft.

Similarly, if cholesteatoma matrix is lying on exposed dura, sigmoid sinus or eroded fallopian canal, one has to decompress the healthy bone along these important structures with diamond burr and get a plane of cleavage between dura, sigmoid sinus or facial nerve and the matrix.

Bone work after removal of the cholesteatoma in canal wall down technique

After cholesteatoma is removed, drilling is further continued to remove all sinodural, perilabyrinthine, retrolabyrinthine, retrofacial and mastoid tip cells which are lying exposed after removal of cholesteatoma sac. The residual anterior buttress is drilled out so as to align the anterior canal wall to anterior attic wall (Fig. 4.13A).

The facial ridge is further lowered depending on the depth of cavity posterior to it and if required up to fallopian canal. The floor of the EAC is drilled to match the floor of mastoid cavity (Fig. 4.13B).

If the disease is extending upto the mastoid tip, then tip should be excised which helps in reducing the size of cavity (Fig. 4.14).

Similarly, the tegmen is smoothened completely. The cavity is then polished by exteriorizing any residual cells and removal of mucosa so that the mastoid cavity looks milky white all around.

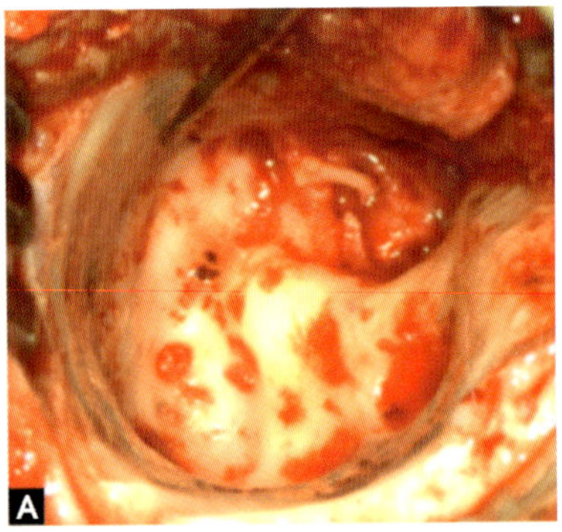

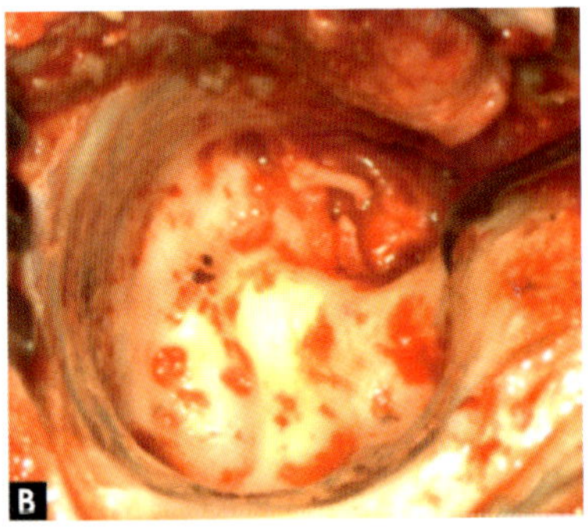

Fig. 4.13 A & B. (A) Alignment of anterior canal wall to anterior attic wall. (B) Floor of EAC aligned with floor of mastoid cavity.

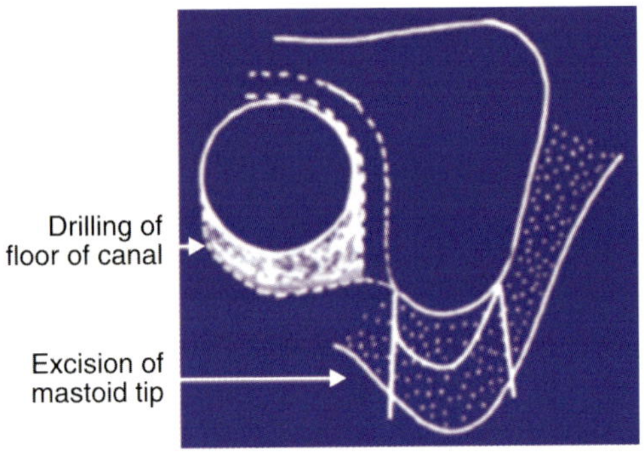

Fig. 4.14. Excision of mastoid tip.

Ossiculoplasty is preferred at this stage or after placing the fascia graft. The preferred material for ossiculoplasty is cartilage with intact perichondrium, preferably on both sides but on at least one side. Second preference is ossicle itself.

The synthetic materials are frequently used at various centres all over the world with reasonably good hearing results and most often cartilage is used between synthetic materials and drum. Some surgeons have reservation for use of cartilage for ossiculoplasty as they claim that it may get absorbed. But most of these centres do use cartilage over the synthetic implant to protect the prosthesis to prevent its extrusion.

Ossiculoplasty, different situations

Suprastructure stapes present

Either use reshaped incus (Fig. 4.15A, B, C & D) or floor cartilage between stapes head and annulus (Fig. 4.16A, B & C).

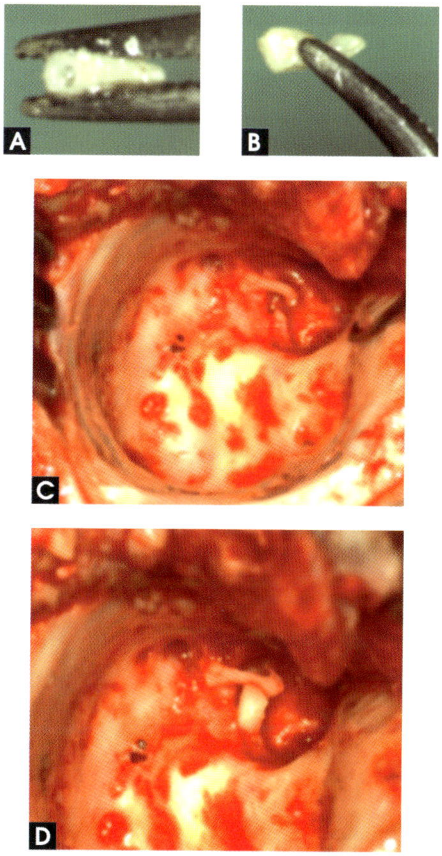

Fig. 4.15A, B, C & D. Right ear. Incus Ossiculoplasty with incus interposition. (A) Incus reshaped, fit for stapes. (B) Groove on short process incus for handle of malleus. (C) Handle of malleus and stapes suprastructure. (D) Final placement of incus.

Suprastructure of stapes absent

Either use incus after reshaping it (Fig. 4.17) or use boomerang-shaped cartilage with perichondrium between FP and annulus (Fig. 4.18).

When we place the cartilage between either head of stapes/footplate and annulus, we give better and larger contact area with tympanic membrane, maintain middle ear space and chances of post-op retraction pocket reduce to minimum.

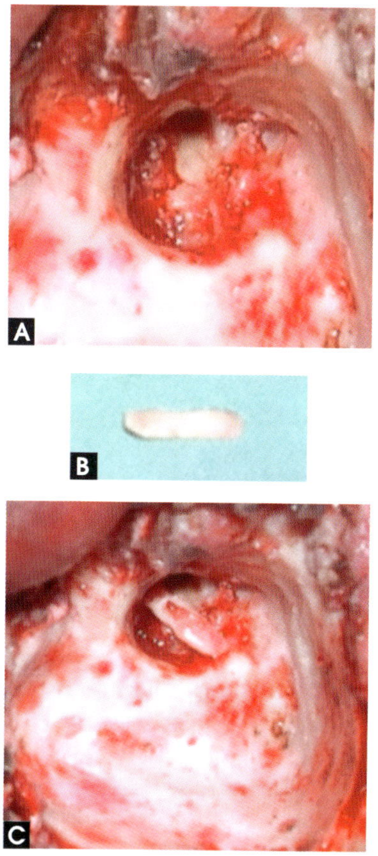

Fig. 4.16. Left ear. Ossiculoplasty using floor cartilage between stapes head and malleus. (A) Only suprastructure stapes +nt. (B) Floor cartilage graft with perichondrium. (C) Graft placed between stapes head and annulus.

Obliteration of bony socket and depth of cavity

The bony sockets are evened out using bone dust collected earlier while drilling the cavity. The areas that commonly require obliteration are retrofacial cell area, mastoid tip area, solid angle and area superior to horizontal portion of FN canal. The sockets can alternatively be obliterated using cartilage with perichondrium on both sides, or at least on one side or small pieces of free muscle with periosteum (Figs. 4.18 to 4.23).

Depending on the size of cavity obliteration can be:

- Partial obliteration, by just filling the bone dust collected earlier, free muscle with periosteum, floor cartilage with perichondrium and inferiorly based post aural muscle flap.
- In extensively big cavity, the obliteration is performed by rotating pedicle of temporalis muscle flap (Fig. 4.22).

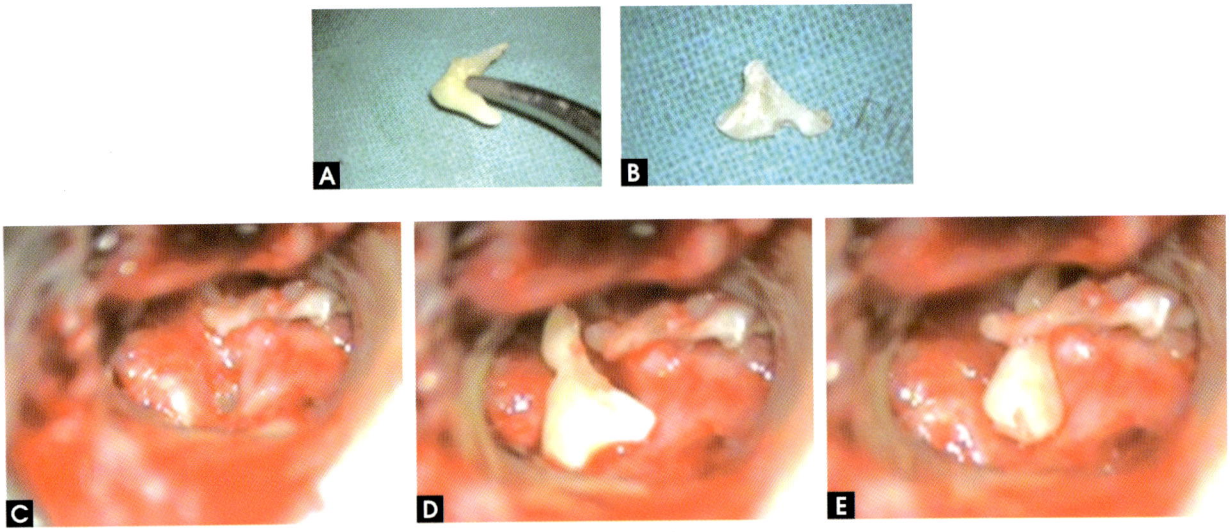

Fig. 4.17. Left ear. Ossiculoplasty with incus reposition between footplate and malleus. (A, B) Reshaping incus – Prominence for footplate; Groove for handle of malleus. (C) Handle of malleus +nt; Stapes suprastructure –nt. (D, E) Final placement of incus.

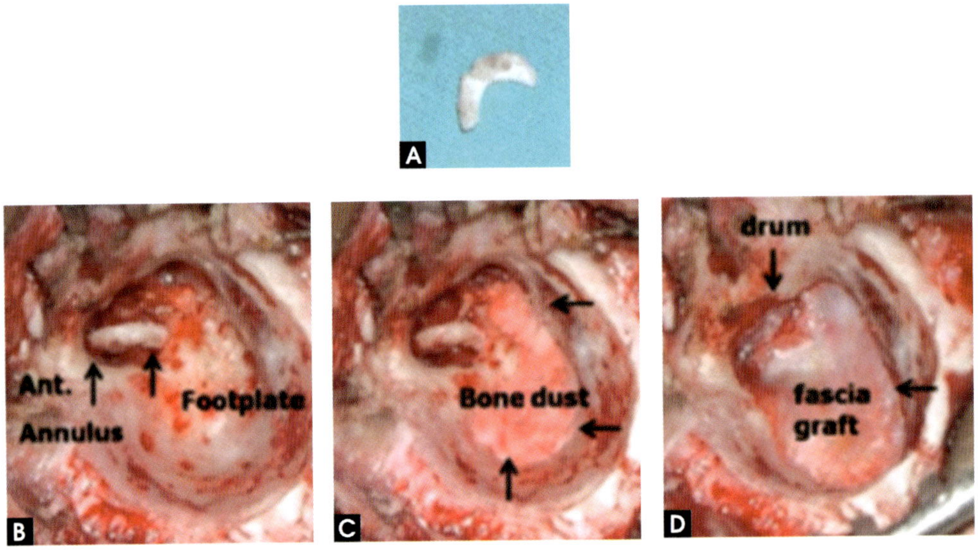

Fig. 4.18. Left ear. Boomerang-shaped cartilage ossiculoplasty between footplate and annulus. (A) Boomerang-shaped floor cartilage with perichondrium. (B, C, D) Floor cartilage graft between footplate and annulus.

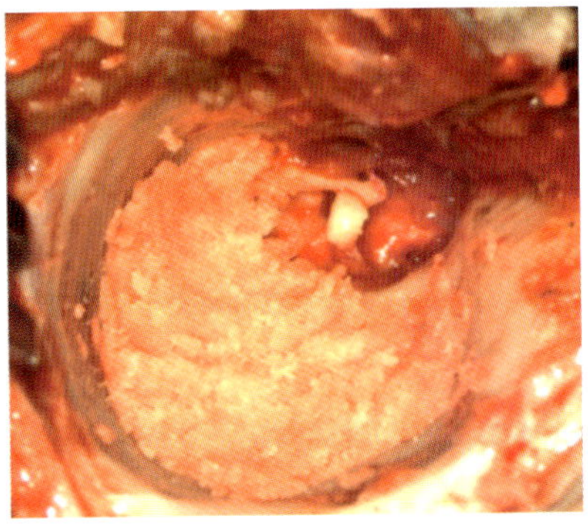

Fig. 4.19. Obliteration of bony sockets with bone dust and cartilage with perichondrium.

In very big cavity PCW is reconstructed with cartilage and the cavity posterior to it is filled with bone dust, cartilage and small pieces of muscle with periosteum as shown in Fig. 4.23).

Drum reconstruction

The defect in the drum as well as the mastoid cavity is covered with underlay fascia graft after performing necessary ossiculoplasty.

In case of mastoid fistula

As mentioned earlier we believe in following disease, in cases of fistula we perform canal wall

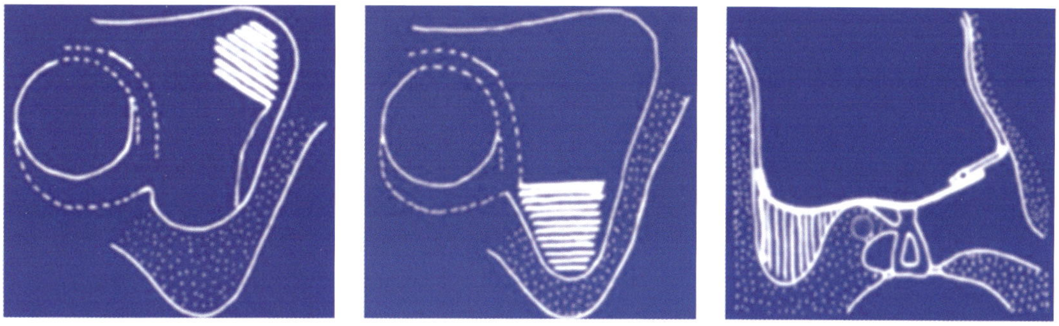

Fig. 4.20. Bony sockets which need to be obliterated.

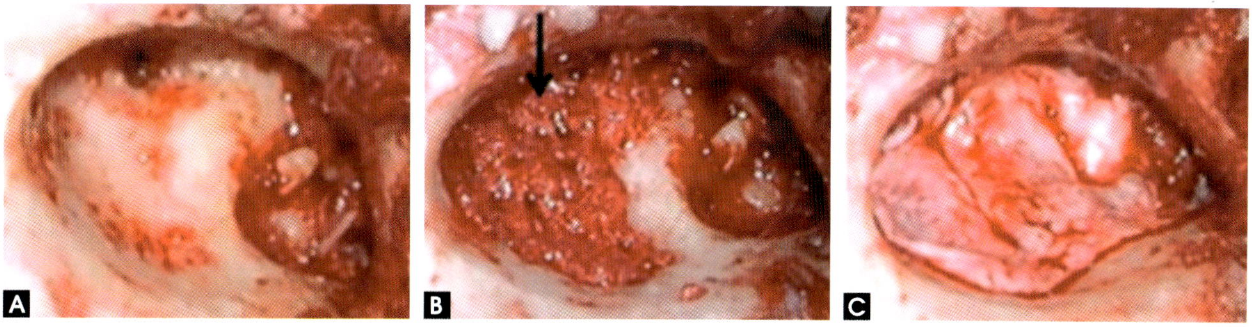

Fig. 4.21. Partial obliteration of mastoid cavity with bone dust.

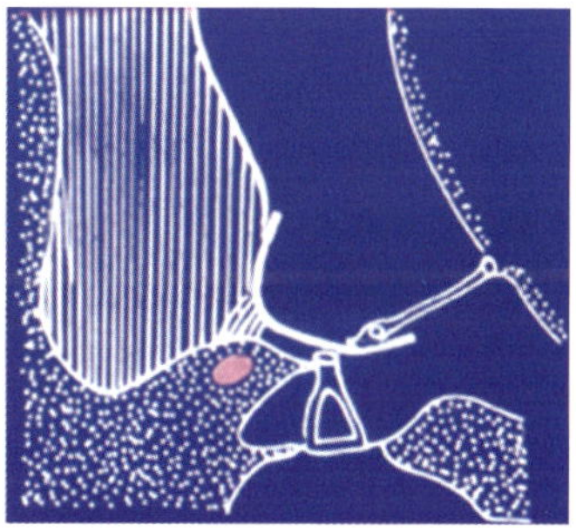

Fig. 4.22. Obliteration of mastoid cavity with temporalis muscle rotation flap.

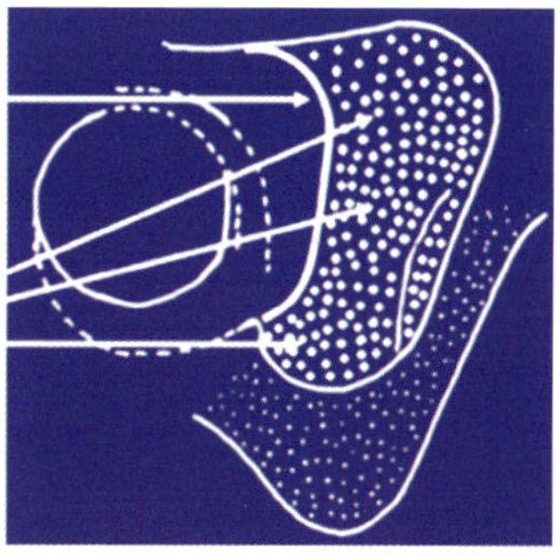

Fig. 4.23. Reconstruction of posterior canal wall and obliteration of mastoid cavity.

down technique following the disease from mastoid cortex, rest of the surgical procedure is same as described earlier (Fig. 4.24).

Meatoplasty

Meatoplasty involves soft tissue, cartilage and bone work.

The soft tissue dissection involves separating the skin and subcutaneous tissue of canal from the subcutaneous tissue of the pinna up to conchal cartilage laterally in 3/4th of circumference. Then the posterior canal wall is split vertically starting from annulus extending upto edge of conchal cartilage. Two horizontal incisions are given along the margins of conchal cartilage. Thus, the canal is opened like a book, creating superior and inferior flaps which are sutured to adjacent soft tissues (Fig. 4.25).

The cartilaginous dissection of meatoplasty involves excision of the floor cartilage and if the cavity is very large, a part of conchal cartilage is excised. It is important not to leave behind exposed cartilage as it may give rise to perichondritis with subsequent cicatrisation of the meatoplasty.

4

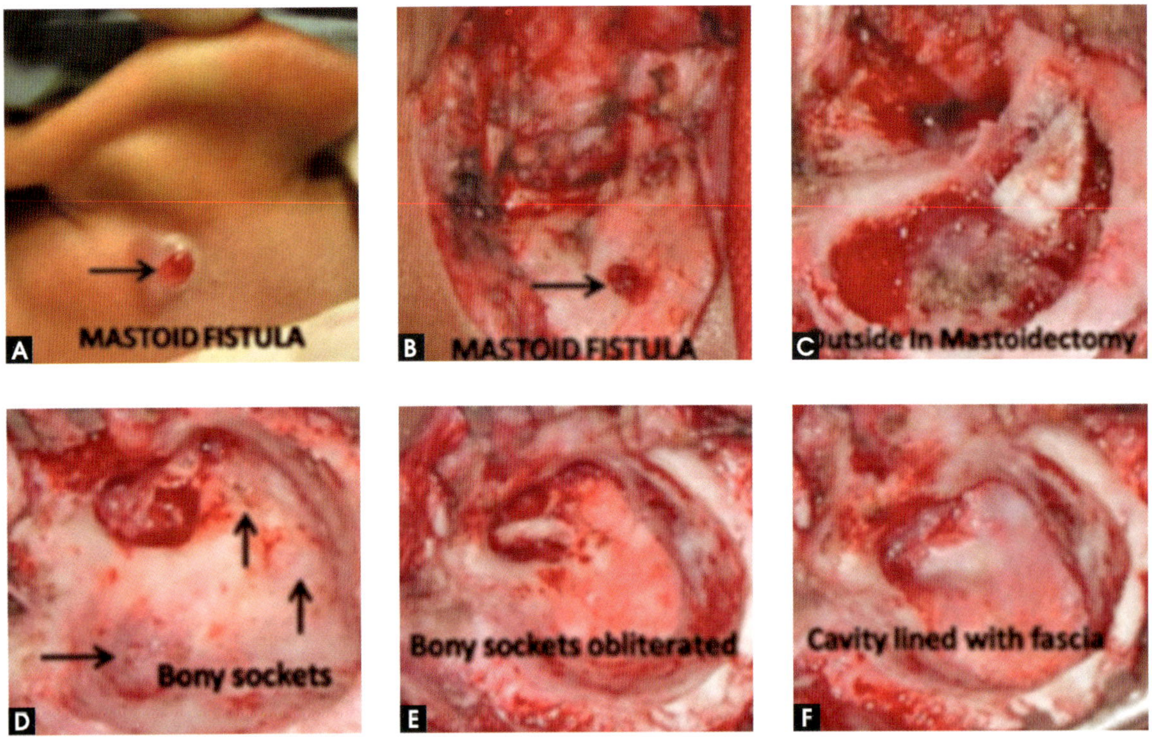

Fig. 4.24. Outside-in canal wall down mastoidectomy in LSSC fistula repair.

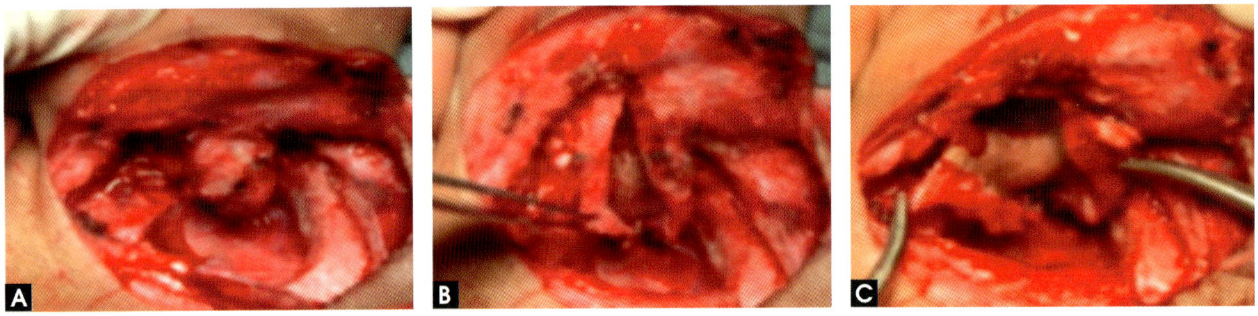

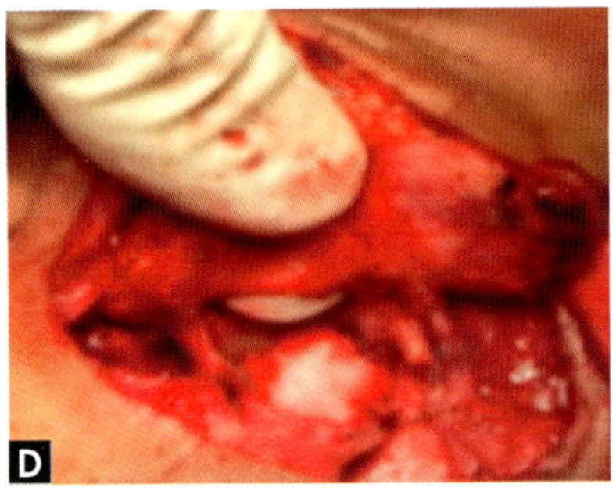

Fig. 4.25. Steps of meatoplasty. (A) Subcutaneous tissue of external canal denuded of cartilage and mobilized right upto concheal cartilage. (B) Posterior canal incised vertically. (C,D) Two horizontal incisions given superiorly to open the canal like a book.

Bony meatoplasty involves drilling the floor of the external canal which has been already mentioned earlier. Sometimes the anterior canal wall bulge may also have to be drilled as mentioned earlier.

Now we suture the meatoplasty flaps to the margins of muscles (Fig. 4.26A, B & C).

Cavity is then filled with gel foam only. No roller gauze pack is used. Musculoperiosteal layer is sutured (Fig. 4.26D, E & F). Skin and subcutaneous layers are sutured in single layer.

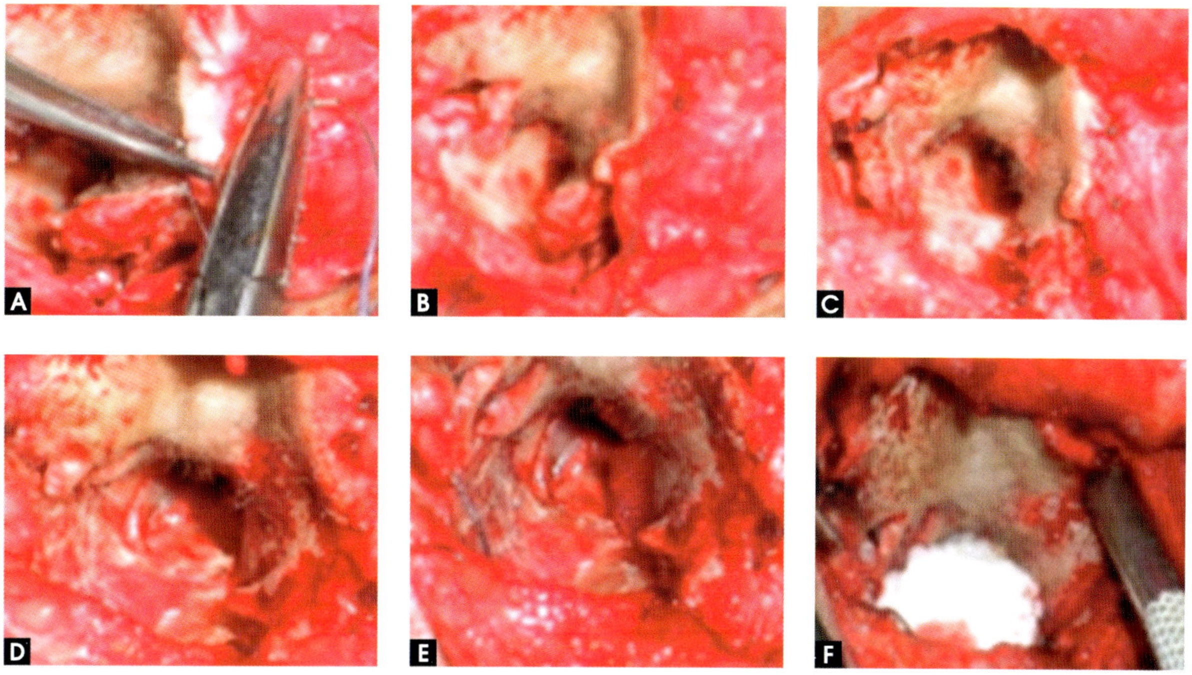

Fig. 4.26A–F). (A, B, C) Suturing of meatoplasty flap. (D) Cavity lined with with F graft. (E) Replacement of TM flap. (F) Cavity packed with gel foam.

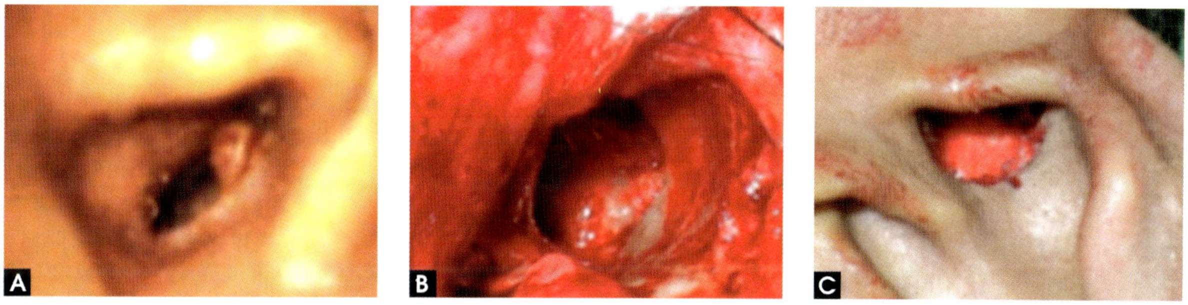

Fig. 4.27. Excision of scar tissue, cartilage and widening of the bony canal (revision meatoplasty)

Outside-in technique

As discussed earlier, only in cases of mastoid fistula with cholesteatoma we follow outside-in technique again we follow the principle of starting drilling directly at the fistula.

RESULTS

In U.K. under National Health Scheme the operated patient is called for the rest of their life for follow-up after cholesteatoma surgery. Compared to that, less than 5% of cases, operated by above explained technique, require prolonged follow-up.

By above explained technique, success rate of surgery – **97.5%** of the total operated cases. Rest **2.5%** cases have either residual cholesteatoma (0.5%), residual perforation, fungal infection, wax or **cicatrisation of meatoplasty** (1%) (Figs. 4.26 & 4.27).

Cause for cicatrisation of meatoplasty

- Exposed cartilage
- Improper mobilization and suturing
- Excessive granulations
- Bone wax
- Tight roller gauze packing
- Improper post-op care

In later years, we have started giving more attention to reduce the size of cavity by performing

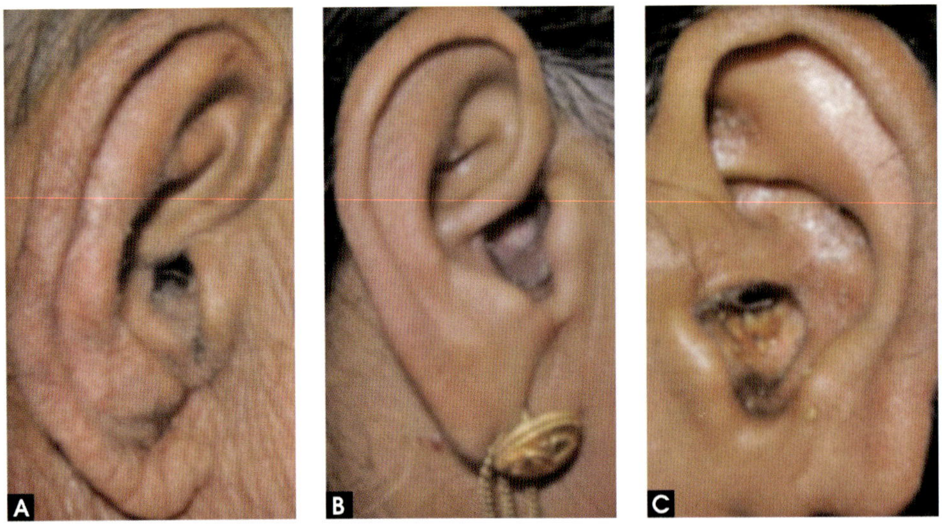

Fig. 4.28. Adequate meatoplasty.

various partial obliteration procedures and this has led to cosmetically acceptable meatoplasty rather than a disfiguring conchoplasty (Fig. 4.28).

In residual perforation, if perforation is small, chemical cautery is done, if bigger additional procedures can be performed through permeatal approach. Preference of graft in these cases will be split thickness cartilage graft with perichondrium from subtragal area.

After performing atticoantrostomy procedure, > 85% cases had hearing loss < 25 dB.

In canal wall down cases, in 70% cases hearing deficit was < 30 dB.

In ossiculoplasty procedure, hearing is better when suprastructure of stapes is present.

Revision mastoidectomy

In most of the revision surgeries the recurrent cholesteatoma is most often due to residual disease rather than recurrence of cholesteatoma. In canal wall down mastoidectomy, whether performed for the second or third revision, similar rewarding results were obtained. In most of the revision cases it was observed that previous surgeon had performed inadequate bone work or not removed cells deeper to cholesteatoma cavity.

4

Key point of the technique

The four D's described in the past following a cholesteatoma surgery i.e. discharge, deafness, doctor dependent cavity and dizziness were the symptoms of last century when the surgeons most often performed the surgery without fine microscope, drill machines, instruments and indequate knowledge and training about the subject. Today, with better facilities as well as better training programmes including various temporal bone surgical workshops conducted all over the country, any one of the four D's of the past should not occur in more than 10% of cases.

In inside-out mastoidectomy, we follow the principle of chasing the disease. It is advantageous in cases of disease limited to the attic or antrum, where with this technique we can avoid a cavity formation, or create a small cavity. In cases of extensive disease, a single cavity is created from beginning.

The most common site for residual or recurrent disease in the middle ear cleft is the tympanic and facial recess and anterior attic. The thinning of the facial ridge and lowering it adequately helps to expose the tympanic and facial recess. Early identification of the facial nerve and ossicles in attic prevents damage to these important structures.

Low lying dura and forward placed sigmoid sinus, which become a hazard in outside-in technique, do not cause any hindrance in inside-out technique.

Due to higher incidence of no or small cavities (good obliteration of cavity), the size of meatoplasty required is smaller, hence cosmetically acceptable.

In revision surgeries where the posterior canal wall has been lowered inadequately, there is a possibility of reconstructing the posterior canal wall, after clearing the residual disease, by using tragal, conchal or the floor cartilage, leaving adequate pathway in attic and aditus for ventilation and drainage.

Following the basic principles of open cavity mastoidectomy even in revision cases, a dry cavity and satisfactory functional results are obtained.

CONCLUSION

The most important points to be kept in mind:

1. **In atticotomy and atticoantrostomy:** Repair of outer attic wall is mandatory. Pieces of cartilage used for reconstruction of outer attic or atticoantral wall should be adequately thin so as not to obliterate the attic or atticoantral pathway posterior to it. It should be broad enough to snugly fit into outer attic or attico-antral defect and in depth i.e. medially enough space should be left for ventilation.

2. **Open cavity mastoidectomy:** Failure is mainly because of poor execution of the surgical technique. Inadequate removal of cells under cholesteatoma matrix, incomplete bone work of not lowering and thinning the facial ridge, not clearing the anterior buttress enough to align anterior attic wall to anterior canal wall, not lowering the floor of canal to match the floor of the cavity, leaving bony sockets without obliteration with bone dust and inadequate meatoplasty or cicatrisation of the meatoplasty opening are the main reasons for the failure of surgery. A perfectly performed open cavity mastoidectomy with tympanoplasty not only results in a trouble-free and water-tolerant ear, but also yields results comparable to intact canal wall mastoidectomy.

SUGGESTED READING

1. Tos M. Manual of Middle Ear Surgery: Mastoid Surgery and Reconstructive Procedures. Thieme, New York, 1995: 275–82.
2. Gulya AJ, Minor LB, Poe DS. Glasscock's Shambaugh Surgery of the Ear, 6th ed. PMPH-USA Ltd., 2010: 517–28.
3. Roth Niklaus T, Haeusler Rudolf. Inside-out technique cholesteatoma surgery: A retrospective long-term analysis of 604 operated ears between 1992 and 2006. *Otol Neurol*, 2009; 30: 59–63.
4. de Aquino JEAP, Filho NAC, de Aquino JNP. Total reconstruction after canal wall down mastoidectomy with posterior wall of the external auditory canal and allograft ossicular ear drum – Long-term observation. *Int Arch Otorhinolaryngol*, 2007; 11: 116–27.
5. Pensak ML. Controversies in Otolaryngology. Thieme, New York, 2001: 203–17.
6. Facek RR. Ear Surgery. Springer-Verlag, Berlin, Heidelberg, 2008: 55–60.
7. Sanna M, Kharaist T, Falcioni M, Russo A, Taibah A. The Temporal Bone: A Manual for Dissection and Surgical Approaches. Thieme, Stuttgart, New York, 2006: 22–38.

CHAPTER 5

Management of Glomus Tumours

K.P. Morwani, Narayan Jayashankar, Rahul Agrawal, Madhuri Mehta

Glomus means a small circumscribed structure in which arterioles connect directly to veins.

DIAGNOSIS

A patient of glomus tumour may present with varying symptoms hence a detailed history and a careful clinical examination is a must.

Glomus tympanicum (Fig. 5.1)

Patient usually presents with a pulsatile tinnitus. On examination a reddish glowing pulsatile mass can be seen behind the drum. As the tumour grows in size, it can erode the ossicular chain or block round window, leading to conductive hearing loss. Haziness seen in mastoid air cell in a case of glomus tympanicum is due to blockage of antrum. CT scan bone window with contrast enhanced CT scan will be able to differentiate between fluid and glomus tympanicum.

Glomus mastoidalis

Patient suffering from glomus mastoidalis may also present with the above complaints, same as glomus tympanicum. If there is secondary infection, patient can also present with signs of mastoiditis.

Glomus jugulare (Figs. 5.2 & 5.3)

Patient usually presents with bleeding polyp or pulsatile mass behind the drum with conductive deafness, pulsatile tinnitus, facial or lower cranial nerve paresis/palsy. Rarely patient may present with paresis of an isolated LCN or palsy of branch of any CN, e.g., as unilateral vocal cord palsy.

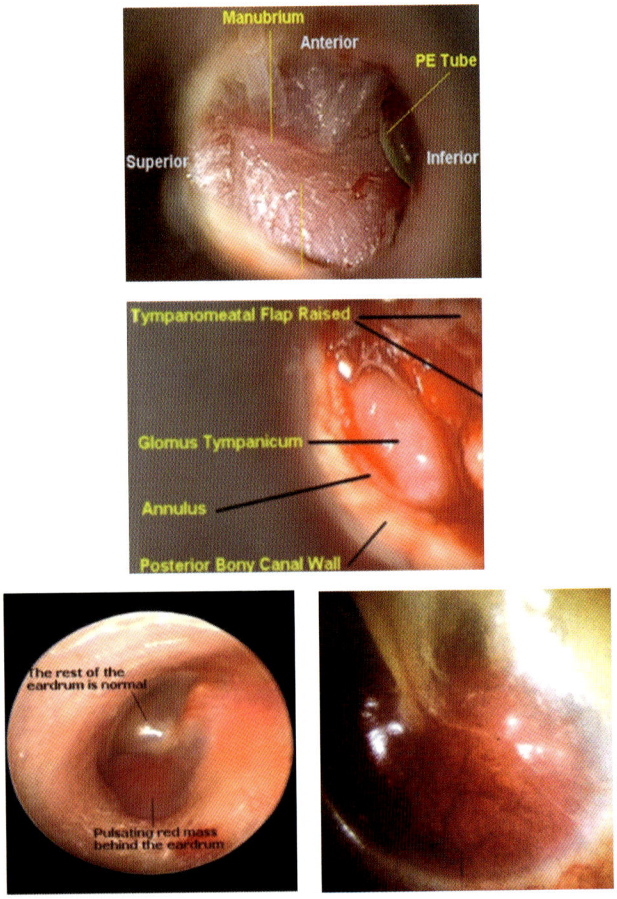

Fig. 5.1. Glomus tympanicum.

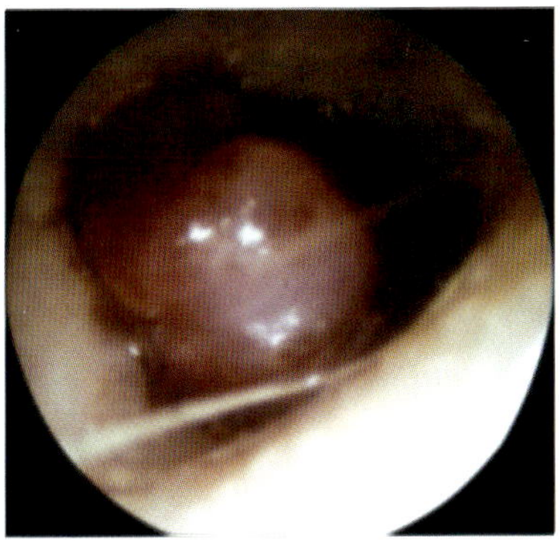

Fig. 5.2. Bleeding polyp.

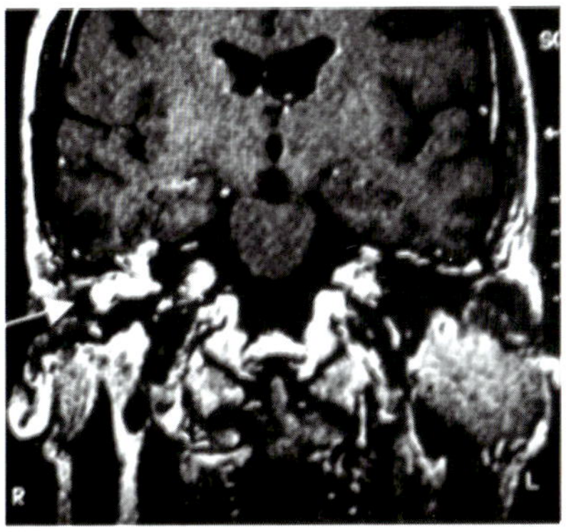

Fig. 5.3. Polyp in EAC extending in middle ear, attic and antrum.

For all the above, definite diagnosis is made on CT scan bone window plus contrast CT. Two important differential diagnoses which should always be kept in mind are high jugular bulb (Fig. 5.4) (differential for glomus jugulare) and dehiscent carotid artery (Fig. 5.5) (differential for glomus tympanicum).

INVESTIGATIONS

In a case of glomus jugulare, biopsy should be deferred. Two investigations which will determine the diagnosis and further management of the lesion are CT scan and also a contrast enhanced MRI if needed. An HRCT of temporal bone with additional contrast enhanced sequences should be asked for. This would enable us to know the relationship of glomus jugulare with middle ear, attic, antrum, mastoid, horizontal and vertical portion of facial nerve and also carotid canal. MRI is needed particularly in two conditions: firstly, to know the extension of tumour from jugular bulb into IJV in neck and its relation with the great vessels; secondly, for intracranial extensions to know whether the tumour is intradural or extradural.

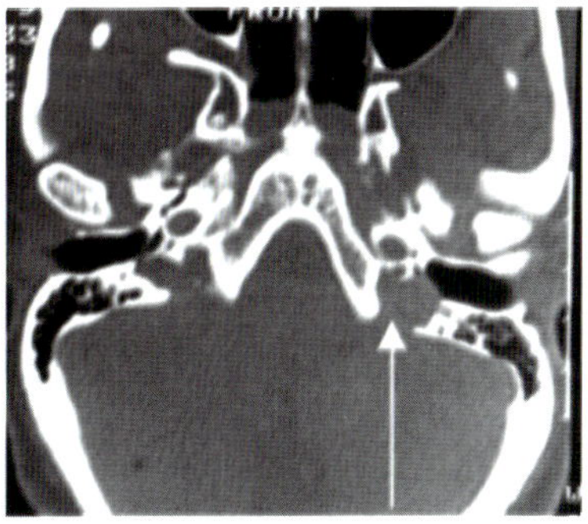

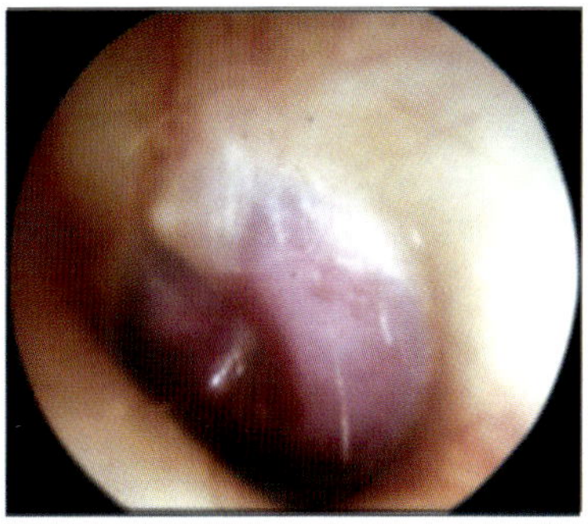

Fig. 5.4. High jugular bulb.

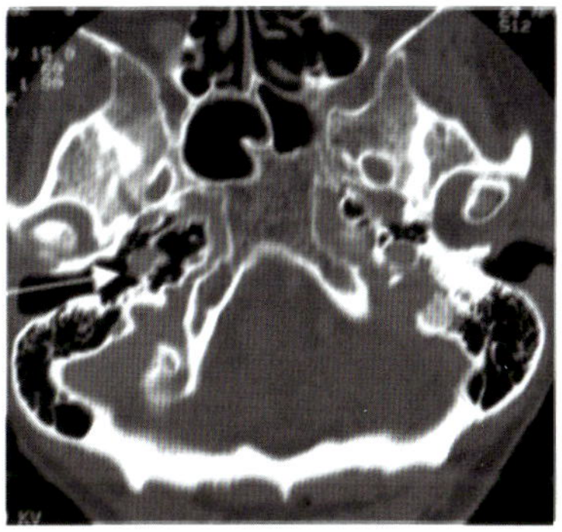

Fig. 5.5. Dehiscent ICA.

FISCH CLASSIFICATION

Type A – Glomus tympanicum (Transcanal) (Fig. 5.6)

A1 Visible on otoscopy

A2 Extends beyond

Type B – Glomus mastoidalis (Transmastoid ICW) (Fig. 5.7)

B1 Limited to tympanomastoid portion

B2 Hypotympanum

Dr. K.P. Morwani has added two additional variants (Fig. 5.8):

B3 Tumour going along eustachian tube parallel to horizontal petrous carotid without bony destruction

B4 Tumour eroding bone of horizontal petrous carotid going into nasopharynx

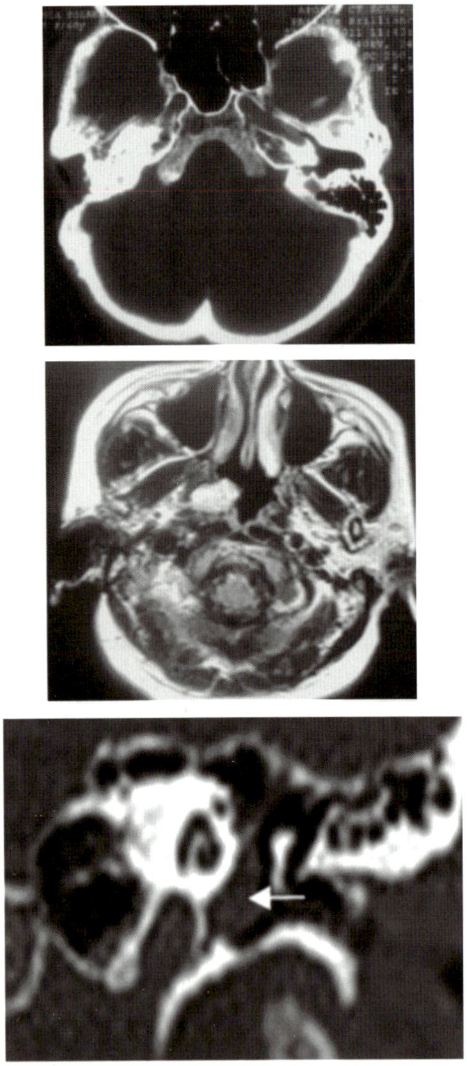

Fig. 5.6. Glomus tympanicum.

Type C – Glomus jugulare

C1 Eroding the carotid foramen (Infrafacial approach) (Fig. 5.9)

C2 Eroding the vertical carotid canal (Infratemporal fossa Type A approach)

C3 Grows along the horizontal portion of ICA (Infratemporal fossa Type A approach) (Fig. 5.10)

C4 Extending to cavernous sinus (Infratemporal fossa Type B approach)

Type D Intracranial extension

De Intracranial extradural extension

1. Tumour displacing posterior fossa dura and < 2 cm in size
2. Tumour displacing posterior fossa dura and > 2 cm in size

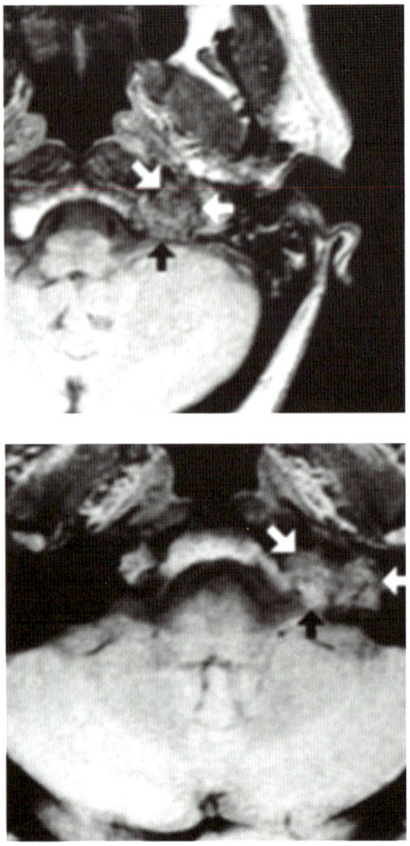

Fig. 5.7. Glomus mastoidalis.

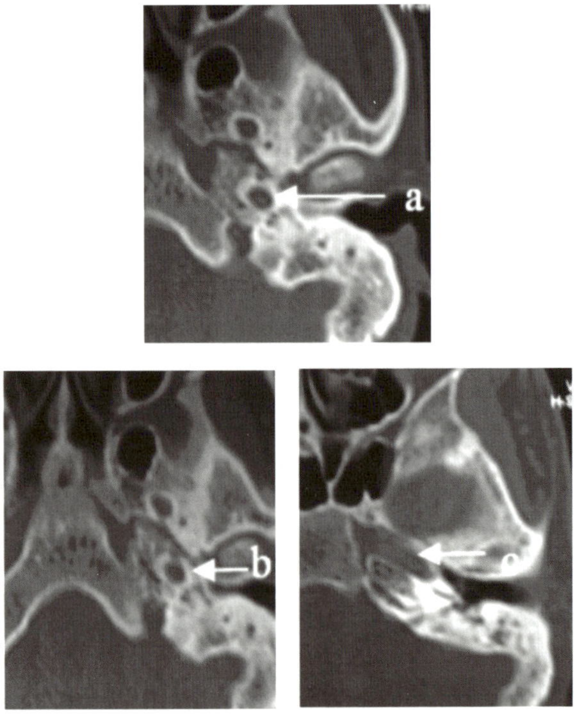

Fig. 5.8. Normal anatomy of ICA – Carotid foramen (A), Canal (B), and Horizontal portion of ICA (C).

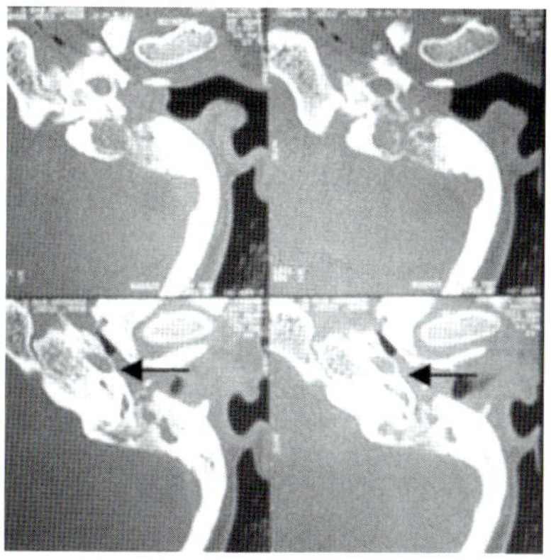

Fig. 5.9. Glomus jugular C1 (intact carotid canal).

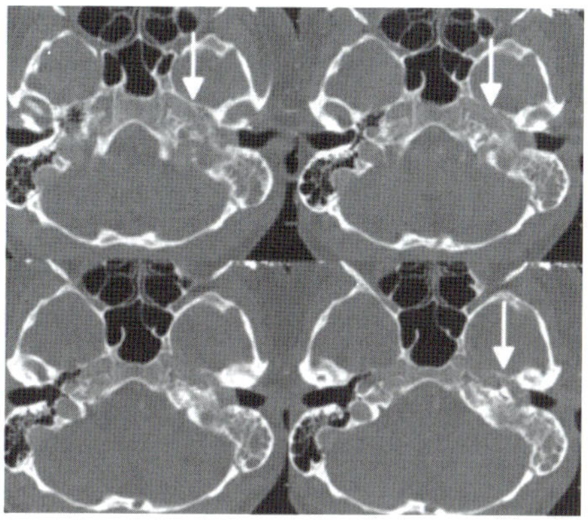

Fig. 5.10. Glomus jugular C3 (arrow – horizontal portion of ICA).

Di Intracranial intradural extension (Fig. 5.11)

1. Intradural extension of < 1 cm in size (Single stage surgery)
2. Intradural extension of > 1 cm in size (Two stage surgery)
3. Extensive tumours

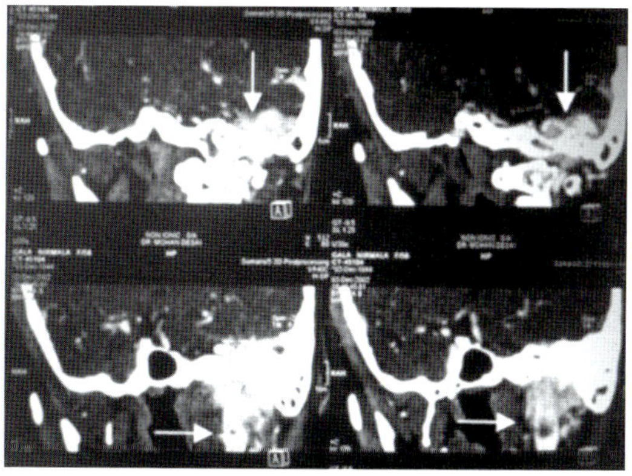

Fig. 5.11. Glomus jugular Di 2 – Intracranial extension (vertical arrow), extension along IJV (horizontal arrow).

SURGICAL MANAGEMENT

Embolization (Fig. 5.12)

Routinely done for all glomus jugulare tumours, i.e., class C and above. Unfortunately not available easily in smaller towns in India. Cost is another limiting factor for embolization. In cases where embolization is not done for whatever reason, we suggest temporary ligation of the external carotid artery above the superior thyroid branch just after complete exposure but before tumour removal. Umbilical tape or tubing of the scalp vein (minus the needle and flanges) are used for temporary occlusion of the artery. Once the tumour is excised, the ligature is released. Of course, this attempt may be unsuccessful if the tumour receives blood supply from internal carotid artery.

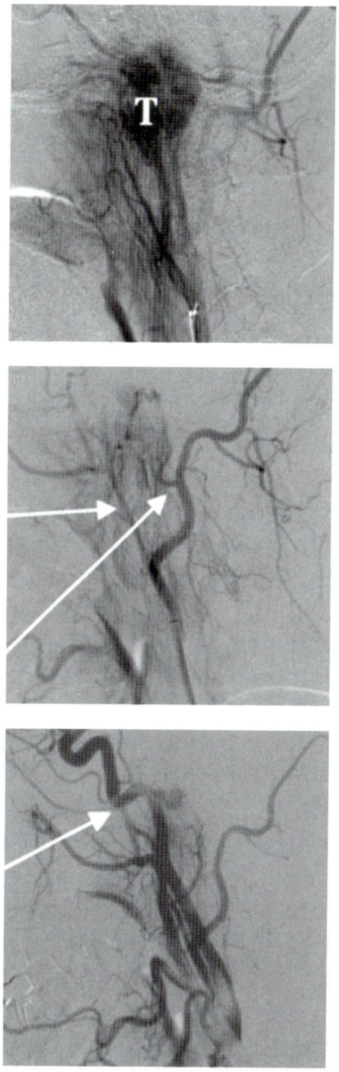

Fig. 5.12. Embolisation of C3 tumour.

Glomus tympanicum

In cases of glomus tympanicum and mastoidalis we do not require either embolisation or ligation of external carotid artery (ECA). To check bleeding in these tumours we depend on hypotensive anesthesia, wide exposure of the tumour, bipolar coagulation, use of adrenaline-soaked cotton, and packing with surgicel.

We approach these tumours permeatally as a case of exploratory tympanotomy. If the tumour extends, e.g., in attic, hypotympanum, tympanic recess, a permeatal widening or canal-plasty is done to expose it completely. Complete exposure of the tumour before handling it is key to a successful surgery. Once the tumour is exposed it should be bipolarized before we proceed to remove it either piecemeal or en-bloc in a single piece. In glomus tympanicum extending to the hypotympanic air cells, it is necessary to clear the cells widely after removal of tumour. Ossicular reconstruction with reinforcement of tympanic membrane can be done after tumour removal if needed.

Glomus mastoidalis

We approach this tumour with intact canal wall mastoidectomy with canal-plasty. Exposure of the hypotympanic air cells as also the infrafacial area may be required. Similarly, in extensive glomus tympanicum and hypotympanicum, the tumour erodes the bone over the vertical tympanic segment of the carotid artery and sometimes goes under the horizontal petrous segment of the internal carotid artery destroying the bone between the carotid artery and the eustachian tube. It may also erode the bone between the eustachian tube and tensor tympani canal. In some cases, it travels down the eustachian tube to present in the nasopharynx, presenting as epistaxis. Posterior tympanotomy is described in literature to get better exposure of the tumour, however, we do a widening of the canal to expose the sinus tympani area and do a simple mastoidectomy to expose the mastoid part of tumour. As in glomus tympanicum, ossicular reconstruction with reinforcement of tympanic membrane can be done after tumour removal, if needed.

5

Glomus jugulare

To check bleeding, in addition to preoperative embolization, we also use intraoperative temporary ligation of ECA and meticulous packing of inferior petrosal vessels. As such we have to open the neck to gain control over lower cranial nerves (LCN), ICA and internal jugulare vein (IJV); hence ECA is temporarily ligated higher up in the neck, just before handling the tumour. This should be performed only after the subtotal petrosectomy and neck dissection is complete, just prior to tumour removal, as it could lead to development of collateral circulation.

Incision

"C" shaped incision is given 5 cm behind the post-auricular sulcus. For C4 tumours incision is carried anteriorly as advocated by Prof. Ugo Fisch, for infra-temporal fossa type B approach. A "U" shaped musculoperiosteal incision is given, creating a flap known as Palva's flap, which will be used as a 2nd layer for cul-de-sac closure (Fig. 5.13).

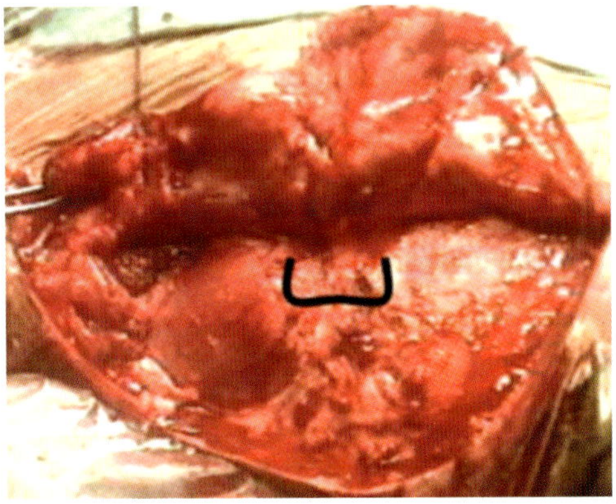

Fig. 5.13. Palva's flap.

Cul-de-sac closure (Fig. 5.14)

Meatotomy is performed in complete circumference between bony and cartilaginous portion of EAC. Skin of EAC is dissected off the underlying subcutaneous tissue and cartilage. Canal skin is then brought out with the help of two sutures at 12 and 6 o'clock positions and excess skin is resected. It is then sutured. 2nd layer of cul-de-sac closure is by Palva's flap. It is brought under EAC and sutured in complete circumference.

Neck dissection (Fig. 5.15)

To start with the great vessels and cranial nerves are exposed in the neck to gain control. Exit of LCN from skull base can roughly be divided in three compartments. In anterior compartment, glosso-pharyngeal nerve is identified as it crosses under

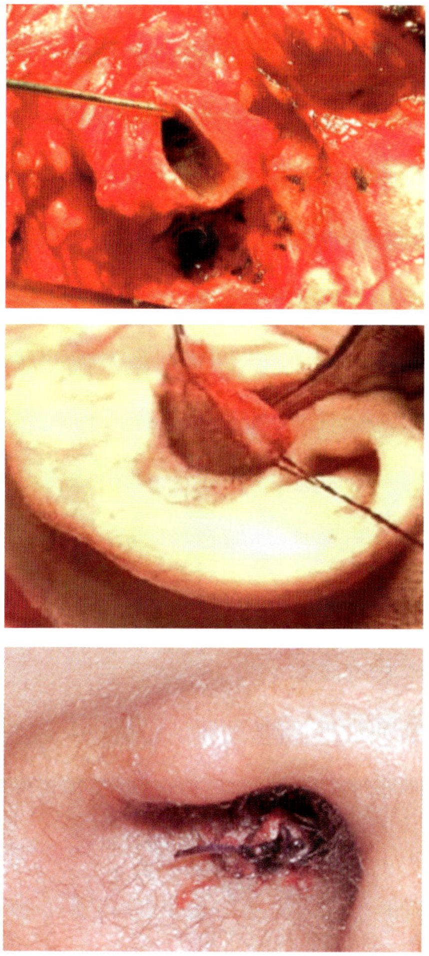

Fig. 5.14. Cul-de-sac closure.

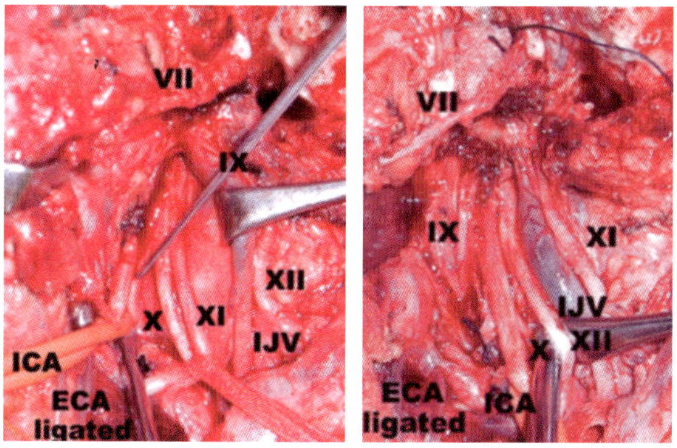

Fig. 5.15. Great vessels and LCN in neck and at their exit from skull base.

the carotid artery and is deeper to posterior belly of digastric muscle. In middle compartment, hypoglossal and vagus nerve can be identified. Hypoglossal nerve emerges from skull under the ICA and lies lateral to ICA in the skull base and the crosses the ECA to lie inferior to submandibular gland in the neck. Vagus nerve runs along the length of ICA and subsequently along the CCA. In posterior compartment, accessory nerve is identified as it emerges deeper to IJV and crosses posteriorly to enter trapezius muscle. IJV and ICA are mobilized in complete circumference. Umbilical tapes are kept around them without tying, as it can be tied later if needed. Facial nerve is exposed as it emerges from stylomastoid foramen and mobilized in parotid gland beyond its bifurcation.

Facial nerve management (Figs. 5.16 to 5.19)

This is followed by a subtotal petrosectomy which would include mastoidectomy with lowering of facial ridge to expose the FN in its vertical course. Drilling should be done posteriorly enough to delineate the sigmoid sinus.

In cases of C1 and limited C2 tumours infrafacial approach is used, in which we mobilize the FN partially maximum up to 2nd genu and temporarily reroute it anteriorly and reposition it back after the surgery. When the FN is rerouted, blood supply at stylomastoid foramen and vertical portion is lost, leading to grades II–III paresis. For better results a vascular bed is created to reposition the FN. For this digastric muscle is mobilized along its length and placed in the depth of the cavity after filling the infracochlear cells with fat or free muscle. FN is repositioned back over the digastric muscle. On top of FN a vascular flap of sternocleidomastoid muscle is placed after splitting it along its length, this flap further gives the needed blood supply and also reduces the dead space in the cavity.

In bigger tumours infratemporal fossa type A approach is used and facial nerve has to be permanently rerouted anteriorly. While rerouting adequate periosteum of stylomastoid foramen is taken with the nerve which is used for suturing it.

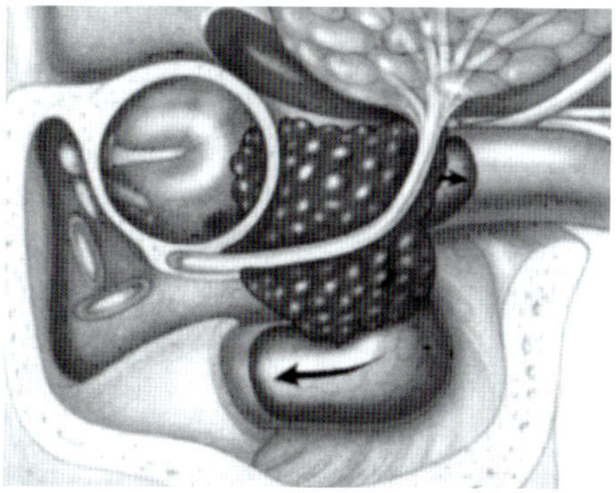

Fig. 5.16. Exposure of facial nerve.

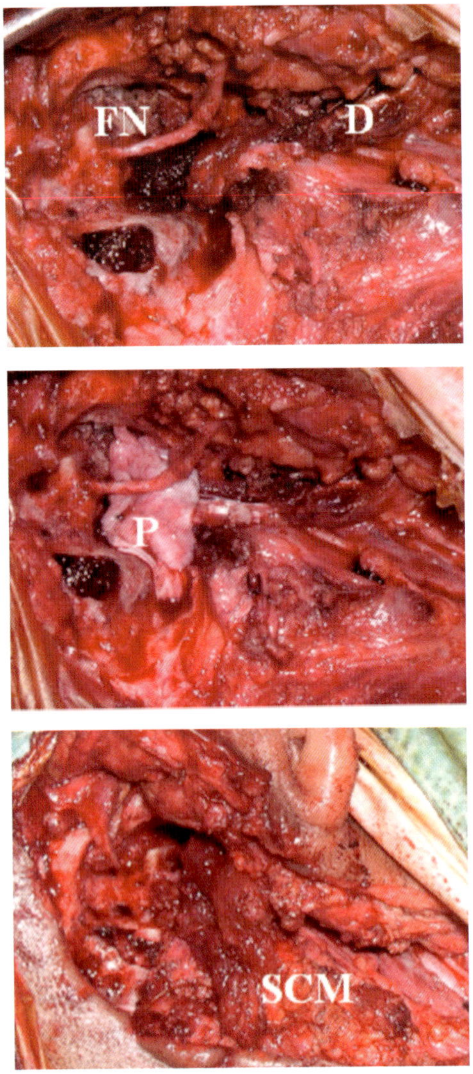

Fig. 5.17. Temporary partially anterior rerouting of facial nerve. Digastric Ms (D), Sternocleidomastoid Ms (SCM), Pericranium (P), Facial nerve (FN).

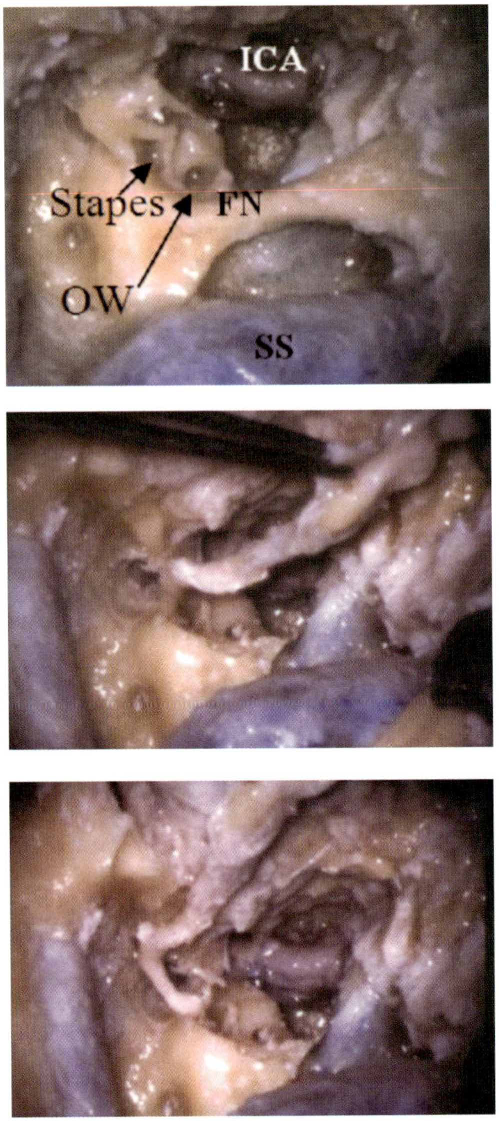

Fig. 5.18. Permanent anterior rerouting of facial nerve.

Another important factor which determines fate of facial nerve is its preoperative status. Firstly, if pre-op FN function was normal then we expect FN to be free of the tumour. Secondly, if patient has FN paresis pre-op then it would suggest either invasion of sheath or nerve tissue by the tumour. There is no harm in excising the nerve sheath and also 20–25% of nerve fibers if needed, along with the tumour. If more then 25% of nerve fibers are found to be involved then it is better to resect the nerve and do a grafting. Thirdly, if the patient presents with pre-op FN palsy, it suggests definite invasion by the tumour, hence further management will depend upon length of invasion. Most often it is feasible to do grafting with greater auricular nerve. In Di tumours where FN is invaded not only in temporal bone but also in CP angle, the distal end of FN may not be available, the options would be a lid loading surgery and facial-hypoglossal anastomosis. In cases where hypoglossal nerve is also not available, either due to invasion by the tumour or patient presents with pre-op hypoglossal nerve palsy, we will rely on lid loading surgery and if needed a sling procedure.

Bone work (Fig. 5.20)

After rerouting FN, bone deeper to fallopian canal, posterior-inferior (mastoid tip) and anterior-inferior (tympanic bone) and infracochlear cells are drilled out completely to expose the jugular bulb and ICA.

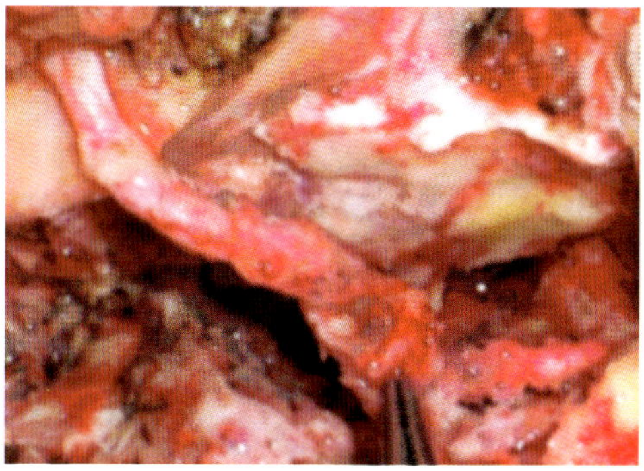

Fig. 5.19. Tumour over FN.

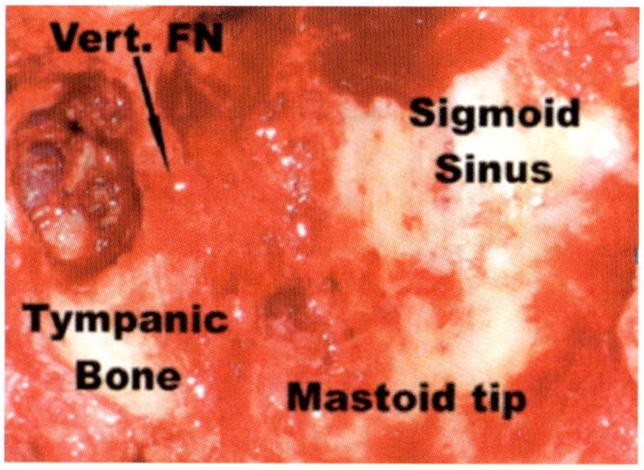

Fig. 5.20. Bone work.

Styloid process is identified, muscular attachments taken off and then excised. All the muscles attached to styloid process are separated by either bipolar diathermy or subperiosteal dissection.

Internal carotid artery

It is covered with thick periosteal layer from carotid canal onwards. Periosteal layer can be excised if involved, whereas if tumour is found over the carotid artery it can be cauterized with the help of a bipolar diathermy. In cases where tumour is found under and anterior to ICA, the artery should be mobilized from neck onwards. Extent of mobilization is decided preoperatively, based on CT scan. Once ICA is mobilized it can be lifted with the help of umbilical tapes, making it easier to remove the tumour all around it.

Tumour removal

At this point, ECA is ligated. Tumour mass is debulked from mastoid cavity, middle ear cleft and jugular bulb after bipolarizing it and leaving the tumour which is attached to jugular bulb and sigmoid sinus. Sigmoid sinus is now blocked extraluminally (surgicel under the bone).

Further dissection can be carried out from IJV upwards or from sigmoid sinus downwards. IJV is ligated in neck beyond tumour and dissected upwards taking care not to damage LCN. At jugular bulb outer wall of jugular vein along the tumour is excised, thus exposing inferior petrosal sinus (3–4 openings) which bleeds torrentially. Individual opening is to be packed with surgicel again taking care not to damage the LCN. Now dissection is carried from upwards by taking sigmoid sinus in complete circumference without damaging the dura deeper to it. Any small dural infiltration (< 1 cm) can be excised in same sitting. Dural defect, if any, is then repaired and hemostasis is achieved. At this stage ECA ligation can be released.

Eustachian tube blockage (Fig. 5.21)

Once the tumour is removed ET should be blocked carefully in three layers. All the mucosa of ET is stripped off as far as possible and it is blocked with free muscle followed by bone piece (styloid process is readily available) and bone dust and lastly by bone wax.

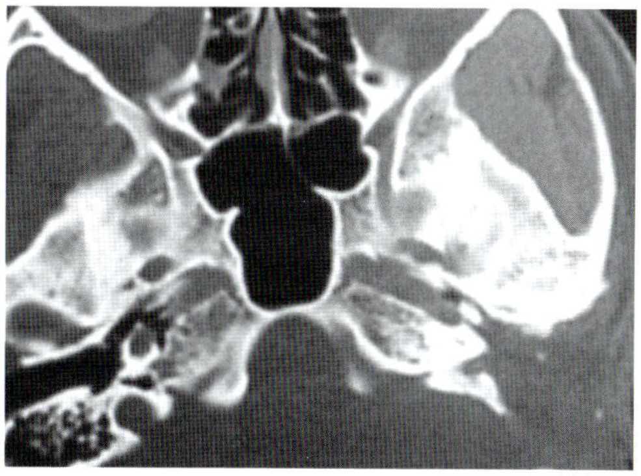

Fig. 5.21. Bone chip in ET.

Closure

Infra-labyrinthine area is packed with fat. The cavity is over-filled with fat over which we place a rotated temporal muscle flap by splitting it horizontally, thereby maintaining its blood supply (Fig. 5.22). In cases of dural defect, use of tissue glue should be considered.

Prevention of CSF leak

Few points to be remembered to prevent CSF leak are:

1. The vertical limb of the skin incision should be over occipital bone.

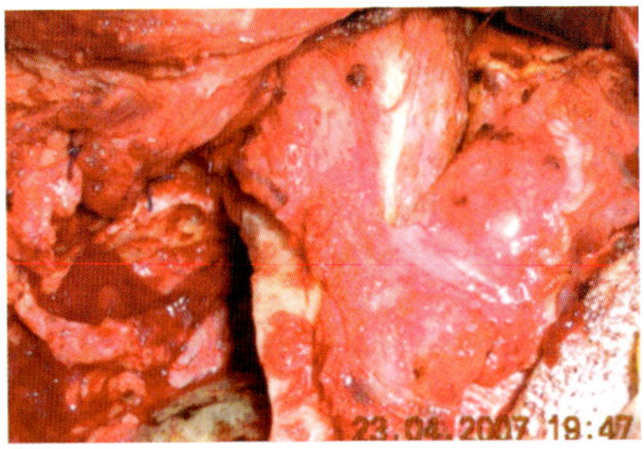

Fig. 5.22. Temporalis muscle split.

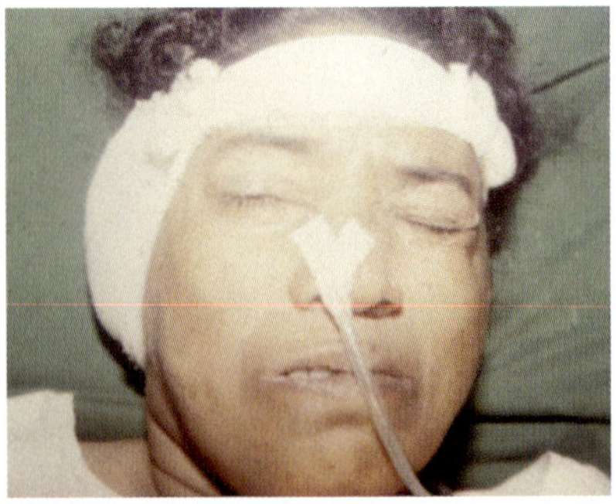

Fig. 5.23. Post-op grade III FN paresis with paresis of LCN.

2. Cul-de-sac closure of external canal in two layers.
3. Proper obliteration of ET with bone chip, pâté and wax.
4. Packing of sigmoid sinus instead of ligation.
5. Infracochlear area and any dural defect should be tightly sealed in multiple layers. Use of tissue glue does help in giving a better seal.
6. Temporalis muscle flap to obliterate cavity.
7. Do not use Ready-Vac drain. Incision sutured in layers, with mattress stitches.
8. Firm mastoid bandage.
9. Big intradural tumours are to be removed in two stages. Decision on which part to remove first, temporal or intradural, depends on symptoms of the patient.

POSTOPERATIVE MANAGEMENT

Antibiotics and analgesics are to be continued. To avoid CSF leak guidelines to be followed are:

1. Strict bed rest.
2. Head up position.
3. Oral Diamox, Syp. Potchlor, to reduce intracranial tension.
4. Avoid use of steroids.
5. Lumbar puncture, if needed. Repeat LP in cases of post-op CSF leak.
6. In extensive leak or large dural defect a continuous lumbar drain should be kept for 5–7 days, electively.

Patient is advised to do passive massage of face. Facial nerve stimulation has a limited role and can be performed for 2–3 weeks only. In spite of preserving the FN, if patient does not show any signs of improvement in FN function in 9 months, faciohypoglossal anastomosis with lid loading surgery should be considered (Fig. 5.23).

Lower cranial nerves (LCN)

More important than facial nerve is the preoperative functional status of lower cranial nerves. For example, it is better to defer surgery for an elderly patient with poor general condition who presents with a glomus jugulare and lower cranial nerve palsy. It is rather better managed by embolisation followed by radiotherapy. Patients with pre-operative LCN paresis have more chances of going up to palsy.

As with FN, prognosis of LCN depends upon their pre-op functional status. Most patients with paresis learn to adjust and are able to swallow without aspiration within 3–4 months. Aspiration has to be checked or it would lead to serious complication, at times requiring tracheostomy, more so in debilitated elderly patients.

If function of LCN does not improve within few weeks, a gastrostomy should be done to improve the general condition. If the function does improve even after 3–4 months type I thyroplasty should be done (Fig. 5.24). Thyroplasty improves quality of voice and reduces aspiration, hence tracheostomy can be closed. It also improves deglutition due to absence of aspiration and better intrathoracic pressure, this is further facilitated by cricopharyngeal myotomy done at the same time. Cricopharyngeal myotomy is done from cricoid to thoracic inlet of cervical esophagus. It should be kept in mind that length and depth of myotomy is very important for effective results (Fig. 5.25).

OUR EXPERIENCE

Cases managed from 1990 to 2011

- Glomus tympanicum – 24 cases
- Glomus hypotympanicum – 28 cases
- Glomus jugulare – 35 cases (Figs. 5.26 & 5.27)

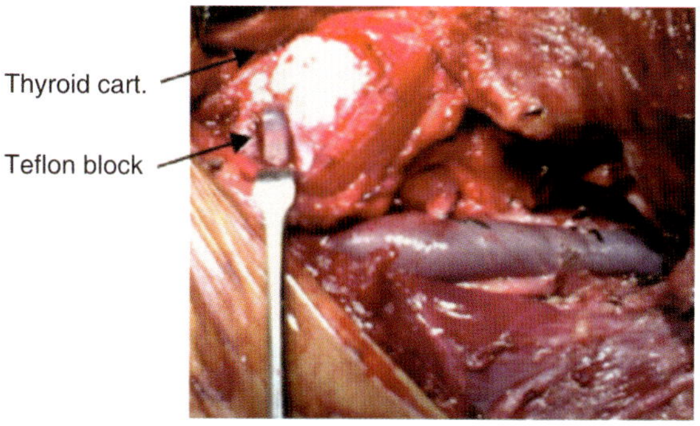

Fig. 5.24. Thyroplasty type I.

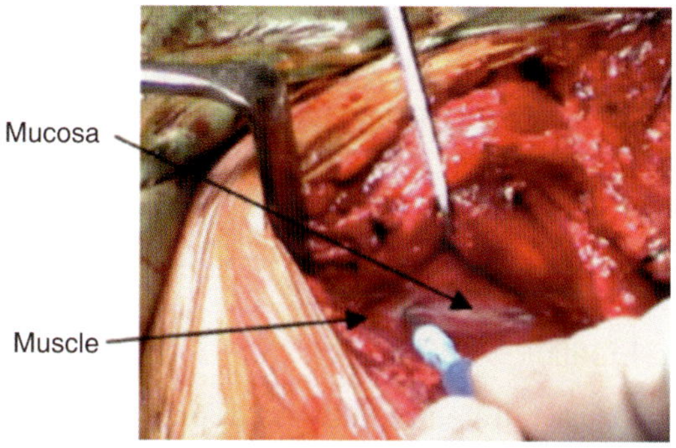

Fig. 5.25. Cricopharyngeal myotomy.

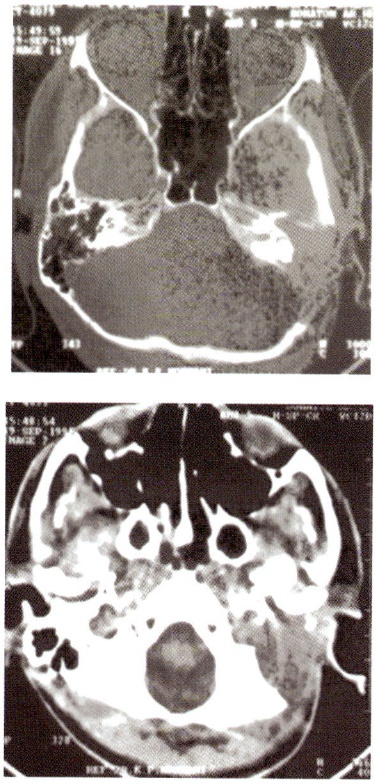

Fig. 5.26. Glomus jugular C1 – pre-op and post-op.

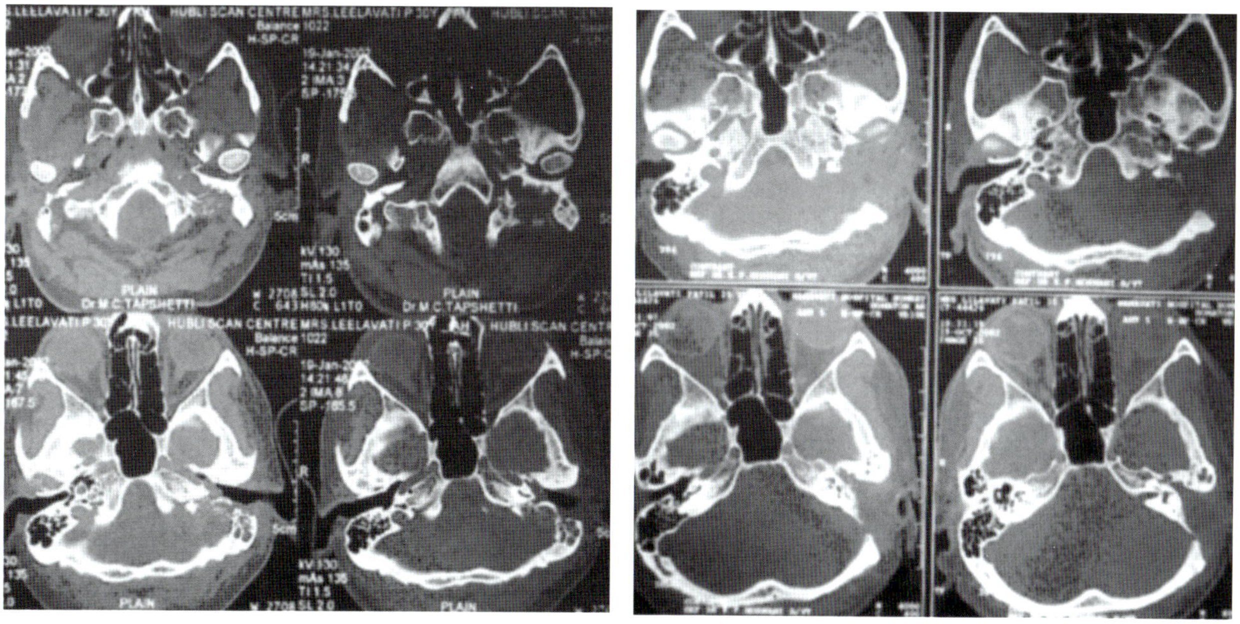

Fig. 5.27. Pre-op and post-op scan of C2 lesion.

Out of 35 cases of glomus jugulare

- Embolisation – 21 patients
- Temporary ligation of ECA in rest of the cases
- In first 5 years blood transfusion given was 1–5 bottles with an average of 2.7 bottles. Subsequently 0–3 bottles, with an average of 1.6 bottles, were used.

Facial nerve status in glomus jugulare cases (1990–2011) (Figs. 5.27 & 5.28)

	Pre-op	*Post-op (1 year)*
Normal FN	25 cases	2 cases
Paresis	7 cases (II–V)	28 cases (II–III)
Palsy	3 cases	5 cases

Lower cranial nerve status in glomus jugulare cases (1990–2011)

	Pre-op	*Post-op*
Normal XN	30 cases	15 cases
Paresis	1 case	15 cases
Palsy	5 cases	5 cases

Out of 5 palsies 1 patient required tracheostomy and 4 patients required type I thyroplasty and crico-pharyngeal myotomy.

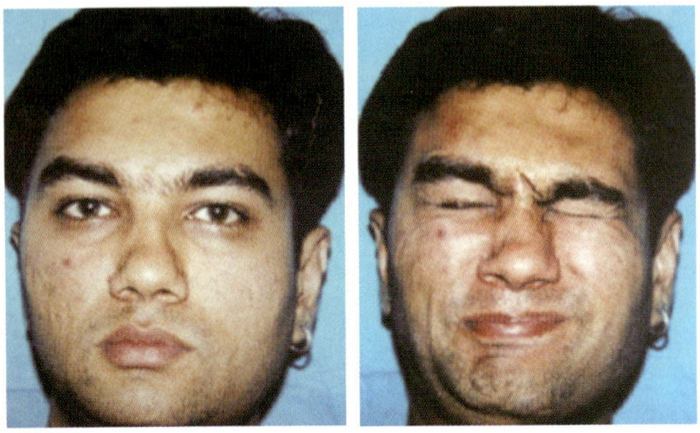

Fig. 5.28. Post-op normal facial nerve.

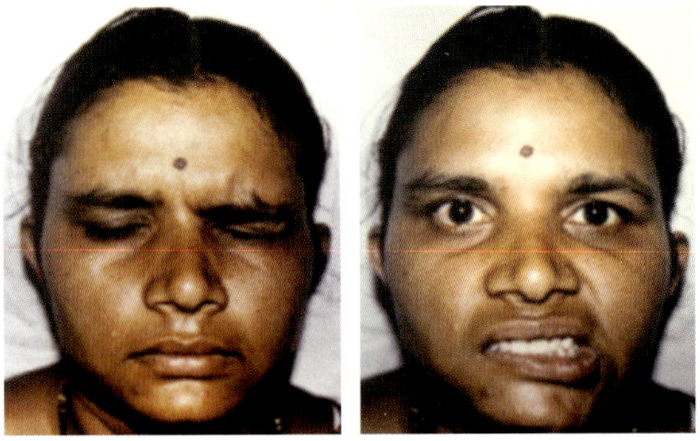

Fig. 5.29. Post-op FN weakness Gr II–III.

"THIS OPERATION IS NOT TO BE ENTRUSTED TO THOSE WHO HAVE MADE NO SERIOUS EFFORT TO ACQUIRE AN ACCURATE ANATOMICAL AND PATHOLOGICAL KNOWLEDGE OF THE FIELD OF ACTION. "

– Charles A. Balance

SUGGESTED READING

1. Fisch U. Infratemporal fossa approach for glomus tumours of the temporal bone. *Ann Otol Rhinol Laryngol*, 1982; 91: 474–9.
2. Fisch U, Fagan P, Valvanis A. The infratemporal fossa approach for the lateral skull base. *Otolaryngol Clin North Am*, 1984; 17: 513–52.
3. Murphy TP, Brackmann DE. Effects of preoperative embolization on glomus jugulare tumours. *Laryngoscope*, 1989; 99: 1244–7.
4. Brackmann DE. The facial nerve in the infratemporal approach. *Otolaryngol Head Neck Surg*, 1987; 97: 15–7.
5. Leonetti JP, Brackmann DE, Prass RC. Improved preservation of facial function in the infratemporal fossa approach to the skull base. *Otolaryngol Head Neck Surg*, 1989; 101: 74–8.
6. Sanna M, Shin SH, De Donato G et al. Management of complex tympanojugular paragangliomas including endovascular intervention. *Laryngoscope*, 2011; 121: 1372–82.

CHAPTER 6

Hearing Loss

Arjun Dass, Gaurav Bambha

The ears are one of the important organs of our body and help in hearing, hence communication. Hearing is the sense of detecting sound, receiving information about the environment through vibratory movement communicated via medium such as air, water or ground. It is one of the traditional five senses, along with sight, touch, smell and taste. Human ear can hear sounds with frequencies between 20 and 20,000 cycles per second (20 Hz to 20 kHz). Human hearing has ability to discriminate small differences in loudness (intensity) and pitch (frequency) over that large range of audible sound. This healthy human range of frequency detection varies from individual to individual, and depends significantly on age, gender and occupational hearing damage. The ears can be affected by various disorders leading to hearing loss. This chapter will be discussed under following headings:

- Basic physiology of hearing
- Definition of hearing loss
- Types of hearing loss
- Etiology of hearing loss
- Assessment of hearing loss
- Treatment of hearing loss
- Social aspects of hearing

BASIC PHYSIOLOGY OF HEARING

The sound in the environments is collected by pinna and reaches the inner ear via external auditory canal and middle ear. From there, the sound reaches to the brain through auditory pathway. The following mechanisms work in the physiology of hearing:

- Mechanical conduction of sound (conductive apparatus)
- Transduction of mechanical energy to electrical impulse (sensory system of cochlea)
- Conduction of electrical impulses to the brain (neural pathway)

Conduction of sound

The pinna and external auditory canal act passively to capture the acoustic energy and direct it to the tympanic membrane, the sound waves strike the tympanic membrane causing it to vibrate. These mechanical vibrations are then transmitted via the ossicles to the perilymph of the inner ear. The perilymph is stimulated by the mechanical (vibrations) energy to form a fluid wave within the cochlea. The middle ear acts as an impedance-matching device. Sound waves travel much easier through air (low impedance) than water (high impedance). If sound waves were directed at the oval window (water) almost all of the acoustic energy would be reflected back to the middle ear (air) and only 1% would enter the cochlea. To increase the efficiency of the system, the middle ear acts to transform the acoustic energy to mechanical energy which then stimulates the cochlear fluid by following mechanisms:

- **Lever action of ossicles:** Handle of malleus is 1.3 times longer than long process of incus, providing a mechanical advantage of 1.3.

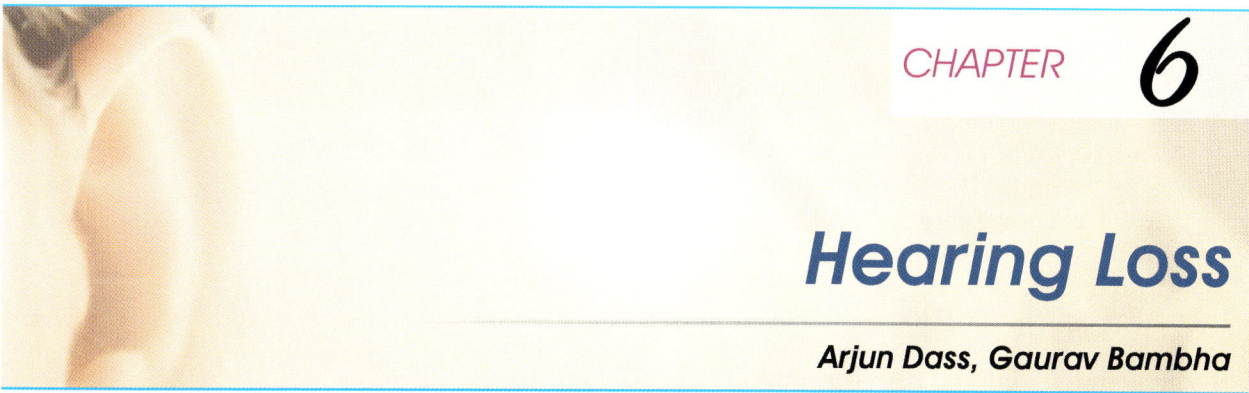

- **Hydraulic action of tympanic membrane:** The area of tympanic membrane is much larger than the area of stapes footplate, average ratio being 21 : 1. As effective vibratory area of tympanic area is only two-thirds, the effective area ratio is reduced to 14 : 1 but according to certain studies, out of the 90 mm^2 only 55 mm^2 is functional, given area of stapes footplate is (3.2 mm^2), the area ratio 17 : 1 and the total transformer ratio (17 × 1.3) is 22.1.
- **Curved membrane effect:** Movements of tympanic membrane are more at the periphery than at the centre where the handle of malleus is attached. This too provides some leverage.

Transduction of mechanical energy into electrical impulse

The cochlea consists of a fluid-filled bony canal within which lies the cochlear duct containing the sensory epithelium. Energy enters the cochlea via the stapes footplate at the oval window and is dissipated through a second opening (which is covered by a membrane) the round window. Vibrations of the stapes footplate cause the perilymph to form a wave. This wave travels throughout the length of the cochlea. It takes approximately 5 sec to travel the whole length of the cochlea. As it passes the basilar membrane of the cochlear duct, the fluid wave causes the basilar membrane to move in a wave-like fashion (i.e., up and down). The wave form travels the length of the cochlea and is dissipated at the round window. Due to changes in the mechanical properties of the basilar membrane, the amplitude of vibration changes as the wave travels along the basilar membrane. Low frequency stimuli cause maximum vibration of basilar membrane at its apex, while high frequency stimulate at its base.

Neural pathway

As the basilar membrane is displaced superiorly by the perilymph wave, the stereocilia at the apex of each inner and outer hair cell, which are embedded in the tectorial membrane, undergo a shearing force (i.e., they are bent). This shearing force causes a change in the resting membrane potential of the hair cell which is transmitted to its basal end and a synapse is formed with a dendrite of the auditory nerve. The hair cell membrane potential change is transmitted across this synapse causing depolarization of the nerve fibre. This neural impulse is then propagated to the auditory centres of the brain.

DEFINITION OF HEARING LOSS

Hearing loss as defined by WHO is the reduced ability of a person to hear in a noisy and quiet environment as compared with the hearing of a normal person. Deafness is a condition wherein the ability to detect certain frequencies of sound is completely or partially impaired.

CLASSIFICATION AND TYPES OF HEARING LOSS

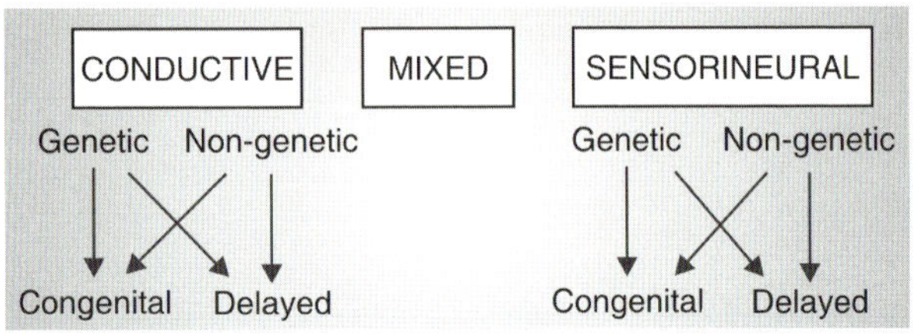

Congenital hearing loss

It implies that the hearing loss is present since birth. It includes hereditary hearing loss or the hearing loss due to other factors present either in utero (antenatal) or at the time of birth (natal) and can be broadly classified into genetic and non-genetic factors.

Genetic

Genetic factors are thought to cause more than 50% of all incidents of congenital hearing loss. Genetic hearing loss could be autosomal dominant, autosomal recessive, or X-linked (related to the sex chromosome).

Non-genetic

Congenital rubella syndrome, congenital syphilis, intrauterine infections including German measles, cytomegalovirus, and herpes simplex virus, complications associated with the Rh factor in the blood, prematurity, hyperbilirubinemia, maternal alcohol/drug/smoking.

Acquired hearing loss

Conductive hearing loss

A conductive hearing impairment is the result of dysfunction in any of the mechanisms that normally conduct sound waves through the outer ear, the ear drum or the bones of the middle ear. Any disease process which interferes with conduction of sound to reach cochlea causes conductive hearing loss. The lesion may lie in the external ear and tympanic membrane, middle ear or ossicles upto the stapedio-vestibular joint and is characterized by the following features.

- Rinne test is negative, i.e., bone conduction (BC) > air conduction (AC).
- Weber is lateralised to poorer ear.
- Absolute bone conduction is normal.
- Pure tone audiometry (PTA) shows bone conduction better than air conduction with air bone gap not more than 60 dB.
- Speech discrimination is good.

Aetiology

Congenital causes:

- Congenital meatal atresia.
- Fixation of stapes foot plate.
- Fixation of malleus head.
- Ossicular discontinuity.
- Congenital cholesteatoma.

Acquired causes:

External ear: Atresia of canal, wax, foreign body, furuncle, acute inflammatory swelling, otomycosis benign or malignant tumours.

Middle ear: Perforation of tympanic membrane, fluid in the middle ear, mass in the middle ear, destruction or fixation or disruption of ossicles and eustachian tube blockage.

Sensorineural hearing loss (SNHL)

It is a type of hearing loss in which the root cause lies either in the vestibulocochlear nerve (CN VIII), the inner ear, or central auditory pathway connecting to the brain. The great majority of human sensorineural hearing loss is caused by abnormalities in the hair cells of the organ of Corti in the cochlea. Rare and unusual sensorineural hearing impairments may be due to involvement of the VIII cranial nerve and the auditory cortex of the brain. SNHL is characterized by the following features:

- Rinne test is reduced positive, i.e., air conduction is better than bone conduction (AC > BC).
- Weber is lateralized to the better ear.
- Bone conduction is reduced on absolute bone conduction and Schwabach test.
- Pure tone audiometery does not show any gap between air and bone conduction.
- Hearing loss may exceed 60 dB.
- Speech discrimination is poor.

Aetiology

Congenital:

- Developmental anomalies of the cochlea
- Chromosomal syndromes
- Congenital cholesteatoma

Acquired:

- *Inflammatory:* Measles, mumps, viral, suppurative labyrinthitis, meningitis and syphilis.
- *Physical trauma:* Either due to fractures of the temporal bone (80% transverse fractures) affecting the cochlea and middle ear, or a shearing injury affecting eighth cranial nerve.
- *Noise-induced:* Prolonged exposure to loud noises (> 90 dB) causes hearing loss which begins at 4000 Hz (high frequency).
- *Ototoxic drugs:* Aminoglycosides (most common cause, e.g., streptomycin), loop diuretics (e.g., furosemide), antimetabolites (e.g., methotrexate), salicylates (e.g., aspirin) quinine and cytotoxic drugs.
- *Ménière's disease:* Causes sensorineural hearing loss in the low frequency range (125 Hz to 1000 Hz). Ménière's disease is characterized by episodes of vertigo, lasting minutes to hours preceded by tinnitus, aural fullness, and fluctuating hearing loss.
- *Cerebellopontine angle tumour:* The cerebellopontine angle is the exit site for both the facial nerve (CN7) and the vestibulocochlear nerve (CN8). Patients with these tumours often have symptoms and signs corresponding to compression of both nerves.

  Acoustic neuroma (vestibular schwannoma): This is a schwannoma (benign neoplasm of Schwann cells).

  Meningioma: Benign tumour of the pia and arachnoid maters.
- *Presbyacusis:* As the age advances, the ear is also affected by the physiological aging process, leading to sensorineural hearing loss known as presbyacusis. It usually manifests after the age of 65 but may occur early also depending upon the hereditary or environmental predisposition.

Sudden sensorineural hearing loss

6

The sensorineural hearing loss which has developed over a period of few hours or days is included in sudden sensorineural hearing loss (SSNHL). This loss is usually complete but can be partial also. Usually one ear is involved. Very rarely the cause is known, and hence most of the time it is labeled as idiopathic sudden sensorineural hearing loss (ISSNHL). The etiological factors are either viral or vascular (ischemia of the inner ear or the eighth cranial nerve). It may also be caused by rupture of the oval or round window. A history of an event that increased intracranial pressure or caused trauma is usually present. Besides the hearing loss, the patient may experience tinnitus or vertigo.

Noise-induced hearing loss

Noise-induced hearing loss is a sensorineural hearing deficit that begins at the higher frequencies (3,000 to 6,000 Hz) and develops gradually as a result of chronic exposure to excessive sound levels. Although the loss is typically symmetrical, noise from such sources as firearms or sirens may produce an asymmetric loss. Acoustic trauma, a related condition, results from an acute blast. Noise can be described in terms of intensity (perceived as loudness) and frequency (perceived as pitch). Both the intensity and the duration of noise exposure determine the potential for damage to the hair cells of the inner ear. Even sounds perceived as "comfortably" loud can be harmful. Noise can cause permanent hearing loss on chronic exposure equal to an average sound pressure level (SPL) of 85 dB or higher for an eight-hour period. Based on the logarithmic scale, a 3-dB increase in SPL represents a doubling of the sound intensity. Therefore, four hours of noise exposure at 88 dB is considered to provide the same noise "dose" as eight hours at 85 dB, and a single gunshot, which is approximately 140 to 170 dB, has the same sound energy as 40 hours of 90-dB noise.

Pathophysiology

To be perceived, sounds must exert a hearing force on the stereocilia of the hair cells lining the basilar membrane of the cochlea. When excessive, this force can lead on to cellular metabolic overload, cell damage and cell death. Noise-induced hearing loss therefore represents excessive "wear and tear" of the delicate inner ear structures. Concurrent exposure to ototoxic substances, such as solvents and heavy metals, may increase the damage potential of noise. Once exposure to damaging noise levels is discontinued, further significant progression of hearing loss stops. Individual susceptibility to noise-induced hearing loss varies a lot, but the reason that some persons are more resistant to it while others are more susceptible is not well understood.

6

DEGREE OF HEARING LOSS

Degree of hearing loss refers to the severity of the loss. The table below shows one of the more commonly used classification systems. The numbers are representative of the patient's hearing loss range in decibels (dB).

Degree of hearing loss	*Hearing loss range (dB)*
Normal	0 to 25
Mild	26 to 40
Moderate	41 to 55
Moderately severe	56 to 70
Very severe	71 to 90
Profound	Above 90

ASSESSMENT OF HEARING

Clinical tests

- **Finger friction test:** It is one of the screening tests, rough but quick method and consist of rubbing or snapping of finger against patient's ear.
- **Watch test:** A clicking watch is brought near to the patient's ear and the distance at which it is heard is measured. It is not done now-a-days.
- **Speech test:** Normally, a person hears conversational voices at 40 feet and whispers (with residual air after normal expiration) at 20 feet. For the purpose of tests, 20 feet is taken normal for both conversation and whisper.
- **Tuning fork tests:** Tuning fork tests are done to know the types of hearing loss, i.e., conductive or sensorineural hearing loss. Tuning fork should be of 256 Hz, 512 Hz (preferred) and 1024 Hz (Fig. 6.1).

Rinne test

Procedure

- Explain the procedure to the patient.
- Hit the prongs of the tuning fork gently against the examiner's elbow or a rubber piece to make it vibrate.
- Base of the vibrating tuning fork is placed against the mastoid of the patient.
- When the sound ceases, patient will give signal.
- Bring the tuning fork in front of the external auditory canal approximately 2.5 cm away.
- Ask the patient whether he/she still hears the sound. If yes then AC > BC.
- Reverse the procedure and confirm.

Result

- **Normal:** Air conduction is better than bone conduction.

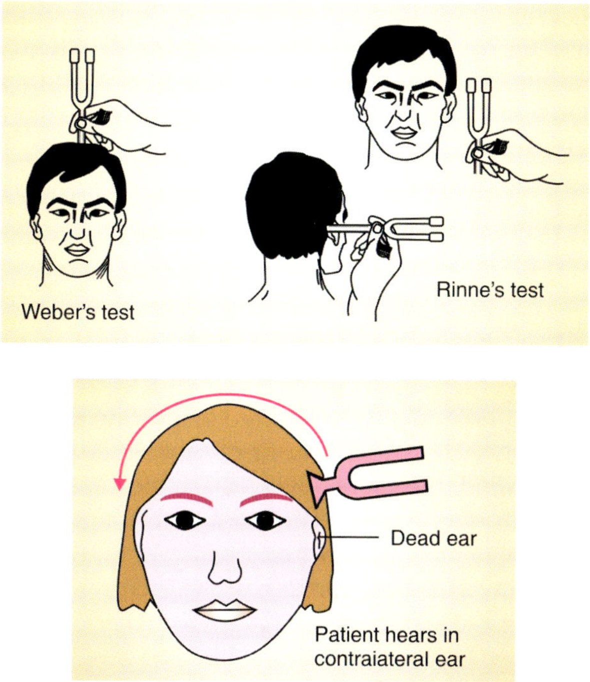

Fig. 6.1. Tuning fork tests.

Air conduction usually persists twice as long as bone conduction, referred to as "positive Rinne test".

SNHL shows reduced positive Rinne test.

- **Abnormal:** Bone conduction better than air conduction.

  Suggests conductive hearing loss.

  Referred to as "negative Rinne test".

Weber test

Procedure

- Explain the procedure to the patient.
- Hit the prongs of the tuning fork gently against the examiner's elbow or a rubber piece to make it vibrate.
- Place the base of the vibrating tuning fork on top of the patient's head or in the middle of the forehead.
- Ask the patient where he/she hears the sound.

Result

- **Normal:** This is in the middle or equal on both the sides.
- **Abnormal:** Sound lateralizes to one ear.

In case of conductive hearing loss, it laterlises to the poorer ear, whereas, in sensorineural hearing loss sound goes to better ear.

Absolute bone conduction (ABC) test

Pre-requisite: The examiner's hearing should be normal.

It is a measure of cochlear function. External meatus of both the patient and the examiner are occluded (by pressing the tragus inward) to prevent ambient air entering through AC route.

In conductive deafness, the patient and the examiner hear the fork for the same duration of time, whereas, in sensorineural deafness, the patient hears the fork for shorter duration.

Schwabach's test

Pre-requisite: The examiner's hearing should be normal.

This test has the same significance as the absolute bone conduction test. In this, bone conduction of patient is compared to that of a normal person but meatus is not occluded. Schwabach is reduced in sensorineural deafness and lengthened in conductive deafness.

Bing test

A vibrating tuning fork is placed on mastoid while the examiner alternatively closes and opens the ear canal by pressing the tragus inward. A normal person or the one with sensorineural hearing loss hears louder when ear canal is occluded and softer when canal is open (bing positive). A person with conductive deafness will appreciate no change (bing negative).

Gelle's test

This test was carried out before the advent of impedance audiometer and was used to find out stapes fixation in otosclerosis or otherwise. This test examines the effect of increased air pressure in air canal. When air pressure increases with Siegle's speculum, it pushes the tympanic membrane and ossicles inward, raises the intralabrynthine pressure and causes immobility of basilar membrane and decreases hearing, but no change is observed when ossicular chain is fixed or disconnected. Gelle's test is performed by placing a vibrating fork on the mastoid while changes in air pressure in the external auditory canal is brought about by Siegle's speculum. Gelle's test is positive in normal person and those with sensorineural hearing loss. It is negative when ossicular chain is fixed or disconnected.

AUDIOMETRY

Audiometry is the testing of hearing ability. Typically, audiometric tests not only determine a subject's hearing level with the help of an audiometer, but may also measure ability to discriminate between different sound intensities, recognize pitch, or distinguished speech from background noise. Acoustic reflex and otoacoustic emissions may also be measured. Results of audiometric tests are used to diagnose hearing loss or diseases of the ear, and often make use of an audiogram.

Pure tone audiometry (PTA)

It is the key hearing test used to identify hearing threshold levels of an individual, enabling determination of the degree, type and configuration of a hearing loss, thus providing the basis for diagnosis and management. PTA is a subjective, behavioural measurement of hearing threshold, as it relies on patient response to pure tone stimuli. Therefore, PTA is used in adults and children old enough to cooperate with the test procedure. As with most clinical tests, calibration of the test environment, the equipment and the stimuli to ISO standards is needed before testing proceeds. PTA only measures thresholds, rather than other aspects of hearing such as sound localization. However, there are benefits of using PTA over other forms of hearing test, such as click auditory brainstem response. PTA provides ear specific thresholds, and uses frequency specific pure tones to give place specific responses, so that the configuration of a hearing loss can be identified. As PTA tests both air and bone conduction, the type of hearing loss can also be identified via the air-bone gap. Although PTA has many clinical benefits, it is not perfect at identifying all losses, such as 'dead regions'. This raises the question of whether or not audiograms accurately predict someone's perceived degree of disability.

The most commonly used assessment of hearing is the determination of the threshold of audibility, i.e., the level of sound required to be just audible. This level can vary for an individual over a range of up to 5 dB from day-to-day and from determination-to-determination, but it also provides an additional and useful tool in monitoring the potential ill effects of exposure to noise. Before carrying out a hearing test, it is important to obtain information about the person's past medical history, not only concerning the ears but also other conditions which may have a bearing on possible hearing loss detected by an audiometric test. The hearing loss is usually bilateral, but variations in each ear have been observed. Wax in the ear can also cause hearing loss, so the ear should be examined to see if wax removal is needed; also to determine if the ear drum has suffered any damage which may reduce the ability of sound to be transported to the cochlea. The audiometric test can be carried out using automatic or manual audiometers, but the essential test procedure is the same.

- The subject is asked to remove anything which might alter the test results, e.g., spectacles, ear rings, hearing aids, etc.
- Instructions are given about the test procedure and the subject is required to indicate whether he/she can just hear or cannot hear a certain sound (the sound level may be increased from a very low level or reduced from a high level).
- Earphones are fitted carefully over the ears and the test is then carried out on each ear.
- First, a threshold test is undertaken in which each ear is subjected to sound at a frequency of 1 kHz at varying levels of intensity ranging from low to high and high to low. The procedure is repeated several times so that an average threshold can be derived for the test. Thresholds can vary due to slight changes in the procedures adopted in setting up the test, e.g., variation of the position of the earphone on the ear. Following this pre-check, both of the subject's ears are tested through a range of frequencies (usually 0.5, 1, 2, 3, 4, 6 and 8 kHz) and hearing loss recorded for each frequency, again via a series of sound exposures. Following that an average result can be computed.
- When the test is completed, a second threshold check should be carried out to see that no errors have crept in during the test. Both threshold checks should vary to each other with a maximum of 10 dB. If they do not, a re-test must be performed.

The accuracy of audiometry can be affected by four main factors:

- Technical limitations: How accurately can either the frequency or the hearing level be determined?
- Learning effect: The first ear tested sometimes appears worse than the second one since the individual becomes more proficient at detecting the threshold.
- Headphone fit: Some of the variation in threshold measurement has been attributed to

differences in the location of the headphones, which in turn affect the detection of the threshold.

- Background noise: Audiometric tests should be carried out in a sound-proof chamber to eliminate external sounds from influencing the test.

Limitation of PTA testing is that it is subjective and relies on the cooperation of the subject. If the subject doesn't cooperate with the test then unrepresentative results will be obtained.

The technique described above enables a comparison between the threshold of hearing of the individual undergoing audiometry with a reference value at a range of octave band frequencies (125, 250, 500, 1000, 2000, 4000, 8000 Hz). From this data a pictorial representation, an audiogram, of hearing loss at various frequencies is produced.

Cross hearing and interaural attenuation

When sound is applied to one ear the contralateral cochlea can also be stimulated to varying degrees, via vibrations through the bone of the skull. When the stimulus presented to the test ear stimulates the cochlea of the non-test ear, this is known as cross hearing. Whenever it is suspected that cross hearing has occurred it is best to use masking. This is done by temporarily elevating the threshold of the non-test ear, by presenting a masking noise at a predetermined level. This prevents the non-test ear from detecting the test signal presented to the test ear. The threshold of the test ear is measured at the same time as when presenting the masking noise to the non-test ear. Thus, thresholds obtained, when masking has been applied, provide an accurate representation of the true hearing threshold level of the test ear.

A reduction or loss of energy occurs with cross hearing, which is referred to as interaural attenuation (IA) or transcranial transmission loss. IA varies with transducer type. It varies from 40 dB to 80 dB with supra-aural headphones. However, with insert earphones it is in the region of 55 dB. The use of insert earphones reduces the need for masking due to the greater IA which occurs when they are used (Fig. 6.2).

Air conduction results in isolation, give little information regarding the type of hearing loss. When the thresholds obtained via air conduction are examined alongside those achieved with bone conduction, the configuration of the hearing loss can

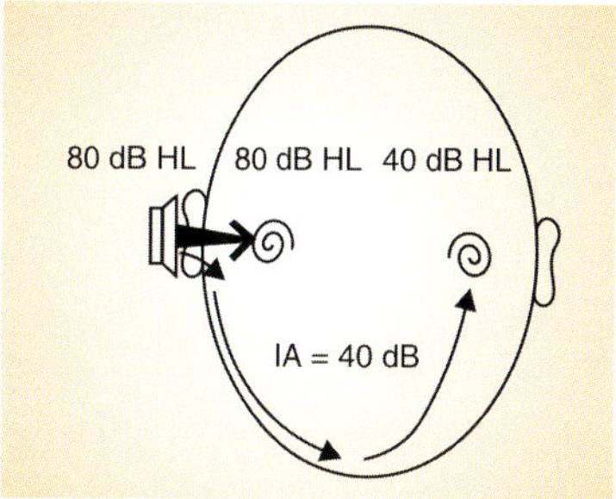

Fig. 6.2. Interaural attenuation with air conduction.

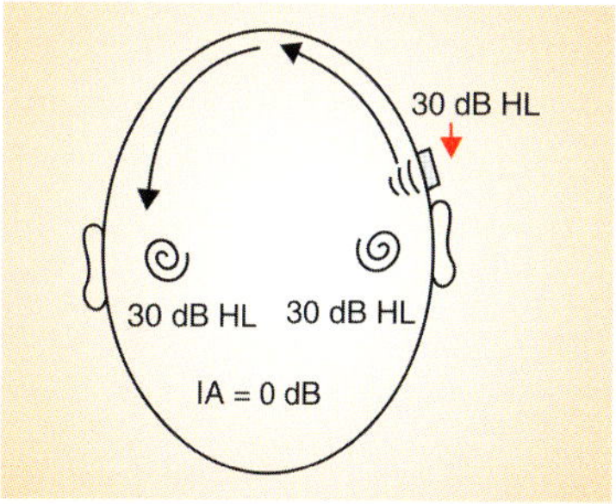

Fig. 6.3. Interaural attenuation with bone conduction.

be determined. However, with bone conduction (performed by placing a vibrator on the mastoid bone behind the ear), both cochleas are stimulated. IA for bone conduction ranges from 0–20 dB (Fig. 6.3). Therefore, conventional audiometry is ear specific, with regards to both air and bone conduction, when masking is applied.

Speech audiometry

In speech audiometry the hearing sensitivity of the subject for the speech is assessed. The main use of the speech audiometry to the neurootologist is in the identification of neural type of hearing loss, in which both the reception as well as the discrimination of speech is impaired more markedly than in cochlear or conductive hearing loss. It includes:

Speech reception threshold (SRT)

It is the lowest intensity level in dB at which 50% of a list of spondee words are correctly identified by a subject. A spondee is a two-syllable word with equal stress on each syllable, e.g., red light.

6

Speech discrimination score (SDS)

It is the percentage of correctly identified words, when words from a specifically prepared list called phonetically balanced word list is presented to the subject. To ascertain the speech discrimination score, fifty words from the phonetically balanced word list is presented to the subject at 35 dB above the

SRT. The SDS is normally between 90% to 100% but in neural lesions the SDS is considerably low.

Impedance audiometry

Impedance audiometry, also known as tympanometry, is acoustic immitance test. It is used to test the condition of the middle ear and mobility of the tympanic membrane by creating variations of air pressure in the ear canal. It measures the sound reflected from the ear drum, when probe tone is presented typically at 226 Hz into the ear canal while the air pressure of the canal is altered between +200 and –400 decapascals. It aids in the assessment of outer ear, middle ear and the functioning of eustachian tube and eliciting acoustic reflex thresholds. The classification system introduced by Jerger is commonly used to classify various types of tympanograms which includes Type A curve, Type As curve, Type Ad curve, Type B curve, Type C curve. Type of tympanometric data cannot be used as a diagnostic indicator as it is description of shape and can be used in conjunction with pure tone audiometry.

Otoacoustic Emission

An otoacoustic emission (OAE) is a sound which is generated from the inner ear. Predicted by Thomas Gold in 1948, its existence was first demonstrated experimentally by David Kemp in 1978. Otoacoustic emissions are acoustic signals generated by the normal inner ear, either in the absence of acoustic stimulation (spontaneous emissions) or in response to acoustic stimulation (acoustically-evoked emissions) or electrical stimulation (electrically-evoked emissions). There are three types of otoacoustic emission testing: Spontaneous, Transient, and Distortion Product. It can be used in neonatal screening, also assist in differentiation of cochlear and retrocochlear hearing losses (e.g., auditory neuropathy). This test can detect blockage in the outer ear canal, as well as the presence of middle ear fluid and damage to the outer hair cells in the cochlea. However, they are absent in cases with hearing loss greater than 25–30 decibels.

Brain stem evoked response audiometry

Brain stem evoked response audiometry also called auditory brain stem response, ABR audiometry, BAER (brainstem auditory evoked response audiometry) first described by Jewett and Williston in 1971 is an objective way of eliciting brain stem potentials in response to audiological click stimuli or tone tip from an acoustic transducer in the form of an insert earphone or headphone. The standard electrode configuration for BERA involves placing a non-inverting electrode over the vertex of the head, and inverting electrodes placed over the ear lobe or mastoid prominence. One more earthing electrode is placed over the forehead. A series of seven waves may be recorded from the scalp vertex during the first 10 msec following sound stimulation which represent successive synapses in the auditory pathway. Wave V is the most consistent and is used in estimation of hearing threshold. Audiological application includes investigation of hearing loss, screening deafness in infants, diagnosing brain stem diseases, estimation of hearing threshold. BERA is resistant to the effect of sleep, sedation, and anesthesia. Its threshold has been found to be within 10 dB as elicited by conventional audiometry. Limitations of BERA are patients with strictly low frequency hearing loss (less than 1 kHz) as it is dominated by the activity of high frequency nerve fibres. Interpretation of waveform whose abnormal morphology renders unequivocal identification of response component is impossible. Excessive myogenic activities can contaminate the evoked response.

MANAGEMENT OF HEARING LOSS

Management of hearing loss depends on the degree of hearing impairment, irrespective of whether the impairment is sensorineural, conductive or mixed.

Surgical management

- **Myringotomy with grommet insertion:** To clear the fluid from the middle ear myringotomy is performed and grommets are placed in the anteroinferior quadrant of the tympanic membrane.
- **Myringoplasty:** Surgical procedure involving the repair of a defect in the tympanic membrane.
- **Tympanoplasty:** Surgical repair of the tympanic membrane with clearance of disease from the middle ear, with the reconstruction of ossicular chain with or without mastoid exploration.
- **Stapedotomy:** It is the surgical procedure in which the fenestra is made in the fixed stapes footplate and piston is placed to enable the movement of the inner ear fluids and stimulation of the hair cells.

Hearing aids

A hearing aid is a device to amplify the sounds reaching the ear.

A hearing aid is an electroacoustic device which typically fits in or behind the wearer's ear, and is designed to amplify and modulate sound for the wearer. There are three basic and essential parts of hearing aids which can be considered as the building blocks for a hearing aid.

- a microphone
- an amplifier
- a receiver

The components of the hearing aid are extremely customized in such a manner that the individual components are selected for each patient and are located in the situation that is best for each ear. Hearing aids can be divided into the following types:

Body worn type (Fig. 6.4)

Behind the ear type (BTE)

BTE can be used for mild to profound hearing loss. BTE aids consist of a case, a tube and an earmold. The case is small and made of plastic. Generally, the case sits behind the pinna (ear) with the tube coming down in the front into the earmold. The case contains the amplification system. The sound is routed from the hearing aid case to the earmold via the tube. The sound can be routed acoustically or electrically.

Spectacle type

Fitted in the spectacle rather than behind the ear.

In the ear type

These devices fit in the concha; they are sometimes visible when standing face to face with someone. These hearing aids are custom made to fit each individual's ear. They can be used in mild to some degree of severe hearing loss.

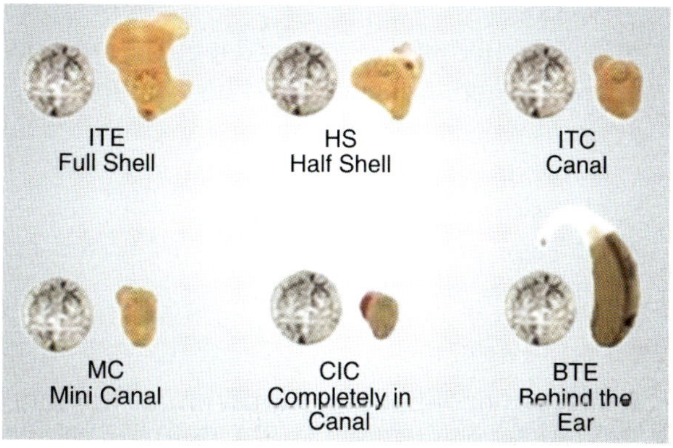

Fig. 6.4. Hearing aids.

In the canal (ITC) and completely in the canal (CIC)

ITC aids are smaller, filling only the bottom half of the external ear. The aid cannot be seen when face to face with the wearer. ITC and CIC aids are generally not visible unless the viewer looks directly into the wearer's ear.

Implantable hearing aids (Fig. 6.5)

Bone anchored hearing aids (BAHA)

It consists of a titanium screw that becomes osseo-integrated in the skull bone behind the ear. To this a transcutaneous titanium abutment is subsequently fitted to which a bone conduction vibrator can be coupled and is indicated in bilateral canal atresia, canal stenosis, persistently discharging ears, conductive or mixed hearing losses not managed with surgery, unilateral sensorineural hearing loss. This is specially useful in infants and young children.

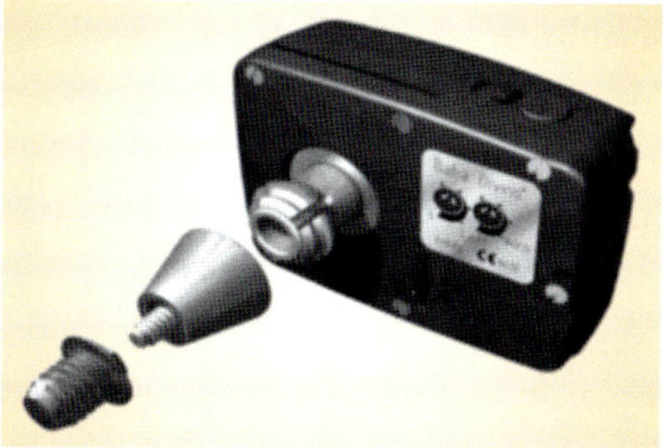

Fig. 6.5. BAHA with its components.

An osteointegrated implant with a titanium abutment is fixed to the skull. The hearing aid is then coupled to the abutment to carry the sound directly to the cochlea via the bone conduction eliminating the soft tissues between the skull bone and bone vibrator of the conventional bone aid. Complications of the procedure include failure of the osteointegration, damage to the dura in children with craniofacial anomalies, crusting and inflammation around the peg.

Cochlear implantation

Cochlear implantation has now become as an established means of auditory rehabilitation. In the past, there was very little that anybody could give any kind of hope to candidates with bilateral

6

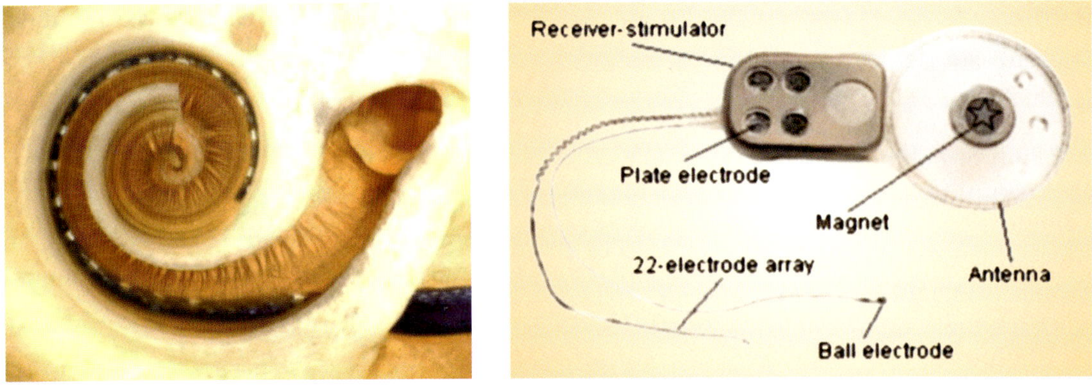

Fig. 6.6. Cochlear implants with the positioning of the electrodes in the cochlea.

profound sensorineural hearing loss, but now the cases of sensorineural deafness are managed successfully. A cochlear implant consists of microphone, speech processor, transmitter, receiver/stimulator and electrode array (Fig. 6.6). A candidate can be postlingual, perilingual or prelingual deaf. It is a team approach and involves various specialists trained in this field. A proper counseling of the parents with the help of the audiometrist and introducing them to other cochlear implantees.

Middle ear implants

There are certain shortcomings associated with the use of conventional aids such as the sound quality, occlusion effects and acoustic feedback. Wax and recurrent otitis externa also forms another significant problem for the users. In a conventional aid the amplified signal is presented to the ear via a miniature loudspeaker situated at a distance from the middle ear. In a middle ear implant the transducer is directly coupled to one of the ossicles or the cochlear window. These devices have predominantly used either a coil and magnet (electromagnetic) or a piezoelectric mode of transmission. The piezoelectric transducer works on the principle that when a voltage is applied to a particular ceramic it causes a proportional deformation and hence displacement of that ceramic. The voltage dependent displacement can then be coupled to the ossicles to drive them.

Vibrant sound bridge

It consists of an internal, surgically implanted part – the vibrating ossicular prosthesis (VORP) and an external radio processor.

PREVENTION OF HEARING LOSS

Health for all is a major target of Govt. of India, as it leads to severe loss of productivity, both physical and economic. Most causes are treatable and in others rehabilitation is possible. Over 50% of causes of hearing loss are preventable. For example, acute suppurative otitis media, chronic suppurative otitis media, secretory otitis media, traumatic, rubella deafness, noise-induced hearing loss and ototoxicity. Prevention of hearing is done at 3 levels.

Primary prevention

It involves elimination or inhibition of onset and development of the problem itself. This is done by educating people, provide services to target group (medical and paramedical assistance), hand bills, pamphlets and posters regarding prevention of hearing impairment to schools, teachers, social workers, etc.

Secondary prevention

This involves screening by specialists, audiologists, ENT specialists to identify individuals suspected of having hearing problems.

- Newborn screening should be done as a routine.
- School children are screened regularly to detect any congenital or acquired hearing loss.
- Employees and employers are educated for noise-induced hearing loss specially in factories.
- Old-age people are regularly educated and screened.

Tertiary prevention

It involves rehabilitation of individuals identified as having hearing loss so that they are able to communicate effectively.

Hearing aids are distributed free of cost. There is AIDS and APPLIANCE scheme of Govt. of India to those who are eligible.

Eligibility

Adequate bone conduction pure tone threshhold such that bone conduction threshold over 0.5, 1 and 2 kHz should be equal to or better than 45 dB HL.

SOCIAL AND MEDICO LEGAL ASPECTS OF HEARING LOSS

Social effects of hearing loss include strain with family and personal relationships. Persons will often experience frustration because they do not hear speech or instructions. They make mistakes that could hurt them or others. They are tense, fearful and are more prone to anger and depression. Social withdrawal and sometimes the family may misinterpret these changes as signs of cognitive or psychological deterioration.

The social disability from hearing loss affects not only the disabled but their families, friends, and associated social and political networks also. Disabled people affirm that the design of the environment often disables them. In better-designed environments, they are disabled less, or not at all. This affirmation arises in part from the understanding that while medical intervention can improve the health issues inherent in certain forms of disability, it does not address societal issues that prevail regardless of the extent or success of medical intervention. In conjunction with this view of changing the environment from a disabling to an enabling atmosphere de-institutionalization of disabled persons by encouraging maximum integration with non-disabled peers.

Medicolegal problems arise if impairment of the sense is the result of trauma, occupation-related or caused by mistreatment and workmen compensation. Other medicolegal problems include restriction to certain education or job opportunity and restrictions for obtaining driving license. Other important issues are regulation for companies to hire certain percentage of the employees who are disabled. Regulation for the workplace to have proper preventive measures to avoid or diminish impairment.

CONCLUSION

In the past there was little anyone could offer to alleviate hearing loss and the deaf person had to learn to cope up as normally as possible in the absence of hearing. With the advent of newer investigative techniques and treatment modalities it has become possible for an otolaryngologist to curb the burden deafness poses on the society. In this chapter we have discussed various etiological factors leading to preventable causes of hearing loss and the way to prevent, investigate and cure it. In brief we have tried to discuss the newer surgical modalities such as cochlear implantation with bilateral profound SNHL, bone anchored hearing aid and middle ear implants, etc. With the wide variety of audiological techniques available the otologist plays a pivotal role along with the help of audiological diagnostic test for the primary candidate selection and audiological rehabilitation.

Suggested Reading

1. Moller, Aage R. An experimental study of acoustic impedance of middle ear and its transmission properties. *Acta Otolaryngol*, 1965; 60: 129–49.
2. Glasscock ME, Jackson CG, Josey AF, Dickin JR, Wiet RJ. Brain stem evoked response audiometry in clinical practice. *Laryngoscope*, 1979; 89: 1021–35.
3. Biswas A. Clinical audio-vestibulometry, 4th ed. Bhalani Publisher, Mumbai, 2009.
4. Dhillon RS, East CA. Ear, nose and throat and head & neck surgery, 2nd ed. Churchill Livingstone, UK, 1999.
5. Kerr A, Smyth G.D.L. Routine speech discrimination test. *J Laryngol Otol*, 1972; 86: 33–41.
6. Probst R, Grevers G, Iro H. Basic otorhinolaryngology: A step-by-step learning guide. Thieme, New York, 2006.
7. Roeser RJ, Valente M, Dunn HH. Audiology diagnosis. Thieme, New York, 2000.
8. Clark G. Cochlear implants: Fundamentals and applications. Springer, New York, 2003.
9. Liden G, Bjorkman G, Nyman H, Kunov H. Tympanometry and acoustic impedance. *Acta Otolaryngol*, 1977; 83: 140–45.
10. Kiefer J, Pok M, Adunka O, Stuerzebecher E, Baumgartner WD, and Schmidt M. Combined electric and acoustic stimulation of the auditory system: Results of a clinical study. *Audio Neuro-otol*, 2005; 10: 134–44.
11. Tyler RS, Dunn CC, Witt SA, et al. Update of bilateral cochlear implantation. *Current Opinion Otolaryngol Head Neck Surg*, 2003; 11: 388–93.

CHAPTER 7

Stapes Surgery

A. Mahadevaiah

Otosclerosis is a primary disease of the labyrinth. The term otosclerosis is obtained from the Greek words meaning hardening of ear bones. The condition was first recognized as a pathological entity by Valsalva in the early eighteenth century. Later, in the nineteenth century, Magnus, Von Troltsch, Politzer and Toynbee were responsible for describing the clinical presentation. During the 20th century, it was recognized as a primary disease of the endochondrial bone of the otic capsule. The normal lamellar bone is replaced by irregular spongy cancellus bone mostly in the stapes region resulting in fixation of the stapes bone and conductive hearing loss.

Incidence

Otosclerosis is more prevalent in Caucasians and less common in African Americans in U.S.A. In India, South Indians are more prone to the disease when compared to North Indians. Though occurring in all age groups, the clinical presentation varies from second to fifth decade of life. Females are more affected, the ratio being 2 : 1, and bilateral ear, in 80% of cases. And about 20 to 30% of patients with progressive sensory neural hearing loss.

Histopathology

The otosclerotic process is divided into two phases. Bone resorption and increased vascularity is seen in the early phase. When the reduction of the matured collagen takes place, the bone acquires a spongy appearance (otospongiosis). The reabsorbed bone is then replaced by the dense sclerotic bone in the later phase. Otosclerosis usually starts from the fistula antefenestrum, occasionally the involvement of posterior ligament is also seen. As disease progresses, the entire footplate may be involved, and in more advanced cases, the entire oval window niche is filled (obliterative otosclerosis). In few cases, we have seen a flat of bone over the facial canal, oval window and extending over to promontory, where it is difficult to identify the oval window and footplate. The cochlear involvement results in sensorineural hearing loss.

Etiology

The exact cause is not known. However well-established causative factors have been reported. The genetic factor has been well recognized. About 50% of patients have positive family history of otosclerosis. Current genetic studies have shown autosomal dominant transmission with incomplete penetrance and known marked heterogenicity of the genetic pattern. There are six different loci which have been identified. The sites which are identified are associated with genes involved in regulation of collagen, cartilage, bone homeostasis, growth suppression and intracellular communications. In Van der Hoeve's syndrome, triad of osteogenesis imperfecta, blue sclera with otosclerosis is seen. Current studies have shown potential role of infective agents in otosclerosis. The measles viral particles, antigens and RNA are found in active cases. A possible relation of typhoid bacterial infections leading to otosclerosis has also been seen in many cases. In many cases, it may be initiated or worsened by pregnancy.

Clinical features

History of progressive hearing loss is the common symptom in adults, usually starts in early twenties. In about 50% of cases family history of otosclerosis has been seen. Most often it is bilateral disease, and unilateral in 15% of cases. Some patients feel that they hear better in noisy environment, known as paracusis of Willis, in sharp contrast to those having sensorineural hearing loss. Complaints of tinnitus especially in early cases which gradually disappears as the lesion matures in most of cases is seen. In small percentage of people vertigo along with conductive hearing loss is seen, it may be due to associated hydrops. Also in many patients after the age of 45 years, an associated sensorineural hearing loss is seen (mixed hearing loss), may be indicator of cochlear otosclerosis. A history of deterioration of hearing during pregnancy is cited in up to 50% of patients.

Physical examination shows normal appearance of tympanic membrane in 90% cases. And in few cases we may see healed perforation due to prior otitis media or grommet insertion in childhood. A Schwartz sign, a reddish hue over promontory due to increased vascularization over the bone under mucoperiosteum may be seen in early stage of disease in absent 10% cases, but not present in all cases.

Clinical diagnosis

Tuning fork tests: Tuning fork tests are useful for clinical diagnosis of type of hearing loss. In conductive hearing loss, Weber test is lateralized to the affected ear in unilateral and more affected side in bilateral cases. Negative Rinne's test is significant in conductive hearing loss. These tests are more reliable with a 500 kHz tuning fork.

Audiometry: Pure tone audiometry will be required to confirm the presence of conductive hearing loss. The air bone gap is widened at lower frequencies. In many advanced cases, we see mixed hearing loss which involves high frequencies. Carhart's notch is seen which is a dip at 2000 Hz in bone conduction curve due to loss of inertial component of stapes vibration.

In unilateral otosclerosis, masking is very essential. In absence of masking, false lateralization may be produced causing serious errors.

Air bone gap is the most important consideration for selection of patient for stapes surgery. A gap of 15–20 dB with speech discrimination scores of 60% is mandatory.

Impedance audiometry: It may be normal in early stages but later shows 'As' curve which is characteristic of ossicular stiffness. Stapedial reflex becomes absent in fixed stapes.

Tympanometry has high value in unilateral cases where hearing losses are so great that contralateral ear is ineffective. Compliance measurements may also help in estimating footplate thickness. If compliance less than 0.2 cm square there is likelihood that footplate is thick or obliterated.

Radiology: Radiology in general does not aid in diagnosis of otosclerosis. However, high resolution CT scan aids in pre-surgical evaluation to define potential complications such as dehiscent facial nerve or jugular bulb.

It may also be helpful in disclosing post-stapedectomy complications such as protrusion of prosthesis, incus necrosis or reobliteration of oval window on high resolution coronal cuts. CT densitometry reading aids in diagnosis of cochlear otosclerosis where double ring effect is seen due to formation of spongiotic foci within dense otic capsule.

Differential diagnosis

It should be differentiated form other causes such as:

- Tympanosclerosis
- Ossicular discontinuity
- Congenital stapes fixation
- Adhesive otitis media
- Attic fixation of head of malleus
- Paget's disease

Management

1. Medical

No medical treatment at present to improve the conductive hearing has been tried. It is given primarily to mature the involved bone and to decrease the osteoclastic activity.

Shambaugh and Scott advocated the use of sodium fluoride as a treatment used on its success in osteoporosis. However, this required high doses and there is no strong evidence to support this efficacy after the treatment.

Hearing aids: Hearing aids are very useful in management. Hearing aid offers an effective means of non-surgical management of the hearing loss in otosclerosis.

2. Surgical management

Stapedectomy – with placement of prosthesis is a treatment of choice.

INDICATIONS OF STAPES SURGERY

- Otosclerosis: Unilateral or bilateral conductive hearing loss with air-bone gap of more than 25 dB or negative Rinne test with 512 Hz tuning fork.
- Stapes tympanosclerosis (with ossification of annular ligament).
- Congenital fixation of stapes footplate.

CONTRAINDICATIONS OF STAPES SURGERY

Absolute

- Only hearing ear.
- Second ear surgery if the operated opposite ear had perilymph gusher intraoperatively or has developed rapidly deteriorating hearing postoperatively.

Relative

- Acute or chronic otitis externa.
- Chronic otitis media with perforation or cholesteatoma – procedure is staged.
- Congenital stapes fixation, especially if associated inner ear, facial nerve or ossicular anomaly.

PREOPERATIVE MEDICATIONS FOR STAPES SURGERY

- Alprazolam 0.25 mg tab per oral 2 hours before surgery.
- Pethidine 100 mg with phenargen 50 mg is given intramuscularly about 45 minutes before surgery.
- Betamethasone 4 mg given intramuscularly to prevent peroperative vestibular shock.
- Appropriate oral broad-spectrum antibiotic is given 2 hours before surgery. We prefer ceftazidime and gentamicin I/V immediately before surgery to combat Pseudomonas infection. This helps to maintain antibiotics level in the blood and minimizes immediate postoperative infection and reparative granuloma.

Anaesthesia

- Stapes surgery is always preferred under local anesthesia with sedation.
- General anesthesia may be necessary in children less than 14 years.

Technique

- 2.2 ml of 2% lignocaine is mixed with 0.3 ml of 1 : 1000 adrenaline to form 2.5 ml solution with approximately 1 : 25000 adrenaline.
- The above-prepared solution is taken in a 2.5 ml disposable syringe with 25 gauge needle and is injected 0.5 ml each at four quadrants.
- 0.3 ml of this solution is injected in the post-aural groove to harvest soft tissue for seal. The remaining 0.2 ml is instilled in the middle ear after elevation of tympanomeatal flap.

Advantages of Local Anesthesia

- Warns injury to inner ear.
- Intraoperative hearing assessment.
- Less bleeding during surgery.

SURGICAL TECHNIQUE

The local area is painted with povidone iodine and spirit and draped. The canal is thoroughly washed with saline to clear all the wax and debris. We prefer to use self-retaining Mahadevaiah canal retractor with/without stand (Fig. 7.1).

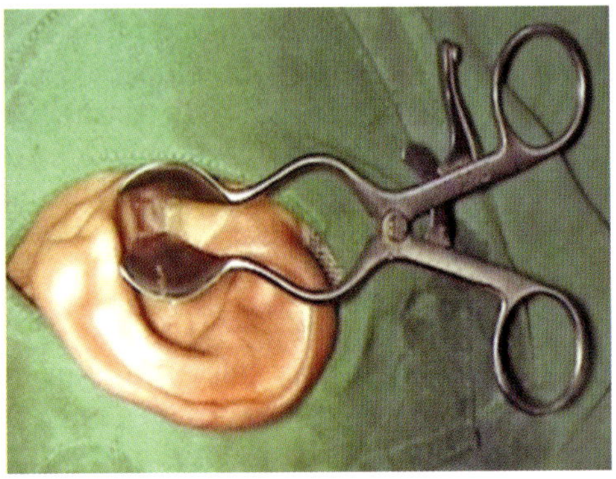

Fig. 7.1. Self-retaining Mahadevaiah canal retractor with/without stand gives good exposure and helps to perform the stapes surgery with both the hands free (left ear).

STEPS

1. Rosen's incisions.
2. Elevation of tympanomeatal flap.
3. Mobilizing the chorda tympani nerve.
4. Removal of overhang.
5. Assessment of ossicular mobility.
6. Making a control fenestra.
7. Cutting of stapedius tendon.
8. Disarticulation of incudostapedial joint.
9. Removal of stapes superstructure.
10. Widening of fenestra and removal of posterior third of footplate, if necessary.
11. Estimation of length and width of piston.
12. Insertion of piston and its crimping.

13. Harvesting of tissue and tissue seal of the fenestra.
14. Replacement of tympanomeatal flap.
15. Evaluation of intraoperative hearing.
16. Closure of wound.

Rosen's Incision (Magnification: 6 times)

A "U" shaped incision (Fig. 7.2) involves two curvilinear incisions (superior and inferior) starting 1–2 mm lateral to the annulus and meeting each other 7 to 8 mm lateral to the annulus close to bony cartilaginous junction.

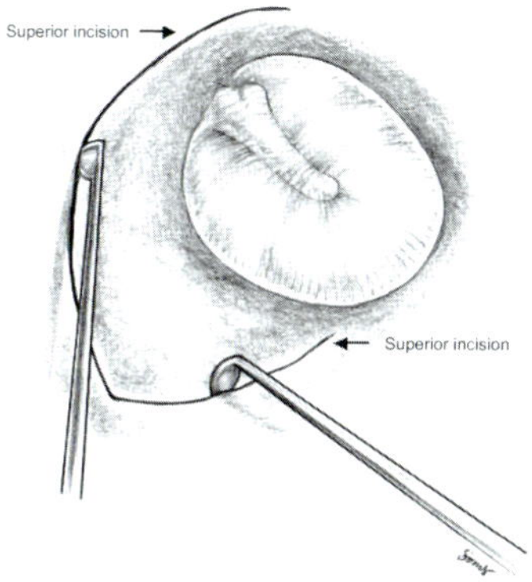

Fig. 7.2. Diagrammatic picture showing a "U" shaped Rosen's incision (right ear). The inferior incision starts 1–2 mm lateral to the annulus from 7 o' clock position and runs in a slanting fashion 7 to 8 mm laterally to reach to 10 o' clock position using angular oval knife. The superior incision is made using Plester's side knife and starts at 1 o' clock position about 2 mm above the lateral process of malleus and runs along the superior and posterior bony canal wall intercepting the inferior incision at 10 o' clock position.

Right ear: The inferior incision starts 1–2 mm lateral to the annulus from 7 o' clock position and runs in a slanting fashion 7 to 8 mm laterally to reach to 10 o' clock position using angular oval knife. The superior incision is made using Plester's side knife and starts at 1 o' clock position about 2 mm above the lateral process of malleus and runs along the superior and posterior bony canal wall intercepting the inferior incision at 10 o' clock position. The superior incision requires sharp dissection using cutting and crushing strokes, especially if there is substantial subcutaneous tissue as found in patients with prominent tympanosquamous suture.

Left ear: The inferior incision starts 1–2 mm lateral to the annulus from 5 o' clock position and runs in a slanting fashion 7 to 8 mm laterally to reach to 2 o' clock position using Plester's side knife. The superior incision is made using same Plester's knife and starts at 11 o' clock position about 2 mm above the lateral process of malleus and runs along the superior and posterior bony canal wall intercepting the inferior incision at 2 o' clock position.

Guidelines and Precautions

- Note that the instrument used for making inferior and superior incisions are for the right-handed surgeon. It changes with the side of ear to be operated to ease the placement of incision. The inferior incision is made with an angular oval knife and superior incision is made with Plester's side knife in right ear. In the left ear both the superior and inferior incisions are made by Plester's side knife.
- If the anterosuperior canal skin is not visible directly due to narrow canal or there is substantial overhanging soft tissue due to prominent tympanosquamous suture, the exposure can be improved by making helico-tragal (endaural) incision between the cartilage of crus of helix and tragus using 15 number blade up to the bony cartilaginous junction.
- It is important to extend the anterosuperior limb of incision at least 5 mm lateral to the fibrous annulus, so that the removal of attic wall in cases of occasional accompanying anterior malleolar fixation (when the malleus head/anterior process is fixed to the anterior attic wall) can be dealt using the same incision without the risk of tear of the tympanic membrane anteriorly. A wide tympano-meatal flap anterosuperiorly helps to adequately cover the bony defect i.e. attic defect after removal of attic wall.

Elevation of Tympanomeatal Flap (Magnification: 6 Times)

The canal skin between the above mentioned incisions is elevated gently using the oval canal elevator by remaining close to the bone using adequate pressure. The canal skin flap may remain attached to the superior incision margin due to fibrous attachments at tympanosquamous suture. These attachments need to be severed by sharp dissection using micro-scissors. The flap is elevated till the fibrous annulus is reached. The annulus is elevated from its sulcus using Rosen's elevator (Fig. 7.3) and the mucosa thus exposed is incised below 9 o'clock position for right ear (3 o'clock for left ear)

7

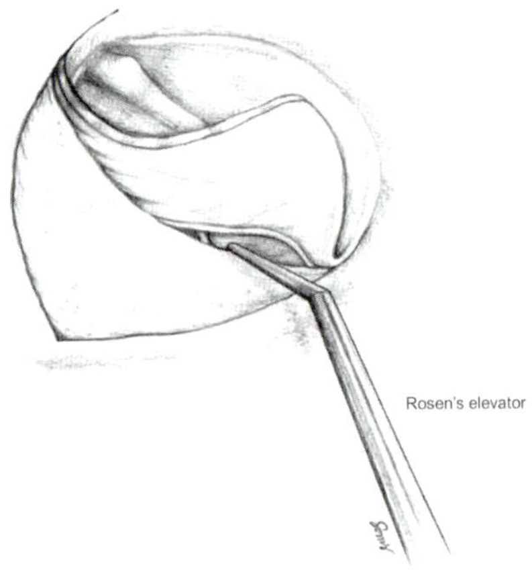

Fig. 7.3. Diagrammatic picture showing elevation of annulus from its sulcus using Rosen's elevator (right ear).

using a sickle knife to enter the middle ear. The inferior part of tympanomeatal flap below notch of rivinus is elevated up to 7 o'clock position for right ear (5 o'clock for left ear) using Rosen's elevator. The superior part of tympanomeatal flap above the posterior notch of Rivinus is elevated initially by Rosen's elevator and later the tympanic membrane is freed from its attachments with mucosal folds by sharp dissection using sickle knife. Posterior malleolar ligament (Fig. 7.4) is resected by sickle knife while taking care to avoid injury to underlying chorda tympani. After complete elevation of the tympanomeatal flap, it is folded over the anterior part of tympanic membrane to avoid it interfering in the latter steps. The malleus handle and the round window niche should be easily visible. The middle ear is filled with the previously prepared anesthetic solution for a few seconds and then it is suctioned out at round window niche. The solution at the oval window area should be sucked before making

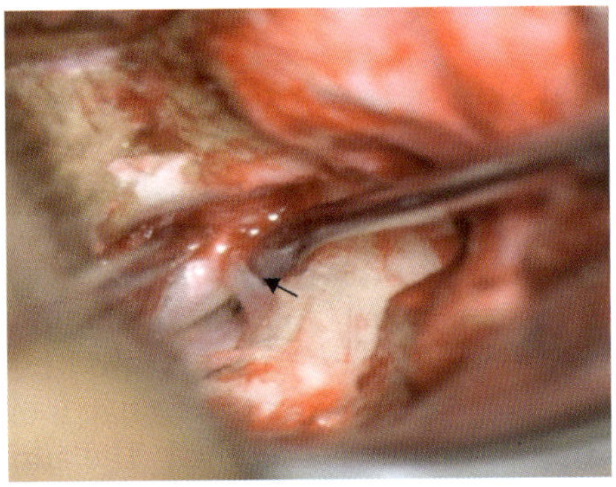

Fig. 7.4. Posterior malleolar ligament (arrow) is attached at posterior notch of Rivinus is cut with sickle knife (left ear).

7

fenestra in the footplate. This helps to anesthetize the middle ear mucosa as well as to reduce bleeding from mucosa over the footplate during later steps.

Guidelines and Precautions

- Remaining close to the bone while elevating the flap, avoids tearing of the flap and over-running the annulus to tear the tympanic membrane.
- The bleeding from the margins of incision should be controlled with pressure using gelfoam/cotton ball (may be dipped in adrenaline if required) or injecting again in the canal lateral to the bleeding point. Bleeding should be controlled completely before the middle ear is entered.
- If the elevation of tympanomeatal flap is continued without including the annulus with it and only the superficial squamous layer of the tympanic membrane is lifted, there are chances of tear in the tympanic membrane. Avoid tearing of the tympanic membrane close to annulus by gently elevating the annulus from its sulcus.
- It is always safe to enter the middle ear in inferior quadrant to avoid injury to ossicles and chorda tympani nerve.
- It is important to anesthetize the middle ear mucosa to prevent sudden movements by patient due to pain while performing fenestra over the footplate.

Mobilizing the Chorda Tympani (Magnification: 6 times)

Chorda tympani nerve emerges from chordal eminence usually at 3 o'clock position in the left ear (9 o' clock position in the right ear). The nerve is identified, and separated from its attachments to tympanic membrane by mucosal folds using smooth blunt curved pick. The nerve is pushed antero-inferiorly, to prevent its injury while removing bony overhang. Its mobilization also helps to achieve adequate working space around the oval window area and prevents it from interfering in subsequent steps. Occasionally the chorda tympani is covered completely by the bony overhang and is identified after removal of the overhang.

Removal of Bony Overhang (Magnification: 6 times)

The medial part of posterosuperior canal wall (also called scutum) between the posterior notch of Rivinus and chordal eminence (also known as iter chordae posticus) forms the bony overhang (Fig. 7.5) that covers the incus and stapes for a variable

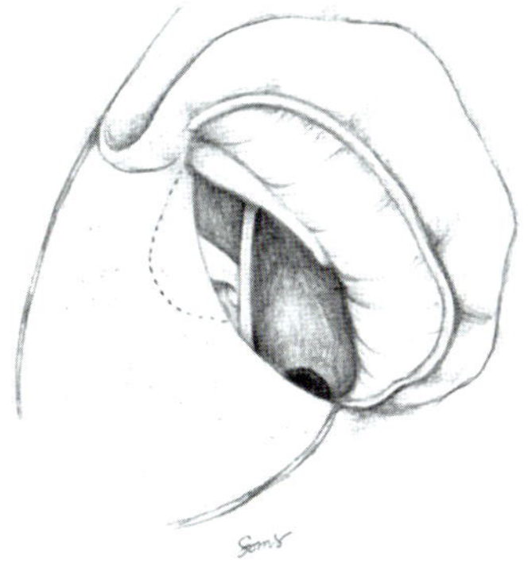

Fig. 7.5. Diagrammatic picture showing the amount of bone to be removed to achieve adequate exposure of the oval window (right ear).

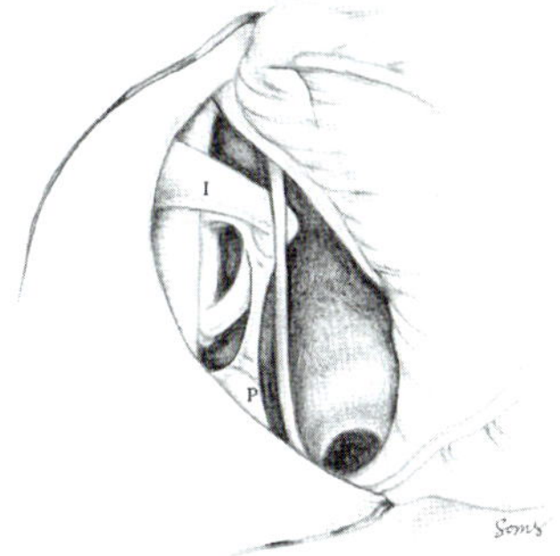

Fig. 7.6. Diagrammatic picture showing adequate exposure after removal of overhang. This includes visualization of the entire stapes with its footplate, long process of incus, horizontal segment of facial canal above the oval window and stapedius tendon with pyramidalis process (right ear).

distance. This bony overhang needs to be removed for adequate exposure of the oval window and to prevent hindrance at maneuvering the instruments while working over the footplate. The overhang is removed using sharp strong House double-ended curette of appropriate size depending upon the working space available. It is easier to start curetting the overhang beginning from the posterior notch of Rivinus, which provides the groove to engage the curette initially and thus avoids slipping of the curette unintentionally. After firmly engaging the curette in the notch, the direction of movement of curette should be rotatory from medial to lateral and away from chorda tympani. In cases of thick posterior bony overhang, it is better to thin out by drilling the thick bone using 1 mm burr tip. Once it is thinned out remaining amount of bony overhang is removed by curette. One should be careful about the chorda tympani nerve. During drilling middle ear and tympanomeatal flap is covered by a cotton ball to prevent bone dust going into the middle ear. Finally, all the bone chips are removed by using large bore suction cannula. The adequate exposure after removal of overhang implies visualization of the entire stapes with its footplate, long process of incus, horizontal segment of facial canal above the oval window and stapedius tendon with pyramidalis process (Fig. 7.6).

Guidelines and Precautions

- The direction of curetting should be away from the ossicles (especially incus) and chorda tympani to avoid accidental injury to it.
- The edges of the curette should always be sharp to enhance bony removal and to prevent its slippage. If the bony wall is thick and cannot be curetted in one go, curette lateral to the edge of overhang to thin it before attempting to curette medial edge. This helps to prevent use of excess pressure or sudden slippage of curette and injury to chorda tympani and incus.
- Lowering the head by 30 degrees may be required to improve the exposure, if the oval window and the footplate are not visualized clearly due to narrow or tortuous canal or facial nerve overhang.
- Improper exposure due to inadequate overhang removal will hamper instrumentation at the footplate and if not corrected will be troublesome throughout the procedure.

Assessment of Ossicular Mobility (Magnification: 6 times)

The mobility of the each of the ossicles is checked individually (Fig. 7.7). The malleus is moved from its undersurface using smooth curved pick and the associated mobility of the incus and stapes is

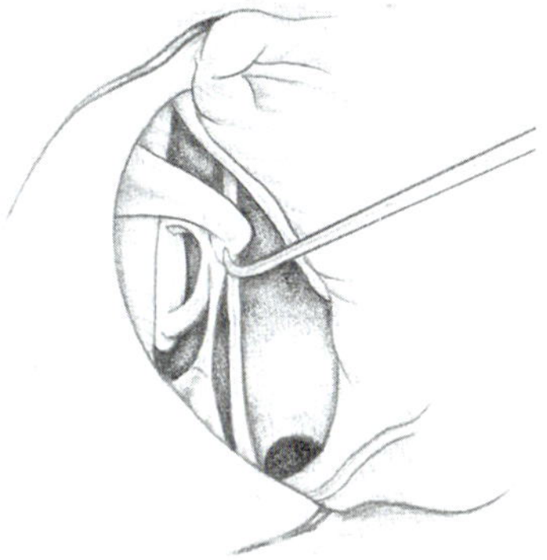

Fig. 7.7. Diagrammatic picture showing assessment of ossicular mobility (right ear).

visualized. The round window reflex is seen simultaneously. When the stapes is fixed as in otosclerosis and the incus is mobile, the movement can be appreciated at the incudostapedial joint but not at stapes footplate. Similarly incus mobility can be confirmed by applying pressure on long process of incus. Lastly the stapes superstructure is palpated directly to check for its mobility.

Guidelines and Precautions

- The associated anterior malleolar fixation is found in around 1 percent of our patients that is missed if all the ossicles are not palpated individually for its mobility.
- Sometimes immobility of incus may be seen till the incudostapedial joint is dislocated; it may be due to partial ankylosis of the incudostapedial joint. In such cases, one should be careful not to fracture lenticular process while dislocating incudostapedial joint. Intact lenticular process is required to prevent dislocation of the piston postoperatively.

Making a Control Fenestra (Magnification: 16 times)

The footplate is now visualized under higher magnification (Fig. 7.8) to confirm the focus of otosclerosis (anterior/posterior/diffuse/biscuit type/obliterative), the condition of facial canal (whether dehiscent or overhanging), promontory and any other associated anomaly. A control fenestra is made over the posterior third of stapes footplate in the inferior part (sometimes superior depending on the space available) using a straight sharp pick (Figs. 7.9, 7.10). The fenestra is made by to and fro rotatory movement of the pick between the index finger and the thumb after gently scratching over the footplate. Fenestra is widened with 0.3 mm Fisch perforator. Be gentle and avoid any undue pressure over the footplate.

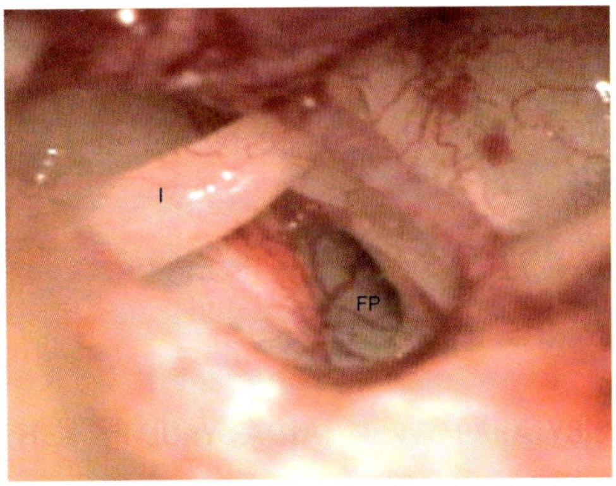

Fig. 7.8. Visualization of footplate (FP) under high magnification to look for the focus otosclerotic focus over facial canal.

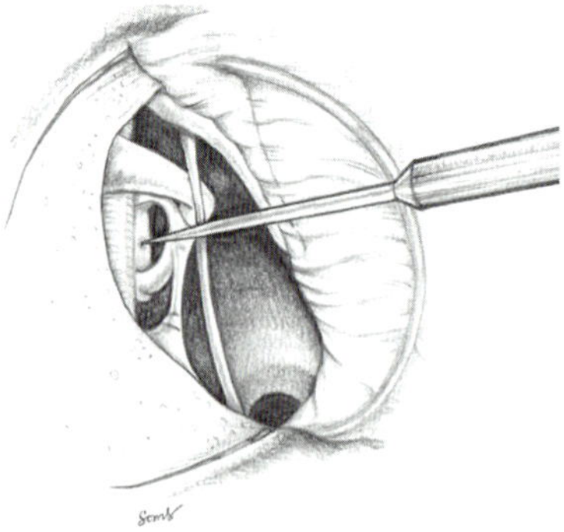

Fig. 7.9. Diagrammatic picture showing making a control fenestra using a straight sharp pick (right ear).

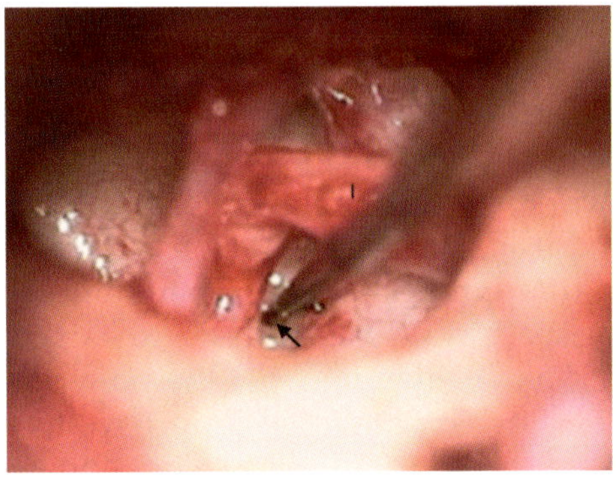

Fig. 7.10. Making a control fenestra using a straight sharp (arrow) pick (right ear).

Guidelines and Precautions

- The posterior third of stapes footplate is fenestrated as the saccule that lies more superficial in the vestibule is located anteriorly. Utricle lies posteriorly about 1 mm below the footplate.
- The purpose of this control fenestra is for early identification of any perilymph gusher and to prevent vestibular "shock" (sudden increase in vestibular pressure causing vertigo and acoustic trauma due to accidental fracture of the footplate while removing the stapes superstructure). The procedure may be abandoned if a profuse perilymph gusher is identified after sealing it with fibrous tissue and patient advised hearing aid to prevent severe sensorineural hearing loss.
- The 0.3 mm control fenestra also helps to retrieve the footplate using a 0.2 mm right angled pick if it

becomes a floater during subsequent steps of removal of superstructure or widening the fenestra.

- It may not be possible to make a control fenestra in certain conditions like very thick or obliterative footplate or narrow niche, overhanging facial nerve or promontory.
- It is essential to have bloodless operative field before any fenestra is made. All the lignocaine and adrenaline solution is thoroughly suctioned before the fenestra is made. If the bleeding occurs after the fenestra is made, one should wait for a few minutes to allow the bleeding to stop by natural coagulation.
- It is important to explain to the patient to avoid sudden head movement (in unstrapped patients) if there is sudden giddiness or hearing of loud noise while making of initial fenestra in the footplate.

Cutting of Stapedius Tendon (Magnification: 16 times)

Stapedius tendon is now severed close to its junction at pyramidalis process using a sharp sickle knife (Fig. 7.11). Alternatively a micro-alligator scissors may be used.

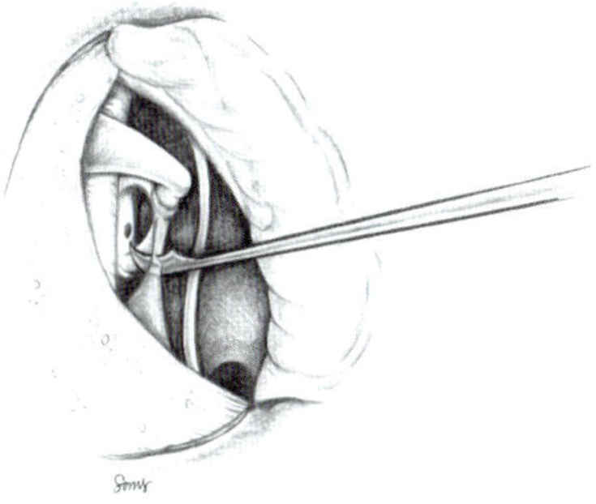

Fig. 7.11. Diagrammatic picture showing cutting of stapedius tendon close to pyramidalis process (right ear).

Disarticulation of Incudostapedial Joint (Magnification: 16 times)

After confirming the exact site of incudostapedial joint capsule by palpating incus over stapes head for a few times while watching for the joint space, the joint is disarticulated using right angled 0.5 mm pick moving back and forth (Fig. 7.12).

Removal of Stapes Superstructure (Magnification: 16 times)

Posterior crus of the stapes superstructure is

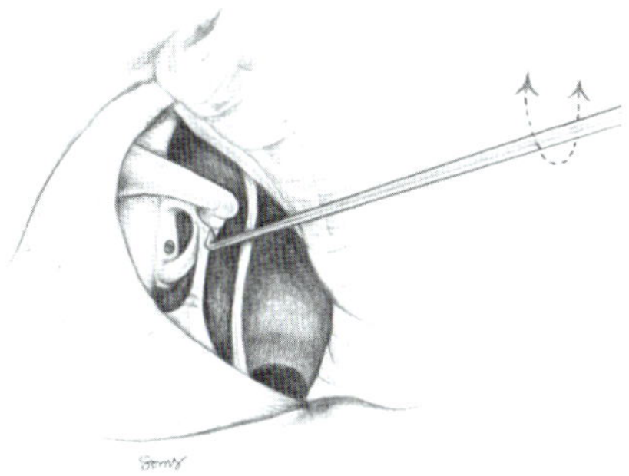

Fig. 7.12. Diagrammatic picture showing disarticulation of incudostapedial joint (right ear).

weakened and then fractured by gently and repeatedly scratching the base of the crus close to its attachment to the footplate using 0.2 mm right angled pick under direct vision (Fig. 7.13). Once the thicker posterior crus is fractured, the anterior crus easily fractures by gentle tilting force over the superstructure downward towards promontory (Fig. 7.14).

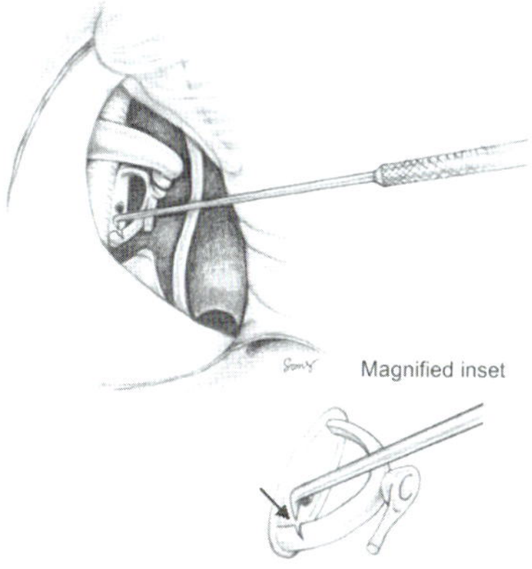

Fig. 7.13. Diagrammatic picture showing removal of stapes superstructure by scratching the base of the posterior crus with 0.2 mm right-angled pick close to its attachment with footplate (arrow) (right ear).

Guidelines and Precautions

- Gently scratch at the posterior crus as close to footplate as possible to prevent fracture and subluxation of the footplate.
- Anterior crus is not seen directly in most of the cases as long process of incus obstructs its vision.
- Posterior crus is thicker and shorter relative to the anterior crus that is thinner and longer. Also the otosclerotic focus is most commonly located anterior to the footplate and thus anterior crus easily fractures without fracturing the footplate once the more sturdy posterior crus is fractured.

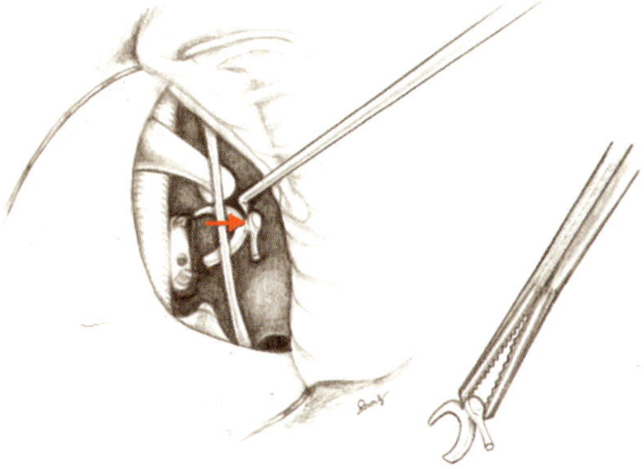

Fig. 7.14. Diagrammatic picture showing removal of stapes superstructure fracturing the anterior crus by gentle tilting force over the superstructure (arrow) downward towards promontory (right ear).

- Occasionally entire footplate may come out while removing the superstructure. In such cases 0.6 mm piston is used with more soft tissue or vein or fascia graft to seal the window.
- Other techniques of fracturing the posterior crus include using crurotomy scissors, skeeter drill or the laser. However, we feel the above-mentioned technique to be easy, safe and can be performed without the need for expensive equipment.

Widening of Fenestra and Removal of Posterior Third of Footplate (Magnification: 16 times)

The posterior third of footplate is then scraped from its undersurface and loose fragments, if any, are removed piecemeal using 0.2 mm right-angled hook (Fig. 7.15). The hook should be inserted just below the medial surface of footplate. Fragments of footplate are removed piecemeal till an adequate size of fenestra is made. We prefer a large fenestra of 0.8 mm or more in size. If this cannot be achieved due to narrow niche, the posterior third of the footplate is removed.

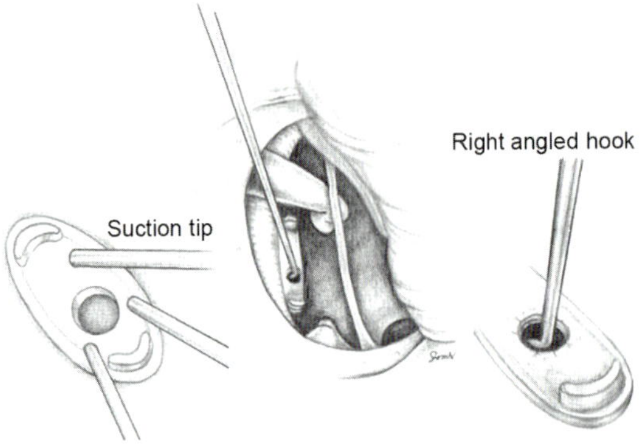

Fig. 7.15. Diagrammatic picture showing widening of fenestra using 0.2 mm right-angled hook. Suction, if required, should be placed on the bone adjacent to the footplate/fenestra and never directly over the exposed vestibule (right ear).

7

Guidelines and Precautions

- Be as atraumatic as possible in widening the fenestra and removing the posterior third of footplate.
- Mucosa over the footplate should not be elevated while enlarging the fenestra as it provides splinting action to occasional fracture fragments and prevents its entry into vestibule.
- When the otosclerotic focus is limited to the anterior part of footplate, the posterior one-third of the footplate may come out while widening the fenestra. Occasionally the whole footplate may come out as mentioned earlier.
- Great care should be taken to avoid dropping the footplate fragments into vestibule.
- Avoid direct suction over the vestibule. Suction, if required, should be placed on the bone adjacent to the footplate/fenestra (Fig. 7.15). Variable on/off thumb control of suction with small suction cannula (22/24 G) is important to remove any blood or fluid around the fenestra. The thumb control is kept open initially and the suction amount increased progressively by covering the hole with thumb.
- We believe that the size of the fenestra should be large enough to allow free frictionless movement of the piston.

Estimation of Length and Width of Piston (Magnification: 10 times)

The distance between the undersurface of the footplate exposed by making a fenestra and the medial surface of the long process of incus is measured using House measuring rod (Fig. 7.16) and is equal to the length of the prosthesis required. The Teflon piston is placed in the measuring jig (Fig. 7.17) and cut as per the measured length (Fig. 7.18).

Note: The measurement protocols given here are for the Teflon piston manufactured in India. The length is measured from the centre of the loop to the end of the shaft of the piston.

The diameter of the shaft of prosthesis varies from 0.4 to 0.6 mm depending on the size of fenestra.

Guidelines and Precautions

- As the thickness of footplate varies considerably in patients of otosclerosis, it is better to estimate

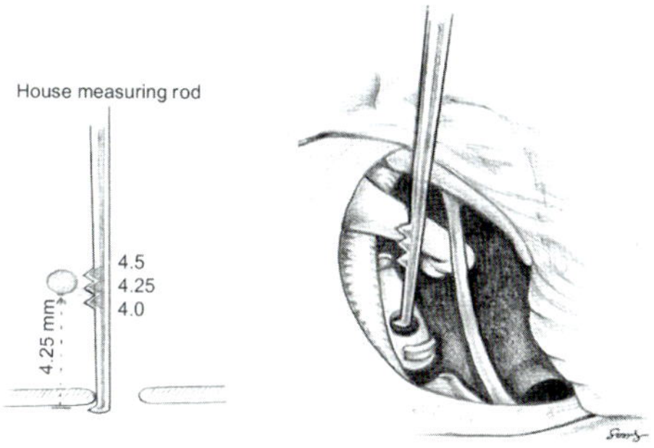

Fig. 7.16. Diagrammatic picture showing estimation of length of piston required using House measuring rod (right ear).

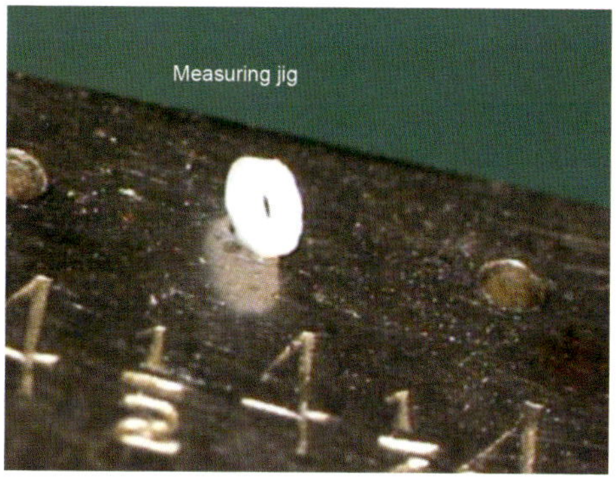

Fig. 7.17. The Teflon piston is placed in the measuring jig as per the measured length.

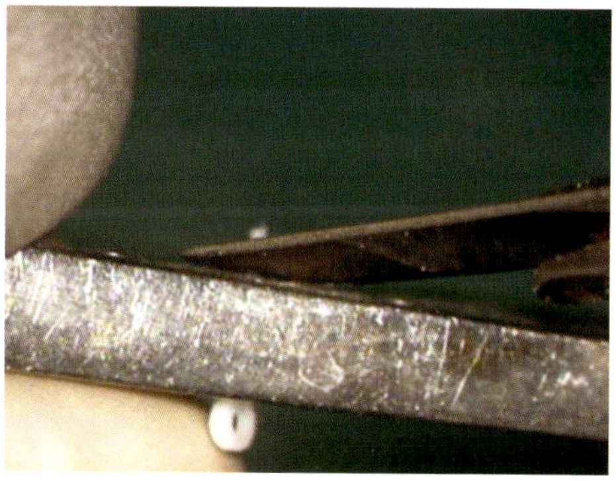

Fig. 7.18. Cutting the excess length of the piston by number 15 blade.

the length of prosthesis after opening the vestibule so that exact length from inner surface of footplate to incus long process can be measured.

- The piston should project approximately 0.25 mm in the vestibule. The length of more than 0.5 mm within the vestibule could be hazardous.

Insertion of Piston (Magnification: 10 times)

- The loop of the Teflon piston is widened and opened up using alligator forceps (Figs. 7.19, 7.20) to enable its placement around long process of incus. The Teflon piston with open loop is held from the back of loop with a slim alligator forceps such that the piston shaft makes an angle of about 135 degrees with alligator forceps (Figs. 7.21, 7.22). The technique of holding the alligator forceps along with the piston should be such that the surgeon should visualize the fenestra, the long process of the incus, the loop and the distal end of the shaft of the piston simultaneously (Fig. 7.23). The shaft of the piston is negotiated into the vestibule and simultaneously the loop is maneuvered around the long process of the incus.

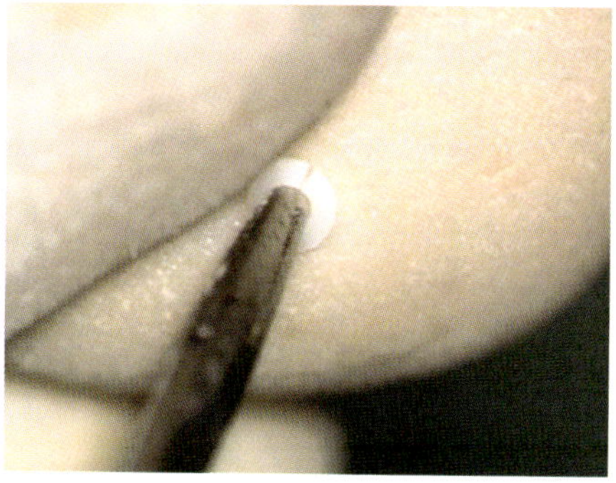

Fig. 7.19. Loop of the Teflon piston is widened using alligator forceps.

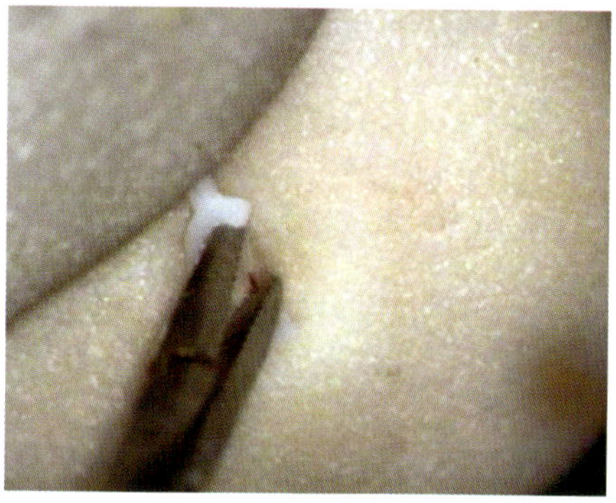

Fig. 7.20. Loop of the Teflon piston is widened using alligator forceps.

- Even after accurate measurement of the length, it is obligatory to re-confirm the length clinically after placement of the piston. The piston is visualized through the vestibular fluid to see if it is not too long (Fig. 7.24).
- "Bending"/Displaceability test: After placement of the piston, its shaft is moved back and forth (anterior to posterior and superior to inferior) (Fig. 7.24). While mobilizing the piston, note whether it tends to come out of the fenestra, which suggests short prosthesis length.

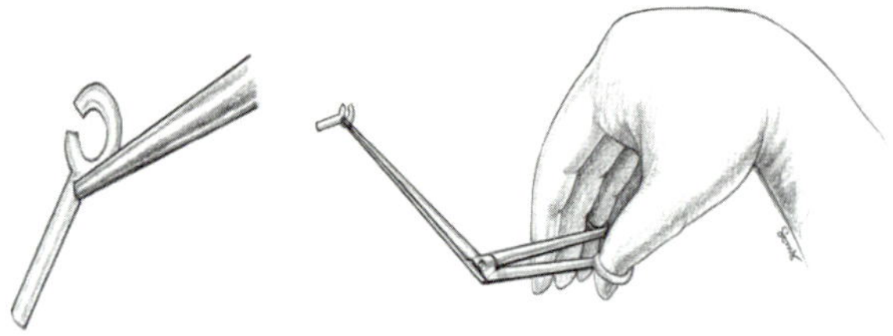

Fig. 7.21. Diagrammatic picture showing technique of holding the alligator forceps along with piston.

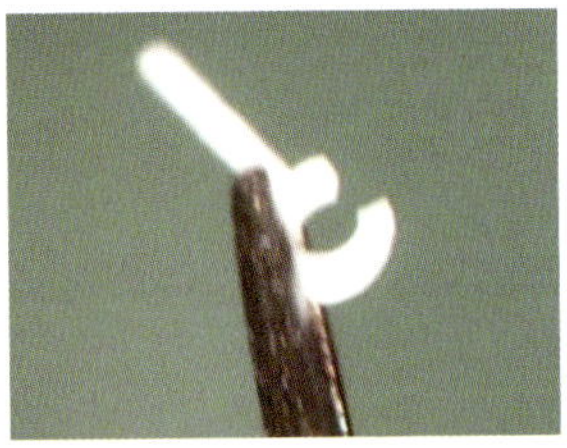

Fig. 7.22. Piston with open loop is hold from the back of loop with a slim alligator forceps.

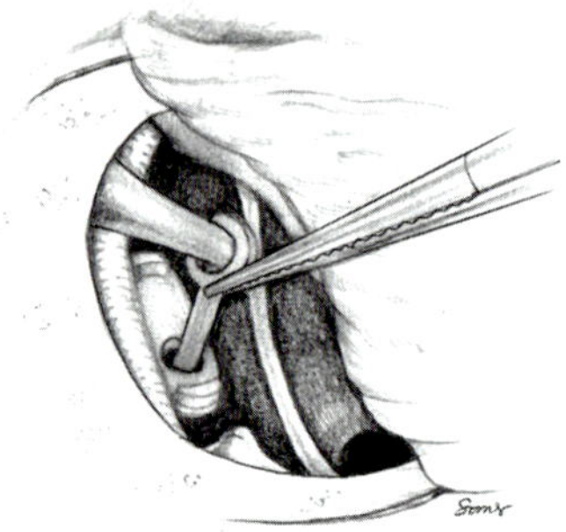

Fig. 7.23. Diagrammatic picture showing visualization of the fenestra, the long process of the incus, the loop and the distal end of the shaft of the piston (right ear).

- "Tilting"/Ballotability test: Gently palpate the incus in medial to lateral direction to mobilize the piston gently in and out of the vestibule to access for any symptomatic vertigo, the presence of which suggests long prosthesis length.
- The prosthesis may need to be removed and reinserted if it is found to be too short or long. If the prosthesis is long, it is removed, shortened appropriately and reinserted. If the prosthesis is short, replace it with a new longer prosthesis of adequate length.
- The final position of the prosthesis is adjusted using right-angled hook such that it lies perpendicular to the footplate and incus long process.
- The widened loop is next crimped over the long process of the incus using the same alligator forceps (Fig. 7.25) or with a specially designed 'crimper'. The crimping process requires extremely minute manipulation and so the

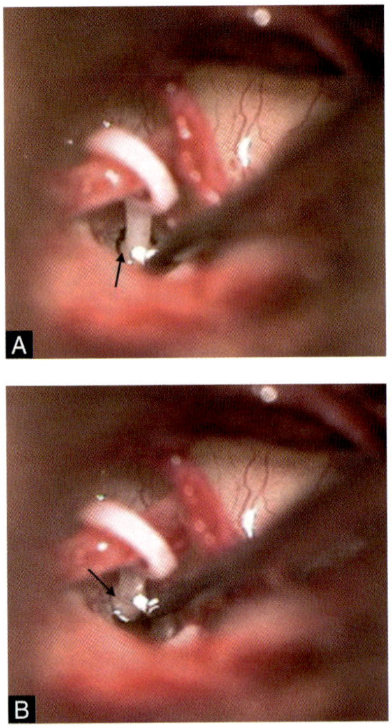

Figs. 7.24A and B. (A) The piston is visualized through the vestibular fluid (arrow) to see if it is not too long (right ear). (B) The piston shaft is moved posterior to anterior and see whether it tends to come out of the fenestra (right ear).

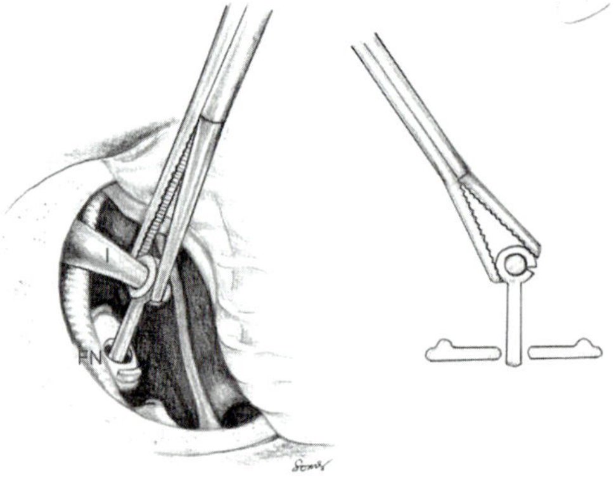

Fig. 7.25. Diagrammatic picture showing crimping of the piston loop (right ear).

alligator forceps may be held with both hands supported over the patients' head to avoid physiological tremors.

Guidelines and Precautions

- Balance the need for magnification (as working on the footplate) with need for depth perception (as during placement or crimping of the prosthesis) and change magnification accordingly throughout the procedure.

- It is important to turn to lesser magnification (from 16 times to 10 times) while insertion of piston so that one can focus both the fenestra as well as long process of incus in same visual field.
- If it is not possible to negotiate the piston into the vestibule and incus simultaneously using alligator forceps, place the piston shaft over the fenestra and pass the upper part of loop of the piston over the incus using 0.2 mm right angled pick while supporting the lower end of the loop against the incus using the suction tip. Avoid excessive movement of the incus to prevent its disarticulation from incudomalleolar joint.
- Crimping of the piston avoids loose prosthesis. The tight crimping of Teflon prosthesis helps to move both incus and the piston as a single unit and usually does not cause any damage to the long process. However, if the prosthesis is loose due to inadequate crimping, it will lead to repeated friction with the mobile incus and cause necrosis of long process of incus.

Harvesting of Tissue to Seal the Fenestra (Magnification: 6 times)

The fenestra is sealed with various types of tissues like lobule fat, vein graft, gelfoam and free fibrous tissue. The subcutaneous fibrous tissue is an excellent material for sealing the defect as it immediately adheres to the piston and seals the vestibule completely (Fig. 7.26). The displaced chorda tympani is replaced under the loop of piston (Fig. 7.27).

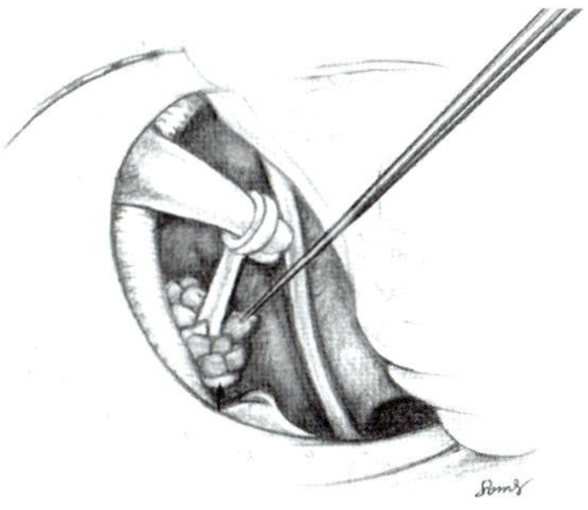

Fig. 7.26. Diagrammatic picture showing sealing the fenestra over the vestibule by fibrous tissue (arrow) around the shaft of the piston.

Guidelines and Precautions

- During the entire process of harvesting and placement of tissue seal neither the instruments nor the harvested tissue should touch the drapes or canal skin to avoid contamination with foreign material. We believe that contamination of the tissue seal due to infection or foreign material is the major cause for occasional (rare) poststapedectomy reparative granuloma, which could lead eventually to severe sensorineural hearing loss.
- The curved pick is usually used to push the piece of fibrous tissue anterior to the piston to seal the fenestra anteriorly.

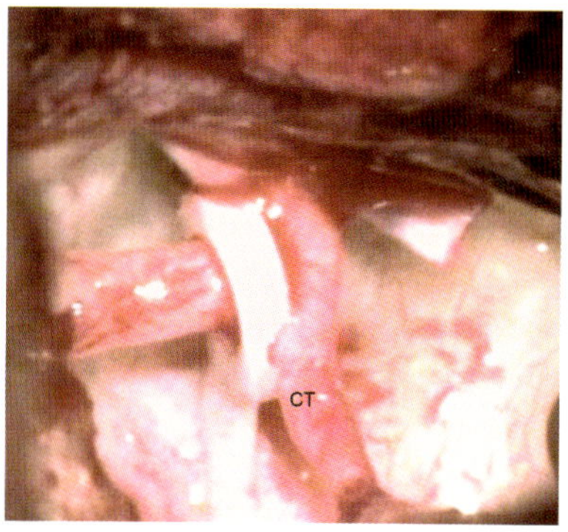

Fig. 7.27. Chorda tympani (CT) is replaced below the loop of piston (right ear).

Replacement of Tympanomeatal Flap (Magnification: 6 times)

The tympanomeatal flap is replaced and the edges of the incisions adjusted against each other.

Guidelines and Precautions

- The edges should be closely approximated otherwise it leads to postoperative healing in a retracted position with the tympanic membrane touching the incus and thus leading to possibility of perforation of the tympanic membrane and extrusion of the prosthesis.

Evaluation of Intraoperative Hearing

We prefer assessment of improvement in hearing intraoperatively by asking the patient to repeat the numbers that the surgeon speaks in patient's vernacular language with lowering intensity till the patient can reply the softest of the murmurs. It gives subjective evidence of improvement in hearing and adequacy of prosthesis length. However, final hearing assessment is done audiologically one month after surgery.

Closure of Wound

A rolled piece of cotton impregnated with antibiotic ointment is placed in the canal to absorb any blood oozing. The post-aural stab incision placed to harvest the tissue for sealing the oval window need not be sutured. Both external auditory meatus and postauricular stab wound covered by gauge pieces which will be removed in 24 to 48 hours before discharge. Again a piece of cotton ball impregnated with antibiotic ointment is placed in the canal, which will be removed by the patient himself after a week. This will help to prevent immediate postoperative infection in the canal.

DIFFICULT SITUATIONS AND PROBLEMS DURING STAPES SURGERY

Very Narrow Canal

The external auditory canal is rarely so narrow as to prevent the procedure through transcanal approach. In most of such cases, the exposure is improved by keeping an endaural (helicotragal) incision. In an extremely rare case one may require post-aural approach along with canalplasty.

Tympanic Membrane Perforation

A pinpoint perforation is approximated and supported by underlying gelfoam. Small tympanic membrane tear requires repair by underlay fibrous tissue (compressed in a graft press) harvested through post-aural stab incision (Fig. 7.28).

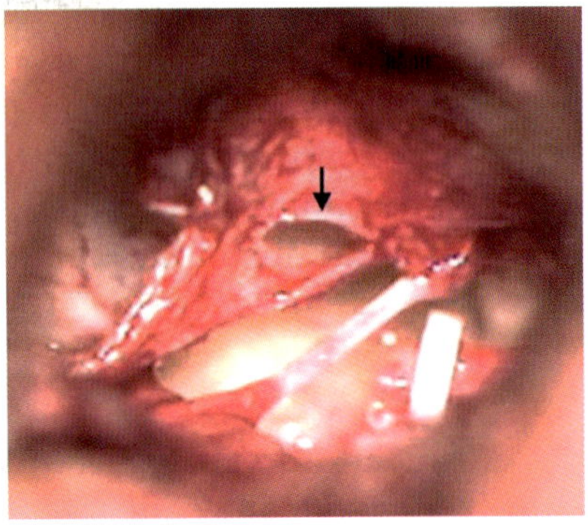

Fig. 7.28. Perforation (arrow) seen before replacing the tympanomeatal flap (left ear).

7

Atrophic Tympanic Membrane

Thin atrophic tympanic membrane may be repaired in the same stage by augmenting the drum with underlay fascia/soft tissue.

Incus Necrosis

The incus long process may be partially or completely necrosed with the lenticular process absent. The lenticular process of incus is necessary to support the piston from disarticulating (Fig. 7.29A). Due to necrosis of lenticular process, the loop of piston tends to dislocate from the incus when the patient is in sitting position (Fig. 7.29B). In partial necrosis of incus, the usual Teflon prosthesis is placed slightly above the level of necrosis and the necrosed part of incus is reinforced using a roll of soft tissue over it. If the loop of the piston is loosely fitting because of thin incus long process, some fibrous tissue is placed between the loop and the incus. Alternatively, we can use wire-teflon piston.

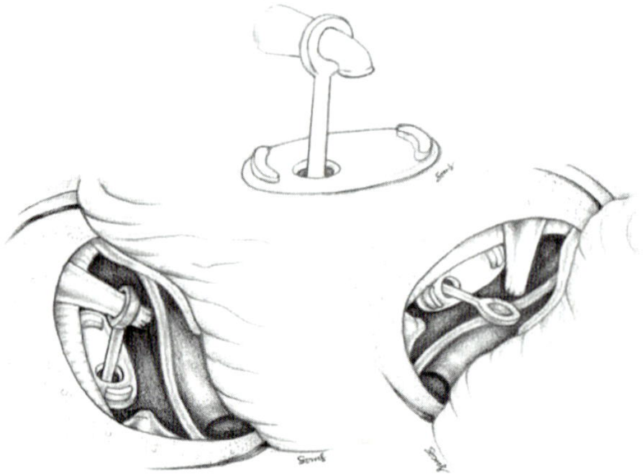

Figs 7.29A to C. (A) Diagrammatic picture showing position of Teflon piston with lenticular process intact. (B) Position of teflon piston with lenticular process necrosis when patient is in supine position. (C) Teflon piston tends to dislocate from the incus with lenticular process necrosis when the patient is in sitting/standing position.

Incus Dislocation

Incus may be dislocated during curetting of overhang, disarticulating I-S joint, removing the superstructure, or while placing/crimping the prosthesis. Usually the incus becomes hypermobile or loose but is not completely disarticulated from the malleus. In such cases, one may abandon the surgery and re-explore after six months when the loose incus is usually fixed to malleus.

If the incus is completely disarticulated or is still loose after re-exploration, it has to be removed and prosthesis (also known as incus replacement prosthesis) kept from malleus handle to the vestibule (malleovestibulopexy) using wire-teflon prosthesis or a special malleus teflon piston with the loop diameter of 1.2 mm and length of 6 to 6.5 mm (normal teflon piston that is used between incus and the vestibule has loop diameter of 0.9 mm). In this situation we feel it is better to make a groove in the malleus handle below the lateral process to stabilize the loop of the piston (Fig. 7.30). The tympanic membrane that is attached to the handle of malleus is elevated by sharp dissection using sickle knife. After supporting the elevated tympanic membrane and malleus handle with suction tip, a shallow groove is made below level of lateral process of malleus using a 0.6 diamond burr that is just enough to place the piston or wire loop. The loop of malleus Teflon piston is passed through the sulcus (Figs. 7.31, 7.32) and then inserted into the vestibule after measuring the length required. Fibrous tissue is placed between the loop of piston and tympanic membrane. This minimizes the chances of extrusion of the piston loop. All these steps of anchoring the piston should be done preferably before making the control fenestra in the stapes footplate to prevent any damage to the vestibule. Similarly malleovestibulopexy can be done using wire-teflon prosthesis.

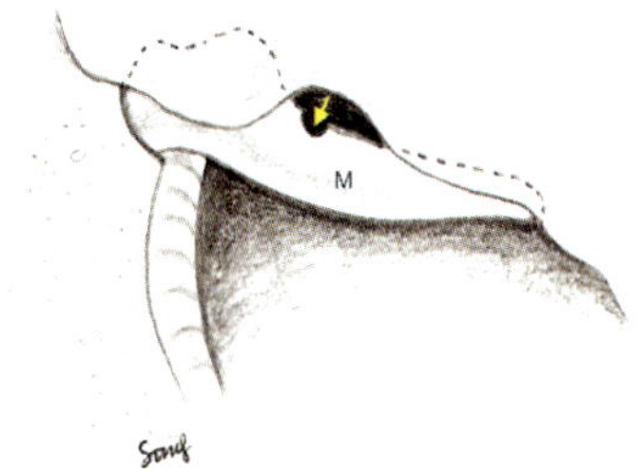

Fig. 7.30. Diagrammatic picture showing making a groove (arrow) over the handle of malleus (M) after elevating tympanic membrane over it (right ear).

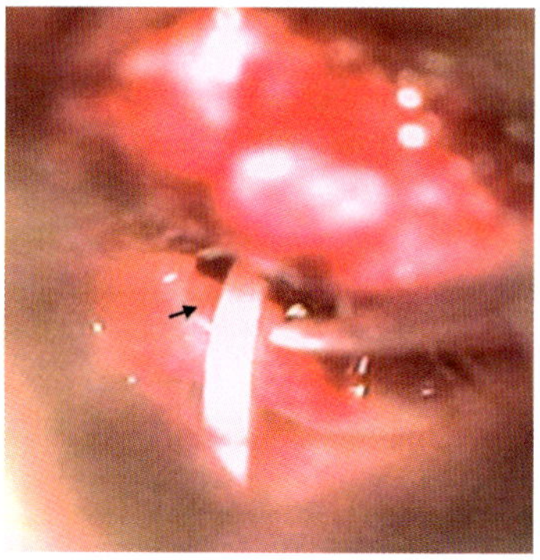

Fig. 7.31. Malleus Teflon piston placed in the sulcus (arrow) over the malleus (right ear).

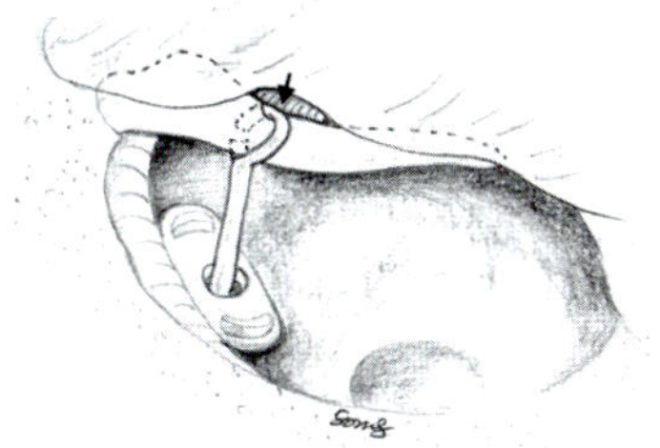

Fig. 7.32. Diagrammatic picture showing separating the loop of piston from the tympanic membrane using free fibrous tissue (arrow) (right ear).

Guidelines and Precautions

- Placing incus replacement prosthesis of ideal length and angulation from malleus handle to vestibule is difficult. In such a situation malleus is pushed more posteriorly by cutting the anterior malleolar ligament.
- In these cases where incus long process is necrosed and cannot be utilized for engaging the prosthesis, the remaining long process is removed using micro-scissors or malleus nipper. The incus should not be removed completely as it helps to stabilize the malleus and prevents its excessive movement that could be transferred to the vestibule.
- The closure of AB gap is poorer in incus replacement prosthesis (malleovestibulopexy) compared to normal Teflon loop prosthesis (stapedotomy).

Malleus/Incus Fixation

Associated malleolar fixation is seen in about 1% of our cases. The commonest site of fixation in our experience is between the anterior process of malleus and bony rim near anterior notch of Rivinus. It is usually due to ossification of anterior malleolar ligament. The diagnosis of associated malleus fixation is confirmed by palpating it after disarticulating the I-S joint. The exposure of the anterior notch of Rivinus and neck of malleus is improved adequately extending the tympanomeatal flap anteriorly. The anterior bony rim is drilled (using a 0.6 mm long diamond burr on contra-angled hand-piece) to widen the gap between the rim and the neck of malleus. The ossified anterior malleolar ligament is severed and the space thus created is filled with soft tissue/gelfoam. While drilling the anterior bony rim and cutting the anterior malleolar ligament one should be careful not to cut the chorda, which passes under it.

Associated attic fixation of malleus and/or incus is very rare. Incus is removed in such cases and head of malleus amputated followed by placement of incus replacement prosthesis from malleus handle to vestibule.

7

Too Short Incus Long Process

A regular Teflon piston can usually be used with a little slanting array. If the incus is too short or abnormally curved, wire-teflon prosthesis with bend is engaged into lower portion of long process of incus as discussed in necrosis of lenticular process of incus.

Obliterative Otosclerosis

Obliterative otosclerosis may range from thick footplate to obliteration of oval window. It is usually not possible to make a control fenestra in cases of obliterative otosclerosis. Therefore the stapes superstructure is removed and the footplate exposed. The footplate is drilled using 0.6 or 0.7 mm diamond burr on contra-angled handpiece using slow rotation drill (around 800 rpm) or skeeter drill. The drilling over the footplate should be performed using gentle strokes thinning it uniformly and the drilling is stopped intermittently to look for blue-lining of the footplate. By using the same burr we can make the fenestra. Alternative the fenestra is made after thinning of the footplate by using a straight pick and widened by using right angle different size picks.

Guidelines and Precautions

- Obliterative otosclerosis is more common in juvenile otosclerosis (otosclerosis in children less than 18 years of age) and in patients with long standing conductive hearing loss especially if initiated in childhood.
- Always warn the patient of hearing loud noise before initiating drilling over the footplate. Otherwise the patient may move suddenly out of fear. Make the footplate uniformly thin and avoid making a straight burr hole in the vestibule.

Overhanging/Dehiscent Facial Nerve

7

There could be variable degree of overhang of the facial canal over the oval window making its exposure narrow. The degree to which a facial nerve is overhanging the oval window niche may range from minimal overhang (that requires no alteration in the procedure) to almost complete coverage of niche (preventing any fenestration). The situation becomes all the more scary/worse if the overlying facial nerve is dehiscent. Occasionally the facial nerve is dehiscent only in its medial part close to footplate, while the lateral facial canal is covered with bone. The management of dehiscent overhanging facial nerve involves making the fenestra in the footplate after removal of superstructure, using routine perforators while retracting the facial nerve with suction cannula. Always avoid direct contact of perforators and hooks with the facial nerve. The direction of movement of hooks should be away from the nerve (towards posterior and inferior side) to avoid injury to unknown dehiscence of facial nerve medially. If there is significant bony overhang of facial canal (Fig. 7.33), the edge of the promontory is drilled till blue-lined to increase the working space (Fig. 7.34). If this does not permit enough exposure, the procedure is abandoned and a hearing aid is considered a safer option. Rarely, the facial nerve may run an abnormal course below the oval window niche over the promontory. Such a condition is mostly accompanied by congenital fixation of stapes and surgery is not continued unless a CT scan is available to rule out associated inner ear anomalies.

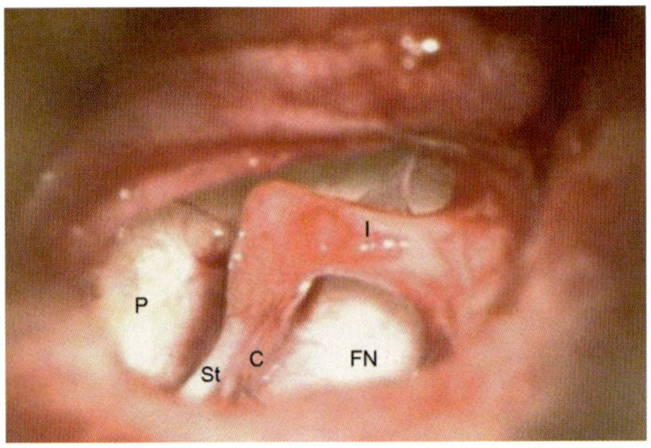

Fig. 7.33. Significant bony overhang of facial canal (FN) with very narrow oval window niche (left ear).

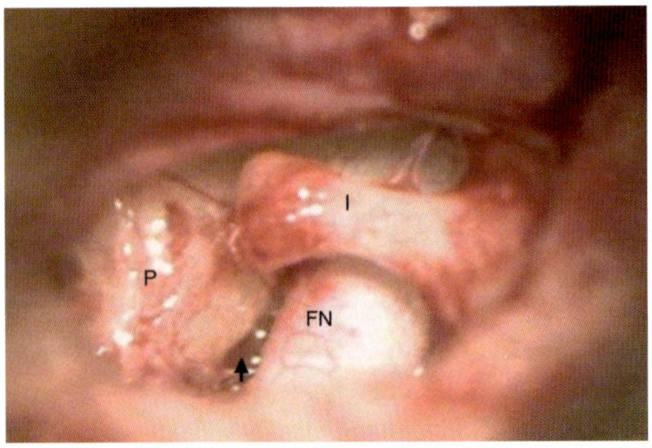

Fig. 7.34. Stapes superstructure is removed (left ear). Very narrow niche (arrow) with overhanging facial nerve (FN) and promontory (P) are seen.

Narrow Oval Window Niche

Narrow niche is a result of overhanging facial nerve/promontory or thick otosclerotic focus over the promontory or facial nerve or both (Fig. 7.35). The focus needs to be removed on either side of the niche to widen it by drilling with a small diamond burr. The management of narrow niche due to overhanging facial nerve is similar to that discussed above.

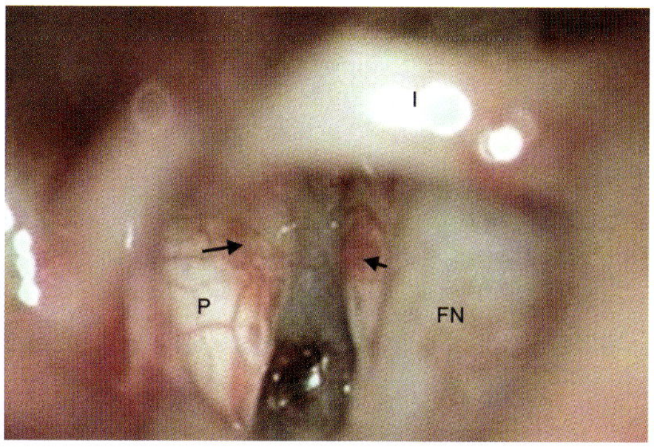

Fig. 7.35. Narrow oval window niche with focus on both the facial canal (FN) and promontory (P) (arrows) (left ear).

Fractured/Floating Footplate

Footplate may fracture or may become "floater" (footplate loses its attachment to annular ligament) (Fig. 7.36) during removal of superstructure or while making/widening a fenestra. Control fenestra of 0.3 mm made prior to removal of superstructure and widening of fenestra helps to provide access to "floating footplate". By passing a 0.2 mm right-angled hook through the fenestra usually the footplate could be retrieved. However, if the control fenestra was not made (due to anatomical reasons such as narrow niche, biscuit footplate or obliterative otosclerosis), the situation is more "critical". In such cases, drill the promontory close to oval window near its posteroinferior part to enable an angled hook to pass under the floater. If it is not possible to remove the fracture fragments/floater, it is better to avoid "fishing" or suctioning in the vestibule, cover the oval window with soft tissue seal and abandon the procedure.

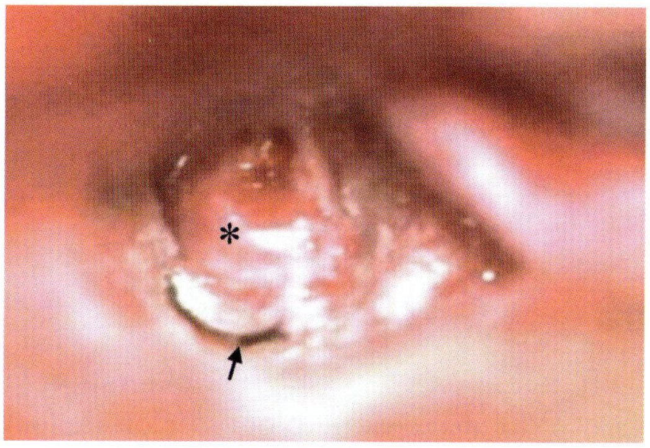

Fig. 7.36. Floating footplate (asterisk) (right ear). The posterior margin of the footplate is medialized into the vestibule (arrow).

Perilymph Gusher

Perilymph (actually cerebrospinal fluid) may start oozing out of the vestibule once the control fenestra is made in occasional cases. Such perilymph gusher may range from mild oozing (mild/moderate gusher) to profuse outflow (severe gusher). Mild to moderate gusher is usually due to abnormally wide cochlear aqueduct while severe gusher is a result of abnormal communication between the subarachnoid space and the perilymph through the defect in modiolus or cribriform plate of cochlea.

Mild gusher does not threaten the hearing outcome and there is no need for any alteration in routine stapes surgery steps. In moderate gusher, intravenous mannitol is started intraoperatively until oozing of cerebrospinal fluid slows down. Once the gusher has slowed, the fenestra is widened. A piece of fibrous tissue is taken from the postauricular sulcus and pressed with vein pressor and is placed over the fenestra after freshening the mucosa around the oval window. The piston is placed into fenestra over the compressed fibrous tissue and hooked to the incus and in addition more pieces of fibrous tissue bits are placed on footplate around the piston. Postoperatively oral acetazolamide and phenobarbitone are given to reduce the cerebrospinal fluid production.

Severe gusher is a potential cause for severe sensorineural hearing loss. A small control fenestra made at the onset of procedure helps to detect severe gusher at an early stage when it could be managed with little risk of sensorineural hearing loss. If detected at this stage, the fenestra is plugged with soft tissue and procedure abandoned. However, if the fenestra is wide or partial footplate has been removed already, it is very difficult to plug the fenestra with soft tissue due to excessive pressure of cerebrospinal fluid. Attempt is made to close the fenestra after allowing adequate cerebrospinal fluid outflow and starting intravenous mannitol. Fenestra is plugged with a larger soft tissue, which extends into the vestibule and is reinforced by prosthesis with/without intact superstructure. Hearing in such cases is usually difficult to preserve and contralateral stapes surgery is absolutely contraindicated.

Persistent Stapedial Artery

Persistent stapedial artery occurs due to persistent communication between middle meningeal artery and internal carotid artery that involutes in early embryonic life. It is a rare condition and we have not encountered stapedial artery covering majority of footplate in over 3500 cases of stapes surgery at our centre. If one does encounter such case, we believe it would be better to abandon the surgery. However, a smaller arterial twig crossing the footplate anteriorly is more frequent and can be usually controlled with small monopolar cautery (applied over a pick which touches the vessel) or laser at both ends followed by its resection. Removal of the mucosa over the footplate and applying adrenaline soaked gelfoam for a few minutes usually controls minimal bleeding.

Revision Stapes Surgery

Stapes surgery is an "all-or-none" phenomenon as regards to hearing improvement. Either the patient regains the conductive component of hearing loss almost completely or he loses all the hearing. However, a few of them have persistent conductive hearing loss or redevelop the hearing loss after initial improvement. Some of the patients develop persistent vertigo with progressive sensorineural hearing loss. These patients require revision surgery. Revision stapes surgery is more challenging and should be attempted by a surgeon with considerable prior experience in primary/revision surgery. Before attempting revision stapes surgery, one should be prepared to deal with all the difficult situations in a meticulous manner with precision.

Never blindly meddle with the neo-membrane over the vestibule and always ask for any vertigo to the patient while removing the previous prosthesis. It is easier to separate the non-wire prosthesis from neo-membrane compared to wire prosthesis, which is often embedded in the scar tissue. Wire prosthesis is fortunately rarely used nowadays. Always go through the previous surgical notes (if available) or contact the previous surgeon (if possible) to know the details and difficulties during previous surgery. If the previous surgeon is a novice and has not caused any further sensorineural hearing loss, the chances for hearing improvement are better. However, if an experienced surgeon has performed the surgery, the possibility is that the condition would not be correctable after re-exploration and hearing aid is always an option.

Common Findings Observed during Revision Stapes Surgery

Prosthesis Related

- Short prosthesis.
- Long prosthesis.
- Loose prosthesis.
- Dislocated prosthesis (prosthesis displaces out of fenestra).
- Disarticulated prosthesis (prosthesis displaces out of incus long process).
- Extrusion of prosthesis through tympanic membrane.

If the prosthesis is found to be short/long or loose and disarticulated from incus long process or dislocated from the healed fenestra, it needs to be removed and replaced with proper length. After dislocation of piston usually fenestra heals by fibrous tissue covering. While refenestration in the healed scar one should be careful about fibrous adhesion with underlying utricle or saccule in the vestibule. Extrusion of the prosthesis may occur if there is postoperative retraction of tympanic membrane that contacts the loop of prosthesis. It is usually caused due to inadequate approximation of the tympanomeatal flap after stapes surgery or due to over-enthusiastic removal of bony overhang.

Ossicular Chain Related

- Incus necrosis.
- Associated malleus/incus fixation.
- Incudomalleolar joint discontinuity.

The management of these conditions is same as discussed in primary surgery.

Oval Window Related

- Re-obliteration of fenestra: Re-obliteration of the fenestra due to re-growth of otosclerotic focus is a rare situation and occasionally occurs due to very narrow fenestra. We therefore prefer to make a fenestra of at least 0.8 mm (approx.).

- Prior fenestra not made due to narrow niche/obliterative otosclerosis: A novice may not be able to manage such difficult conditions and is one of the commonest causes of persistent hearing loss in our revision surgeries.
- Reparative granuloma: The etiopathogenesis of the condition is still unconfirmed and is mainly considered due to foreign body or infective inflammation. Diagnosis of this unfortunate condition is made by onset of vertigo, tinnitus and hearing loss within 2–4 weeks of surgery after initial improvement of hearing. It needs surgical exploration and removal off all the granulations around the vestibule (and sometimes within the vestibule) along with prosthesis and replacing the prosthesis with connective tissue seal. Though the incidence of this condition has drastically reduced in last decade (our incidence is 0.03%), it is one of the common causes for complete hearing loss postoperatively.
- Perilymph leak: Adequate tissue seal of the fenestra intraoperatively is a must to prevent perilymph leak. Absolute bed rest for 24 hours and no air travel or weight lifting within 15 days of surgery is essential to prevent early perilymph leak. We did not have virtually any case of early perilymph leak in any of our patients.
- Facial nerve injury is an uncommon complication of stapes surgery and occurs due to unwarranted manipulation around it while making fenestra using micro drill especially in over hanging facial nerve with facial bony canal dehiscence cases. While widening the fenestra with angled pick in case facial canal is dehiscent, the direction of the pick should be away from the exposed nerve. If there is extensive damage to the nerve cable nerve graft is required.

CONCLUSION

Otosclerosis is unique primary osseous lesion of the temporal bone of idiopathic aetiology with autosomal dominant genetic incomplete clinical penetrance. It is more common in South Indians than North Indians. Tuning fork, PTA and impedance audiometry are carried out along with radiology of temporal bone for diagnosis. Progressive conductive hearing loss from stapes fixation arises from the dual pathologic processes of otospongiosis and otosclerosis. Stapes surgery or fitting of suitaible hearing aid can rehabilitate the hearing. However, stapedectomy with insertion of piston and its crimping have better prospects for management of hearing loss.

SUGGESTED READING

1. Mahadevaiah A, Parikh B. Surgical techniques in chronic otitis media and otosclerosis: Text and Atlas, 2nd ed. CBS Publisher & Distributors Pvt. Ltd., New Delhi, 2011.
2. Merchant S N, McKenna MJ, Browning GG, Rea PA, Tange RA. Otosclerosis. *In:* Gleeson M, Browning GG, Burton MJ, Clarke R, Hibbert J, Lund VJ, Luxon LM, Watkinson JC, editors. Scott-Brown's Otorhinolaryngology, Head and Neck Surgery, Vol 3. Edward Arnold (Publisher) Ltd., London, 2008; 3453–85.
3. Stewart MG. Outcomes and patient-based hearing status in conductive hearing loss. *Laryngoscope*, 2001; 11: 1–21.
4. Shea JJ. Forty years of stapes surgery. *Am J Otol*, 1998; 19: 52–5.
5. Zarandy MM, Rutka J. Otosclerosis in diseases of the inner ear: A clinical, radiologic and pathologic atlas. Springer International edition, New York, 2010; 47–52.
6. Menger DJ, Tange RA. The aetiology of otosclerosis: A review of literature. *Clin Otolaryngol Allied Sci*, 2003; 28: 112–20.
7. Causse JB, Causse JR, Wiet RJ, Yoo TJ. Complication of stapedectomies. *Am J Otol*, 1983; 4: 279–80.
8. de Bruijn AJ, Tange RA, Dreschler WA. Comparison of stapes prosthesis: a retrospective analysis of individual audiometric results obtained after stapedectomy by implantation of a gold and a teflon piston. *Am J Otol*, 1999; 20: 573–80.
9. de Souza C, Glasslock III ME. Otoscerosis and stapedectomy: Diagnosis, management and complication. Thieme, New York, 2004.
10. Parker PM. Otosclerosis: Webster's timeline history 1893–2007. ICON Group International, California, 2009.
11. Sudhoff H, Hildmann H. Stapes surgery. *In:* Hildmann H, Sudhoff H. Middle ear surgery. Springer-Verlag, Berlin, Heidelberg, New York, 2006; 112–8.

CHAPTER 8

Management of Facial Nerve Palsy

Bachi T. Hathiram, Vicky S. Khattar

The facial nerve is a mixed nerve innervating the muscles of facial expression. The otorhino-laryngologists often face the challenge of treating a patient with paralysis of the facial nerve. Treating such a patient is, in the true sense, a challenge since both the patient and the relatives are in great distress with many questions on their minds and putting them at ease can be taxing at the least, to the best of specialists. Facial nerve paralysis often results in great psychological and emotional trauma not only to the patient, but also to the relatives and early management of this would result not only in improving the chances of recovery of the nerve but also in preventing great anguish to the patient.

The facial nerve has been the subject of awe and fascination amongst otologists since time immemorial with debates being conducted on whether or not to fear this magnificent structure which courses within the temporal bone. It is the seventh cranial nerve and is essentially a motor nerve with a sensory and secretomotor branches given out during its course through the middle ear; hence, the term 'mixed' nerve when used for the facial nerve is not incorrect. Over time, several exhaustive studies have been carried out to study the anatomy and functions of this nerve. As the nerve courses through the bony fallopian canal in its tortuous intratemporal course, it is maximally prone to trauma due to its precarious position.

We, as otologists, deal only with the lower motor neuron type of facial palsy. There are more than 40 causes of facial palsy enumerated in literature, but the commonly seen causes in practice are dealt with in this article and their management protocols discussed with the expected prognosis.

Anatomical considerations

The facial nerve or the seventh cranial nerve is a mixed nerve. It is the nerve of the second branchial arch. It exits the brain at the cerebello-pontine angle along with the eighth cranial nerve to run in the internal acoustic canal (IAC). Its pathway can be divided into: the supranuclear and the infranuclear pathway. It is this infranuclear pathway which is of interest to us otologists, since we deal with the nerve in this portion of its course.

The course of the facial nerve has been divided by anatomists into: Intracranial, Intratemporal and Extratemporal.

On exiting at the lower border of the pons, the facial nerve along with the vestibulocochlear nerve enters the internal acoustic canal at the porus (medial opening of the IAC). The nerve comprises of a motor root and a sensory root (nervus intermedius/nerve of Wrisberg); the motor root caries fibres to the muscles of the second branchial arch (muscles of facial expression, stylohyoid, posterior belly of the digastric, and the postauricular muscles), whereas the sensory root comprises of:

- the special visceral afferent carrying taste to the anterior 2/3rd of the tongue via the chorda tympani,

- the special visceral efferent to the facial muscles, and
- the general visceral efferent to the salivary glands via the petrosal nerves.

On entering the IAC, the facial nerve and the nervus intermedius unite to form a common trunk. The facial nerve leaves the IAC at its lateral end (fundus) to run for a short distance (labyrinthine segment) before entering the temporal bone after its first genu. It is in the labyrinthine segment that it gives its first division, the greater superficial petrosal nerve. It then enters the temporal bone bending at an acute angle (the first genu) from where it starts its tympanic segment.

Within the temporal bone, it runs through a narrow bony canal (Fallopian canal) first in its tympanic/horizontal segment and then, after the second genu in its mastoid/vertical segment. It exits the temporal bone through the stylomastoid foramen. Just prior to entering the stylomastoid foramen, the nerve deviates from its vertical course to take a distinct obtuse-angled turn forward; this is termed as the 'third genu' of the facial nerve (Grewal and Hathiram, 2006).

After its exit from the stylomastoid foramen, the nerve enters its extra-temporal course, turning anteriorly in the substance of the parotid gland and dividing into two main branches; the temporofacial which is superior and the cervicofacial which is inferior. From these two main branches, a plexiform arrangement of nerves arise (pes anserinus/parotid plexus) to innervate the muscles of facial expression.

The various branches of the facial nerve include:

1. The greater superficial petrosal nerve, which is the first branch from its labyrinthine segment.
2. Nerve to the stapedius muscle.
3. The chorda tympani nerve.
4. A small sensory branch to the skin of the posterior aspect of the external auditory canal.

Branches 2, 3 and 4 arise from the vertical/mastoid segment of the nerve.

5. The Ansa Haller (inconstant).
6. The posterior auricular branch.
7. The stylohyoid branch.
8. Branch to the posterior belly of the digastric.
9. The lingual branch which replaces the Ansa Haller.

Branches 5, 6, 7, 8 and 9 arise in the neck after the nerve exits the stylomastoid foramen.

10. Temporal branches.
11. Zygomatic branches.
12. Buccal branches.
13. Marginal mandibular branch.
14. Cervical branch.

Branches 10, 11, 12, 13, and 14 form the parotid plexus within the substance of the parotid gland.

Surgical considerations

There are various anatomical landmarks that help to identify this important structure intra-operatively:

- Conley's tragal pointer: the nerve lies medial to and about 1 cm inferior to the tragal cartilage. However, one has to keep in mind that this being a soft-tissue landmark, it tends to get distorted in parotid gland tumours/swellings.
- The tympanomastoid suture: the nerve lies just deep to this.
- The styloid process: the nerve lies lateral to this.
- The nerve can be traced backwards from any one of its terminal branches towards the main trunk.
- The cog is a landmark for the first genu of the nerve in the middle ear.
- The processus cochleariformis lies inferior to the tympanic segment of the nerve.
- The oval window is a landmark for the second genu.
- The lateral semicircular canal lies postero-superior to the second genu – this is a constant and reliable landmark.
- The pyramidal eminence is another important landmark as the nerve turns sharply down-wards at the second genu. The nerve lies posterolateral to this process.
- The chorda tympani and the digastric ridge are useful landmarks for the nerve.

However, it is important to remember that in most cases operated for facial palsy (CSOM, trauma, tumour, etc), the anatomical landmarks are destroyed. Also, there may be anatomical variations which should be kept in mind during surgery on this vital structure.

Causes of facial nerve palsy

The various causes of paralysis of the facial nerve can be classified as Congenital, Traumatic (accidental or iatrogenic), Infective/Inflammatory, Neoplastic and Miscellaneous (including Idiopathic). The common causes seen in clinical practice include; Idiopathic (Bell's) palsy, Traumatic palsy (accidental as well as iatrogenic trauma), Palsy due to ear infection (unsafe chronic suppurative otitis media, acute suppurative otitis media, etc.) and rarely tumours (facial nerve neuroma or vestibular schwannoma). Each of these with their treatment protocols will be subsequently described in this article.

IDIOPATHIC FACIAL NERVE PALSY/BELL'S PALSY

This is the commonest type of facial nerve paralysis and hence, the most frequently encountered in clinical practice. It is characteristically described as the acute, idiopathic lower motor neuron paralysis of the seventh cranial nerve which is unilateral, non-progressive, self-limiting, non-life-threatening and spontaneously remitting by 4–6 months and always by one year. It was described by Sir Charles Bell in 1829 and hence was termed as 'Bell's Palsy'. The diagnosis of this condition is only by exclusion of the other causes of facial palsy.

Patients presenting with Bell's palsy, more often than not, give a history of exposure to a cold draught of wind or washing the face with cold water following which the paralysis of the face was noticed which is usually associated with postauricular pain radiating to the upper neck. Characteristically, the palsy is unilateral, sudden in onset with a sensation of numbness on the affected side of the face. At times, there may be history of viral upper respiratory tract infection at the time of palsy or preceding it by 7–10 days. On otoscopic examination, the tympanic membrane is normal and the chorda tympani nerve may appear red and inflamed if seen within ten days of onset of palsy. Pure tone audiometry reveals hearing sensitivity within normal limits but, testing of the acoustic reflex will reveal an absent stapedial reflex in 90% of patients. An MRI of the facial nerve is mandatory prior to labelling any palsy of the facial nerve as Bell's.

The management of this condition is yet controversial with some otologists in favour of surgical decompression whereas others strongly opposing any surgical intervention.

Treatment protocols and results

Once the diagnosis of Bell's palsy is confirmed, the patient is started on medical therapy without delay. The medical therapy comprises of steroids (Prednisolone 1 mg/kg/day in divided doses) given orally and tapered over three weeks, antiviral agent Acyclovir (200 mg five times a day for ten days), antibiotics, vasodilators (Xanthinol nicotinate) orally, vitamins B_1, B_6 and B_{12}, Ascorbic acid, and eye-care which includes artificial tears, dark glasses in the day and eye-shield with an antibiotic eye-cream at night to prevent corneal damage. Also, the role of physiotherapy, both active and passive, cannot be stressed enough.

Prognostic tests are performed every alternate week to evaluate recovery of nerve function and these include; Nerve Excitability Test, Electromyography and the acoustic reflex. Recovery of the stapedial reflex is considered to be the first sign to signal the return of nerve activity.

Medical management is the first line of treatment in this condition and forms the mainstay of treatment. Majority of the patients show evidence of recovery by the 3rd–4th week of onset of palsy with medical management and complete recovery occurs by the 3rd–6th month. However, poor prognosis has been related to complete paralysis at onset or incomplete paralysis with late onset of recovery, old age, dry eye, absent taste sensation, absent stapedius reflex and postauricular pain (Peitersen, 2002).

Whether or not a patient with Bell's palsy should be treated surgically, and if so, when this decision should be taken is still a topic of great debate. The Marsh and Coker criteria (1991) for surgical decompression of the nerve are as follows:

- Complete denervation.
- Paralysis for more than 4–6 weeks.
- Incomplete return of function in 60 days.
- Recurrent facial palsy.
- Nerve excitability test shows a difference of 3.5 mA on both the sides.

If there are no signs of recovery of function of the nerve within 3–6 weeks of onset of the palsy, as seen by serial documentation of the acoustic reflex and nerve excitability test as well as clinical examination, the facial nerve may be surgically decompressed along its entire course from its labyrinthine segment to its exit from the stylomastoid foramen. This is done keeping in mind the pathophysiology of this condition which shows 'skip lesions'. Also, since the narrowest portion of the Fallopian canal is at the labyrinthine segment, it is advised to decompress the nerve at the fundus, the best approach to which would be via a 'middle cranial fossa approach'. Literature also mentions a 'trans-zygomatic' approach to the labyrinthine segment for the same indication.

Decompression needs to be carried out earlier if there is evidence of worsening of function after a prolonged delay, e.g., paresis progressing to palsy. In such a case, other causes of facial palsy should be looked for and the diagnosis of Bell's, reconsidered. However, beyond two years after the onset of facial palsy, the muscles undergo disuse atrophy and also the nerve fails to regenerate. Hence, we are of the opinion that after two years of onset of palsy, other methods may be employed to regain facial symmetry as decompression of the nerve would be futile.

Our experience

In our series of 240 cases of Bell's palsy, surgical decompression was required only in 10 patients: 9 of whom failed to improve within 12 weeks of starting medical management and 1 patient worsened despite starting medical management. All the other patients showed evidence of recovery clinically within 6–8 weeks of starting medical management. However, complete recovery was seen in 228 patients with 2 patients who came to us after 14–21 days of onset of palsy showing only partial recovery at the end of 6 months.

Hence, there is a definite relationship between time of onset of palsy and time of starting medical management with both being directly proportional to each other. Recovery is best seen in those cases where medical management was started within 10-14 days of onset of palsy. The prognosis is guarded for patients who come after 10–14 days have elapsed.

POST-TRAUMATIC FACIAL NERVE PARALYSIS

In today's age of technology coupled with speed, vehicular accidents and polytrauma with head injury are on the rise. Temporal bone fractures are extremely common with head injuries. In fact trauma is the second most common cause of paralysis of the facial nerve after idiopathic palsy. The risk of injury to the nerve is greatly increased in transverse fractures of the temporal bone, followed by comminuted fractures and then, longitudinal fractures.

The patient is usually admitted in the trauma ward for head injury and presents with a variety of symptoms such as hearing loss, facial paralysis, vertigo, nystagmus and may be even a CSF leak. Occasionally, the skin over the mastoid may be bluish in colour (Battle's sign).

Kettel (1950) believed that an immediate-onset facial paralysis following trauma should be explored as soon as the patient's condition permits. The facial palsy may be due to various reasons; an incomplete or complete transection of the nerve, bony fragments compressing the nerve, oedema of the nerve due to injury, or compression due to the nerve sheath being caught in the fracture fragments.

A high resolution CT scan of the temporal bone with brain cuts is recommended strongly to rule out intracranial lesions in addition to enabling us to pinpoint the exact site of trauma to the nerve (Figs. 8.1, 8.2).

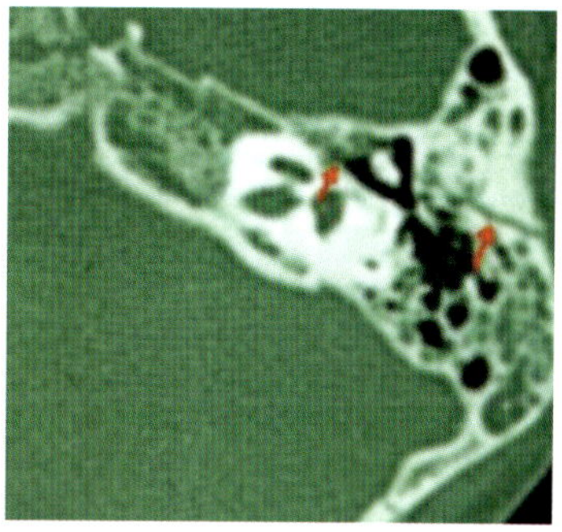

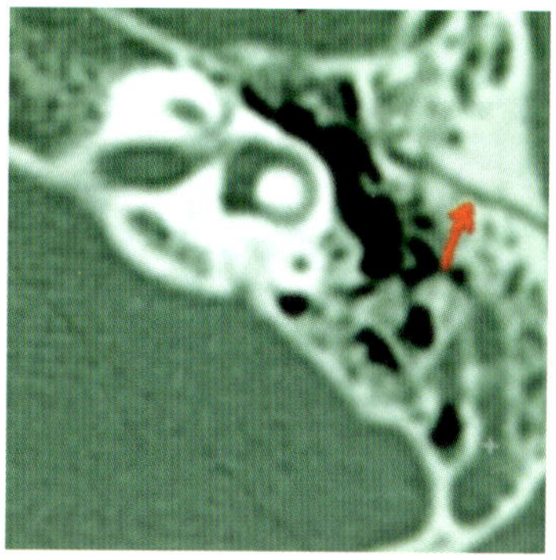

Figs. 8.1, 8.2. Axial view of high resolution CT scan of the temporal bone showing a longitudinal fracture of the temporal bone causing facial palsy. Note the line of fracture going towards the first genu and tympanic segment of the facial nerve. The longitudinal fractures are less likely to cause facial nerve palsy as compared to their transverse fracture counterparts.

As soon as the general condition of the patient permits, preferably within 72 hours after the injury, the nerve needs to be decompressed and the fracture fragments removed. According to McCabe (1972), if 72 hours after injury have passed, the optimum time for surgery to decompress the nerve is on the 21st day as the nerve cell body is maximally capable of passing the axoplasmic filaments across the neuronal gap. The nerve is decompressed in its entire length after evacuating the haematoma within the middle ear cleft (Figs. 8.3 A & B). A posterior tympanotomy is preferred if the posterior canal wall is intact (Fig. 8.4) or if hearing is good. Any associated damage to the other structures in the ear such as the ossicular chain, labyrinth, oval/round windows or a CSF leak is treated at the same time. Recovery is good if the decompression is performed early (Figs. 8.5 to 8.10).

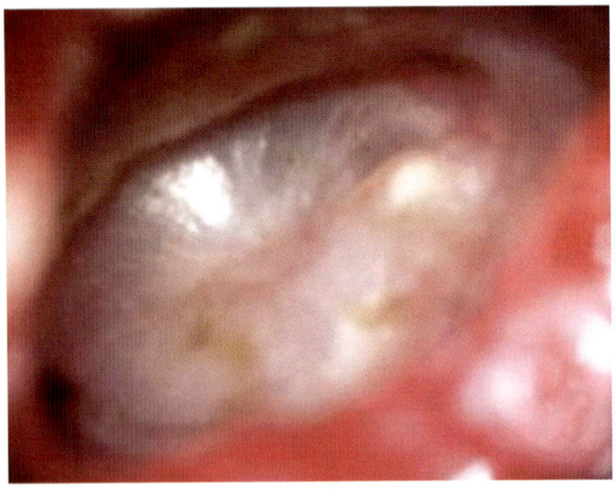

Fig. 8.3A. Intraoperative microscopic view showing a haemotympanum, which often accompanies patients with head trauma and facial nerve weakness.

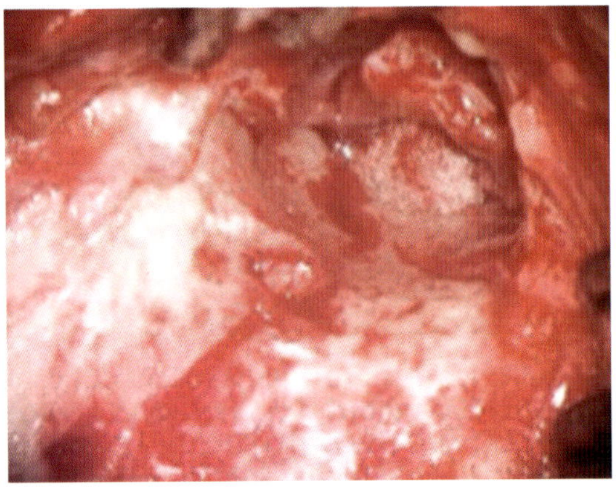

Fig. 8.3B. Intraoperative microscopic view showing the longitudinal temporal bone fracture line running across the mastoid cortex towards the external auditiory canal.

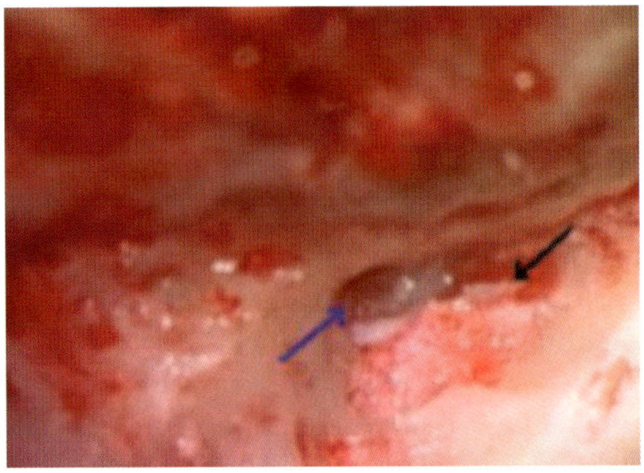

Fig. 8.4. Intraoperative microscopic view of a patient with traumatic facial nerve paresis. A posterior tympanotomy has been performed (blue arrow) and the fractured spicule of bone is seen compressing the facial nerve in the mastoid segment (black arrow).

A cause for controversy is 'delayed' facial palsy occurring in a patient with head injury. We prefer to 'wait and watch' in this group of patients and treat them with the medical line of management which includes systemic steroids in addition to antibiotics and physiotherapy. Most of these show evidence of recovery within 3 weeks and may progress to near-complete recovery of function.

In cases of facial paralysis of iatrogenic aetiology such as seen following ear surgery, it is best to explore the ear and decompress/repair the injured nerve at the earliest to prevent irreversible damage. Only in cases where the surgeon is sure to have identified the nerve and not have injured it during ear surgery, exploration is deferred.

Treatment protocols and results

Facial nerve palsy following trauma (accidental or iatrogenic) needs to be treated as an emergency. Immediate palsy after the trauma merits surgical management along with the medical line of management. There is no role for only medical management in such cases.

A high resolution CT scan of the temporal bone is mandatory prior to planning surgery as it not only helps in identifying the exact site of trauma but also serves as a 'road-map' for the ear exploration.

The facial nerve is traced along its course in the temporal bone and the site of trauma, identified. The nerve is then decompressed proximal and distal to the site of injury after taking care to gently remove all bone fragments around the injured nerve. At times, there may be a fracture fragment impinging

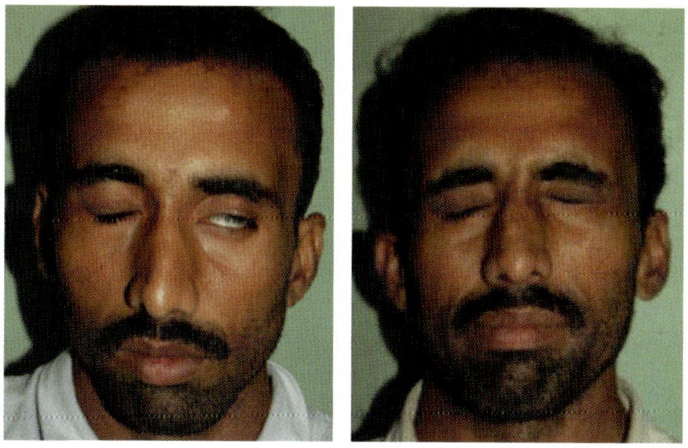

Figs. 8.5, 8.6. Pre- and postoperative clinical photographs showing return of complete closure of the eye after six weeks of facial nerve decompression.

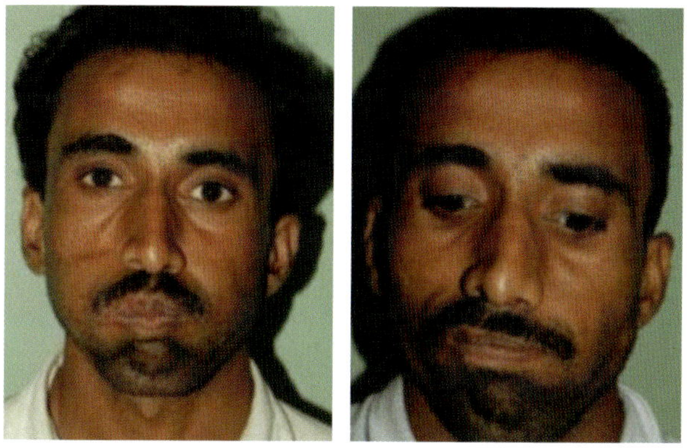

Figs. 8.7, 8.8. Pre- and postoperative clinical photographs showing return of cheek blowing function after six weeks of facial nerve decompression.

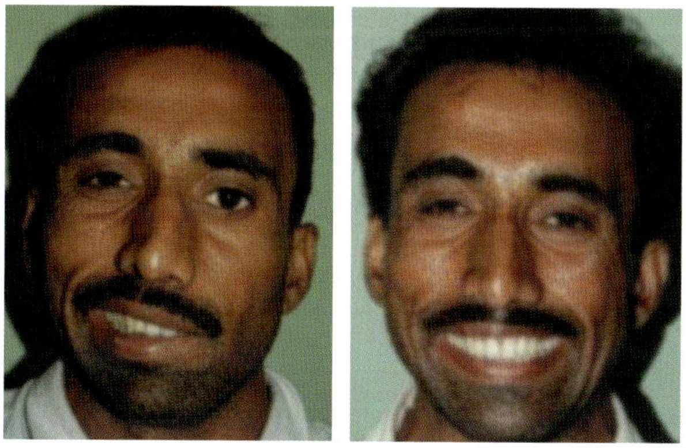

Figs. 8.9, 8.10. Pre- and postoperative clinical photographs showing return of a symmetrical smile after six weeks of facial nerve decompression.

on the nerve, and this should be gently removed taking care not to cause further damage. Repair of the nerve following decompression depends upon the type and extent of injury that has occurred. If there is injury with a sharp instrument such a sickle knife, the cut ends are approximated if the cut is partial and kept in position with a connective tissue graft; if the nerve is transected, the cut ends are kept together with 8-0 Vicryl and this is further augmented with a connective tissue graft. In cases of injury with the burr, the nerve gets sheared-off from its canal, and the cut ends need to be traced. If a short segment of the nerve is missing, re-routing and anastomosis is performed taking care that the suture line is tension-free. If this is not possible, then nerve grafting is performed using the Greater auricular or Sural nerve grafts depending on the length of nerve graft required.

Our experience

Being a tertiary care centre in the heart of the city, we have a well-equipped trauma ward with cases coming from the city as well as those referred from peripheral hospitals. In our series of 186 cases of facial nerve paralysis following trauma, 142 were following accidental trauma and 44 were due to iatrogenic trauma referred to us by the primary surgeon.

Of the 142 patients who came to us with accidental trauma and were operated, 138 showed improvement of the palsy following surgery. 4 patients were referred to us only after 3 weeks of palsy, as they were in a comatose state when admitted and the palsy was noticed only when the general condition improved. These 4 patients, despite decompression, did not show any signs of recovery at the end of 6 months. Of the 138 who showed evidence of recovery following surgery, only 76 recovered completely (Figs. 8.5–8.10) whereas the other 62 showed various grades of recovery from House-Brackman II-IV when assessed at the end of 6 months.

Of the 44 cases who were referred to us following iatrogenic trauma, 36 showed signs of recovery at the end of 4–6 weeks following decompression, probably because these were referred to us within 2–4 days of first surgery. These showed grades of recovery ranging from House-Brackman I-II at the end of 6–9 months following decompresson. Four patients who had complete transection of the nerve, with loss of segment (Fig. 8.11), needed a nerve graft and of these, 2 showed recovery (House-Brackman III) at the end of 12–15 months following surgery, 1 failed to recover whereas, 1 was lost to follow-up. There were 4 patients who came to us after 3–6 months following the first surgery and despite

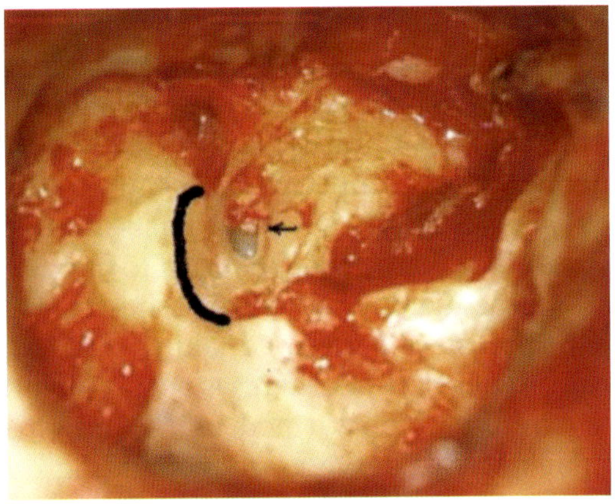

Fig. 8.11. Intraoperative microscopic view (patient with iatrogenic facial nerve palsy) showing a complete loss of a full thickness segment of the right facial nerve caused by a cutting burr (black line) in the region of the second genu of the facial nerve. Note the damage caused to the stapes footplate (arrow).

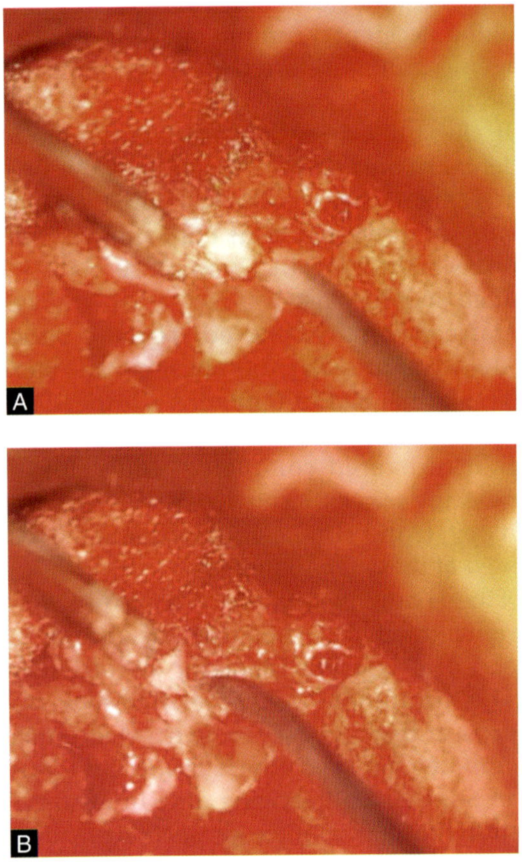

Figs. 8.12A & B. Intraoperative microscopic view of a patient with 'iatrogenic facial nerve paresis' showing a piece of cartilage used for ossicular reconstruction compressing the tympanic segment of the facial nerve (Fig. 8.12A) and subsequently being removed (Fig. 8.12B).

completely decompressing the nerve surgically 2 had cartilage embedded into the nerve (Figs. 8.12 A & B), 1 had a refashioned ossicles compressing the nerve and 1 had partial transaction of the nerve with granuloma formation) they failed to show evidence of recovery at the end of 9 months following decompression.

As is true in any case of injury to any nerve, we believe that the earlier we decompress the injured facial nerve (Fig. 8.13), better are the chances of recovery of function. Also, the prognosis to a great extent depends on the type and extent of injury to the nerve. A neuropraxia recovers faster and completely as compared to a transaction, which will show better recovery than a nerve which requires to be grafted.

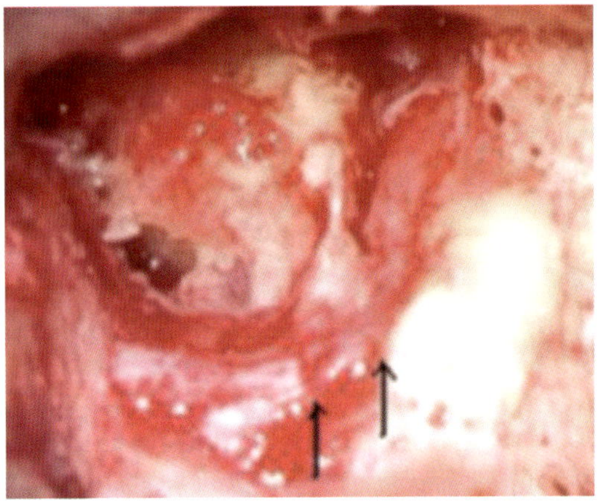

Fig. 8.13. Intraoperative miscoscopic view of another patient with blunt trauma to the left facial nerve in the region of the second genu (black arrows) following ossiculoplasty which had been performed in close proximity to a dehiscent facial nerve. The nerve should be decompressed proximal and distal to the site of neuropraxia for optimal recovery.

FACIAL PALSY DUE TO EAR INFECTIONS

The facial nerve follows a long and tortuous course in a bony canal within the temporal bone and hence, it is very susceptible to injury due to various infections of the ear. Of all cases of ear infections, only 1–2% show evidence of facial nerve palsy (Tonndorf, 1924; Lund, 1929; and Kettel, 1943). Amongst ear infections causing facial palsy the commonest cause in our country is unsafe chronic suppurative otitis media (CSOM) with cholesteatoma or granulations or an aural polyp. This occurs due to the bone-eroding property of the disease process (Fig. 8.14). However, if the bony canal is dehiscent, even safe CSOM or acute suppurative otitis media may cause facial palsy. Tuberculous otitis media usually presents with a complication such as facial palsy, labyrinthitis, labyrinthine fistula, meningitis or intracranial abscess (Grewal and Hathiram, 1999). Facial palsy tends to occur early in tuberculous otitis media due to bone erosion by granulation tissue and formation of bony sequestra.

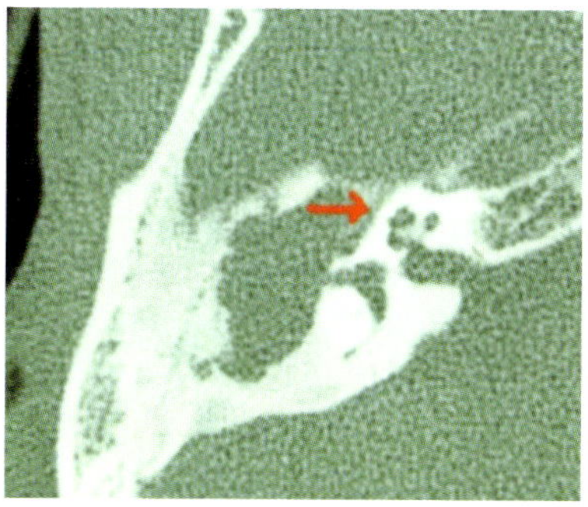

Fig. 8.14. Axial view of a high resolution CT scan of the temporal bone showing erosion of the lateral wall of the tympanic segment of the facial nerve in a patient with chronic suppurative otitis media.

Treatment protocols and results

The management of the facial palsy in such cases would be surgical with complete clearance of the disease in the middle ear cleft and decompression of the injured nerve. A high resolution CT scan of the temporal bone is mandatory prior to surgery since it helps to determine the extent of damage caused by the pathology. However, most anatomical landmarks are destroyed by the disease and hence, the surgery should be performed by a skilled surgeon to prevent residual disease or inadvertent damage to the nerve. Also, the pure tone audiogram may detect a sensorineural hearing loss in the same ear since the disease may have also eroded the bone of the lateral semicircular canal. The results of meticulous surgery with complete clearance of the disease process and decompression of the nerve are gratifying (Figs. 8.15, 8.16). However, the nerve sheath is never slit as the cause of the palsy is infection and the tough sheath acts as a barrier to this preventing further nerve damage by the toxins. Surgery is undertaken at the earliest to prevent irreversible damage to the nerve, however, in the event of life-threatening intracranial complications being present, treatment of these takes a precedence over a mastoidectomy.

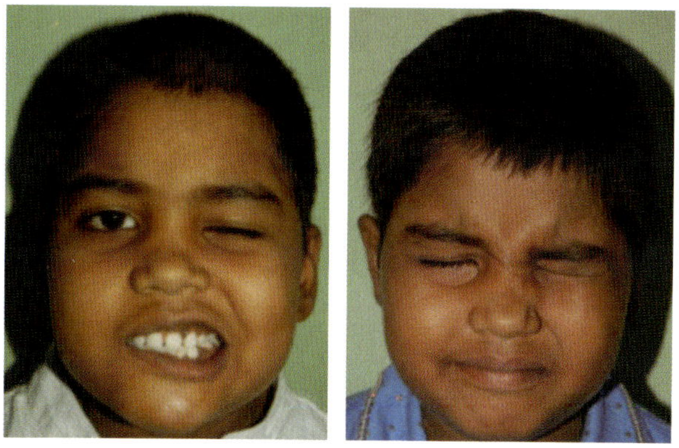

Figs. 8.15, 8.16. Pre- and postoperative clinical photographs showing return of complete facial nerve function after four weeks of facial nerve decompression performed for a patient with chronic suppurative otitis media with cholesteatoma and facial palsy.

Our experience

In our series of 226 patients presenting with facial palsy secondary to unsafe CSOM, all patients were subjected to a canal-wall-down tympanomastoidectomy after a pure tone audiogram and HRCT of the temporal bone, at the earliest. Of these, 189 had cholesteatoma, 29 had granulations and 8 had aural polyp. Of the patients with granulations, 13 patients showed evidence of tuberculosis on histopathology and culture. Of the 8 aural polyps, 2 were malignant whereas 6 were benign on histopathological examination. Recovery of facial nerve function (HouseBrackman grades I-III) was seen in 215 patients. All patients with cholesteatoma showed recovery of facial nerve function, in fact some showed early evidence of recovery even on the 5–7th post-operative day. Of the 11 patients who failed to improve by the 6th month following surgery, 2 had malignancy of the middle ear cleft, 4 were diagnosed as tuberculous otitis media (they failed to improve even after starting anti tuberculous drugs), and 5 were patients who had non-specific granulation tissue on histopathology.

Hence, in our experience, recovery of facial nerve function is good if there is cholesteatoma as compared to the presence of granulation tissue in the middle ear cleft (Figs. 8.17, 8.18).

CONCLUSION

Facial paralysis is a devastating condition with numerous implications. Its etiology is varied and the recent advances in imaging, electrodiagnostic testing, as well as microsurgery have provided great

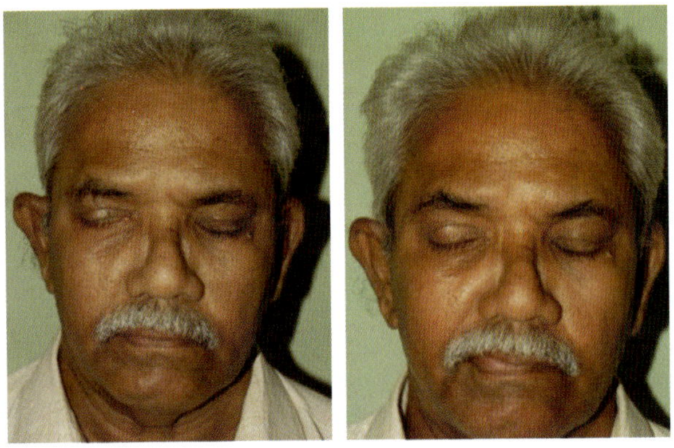

Figs. 8.17, 8.18. Pre- and postoperative clinical photographs showing return of complete closure of the eye after two weeks of facial nerve decompression. Many times in patients with cholesteatoma there is only a paresis of the nerve in the early stages of affliction, and the surgical results of decompression are best if the facial weakness is diagnosed and treated in these 'early' stages, prior to the onset of complete facial palsy.

insight into the pathophysiology, diagnosis, treatment, and rehabilitation of the injured facial nerve.

The management of facial paralysis is one of the most complex areas of reconstructive surgery. The otologist needs a thorough understanding of the surgical techniques available to treat this condition since facial palsy results in a variety of functional and cosmetic deficits in addition to emotional scarring.

ACKNOWLEDGEMENT

We are grateful to our Dean, Dr. Ravi Rananavare for granting permission to publish this article.

SUGGESTED READING

1. Grewal DS and Hathiram BT. Anatomy of the facial nerve *In:* Atlas of Surgery of the Facial Nerve. Jaypee, 2006; p. 3.
2. Peitersen E. Bell's Palsy: The spontaneous course of 2,500 peripheral facial nerve palsies of different etiologies. *Acta Otolaryngol,* 2002; 549: 4–30
3. Marsch MJ, Coker NJ. Surgical Decompression of Idiopathic facial palsy. *Otolaryngol Clin North Am,* 1991; 24: 675–90.
4. Kettel K. Peripheral facial palsy in fractures of the temporal bone. *Arch Otolaryngol,* 1950; 57: 25.
5. McCabe BF. Injuries to the facial nerve. *Laryngoscope,* 1972; 82: 1891–6.
6. Tonndorf W. Facialiskrampfe. Z Hals-usw Hk 1924; 8: 98.
7. Lund R. Die Facialisparese bei den suppurativen Mittelohrleiden mit besonderem hinblick auf ihre Bedeutung als Operationsindikation. Z Hals-usw Hk 1929; 23: 296.
8. Kettel K. Facial palsy of otitic origin. *Arch Otolaryngol,* 1943; 37: 303–348.
9. Grewal DS, Hathiram BT. 'Tuberculous Otitis Media' in ENT Disorders in a Tropical Environment. 2nd ed. Published by MERF publications edited by Prof. S. Kameswaran and Prof. Mohan Kameswaran, Chennai, India. 1999; pp 65–77.

CHAPTER 9

Traumatic Facial Nerve Palsy

K.P. Morwani, Rahul Agrawal

In this chapter we are going to discuss the management of traumatic facial nerve palsy as managed by the senior author and his associates. As an ENT surgeon we should have good knowledge of facial nerve and every teaching institute should have one ENT surgeon dedicated for facial nerve management.

Traumatic facial nerve palsy can be due to:

1. Road traffic accident
2. Otological and cerebellopontine angle surgery
3. Submandibular and temporomandibular joint surgery
4. Parotid surgery.

Management and prognosis of facial nerve paralysis depends upon grading of facial nerve status at the time of trauma and time span between trauma and presentation. At times treatment may differ depending upon other associated symptoms like decreased hearing, giddiness, etc.

Grading of facial nerve at the time of presentation is most important. I have been referred hundreds of facial nerve trauma cases by ENT colleagues. In more than 90% of cases it was labelled as facial nerve paresis or palsy. Only in about 10% of cases it was properly graded. This is in spite of literature emphasizing the importance of grading. I take this opportunity to reemphasize the importance of House-Brackmann grading.

House-Brackmann nerve grading

Grade 1 Normal facial function

Grade 2 Mild dysfunction which includes slight weakness and synkinesis on close inspection; moderate to good movement of forehead muscles; complete closure of eye with minimal effort, slight asymmetry of mouth, but normal symmetry and tone at rest

Grade 3 Moderate dysfunction which has gross but not obvious disfiguring between two sides, noticeable but not severe synkinesis, contracture and/or hemifacial spasm, however, at rest normal symmetry and tone is maintained; movement of forehead slight to moderate, complete closure of eye with effort and slight weakness of mouth even with maximum effort

Grade 4 Moderately severe dysfunction, i.e., facial weakness or asymmetry, but at rest normal symmetry and tone; no movement of forehead, incomplete eye closure and mouth asymmetry with maximum effort

Grade 5 Severe dysfunction having only barely perceptible motion and asymmetry at rest; no forehead movement, incomplete eye closure and slight movement of mouth

Grade 6 Complete paralysis with no movement

As clinician we may differ in grading by one grade either worse or better. Eventually there will be no gross difference if we use it regularly. In my practice of four decades, I have noticed that a patient may not have a uniform grade in whole of his face. Hence face has been subdivided into:

1. Forehead
2. Eye closure
3. Nasolabial fold
4. Angle of mouth

After sacrificing the facial nerve in various skull base procedures the immediate face is most often grade IV or V and it takes 40 to 72 hours for FN weakness to become grade VI. Eye closure with mastoid bandage may be as good as grade III or IV. This is important finding not emphasized in literature. Hence, immediate post-traumatic grade IV or V should be assessed more critically and reassessed at the end of 72 hours before deciding further management.

IATROGENIC FACIAL NERVE PARALYSIS

In post-otological procedures, assessment should be done after 6 to 8 hours, time taken by local infiltration to abate. In post-otological surgery cases referred to us, operating surgeon most often denies that he was anywhere near facial nerve during the surgery. Secondly, he grades the weakness lesser to actually what it is. Moreover, the operating surgeon wants to wait for a longer time hoping against hope that the weakness given by him will improve. The medicolegal problems are going to increase in our country due to literacy rate, internet and adverse reporting and provocation by other physicians. Hence, one has to be very cautious in these cases.

Dictum to be followed in post-otological procedure is to act fast. If injury to facial nerve is recognized intraoperatively then it should be repaired there and then. On the other hand if it is not recognized intraoperatively or the surgeon is not trained enough to deal with facial nerve, then help should be taken from an experienced facial nerve surgeon. The revision surgery is planned at the earliest, i.e., within few days.

POST HEAD INJURY FACIAL NERVE PARALYSIS

The trauma can be intracranial (rarely), intratemporal or infratemporal (associated with facial injury) (Fig. 9.1).

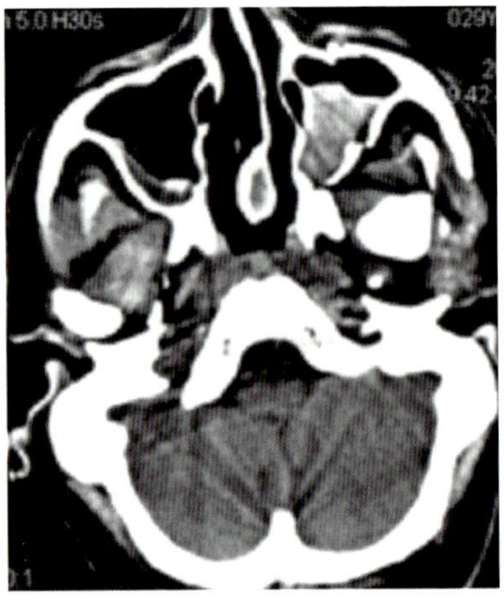

Fig. 9.1. CT scan showing multiple facial fractures.

Classically defined in literature is that post head injury facial nerve paralysis should be divided in acute onset and late onset. But practically this division may be used less frequently, as often patient presents late, mostly due to his neurological condition. Functional as well as cosmetic defects borne by the patient after facial nerve palsy makes it one of the most unacceptable and unsettling to the patient.

Complete otologic history is first step in management. Along with a thorough ENT examination, proper grading of facial nerve status by using House-Brackmann system is a pre-requisite. Author prefers to grade forehead, eye, nasolabial fold and angle of mouth separately as their grades may differ.

Further management depends on following things:

1. Grading of facial nerve.
2. Timing of presentation.
3. Other otological signs.

Now let's consider different situations one by one.

Below is a flowchart (Fig. 9.2) depicting the management depending upon facial nerve status at the time of presentation.

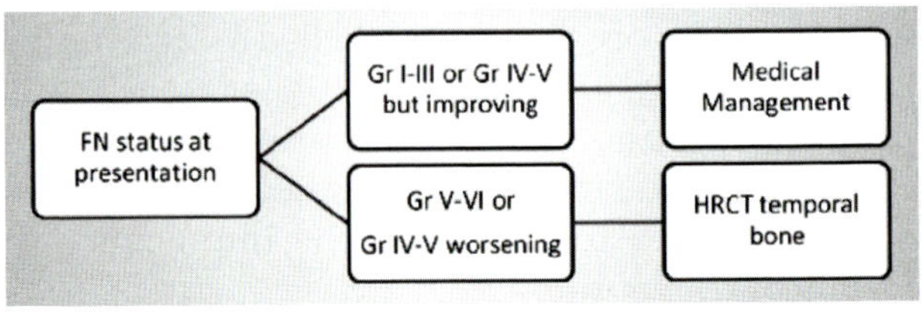

Fig. 9.2. Flowchart depicting the management facial nerve paralysis.

At the time of presentation if patient has grade I to III facial nerve paresis or it is grade IV or V but improving on serial visits, then he should be kept on medical management. It signifies that there is nerve compression but no transaction of nerve. Patient should be started on methyl-prednisolone (1 mg/kg body wt.) in tapering dose spread over three weeks. On the other hand, grade V or VI at the time of presentation or grade IV or V paresis but worsening on serial visits, means significant nerve damage which requires high resolution CT scan of temporal bone (1 mm thick slices in bone window).

Absolute indications for surgery on CT scan are:

1. Fracture line perpendicular to fallopian canal and bisecting it.
2. Boney specule impinging the fallopian canal.
3. Incus and/or malleus medialised and compressing the fallopian canal.

Relative indications for surgery on CT scan are:

1. Haziness in geniculate ganglion area.
2. Highly pneumatised temporal bone.

Advantage of facial nerve surgery can be explained to the patient when surgical intervention is performed for following indications:

1. CSF otorrhea not managed by medical treatment.
2. Conductive hearing loss, tympanic membrane perforation (not healing spontaneously).
3. Vertigo associated with stapes injury.

Late presentation

Facial nerve surgery will not be of any help when patient presents after 1 year. Patient would get best benefit with facio-hypoglossal anastomosis and gold eyelid implant.

As de-nervated muscles atrophy over time, hence even facio-hypoglossal anastomosis would not help after 2 years of facial nerve palsy. In these cases we have to reanimate the eye and the angle of mouth separately. Gold eyelid implant is best suited for eye reanimation. Whereas for angle of mouth we have following options:

1. Static slings
   (a) Fascia lata
   (b) Barbed proline wire
2. Dynamic sling – temporalis muscle transfer

SURGICAL OPTIONS

Facial Nerve decompression / anastomosis

Surgical approaches (Fig. 9.3)

1. Serviceable hearing
   (a) Middle cranial fossa – when injury is associated with CSF leak [IAC, FN (I), GG]
   (b) Transzygomatic, trans-attic – when injury is anywhere from labyrinthine segment to vertical course [FN (t), FN (I), GG]
   (c) Transmastoid – when injury is anywhere from 1st genu to vertical course [FN (m), FN (2G), FN (t), GG]
2. Nonserviceable hearing
   (a) Transmastoid
   (b) Translabyrinthine

When to do grafting?

1. If only 20–25% thickness of nerve fibers are damaged then no grafting is required. Cut ends should be approximated by using 6-0 monofilament.
2. Partial thickness grafting is required when 40–60% thickness of nerve fibers are damaged.
3. Full thickness grafting should be done when damage is above 60–75%.

Preparation of graft bed

1. Excision of end-on neuroma, fibrous nerve.
2. Freshening of edges – done with sharp knife.
3. Removal of soft tissue over the nerve graft.

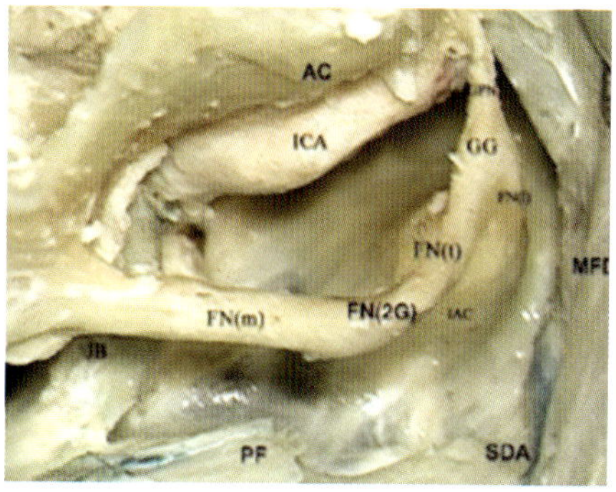

Fig. 9.3. AC – anterior canal wall, ICA – internal carotid artery, MFD – middle fossa dura, SDA – sinodural angle, PF – posterior fossa, FN (m) – facial nerve (vertical segment), FN (2G) – facial nerve (2nd genu), FN (t) – facial nerve (transverse segment), FN (I) – facial nerve (labyrinthine segment), GG – geniculate ganglion, IAC – internal auditory canal, GPN – greater superficial petrosal nerve.

9

Results of facial nerve grafting (Mark May's book)

1. Grade III – 70%
2. Grade IV & V – 15%
3. Grade VI – 15%

Results of facial nerve decompression (Mark May's book)

1. Grade I – 73%
2. Grade II – 12%
3. Grade III – 6%
4. Grade IV – 4%
5. Grade V – 3%
6. Grade VI – 2%

End to side facio-hypoglossal anastomosis

Facial and hypoglossal nerve are exposed via modified parotidectomy incision. Proximal end of facial nerve is identified and sharply cut obliquely. It is dissected upto the bifurcation of facial nerve.

Hypoglossal nerve is identified in the neck and a wedge is created involving 1/3rd of thickness of the nerve (Figs. 9.4 and 9.5). This preserves the function of hypoglossal nerve also.

Proximal end of facial nerve is then rotated inferiorly and anastomosed to hypoglossal nerve. Greater auricular or sural nerve can be used to bridge the gap in between both the nerves.

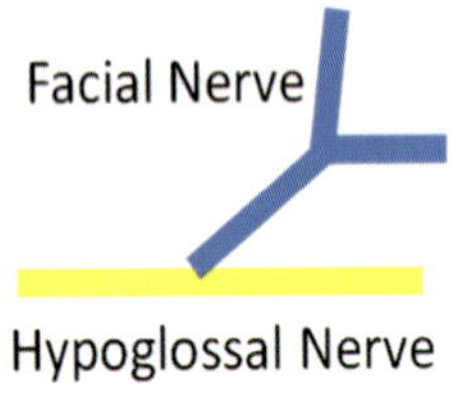

Fig. 9.4. Facio-hypoglossal anastomosis.

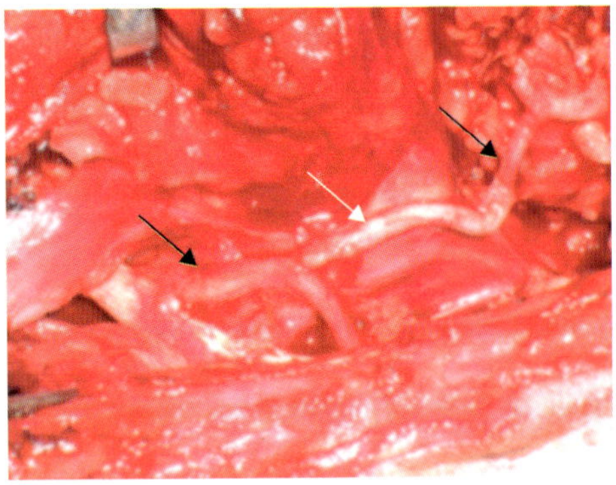

Fig. 9.5. Facio-hypoglossal anastomosis (thick black arrow – hypoglossal nerve, thin black arrow – facial nerve, white arrow – sural nerve graft).

Gold eyelid implant

For gold eyelid implant a curvilinear rectangular gold of 2.0 to 2.2 gm of weight is used. Lateral end is smaller than the medial end (as shown in Fig. 9.6). Weight of the implant has to be determined preoperatively (Fig. 9.7).

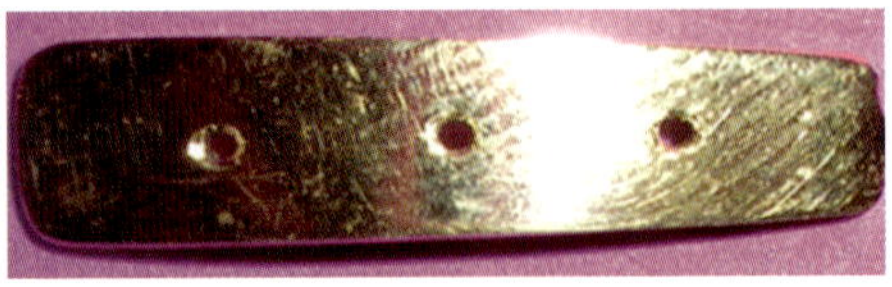

Fig. 9.6. Gold implant.

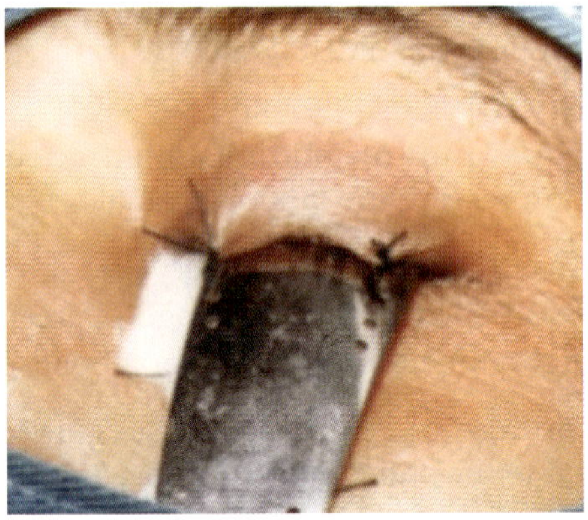

Fig. 9.7. Preoperative preparation.

Incision is given in middle 1/3rd of eyelid (Fig. 9.8) approximately 5 mm away from lid margin. Incision is deepened to expose the tarsal plate which is seen as a white tough layer. Pockets are created in between the muscle layer and the tarsal plate apeneurosis to accommodate the implant keeping in mind not to overdo it.

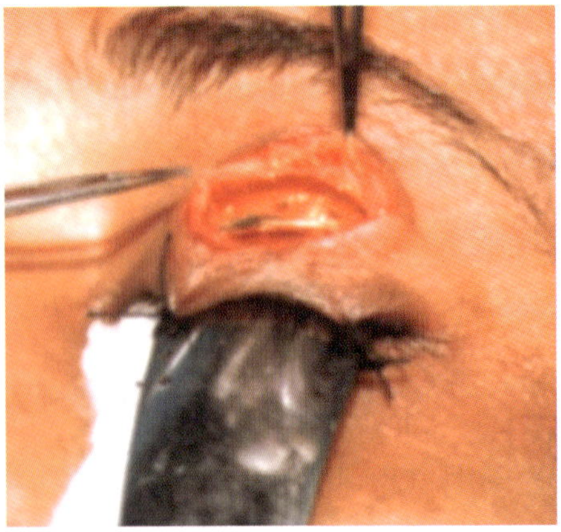

Fig. 9.8. Gold implant in-situ.

Implant is placed on the tarsal plate and sutured with a non-absorbable 5-0 suture. Incision is closed in layers using 5-0 vicryl (Fig. 9.9).

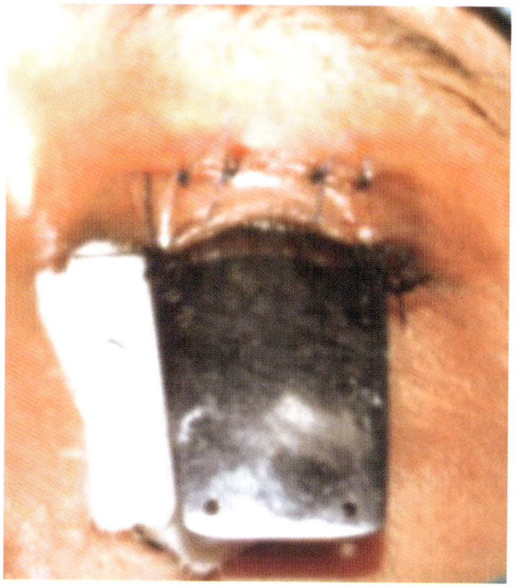

Fig. 9.9. Incision sutured.

Sling surgery

1. Static slings
   (a) Fascia lata
   (b) Barbed proline wire
2. Dynamic sling – temporalis muscle transfer

BILATERAL FACIAL NERVE PALSY

As stated above management depends on following things:

1. Grading of facial nerve.
2. Timing of presentation.
3. Other otological signs.

Parameters discussed above remain valid for bilateral facial nerve paralysis also. Another thing which we need to keep in mind in these cases is the morbidity associated with bilateral facial nerve paralysis. Hence, we need to be more aggressive in treating these cases by giving an option of earlier surgical intervention to the patient.

We would discuss how we managed four cases of bilateral facial nerve palsy to explain our management protocol (Figs. 9.10 to 9.13).

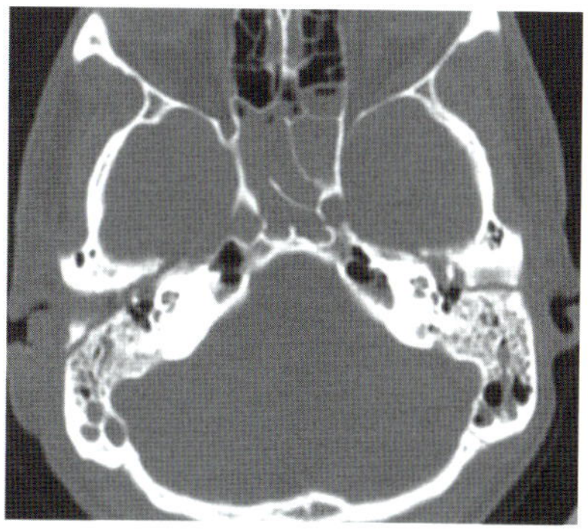

Fig. 9.10. CT scan of bilateral temporal bone fracture with bilateral facial nerve paralysis (case 1).

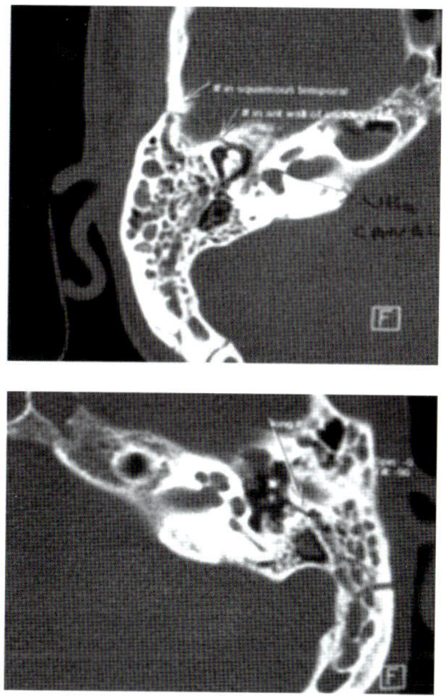

Fig. 9.11. CT scan of bilateral temporal bone fracture with bilateral facial nerve paralysis (case 2).

Intraoperative findings in two cases showed that there was transaction of nerve requiring nerve grafting which meant that side of face would start showing improvement after 6 months and complete recovery might take up to 2 years. Taking in view the prognosis of operated side and the morbidity associated with bilateral facial nerve paralysis, we decided to decompress the opposite side which had grade V palsy in one case and grade IV in other, within two days of operating the first side. The recovery of facial nerve on the 2nd side started within 2 and 4 weeks respectively and recovery finally was grade I. On first side, where grafting was done, total recovery took 15 months and 24 months respectively. The grade of recovery was grade III in one case and grade IV in the other.

Intraoperative findings in other two cases showed that there was pressure due to bone pieces, and inflammation and edema in facial nerve fibers, this required only decompression, along with incision of sheath. There was no sign of transaction

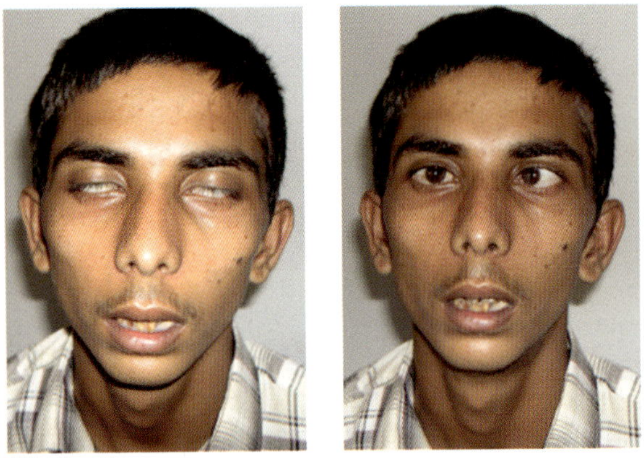

Fig. 9.12. Preoperative bilateral facial nerve paralysis (case 2).

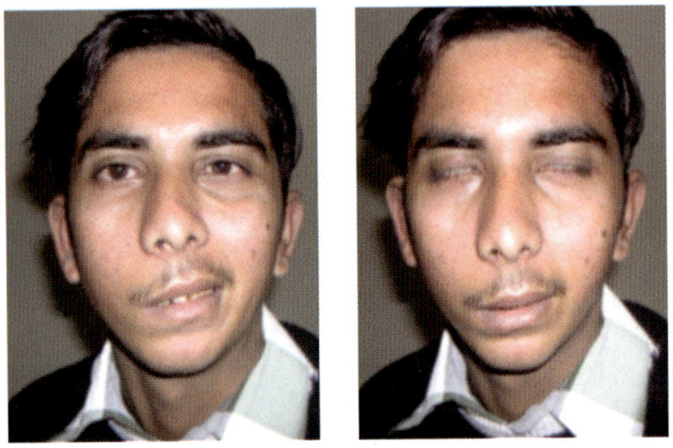

Fig. 9.13. Postoperative bilateral facial nerve paralysis after 4 months (case 2).

of the nerve. Hence, we waited for the other side to recover on its own, which finally it did in both cases. In these patients recovery started much sooner. The operated side recovered up to grade I. The unoperated side also had excellent improvement but only up to grade II. He was left with minimal residual weakness of forehead muscles and negligible weakness of nasolabial fold on the unoperated side.

CONCLUSION

Most common cause of facial nerve paralysis is post road traffic accidents. Early surgical intervention gives better results whether patient has either grade V–VI palsy or grade III–IV palsy but getting worse. For late presentations patient would require some kind of reanimation surgery. Hence, management of every case of facial nerve paralysis has to be individualized.

SUGGESTED READING

1. May M, Schaikin BM. The Facial Nerve, 2nd ed. Thieme, New York, 2000.
2. May M, Schaikin BM. Facial Paralysis: Rehabilitation Techniques. Thieme, New York, 2003.
3. Napoli AM, Panagos P. Delayed presentation of traumatic facial nerve (CNVII) paralysis. *J Emergency Med*, 2005; 29: 421–4.
4. Kinoshita T, Ishii K, Okitsu T, Okudera T, Ogawa T. Facial nerve palsy: Evalution by Contrast-enhanced MRI imaging. *Clin Radiol*, 2001; 56: 926–32.
5. Lichius OG, Streppel M, Stennert E. Postoperative functional evalution of different reanimation techniques for facial nerve repair. *Am J Surg*, 2006; 191: 61–7.
6. Hausamen JE, Samii M, Schmidseder R. Indication and technique for reconstruction of nerve defects in head neck. *J Maxillofacial Surg*, 1974; 2: 159–67.
7. Nosan DK, Benecke JE, Murr RH. Current perspective on temporal bone trauma. *Otolaryngol Head Neck Surg*, 1997; 117: 67–71.
8. Darrouzet V, Duclos JY, Liguoro D, Truilhe Y, Debonfils C, Bebear JP. Management of facial paralysis resulting from temporal bone fracture: Our experience in 115 cases. *Otolaryngol Head Neck Surg*, 2001; 125: 77–84.
9. Maurizio F, Abdelkader T, Alessandra R, Enrico P, Mario S. Facial nerve grafting. *Otol Neurotol*, 2003; 24: 486–9.
10. Hausamen JE, Schmelzeisen R. Current principles in microsurgical nerve repair. *Br J Oral Maxillofacial Surg*, 1996; 34: 143–57.
11. Danner CJ. Facial nerve paralysis. *Otolaryngol Clin North Am*, 2008; 41: 619–32.
12. Kim J, Moon IS, Lee WS. Effect of delayed decompression after early steroid treatment on facial paralysis. *Acta Otolaryngologica*, 2010; 130: 179–4.
13. Fisch U, Mattox D, Aeppli A, Ualavanis A. Microsurgery of the Skull Base. Thieme, New York, 1988.
14. House JW, Brackmann DE. Facial nerve grading system. *Otolaryngol Head Neck Surg*, 1985; 93: 146–7.
15. Gulya AJ, Minor LB, Poe DS. Glasscock's Shambaugh Surgery of the Ear, 6th ed. People's Medical Publishing House, Connecticut, USA, 2010: 619-42.

CHAPTER 10

Ossiculoplasty: Principles and Practice

Gautam Bir Singh

Ossiculoplasty is a very challenging and difficult surgery in otology. This is evident from the fact that the results of ossiculoplasty worldwide vary between 35–70%. The author's personal results are also around 50% only. Despite great advancements in ear surgery, closure of air-bone gap on a consistent basis has proven elusive. The excellent hearing results which are consistently obtained in stapes surgery are not achieved in ossicular reconstruction even in the best of centres. Thus, it is obvious that the factors influencing the outcome of ossiculoplasty are yet to be clearly delineated.

PATIENT SELECTION AND EVALUATION

All the patients with CSOM would qualify as candidates for ossiculoplasty if they audiologically fulfil the following criteria (this I call as rule of 30):

1. An air-bone gap of minimum of 30db
2. Ossiculoplasty is not done if bone conduction is worse than 30 dB and SRT (speech reception threshold) is of 30 dB or less.

   Also ossiculoplasty is avoided if SRT is within 15 dB of the contralateral ear.

No special pre-operative evaluation is required; the author follows the following criteria:

- A dry ear for 4 weeks.
- PTA in accordance with the audiological guidelines defined above.
- Routine investigations for local or general anaesthesia as the case may be.

I exclude the following patients:

- Age below 7 years.
- Patients not meeting audiological guidelines mentioned earlier.
- Patients with only hearing ear.
- Patients with any congenital anomalies like cleft lip, cleft palate or any syndromal diagnosis.

The author would also like to emphasize that no evaluation of 'Eustachian Tube (ET)' is done for any case at any age. The pathophysiology of the ear diseases is now better explained by Jacob and Sade's gas diffusion theory. Moreover there exists no judicious method to accurately measure the functioning and patency of ET. All the tests that have been mentioned in the literature for ET have been refuted scientifically at one time or the other.

In children I tend to avoid ossiculoplasty below 7 years as most of the studies give very poor results in the range of 30–50%. Moreover, anatomical maturity of Eustachian tube takes place at 7 years of age, i.e., there is increase in cartilaginous portion and tensor palati mass thereby aiding the ventilatory function and preventing ascending infection. However, as the role of ET stands challenged, it would be interesting to evaluate results in younger patients.

Finally, a realistic hearing improvement must be offered to the patient. Remember hearing can only be improved to a certain extent, but can never be normal.

PROSTHESIS SELECTION

In 1950–60's when ossiculoplasty was first initiated in the world, autografts like incus, malleus and cortical bones were used. Subsequently homografts were introduced. Interestingly, they have stood the test of time and are still used and give excellent audiological results. They maintain their morphological size, shape and contour for extended periods: as long as 25–30 years. Histologically, they show replacement of nonviable bone by new bone – a process known as creeping substitution. However, these grafts have a tendency to get ankylosed when they come in contact with other bony surfaces in the middle ear. Thus, these grafts require meticulous sculpting so that they fit snugly, this is time-consuming and sculpting with drills leads to thermal injury thereby causing subsequent resorption. On account of this reason copius irrigation is undertaken while sculpting them. There has also been a decline in the use of homografts as they run a risk of transmission of human immunodeficiency virus and prions (i.e., Creutzfeldt-Jakob disease). Moreover such homograft banks are only attached to big medical institutions and thus do not find easy access with all otologists. Nevertheless, they are the most viable ossicular material available till date and may be regarded as a gold standard.

In 1956, Jansen for the first time used cartilage for ossicular construction. Since then this has been widely used worldwide with excellent results. The cartilage also happen to be my ossicular graft of choice. They are readily available: tragal and conchal, conchal cartilage even has a natural curve which aids in their snug fit during surgery. Further, they do not require time for sculpting. However, histological studies have shown that they develop chondromalacia and do have a tendency to undergo resorption over a period of time, but some studies have also shown that cartilage gets calcified as a result of vascularisation.

10

In 1952, Wullstein used artificial material palavit (vinyl-acryl plastic) for the first time for ossiculoplasty. Since then a number of materials like polyethylene, polytetrafluoroethylene, silicone, stainless steel, proplast, plastipore, ceravital, bioglass, carbon, gold, platinum, titanium, hydroxylapatite (HA), tentalium, and aluminium oxide ceramic, have all been used for ossiculoplasty. However, presently only HA and titanium implants are being used and rest have all been abandoned. All these implants elicit foreign body giant cell reactions and biodegradation. In addition, as compared to autografts they also have a high extrusion rate.

HA is a mineral matrix of living bone, used for the first time by Wehrs in 1985 as incus prosthesis. Its disadvantages are that it has a large mass creating high input impedance, it is solid; obstructing the surgeon's view while operating and is brittle (it is thus combined with other materials like polythene to make it malleable and strong). Long-term extrusion rate of HA is 4 to 16%.

Titanium prosthesis for ossicular reconstruction was first reported in Germany in 1993. It has a low mass and thus may provide better hearing at higher frequencies. It is nonmagnetic, has low specific density, and excellent biocompatibility. In addition this prosthesis has an open head, allowing better visualization. Medical literature reports an extrusion rate of 1–3% with follow-up period of 3 years or less for titanium implants.

Synthetic implants are available in the form of PORP (partial ossicular replacement prosthesis) and TORP (total ossicular replacement prosthesis). It would be pertinent to note that synthetic implants require interpolation of a cartilage strip when in direct contact with tympanic membrane, otherwise they have high extrusion rates. However, HA prosthesis can be used without cartilages.

Another material which merits mention is bone cement, especially hydroxylapetite phosphate cement. This is used to bridge gap between distal erosions of incus and intact stapes. Excellent hearing results with no extrusion have been reported in the medical literature with HA cement. Fibrin glue with bone paste too can be used for the same purpose with good results.

From the above account it is clear that no specific graft or biomaterial can be regarded as the ossicular material of choice; all have their own merits and demerits. Presently, in view of their low extrusion rate titanium and HA implants are being aggressively promoted commercially. However, these are newer implants and thus not much scientific literature is available on them: their long term efficacy is yet to be evaluated. An ideal graft or synthetic prosthesis is yet to be discovered or invented.

CLASSIFICATION FOR OSSICULOPLASTY

Medical Literature is replete with many classifications for tympanoplasty, but author follows and recommends "Tos Classification" which is clinically most apt to define tympanoplasties. This is a modified version of "Wullstein Classification":

- **Type I:** Intact chain. Graft is placed on the handle of malleus, i.e., myringoplasty.
- **Type II:** Intact stapes and defective long process of incus. Interposition of an ossicle or any other prosthesis between stapedial arch and malleus handle or ear drum.
- **Type III:** Absent or severely defective stapedial arch. Placement of an ossicle or prosthesis between footplate and the malleus handle or ear drum.
- **Type IV:** Sound protection of the round window with a graft, and formation of an air space in the hypotympanum. The footplate is covered by keratinized epithelium.
- **Type VA:** Fenestration of the lateral semicircular canal in cases with no ossicles and a fixed stapes footplate. In such cases the stapedial arch is usually missing. The round window is protected.
- **Type VB:** Platinectomy. The oval window niche is filled with fatty tissue or fibrous tissue.

The aforesaid classification can also be used in mastoid operations. The said operation is added to the classification, e.g, atticotomy with type II tympanoplasty or MRM (modified radical mastoidectomy) with type III tympanoplasty.

SURGICAL CONSIDERATIONS

Ossicular reconstruction may be done under local anaesthesia or general anaesthesia in accordance with the surgical skill of the surgeon and patient compliance. Local anaesthesia offers the advantage of hearing assessment, absence of gas accumulation in middle ear, alteration of the position of tympanic membrane with respect to the prosthesis and above all it is highly cost effective. General anaesthesia rids the patient of all discomfort and removes the time factor for the surgeon. The middle ear gas factor can be compensated by the use of nitrous oxide.

From a surgical point of view, following conditions may arise on the exploration of the middle ear:

1. Loss of incus (malleus and stapes intact and mobile).
2. Loss of incus and stapes suprastructure (malleus and footplate of stapes intact and mobile).
3. Loss of malleus and incus (stapes intact and mobile).
4. Loss of malleus, incus and stapes suprastructure (footplate of stapes intact and mobile).

1. Loss of incus (malleus and stapes intact and mobile)

This is the commonest condition of ossicular disruption seen by all of us. If the long process of the incus is having a minimum necrosis, i.e., 1 mm or less, the gap may be bridged with bone cement (Fig. 10.1). Bone paste with fibrin glue has also been used with good results. However, if the gap is more it may be bridged by a cartilage, cortical bone or even some specific synthetic prosthesis designed for this type of long process of incus necrosis (Plester/Applebaum prosthesis). If there is considerable necrosis of long process of incus grossly affecting the continuity then certainly some ossicular reconstruction is required. The incus may be removed and resculpted and interpositioned between the handle of malleus and stapes head (Fig. 10.2). I personally use cartilage graft for this purpose

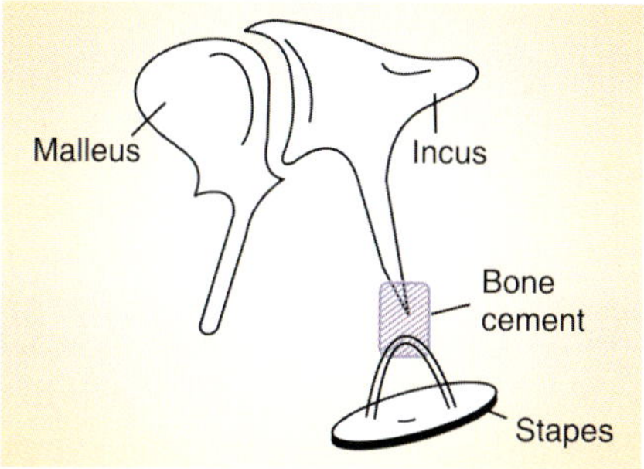

Fig. 10.1. Bone cement bridging gap between necrosed long process of incus and stapes.

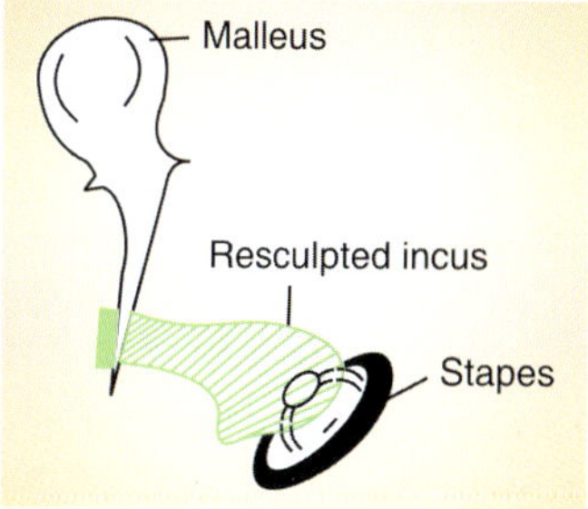

Fig. 10.2. Resculpted incus interpolated between malleus and stapes.

10

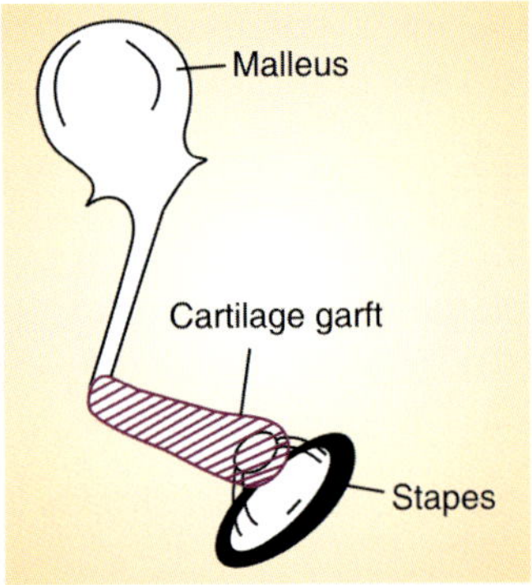

Fig. 10.3. Cartilage graft interpolated between malleus and stapes.

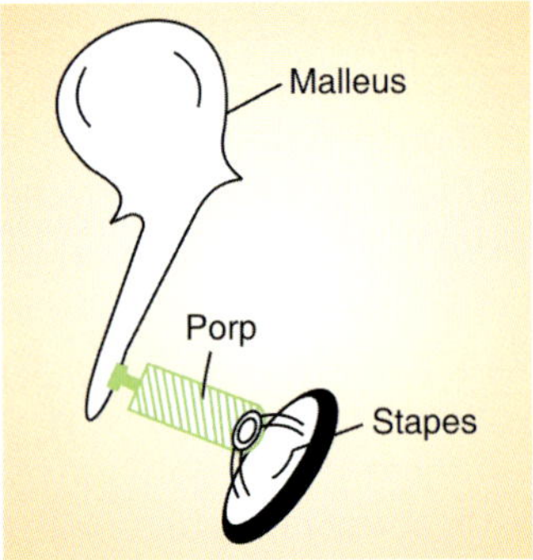

Fig. 10.4. A PORP used for necrosed incus, between malleus and stapes.

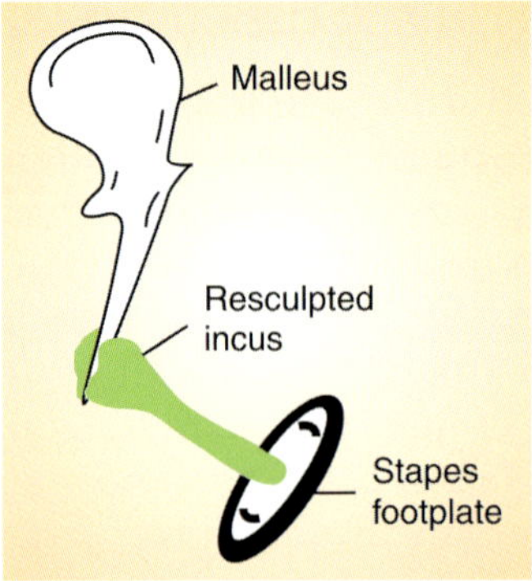

Fig. 10.5. A resculpted incus interpolated between stapes footplate and intact malleus.

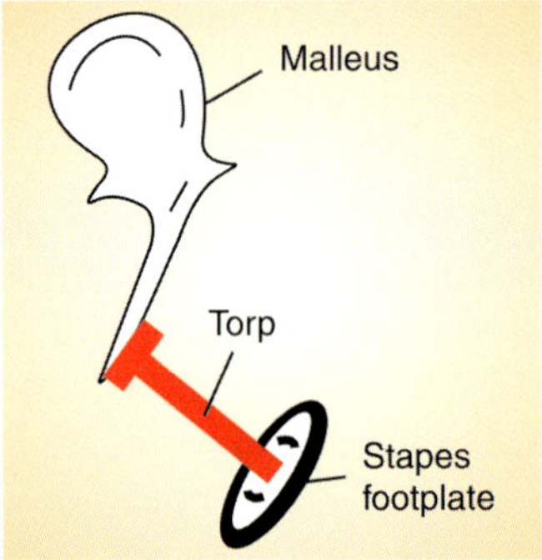

Fig. 10.6. A TORP used for ossicular assembly, placed between malleus and footplate of stapes.

(Fig. 10.3). Cortical bone and PORP can also be used to carry out the said procedure (Fig. 10.4).

2. Loss of incus and stapes suprastructure (malleus and footplate of stapes intact and mobile)

If the stapes suprastructure is also lost with incus then a resculpted incus, cartilage or cortical bone may be used between the malleus and stapes footplate (Fig. 10.5). Synthetic prosthesis in the form of TORP would also serve the same purpose (Fig. 10.6).

3. Loss of malleus and incus (stapes intact and mobile)

10

For this situation, the books recommend that any autograft can be used to construct the assembly line, but my personal experience is that this assembly line is very unstable and I have always had very poor results. I recommend the following procedure with a cartilaginous graft.

We place a cartilaginous graft of about 4 mm in size on the stapes head. One end of the cartilage is in contact with stapes head and the other end is on the anteroinferior bony annulus at about 5 O'clock

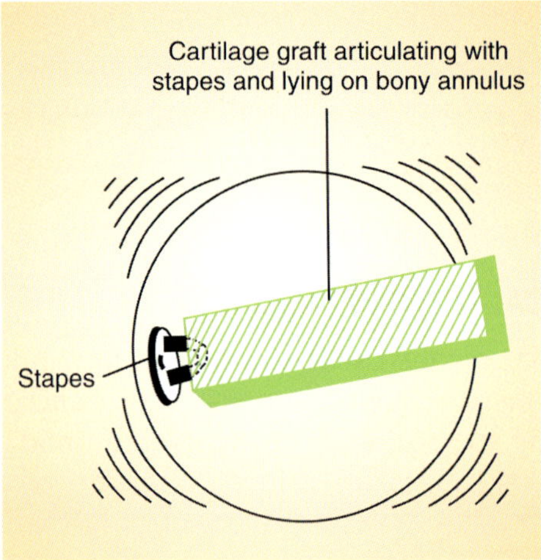

Fig. 10.7. An annulus stapes cartilage plate placed on head of stapes and the bony annulus.

position (Fig. 10.7). Then over this we place a temporalis fascia graft. To the author this procedure has given excellent results.

However, a PORP can also be used, but since the prosthesis comes in direct contact with the tympanic membrane, a cartilage graft has to be interpolated between the tympanic membrane and PORP. This prevents extrusion of the prosthesis. The other end at the stapes head may be secured with bone cement.

4. Loss of malleus, incus and stapes suprastructure (footplate of stapes intact and mobile)

In this condition again the author has had very poor results in placing cartilaginous grafts and resculpted incus between the stapes footplate and tympanic membrane. The assembly line is very unstable. I would recommend the use of TORP in such cases (Fig. 10.8). This prosthesis is to be secured with a horseshoe cartilage at the base and a cartilage strut between prosthesis and the tympanic membrane.

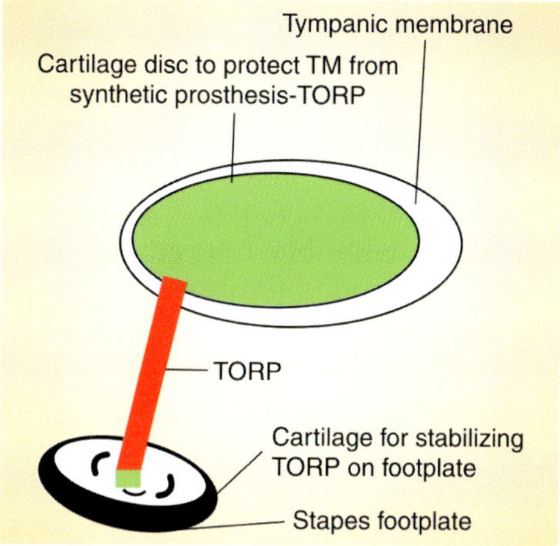

Fig. 10.8. A TORP in contact with tympanic membrane (protected at this end by cartilage disc) and stapes footplate (stabilized by cartilage).

If at any time one encounters a fixed footplate it is needless to say that all such cases would require a stapedotomy and a suitable piston hinged to incus or malleus as the case may be.

Rarely, one may come across total fixation of the ossicular chain (author has no personal experience about this condition). In this condition the incus is removed, after stapedotomy the prosthesis is clipped to the handle of malleus and finally the head is amputated. Recent review of medical literature suggests that in the future this may be supplanted with a round window vibrioplasty, using the floating mass transducer.

I personally use cartilage grafts for all my ossiculoplasty except in condition 4, where I recommend TORP. However, these are my personal experiences blended with all the academic knowledge that I have imbibed over a period of time and thus are not the final word on the surgical technique or ossicular material. The surgical technique and prosthesis is a matter of choice.

POSTOPERATIVE CARE

The patients are discharged on the next day of surgery under antibiotic cover with analgesics and an anti-allergic with nasal decongestant. No special instruction to the patient is given apart from: not to sleep on the operated side, avoid nose blowing, if sneezing is unavoidable then mouth should be open and to prevent water from entering the operated ear. The first postoperative visit thereafter is on the 10th day when stitches (post-auricular) and the ear canal wicks are removed. Thereafter patient is told to avoid water in the external auditory canal for the next 4 weeks and report to us in case some untoward incident occurs like pus discharge from the ear. The author does no manipulations in the operated ear like suction clearance of gel foam. The second postoperative visit is at 6 weeks, where again patient is fully examined. Finally the patient is called at the end of 3 months and 6 months to evaluate the hearing status.

AUDIOLOGICAL OUTCOMES

The results of ossiculoplasty are graded on the basis of closure of air-bone gap as:

ABG (< 10 dB)	Excellent
ABG (11–20)	Good
ABG (21–30)	Fair

However, hearing is essentially a binaural phenomenon, thus the contralateral ear must be given due consideration in order to get good audiological results. Therefore the "Belfast Rule of Thumb" would certainly be good functional audiological criteria. It states that postoperative hearing in the operated ear will be useful to the patient if:

1. The air conduction threshold is less than 30 dB HL (regardless of the hearing in the opposite ear).
2. The air conduction threshold is within 15 dB HL of the air conduction threshold in a better contralateral ear.

In this context ENT surgeons are advised to review the audiological indications for ossicular reconstruction (mentioned in text earlier): ossiculoplasty is avoided if SRT is within 15 dB of the contralateral ear.

10

The author usually gets audiograms at the end of 3rd month and 6th month postoperatively. The hearing certainly improves with time. A repeat audiogram at the end of 1 year would also further aid in analysing the hearing outcomes, but in Indian settings there is a high dropout rate. Patients do not turnup at the end of one year in a tertiary care government hospital, probably as they come from far away places. Last but not the least the author has observed that if one is able to give a 10 dB hearing improvement in two consecutive frequencies compared to preoperative air conduction thresholds, the patient is highly satisfied irrespective of the audiological grading given above.

FACTORS AFFECTING OSSICULOPLASTY

1. Middle ear environment

The middle ear should be free from any type of infection, the hallmark of which is discharge. Further, no pathologies like polyp, granulations or cholesteatoma should be present.

For the long-term success of tympanoplasties a well-aerated middle ear is a must. Most of the otologists believe that aeration of the middle ear is the primary physiological function of Eustachian tube, and thus define an important role for it. However, a healthy mastoid also plays an important role in maintaining aeration. Moreover, once the middle ear is closed as a result of tympanoplasty, the reversal in mastoid pathology including opening and normal functioning of previously blocked ET takes place. All this aids the middle ear cleft to attain near normal physiological function. The author has carried out a prospective controlled trial to evaluate ET function in type I tympanoplasty in paediatric patients, and found no role for it. Our study is consistent with the results reported in medical literature by other otologists on the cited subject. Nevertheless, at this stage it would suffice to state that since no definitive parameter exists to measure the functioning of ET, there may be a contributory role for it in middle ear pathophysiology including tympanoplasties, but certainly it does not play a primary role.

2. Condition of ossicles

To get the best results in ossiculoplasties, it is very important to have an intact and mobile stapes. Even with the loss of stapes suprastructure the audiological results deteriorate.

The role of malleus is disputed. It is widely believed that once malleus is eliminated from the ossicular assembly, the lever mechanism of the ossicular chain is lost, i.e., if a graft or prosthesis is placed directly in contact with tympanic membrane the prosthesis would function as a piston thereby giving audiologically inferior results. However, recent studies on the cited subject report no clinical difference in audiological results whether malleus is present or absent.

3. Surgical expertise

With only 35–70% success rate reported in the world medical literature for ossiculoplasties, it is needless to say that surgical expertise matters a lot. The placement and securing of prosthesis with optimal tension is the key to success. The prosthesis should be snugly fitting: neither under tension, i.e., too tight nor loose. A prosthesis placed tightly won't give good audiological results and a loose fit will fall away from the assembly line getting ankylosed (autografts) or extruded (biomaterial prosthesis).

During ossiculoplasty if malleus is medialized it results in increased angulation of the prosthesis thereby decreasing the efficacy of energy transfer and stability of the reconstruction. Usually, cutting off the tensor tympani tendon allows lateralization of malleus. However, if malleus is significantly lateralized it may be bypassed and the graft may be placed in direct contact with tympanic membrane. The biomaterial prosthesis then has to be secured with cartilage strip to prevent extrusion.

4. Staging of surgery

A considerable controversy also exists regarding ossiculoplasty during cholesteatoma surgery. Most of the otologists stage ossiculoplasty in these cases. The author, however, would like to emphasize that this can be done at the same time along with mastoid surgery, after all a type III tympanoplasty is usually done in all cases at the same setting with very good audiological results. In Indian settings it is also difficult to keep the patients in regular follow-up, especially in government institutions. In addition, a graft/prosthesis assembly uptake certainly works out to be highly cost effective both for the patient and the surgeon as it avoids the second look surgery; moreover no harm is done to the patient if ossiculoplasty is ventured at the first instance.

However, the incus remodelling and reposition

should not be done in cases where the ossicle chain is engulfed by cholesteatoma as there are chances of cholesteatoma implantation, i.e., autograft ossicles are best avoided in such cases. In addition, if a mastoid surgery is being performed for a persistently discharging ear, ossiculoplasty is again best avoided, for such cases do have discharge post-operatively and the graft assembly is extruded out. Most of these cases that the author has operated on have given very poor results in terms of ossiculoplasty and sometimes do require a long-term antibiotic cover to make the ear dry along with an anti-allergic. This is probably due to the allergic component which sets in over a period of time along with the infection.

Further, it would be pertinent to note that type of mastoid surgery, i.e., canal wall up or down has little influence on the outcome of the surgery. It is the extent of the middle ear disease which is a more important factor influencing ossiculoplasty.

5. Audiological status of the other ear

All otologists are advised to give due consideration to the hearing status of the other ear in accordance with the "Belfast Rule of Thumb" (mentioned earlier in text) while selecting patients for ossiculoplasty in order to get functional audiological results. Otherwise they may land in a strange predicament of: surgery audiologically successful, but with no subjective hearing improvement in patient.

COMPLICATIONS

It is not the endeavour of this article to discuss the management of complications of tympanoplasty, thus a brief outline is presented here. Intraoperative bleeding, damage or stretching of chorda tympani, facial nerve palsy, infections, recurrent cholesteatoma (if tympanoplasty is done with mastoid surgery) have all been mentioned in literature.

With the manipulation of the ossicular chain there is always a realistic chance of having sensorineural hearing loss. And accompanying with this, tinnitus is also recorded in some patients. Sometimes it settles down or probably patient becomes oblivious of it once the hearing improves. But these complications along with facial nerve palsy are quite dreadful, both for the patient and operating surgeon, thus a proper counselling is a must. Many-a-time patients also experience dizziness and vertigo which eventually settles down by adequate drug treatment. Last but not the least finally one can have tympanoplasty failure.

In view of all these complications and poor audiological results, the option of hearing aid should always be discussed with patients. This certainly becomes important if patient has bilateral hearing loss or is a child. This also has a medicolegal significance in the modern era. In the author's experience most of our patients in government setup usually refuse hearing aid for there is a stigma attached to using hearing aids especially at young age and good digital hearing aid is costly (operations are usually cost-free).

SUMMARY

The success rate for ossiculoplasty worldwide is only 35–70%. In addition, the results are not reproducible on a consistent basis. Thus the surgery should be approached with caution and guarded prognosis.

A simple rule of 30 is followed for selection of patients on the basis of PTA and SRT:

1. An air-bone gap of minimum of 30 dB.
2. Ossiculoplasty not done if bone conduction is worse than 30 dB and SRT is of 30 dB or less.

Also ossiculoplasty is avoided if SRT is within 15 dB of the contralateral ear.

The final postoperative audiological results are graded on the basis of closure of air-bone gap (ABG) as:

ABG (< 10 dB)	Excellent
ABG (11–20 dB)	Good
ABG (21–30 dB)	Fair

It would be prudent to note that to get better and functional audiological results, "Belfast Rule of Thumb" must be considered and given due importance while selecting and evaluating a patient. It states that postoperative hearing in the operated ear will be useful to the patient if:

1. The air conduction threshold is less than 30 dB HL (regardless of the hearing in the opposite ear).
2. The air conduction threshold is within 15 dB HL of the air conduction threshold in a better contralateral ear.

Autografts and synthetic prosthesis (HA and titanium) are all used worldwide with varying results. The superiority of synthetic implants over autografts is yet to be established.

An intact and mobile stapes is probably the most important factor that influences the outcome of the surgery along with a good surgical technique. Eustachian tube does not play a significant role.

The option of hearing aids must be offered to all patients in view of poor audiological outcomes of ossiculoplasty and keeping in view the medicolegal aspect in modern era.

There are no set rules or guidelines for ossiculoplasty, thus surgical technique and selection of prosthesis is a matter of personal choice, albeit it should give good and persistent audiological results in the best interest of the patient.

SUGGESTED READING

1. Merchant SN, Ravicz ME, Voss SE, et al. Middle ear mechanics in normal, diseased and reconstructed ear. *J Laryngol Otol*, 1998; 112: 715–31.
2. Bahmad F Jr, Merchant SN. Histopathology of Ossicular grafts and implants in chronic otitis media. *Ann Otol Rhinol Laryngol*, 2007; 116(3): 181–91.
3. Sade J, Luntz M. Dynamic measurement of gas composition in middle ear; steady state values. *Acta Otolaryngol*, 1993; 113: 353–7.
4. Manning SC, Cantekin EL, Renne MA, et al. Prognostic value of ET function in paediatric tympanoplasty. *Laryngoscope*, 1987; 97: 1012–6.
5. Chandrashekhar SS, House JW, Devgun U. Paediatric Tympanoplasty: A 10 years experience. *Arch Otolaryngol Head Neck Surg*, 1995; 121: 873–8.
6. Yamamoto E, Iwanaga M, Fukumoto M. Histological study of homograft cartilages implanted in the middle ear. *Otolaryngol Head Neck Surg*, 1988; 98: 546–51.
7. Belal A Jr, Sanna M, Gamelotti R. Pathology as it relates to ear surgery. V Ossiculoplasty. *J Laryngol Otol*, 1984; 98: 229–40.
8. Tos M. Tympanoplasty - general. *In:* Tos M. ed. Manual of Middle Ear Surgery. Vol 1. Stuttgart: Thieme, 1993: 238–44.
9. Heermann J, Heermann H, Kopstein E. Fascia and cartilage palisade tympanoplasty: Nine years experience. *Arch Otolaryngol*, 1970; 91: 228–41.
10. Tos M. Tympanoplasty with handle of malleus missing. *In:* Tos M. ed. Manual of Middle Ear Surgery. Vol 1. Stuttgart: Thieme, 1993: 330–47.
11. Colleti V, Soli SD, Carner M, et al. Treatment of mixed hearing losses via implantation of vibratory transducer on the round window. *Int J Audiol*, 2006; 45: 600–608.
12. Smyth GD, Patterson CC. Results of middle ear reconstruction: do patients and surgeons agree? *Am J of Otol*, 1985; 6: 276–9.
13. Toner JC, Smyth GD, Kerr AG. Realities in ossiculoplasty. *J Laryngol Otol*, 1991; 101: 180–5.
14. Singh GB, Sidhu TS, Sharma A, et al. Tympanoplasty type I in children-an evaluative study. *Int J Paediar Otolaryngol*, 2005; 69: 1071–6.
15. Sade J, Amos AR. The Eustachian tube. *In:* Ludman H, Wright T. Diseases of ear. London: Arnold, 1998: 334–52.
16. Brackmann DE, Sheehy JL, Luxford WM. TORPs and PORPs in tympanoplasty: A review of 1042 operations. *Otolaryngol Head Neck Surg*, 1984; 92: 32–7.
17. Javia LR, Ruckenstein MJ. Ossiculoplasty. *Otolaryngol Clin N Am*, 2006; 39: 1177–89.

ACKNOWLEDGEMENT

I would like to acknowledge the professional support extended to me by my wife Dr (Ms) Nitasha Singh (Junior Consultant, Cardiology, Fortis Escorts Hospital, Faridabad) in drafting the manuscript of this chapter.

CHAPTER 11

Cochlear Implantation

Mohan Kameswaran, S. Raghunandhan

Hearing loss is one of the commonest congenital anomalies to affect children world over. WHO recently reports that nearly 2–3 per 1000 live births are found to have severe to profound hearing loss. This scenario is more predominant in the large populous developing countries like in the Indian subcontinent. Hearing loss at birth is considered a social stigma even in present day society and ends as a double tragedy, as it leads to not only deafness but also language deprivation. However, today hearing loss, both congenital and acquired is the only truly remediable handicap, due to remarkable advances in biomedical engineering and surgical techniques. The advent of numerous implantable hearing devices, which are indicated for a varying types and extent of hearing losses, have successfully broken the acoustic barrier, thus resurrecting individuals from slipping into a deaf world, integrating them into the normal society and providing them with a highly productive quality of life.

Cochlear implants help to restore hearing by integration of an external circuitry with the peripheral hearing apparatus and the central circuitry of the brain. They are safe and extremely effective in restoring hearing both in children and adults with severe to profound hearing loss, who do not receive benefit from conventional hearing aids. These devices electronically stimulate the cochlea/auditory nerve and the higher hearing centers in the brain (Fig. 11.1).

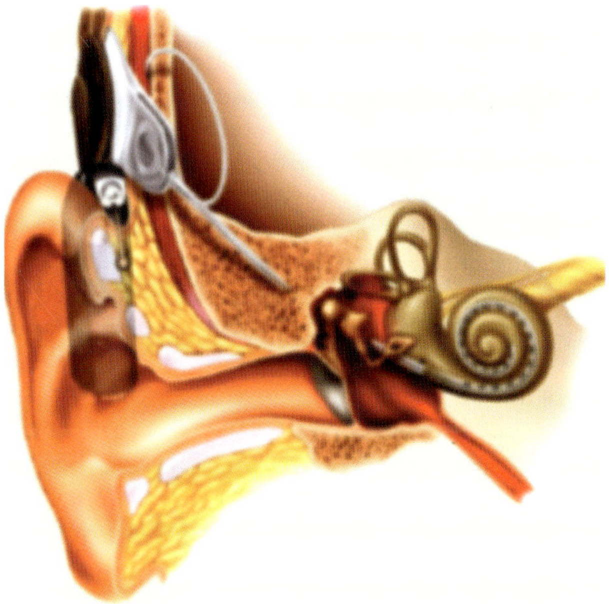

Fig. 11.1. Cochlear implant unit.

The auditory system is unique in its organization and tonotopicity, which gives it the opportunity to receive and integrate external electronic circuits. This is possible because of the low potential for rejection of the device by the ear and nervous system. Thus, hearing restoration is the first successful path-breaking attempt in medical science to integrate an electronic device with the central nervous system, in order to fully restore a lost special sense organ. The cochlear implant represents the

11

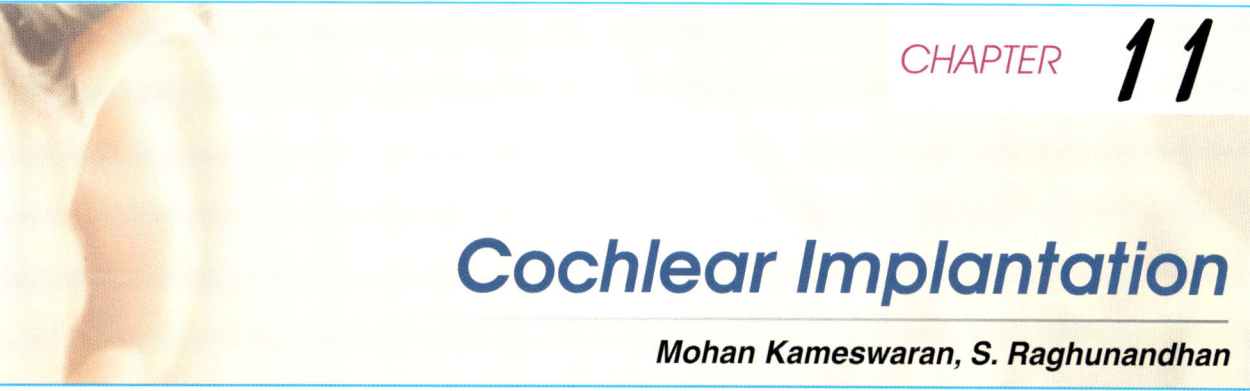

most successful attempt by man to date, to interface a prosthetic device with the nervous system. It has been one of the most significant advancements of the 21st century in the field of otology. The impact of this monumental innovation can be measured by its potential to change the quality of human life. This chapter highlights cochlear implants, enumerating their indications, components, surgical techniques, habilitation protocols and overall outcomes.

SENSORINEURAL HEARING LOSS IN CHILDREN

It is the hearing impairment caused by abnormalities in the structure or functioning of the inner ear and/or the auditory pathways (includes cochlear and retrocochlear deafness). Although 90% of cases of sensorineural deafness are of cochlear origin, conditions like retrocochlear pathology and auditory neuropathy have to be ruled out to confirm a diagnosis of cochlear deafness. Incidence of sensorineural deafness among children is about 1 : 1500 to 1 : 2000 in the Indian subcontinent. Around 50% of these children are born deaf and are not identified until about 18 months old, while 25% are still left undiagnosed at 3 years of age. Such late diagnosis can have a devastating effect on their speech and language acquisition, social skills and communication development, which can last a lifetime. However, if deaf children are identified at an early stage, and appropriate intervention is done, they can develop at the same rate as their hearing peers into normal adults. Now the technology has advanced to the level of objectively determining a child's hearing status shortly after birth. Signs of delayed speech and language development are a strong indicator of hearing loss in children.

Congenital (genetic) deafness

11

Nearly 50% of sensorineural hearing impairment in children is due to genetic factors (congenital deafness). Among the inherited deafness, 75–88% is autosomal recessive (AR), 12–24% is autosomal dominant (AD) and 1% is X-linked. Autosomal recessive is usually stable; autosomal dominant tends toward progression and conductive autosomal recessive HL always exists as part of a syndrome. Mutations in the connexin 26 (Cx26) gene is the most common cause of hearing loss. Connexin-26 is a transmembrane protein that forms channels allowing rapid ion transport between cells of the organ of Corti. This Connexin-26 protein is coded by the Gap Junction Beta 2 (GJB2) gene. Non-syndromic Autosomal Recessive Deafness occurs due a DFNB1 locus mutation defect in the GJB2 gene which disrupts the K+ ion channels in the organ of Corti. Connexin-26 screening among children with congenital hearing loss rules out syndromic associations. Screening provides vital epidemiological data about prevalence of non-syndromic congenital deafness in our society (80% of congenital deafness is non-syndromic) and it helps in counseling the family regarding possibility of deafness among future children.

Cx26 hearing loss is most often seen in a person with:

- Hearing loss that was found at birth or in early childhood.
- Hearing loss that is mild, moderate, severe or profound.
- Hearing loss without any other medical problems (non-syndromic).
- Hearing loss with no identified cause.

Although these are the most common characteristics of hearing loss due to a mutation in Cx26, there can be variations even within a family. There have been several occasions when skin disorders have been found in people with deafness due to dominant Cx26 mutations. Furthermore, there have been instances when a child's deafness was originally thought to be due to non-hereditary factors (e.g., an infection or exposure to antibiotics) and then the child was later found to have mutations in Cx26. In such cases, it is more likely that the child's deafness was caused by the Cx26 mutations than by environmental agents. It should also be noted that many children with Cx26 mutations have no family history of hearing loss. An Autosomal dominant mutation in the EYA1 gene on chromosome 8q13.3 – "Drosophila Eye Absent gene", may also cause congenital hearing loss manifesting as Melnick-Fraser Syndrome or Branchio-Oto-Renal Syndrome.

Acquired Inner Ear Deafness

This is due to maternal ingestion of teratogens/ototoxicity, intrauterine infections (rubella, cytomegalic inclusion disease, toxoplasmosis, influenza, herpes 1 and 2, and syphilis), perinatal causes such as prematurity, anoxia, kernicterus, ototoxic medication, and meningitis. Maternal alcoholism – nutritional disturbances, endocrine disease – maternal thyrotoxicosis, diabetes and immunologic disorders are also etiological factors.

COCHLEAR IMPLANTS (CI)

A cochlear implant is a surgically implantable device that helps restore hearing in patients with severe to profound hearing loss, unresponsive to amplification by conventional hearing aids. Cochlear implants are electronic devices designed to detect mechanical sound energy and convert it into electrical signals that can be delivered to the cochlear nerve, bypassing the damaged hair cells of the cochlea (Fig. 11.1). These electrical signals are processed by an external speech processor and sent via a radio-frequency interface into an array of electrodes implanted surgically within the cochlea. The implant system preserves the tonotopic map of the cochlea as in nature and hence the auditory brain perceives these electrical impulses as sound.

History of implants

Volta, in the year 1790, became the first person to experience and publish the effects of electrical current on the auditory system. He inserted a metal rod in each ear and then subjected himself to approximately 50 volts of electricity. He reported that the sensation was that of receiving a blow to the head followed by the sound of thick soup boiling. Volta was followed by a string of scientists who continued to experiment with electricity and hearing over the next 167 years. It was Djourno and Eyries who reported the first stimulation of the acoustic nerve by direct application of an electrode in a deaf person (1957). The patient was undergoing an operation for cholesteatoma and the auditory nerve was exposed. An electrode was placed on the nerve and an induction coil and ground electrode were placed in the temporalis muscle. The coil could then be stimulated by currents produced by a second coil placed against the overlying skin. On subsequent experimentation with the patient reported hearing sounds like crickets or a roulette wheel when the second coil was applied. He was able to distinguish simple words and noted improvement of his speech reading ability.

This was followed by a string of implantations performed by House, Doyle, Simmons, and others. Advances in microelectronics, biocompatible materials, and microscopic otologic surgery propelled House to produce the first single-channel implant in 1972 which stimulated the auditory nerve via the scala tympani. In 1984 the cochlear implant gained FDA approval for use in adults. This corresponded with the introduction of multichannel implants by Graham Clarke, which significantly improved spectral perception and open-set speech understanding. The 1990's saw significant improvements in speech processor designs. SPEAK and CIS speech processing strategies produced large improvements in recipient's speech recognition. The late 1990's and early 2000's saw technologic improvements such as the peri-modiolar contour electrode, split electrodes, behind-the-ear processors, and implantation for children as young as 12 months. The first paediatric cochlear implantation was done in the U.S. in 1987. Today a spectrum of implants are available along with improved speech processing strategies. Rapid technological advancements in bioengineering and implant manufacturing methods have led to miniaturization of the device, with high quality refinement in sound signals, providing better 'hearing in noise' and music appreciation among cochlear implantees.

Components of a cochlear implant system

The implant has external components, consisting of a microphone which receives and transduces sound into an electrical waveform, a speech processor which divides the signals into components for each of the electrodes and a transmitting coil which sends the signals across the scalp to the internal components (Fig. 11.2).

The internal components include a receiver-stimulator, which receives the signals from the transmitting coil and sends it to the electrode array which is implanted in the scala tympani of the cochlea. Speech processors are currently available as body worn and ear level speech processors. All components play an important part in converting sound to an electrical stimulus. The microphone receives and transduces sound into an electrical representation. This is done in an analog (continuous) fashion. The external speech processor and signal-transfer hardware shapes the electrical signal. This requires amplifying, compressing, filtering, and shaping. Amplification is necessary to increase some signal levels to the point that they can be used in the electrical circuits. Compression is a necessary second step of signal modulation. The normal human ear can hear gradations of sound intensity in a range of 120 dB. Persons with severe to profound hearing loss do not have this same

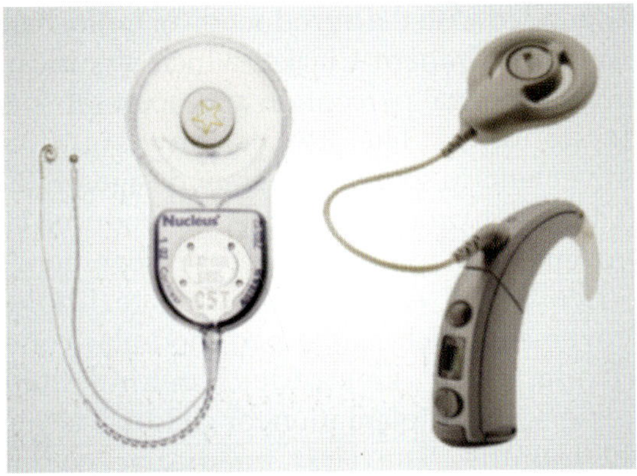

Fig. 11.2. Cochlear implant – internal and external components.

range. In the high frequencies their dynamic range (the difference between their absolute threshold and painful sound) can sometimes be only 5 dB. The range in the lower frequencies is often 10–25 dB. This means that significant compression of the sound energy must take place in order to render it useful. Thus, all cochlear implants employ gain control of one kind or another. These systems monitor the output voltage and adjust the ratio of compression to keep the output in a range where it provides useful, but not painful stimuli.

Filtering of the input signal is the next step. Frequencies between 100 Hz and 4000 Hz are generally those most important for understanding speech. Sound energy is analyzed using several different types of filters. This allows the unimportant frequencies to be removed and the frequencies of interest to be separately modified. Useful sound information is filtered into frequency bands. This information can then be analyzed for speech patterns and channeled to the appropriate portion of the electrode array. The transmitter, or outer coil, is placed on the mastoid (usually held in place by magnets) and sends the processed signal to the receiver via radio-frequency. The receiver, surgically placed in a well over the mastoid, receives the signal and sends electrical energy to one or many electrodes in the array. The electrode array, which lies within the cochlea, delivers the electric signal to electrodes along its length. The electrical field generated at these locations serves to discharge the neural components of the auditory system. The eighth nerve then conveys this stimulus to the central nervous system which decodes and interprets the signal. Just as important as any of the man-made components is the individual's ability to adjust to, interpret and respond to the electrical stimulus. Length of time spent without sound stimulation of the auditory system, presence or absence of previous experience with sound, personal motivation, community or family support, and opportunities for rehabilitation have been shown to be important factors in achieving a good outcome. These factors are important in understanding significant differences in patient outcomes despite similar preoperative auditory deficits, surgical course, and cochlear implant hardware.

Types of cochlear implants

Cochlear implants differ in the way that they process sound and how they present electricity to the hearing nerve. Other than the speech processing strategies discussed below, there are two different ways of encoding sound information. The first form, analog coding, involves continuous coding of the sound signal with subsequent transfer to the receiver in multiple radio-frequency channels. Electrodes are continuously stimulated. The second form, digital coding, requires sampling of the sound waveform and assigning a number to these "bits" of information. These bits of information are then transferred to the receiver where they are decoded. Electrodes are stimulated in a pulse fashion. Interestingly, neither approach is 100% effective for all implant users. Recently, combining the two schemes has seen some success. Cochlear implants can also be distinguished by their use of single vs. multiple channels, the number of electrodes, and their use of either monopolar or bipolar stimulation. The number of electrodes stimulated with different electrical stimuli determines the "channels" used. In other words, an implant may have multiple electrodes, but if the same information is presented to all the electrodes at one time they are essentially functioning as a single-channel system. In contrast, multi-channel devices provide different information to several electrodes or groups of electrodes. Early implants had only one electrode (and one channel); recent advances have lead to the development of implants with multiple electrodes (22) and multiple channels (usually 4–8). Having more electrodes means that multiple channels can be localized to areas of the cochlea that are most responsive, and stray current that is stimulating adjacent structures (facial nerve, vestibular nerve) can be rerouted.

Cochlear implants can employ monopolar or bipolar stimulation. In a monopolar system there is only one ground electrode for all the others. The ground is usually located at or outside the round window. Thus an electrical field is created from the stimulated electrode to the ground. A bipolar arrangement is such that the ground for each electrode is much closer (adjacent to, or a few electrodes away). In the highly conductive environment of the inner ear, monopolar stimulation results in some limitations. As additional electrodes are stimulated with different streams (channels) of information the electrical fields created by stimulated electrodes may interfere with fields at other sites. This makes it difficult to stimulate more than one electrode at a time, or electrodes that are close together. The bipolar configuration was an attempt to limit this interaction by placing a ground near each electrode such that a smaller field would be created with less interference and more discrete stimulation. Once again, one approach does not achieve satisfaction with all patients. As a result, many implants offer both grounding methods.

Speech processing strategies

There are many different ways of processing the auditory signal for presentation at the level of the cochlear ganglia. The most commonly employed are the spectral peak (SPEAK), continuous interleaved sampling (CIS), and compressed analog stimulation. The SPEAK strategy is characterized by filtering sound into 20 different bands covering the range of 200 Hz to 10,000 Hz. Each filter corresponds to an electrode on the array. The outputs for each filter are analyzed and those channels of highest amplitude that contain speech frequencies are stimulated. The stimulus rate is equal to the period of the lowest frequency of speech (F0). The dominant speech frequency between 280 and 1000 Hz (F1) is then identified and the appropriate apical electrode is stimulated. The dominant speech frequency between 800 and 4000 Hz (F2) is then identified and the appropriate basal electrode is stimulated. Three additional high frequency filters measure input in the 2000–2800 Hz, 2800–4000 Hz, and > 4000 Hz ranges. Stimulus is sent to apical electrodes (in order to take advantage of the greater incidence of ganglion cell survival at the apex of the cochlea). These channels provide additional cues for consonant perception and environmental sounds. Electrodes are stimulated sequentially, and at amplitudes specific for each frequency peak.

The continuous interleaved sampled (CIS) strategy is employed by the Clarion and MED-EL systems. This system works by filtering the speech into eight bands. The bands with the highest amplitude within the speech frequencies are subsequently compressed and their corresponding electrodes are stimulated. The CIS strategy uses high-rate pulsatile stimuli to capture the fine temporal details of speech. The advanced combined encoder (ACE) strategy filters speech into a set number of channels and then selects the highest envelope signals for each cycle of stimulation. Stimulation is carried out in a very rapid fashion (much faster than the SPEAK strategy which stimulates at the rate of the lowest frequency of speech—180–300 cycles/second). The simultaneous analog strategy (SAS) closely mimics the normal ear. All incoming sound is compressed and filtered into eight channels. These channels are then simultaneously and continuously presented to the appropriate tonotopic electrode. There is no effort to select for speech frequencies. Intensity is coded by either stimulus amplitude, rate or both. The SAS strategy has met with limited success, whereas the SPEAK and CIS strategies have been relatively successful. It appears that no one system is effective for all recipients. For this reason, recent advances have made it possible for one cochlear implant to offer several speech processing strategies in the same implant. This allows the audiologist and patient to choose what strategy is best for that individual.

Currently, the Nucleus systems are made to employ several processing strategies. These include spectral peak (SPEAK), advanced combined encoder (ACE), and continuous interleaved sampling (CIS). The Advanced Bionics systems use CIS to stimulate in a monopolar fashion as well as simultaneous analog stimulation (SAS). Medical Electronic (Med-El) produces a product with 12 electrode pairs suitable for deep insertion that relies on the CIS strategy with the most rapid stimulation rate of all implants. Recent advances in technologies have included the development of curved electrode arrays which are intended to more closely approximate the modiolus. Studies seem to indicate that electrodes closer to the basilar membrane need less current to stimulate the nerve and may improve spatial specificity of stimulation.

Indications for cochlear implantation

Bilateral profound cochlear hearing loss unresponsive to amplification by the most powerful hearing aids, is the prime indication for a cochlear implant. All children below the age of 6 years who have congenital or acquired profound hearing loss and who will not benefit from conventional hearing aids and all adults who have lost hearing after acquisition of language are ideal candidates. The only true prerequisite is an intact auditory nerve. Post-lingual candidates do extremely well with an implant and in pre- and peri-lingual candidates, an important factor influencing candidacy is neural plasticity and the emphasis is now on implantation as early as possible to maximize speech understanding and perception. In very young children language acquisition is easier, hence the need for early implantation. Owing to the loss of neural plasticity in older pre-lingually deaf people, the response to implantation may not be optimal and extensive pre-op counseling regarding realistic expectations is crucial.

Today, the indications have expanded to include candidates with low frequency residual hearing and those with severe hearing loss. These expanded indications for implantation are related to age, additional handicaps, residual hearing, and special etiologies of deafness. The minimum age for implantation in children has come down and children as young as 6 months of age have been implanted. Because the cochlea is full size at birth, there is no anatomic difficulty with electrode insertion in very young children.

Medical and radiological criteria have expanded to include significant cochlear abnormalities including additional handicaps, as in Syndromic Deafness. The recent trend is towards bilateral simultaneous or sequential implantation, which provides immense benefits of binaural hearing.

Contraindications for cochlear implantation

Cochlear aplasia, absence of auditory nerves, retrocochlear causes of deafness, central deafness, presence of external or middle ear infections, coexistent severe medical illness are contraindications for cochlear implantation.

Not all patients with sensorineural hearing loss are good candidates for cochlear implantation. For example, patients with pure tone thresholds greater than 90 dB with residual hearing through 2000 Hz often do better with hearing aids than with implantation. Computed tomography findings may also preclude implantation. The absence of the cochlea (Michel deformity), and a small internal auditory canal (associated with cochlear nerve atresia) are contraindications to implantation on that side. Other forms of dysplasia are not necessarily contraindications. However, when implantation of a dysplastic cochlea is to be undertaken informed consent is especially important. Cochlear implants in these patients are associated with increased risk of poor result, CSF leak, and meningitis.

The presence of active middle ear disease is a contraindication to surgery. This process should be treated and resolved before implantation. In a study by Luntz otitis-prone patients were treated by protocol (antibiotics, PETs, etc.) before surgery and then implanted (often with PETs in place). No delay was necessary when compared with patients who were not otitis-prone. Several were noted to have inflamed middle ear mucosa on implantation which required removal in order to identify the round window, but did very well with few postoperative episodes of otitis. Children with a history of chronic suppurative otitis media were implanted in a study by El-Kashlan without demonstrable early or late complications. Patients with a history of canal wall down mastoidectomy may need surgery to reconstruct the posterior canal wall or close off the canal before implantation.

Meningitis may lead to hearing loss and ossification of the cochlea. Labyrinthitis ossificans is usually identifiable on CT scan (brightly lit cochlea with obliteration of the basal cochlear duct) and is a relative contraindication when there is a patent contralateral basal turn. MRI is often better at delineating patency of the cochlea and should be pursued if there is any question. Very young children with hearing loss after meningitis should be followed with CT/MRI until they reach implantable age. Early implantation may be indicated if evidence of ossification is noted. Adults and children with acute meningitis should be treated with steroids to avoid hearing loss. Those that do sustain hearing loss secondary to meningitis should be observed for 6 months before implantation due to the substantial number of patients that will regain their hearing in at least one ear.

Advanced otosclerosis can also cause ossification of the basal turn of the cochlea. This finding is most often noted on CT scan. This is not a contraindication as long as the surgeon is prepared to perform a drill out or pursue implantation into the scala vestibuli. Patients with otosclerosis can achieve excellent results from implantation. A diagnosis of neurofibromatosis II (history of progressive hearing loss and suggestive MRI findings), mental retardation, psychosis, organic brain dysfunction, and unrealistic expectations may also be contra-indications.

Pre-operative assessment

Prior to implantation a basic workup including hematological, chest X-ray, ECG, TORCH screen need to be performed. An audiologic assessment is the primary means of determining implant candidacy. Audiological and electrophysiologic investigations include puretone or behavioral audiometry and impedance audiometry, Otoacoustic Emissions (OAE), Brainstem Evoked Response Audiometry (BERA), Auditory steady state response (ASSR), aided audiometry and a hearing aid benefit evaluation. Promontory stimulation testing can be done in older children and adults to assess the response of the cochlea to electrical stimulation.

High resolution CT scans of the temporal bones are done to plan the surgical route for implantation, identify the vital structures like the facial nerve and promontory and also to rule out any evidence of middle ear disease/mastoiditis. Magnetic Resonance Imaging is the gold standard investigation for the assessment of cochlear anatomy and the vestibulocochlear bundle (Figs. 6.3 and 6.4).

It reveals anomalies like Mondini's and Michel's aplasia, labyrinthitis ossificans, or absent eighth nerve. Rapid advances in genetics and molecular biology are revolutionizing our understanding of congenital deafness and Genetic counseling should

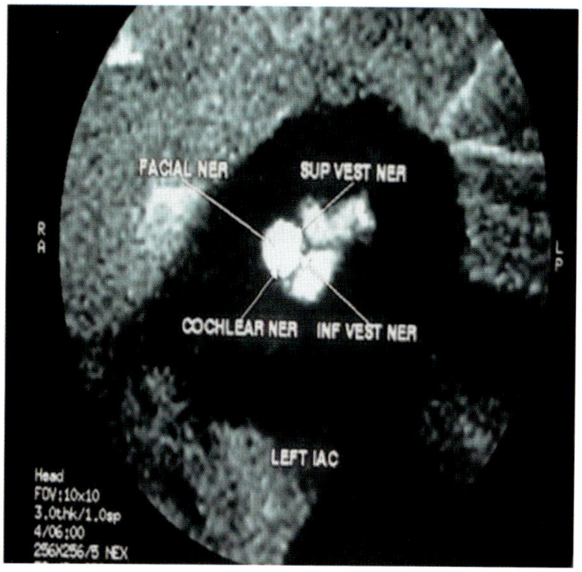

Fig. 11.3. MRI of the internal auditory meatus showing intact cochlear nerve.

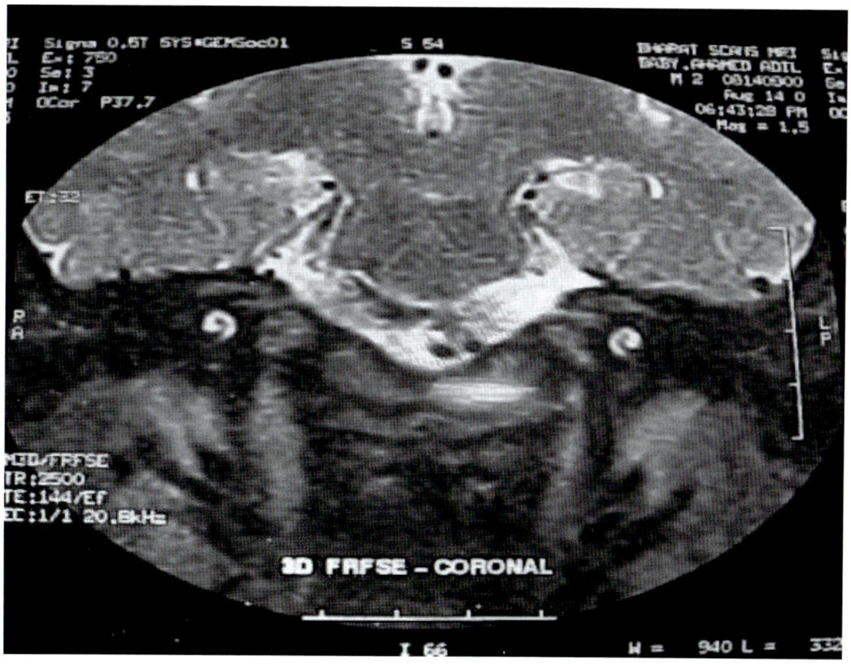

Fig. 11.4. MRI showing bilateral normal fluid-filled coclea – the "Comma" sign.

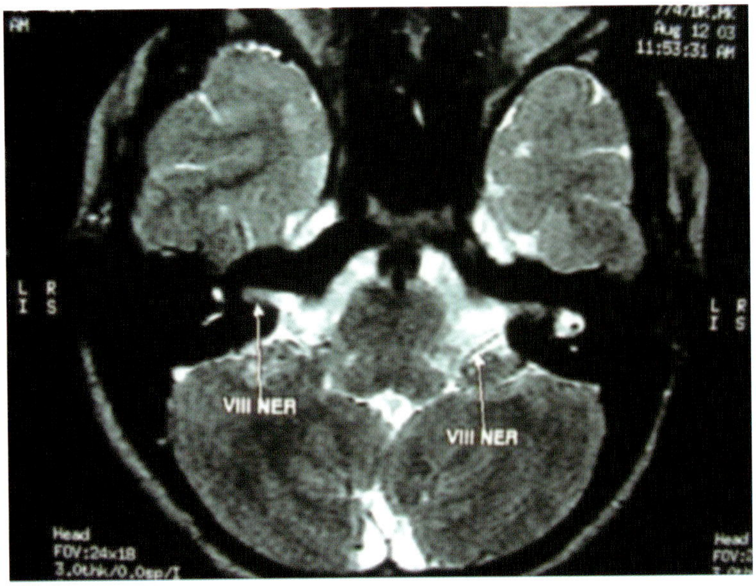

Fig. 11.5. MRI showing bilateral normal vestibulocochlear nerve bundle.

play an important part in prevention. Hence, a genetic specialist's opinion is sought in patients with syndromic etiology of deafness. Children need to get evaluated by a child psychologist for assessment of mental functions and IQ, prior to implantation an ophthalmologist needs to perform a fundus examination to rule out associated visual impairment as seen in Usher's syndrome (Fig. 11.6).

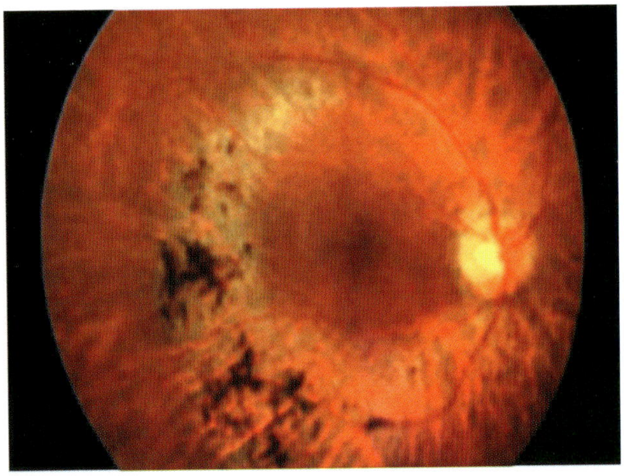

Fig. 11.6. Retinitis pigmentosa in Usher's syndrome.

In children pre-implant meningococcal vaccination is carried out. Pre-op habilitation is important before surgery. Counseling patients and parents prior to implantation to develop realistic expectations of the likely outcome is vital. Hence, candidates and parents need to meet and interact with other cochlear implantees, to have a perspective on the procedure and its outcome.

Cochlear implantation surgical procedure

The goal of cochlear implant surgery is to insert the entire electrode array into the scala tympani with as little damage as possible to the structure of the inner ear. The success of cochlear implantation depends on scrupulous attention to technique at all the various steps of the procedure. Implantation is performed with strict aseptic precautions and is done under general anesthesia. Surgery is essentially the same in children and adults because the anatomic structures are of adult configuration at birth. However, in very young children, there is a slightly increased risk of facial palsy and hypovolemic shock due to blood loss.

The steps of surgery are as follows: Usually an extended post-auricular incision is made to expose the mastoid cortex. The incision should be made more than 1 cm away from the location of the coil of the implant. The mastoid is drilled out to expose the mastoid antrum. Saucerization of the cavity is not done. Posterior tympanotomy is performed, the facial recess is opened and the promontory and round window niche are exposed, without exposing the facial nerve. A well for receiver-stimulator is fashioned in the skull behind the mastoid cavity using a template as a guide and a groove is made to connect it to the mastoid cavity (Fig. 11.7).

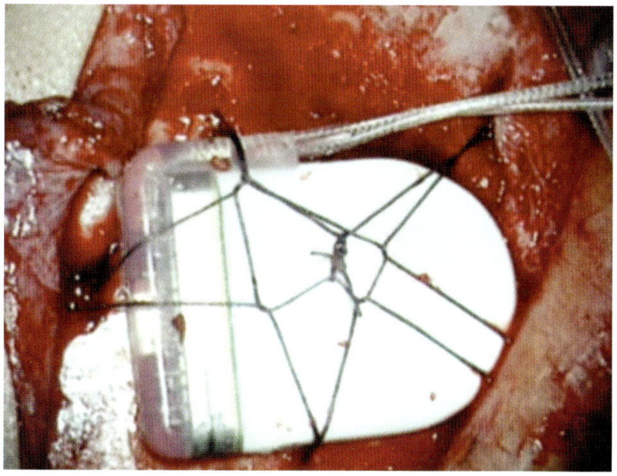

Fig. 11.7. CI Receiver-stimulator coil in-situ.

Tie-down holes are made on either side of the well for securing the implant. Cochleostomy is done at the basal turn of the cochlea which is opened anterior to the round window to make the axis of introduction of the electrode array straight (Fig. 11.8). The electrode array is inserted atraumatically into the scala tympani using a claw. Alternatively, a round window insertion may be performed after drilling out the anterior lip of the RW niche and adequately exposing the secondary tympanic membrane. Once the electrodes are inserted, diathermy should not be used. Fixation of the device and electrode array and wound closure is done. Electrophysiological testing – impedance telemetry,

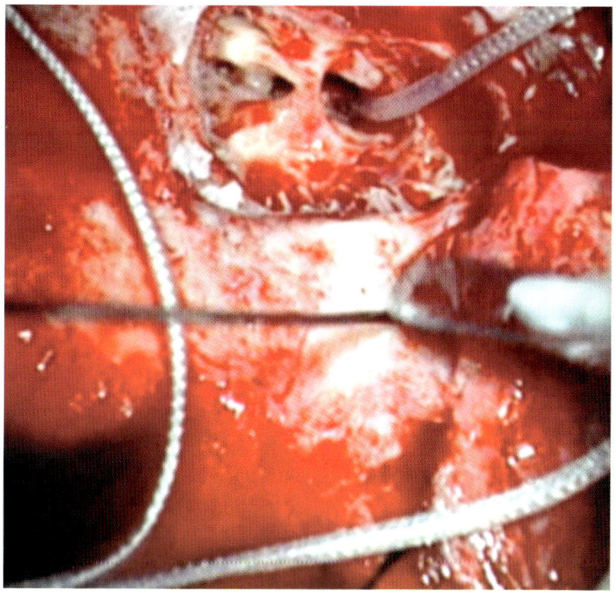

Fig. 11.8. CI electrodes array in-situ.

neural response telemetry and electrically evoked stapedial reflex thresholds are performed intra-operatively to confirm the optimal performance of the implant in-situ. This assures the implant team that the device is functioning and that the patient is receiving an auditory stimulus and responding appropriately.

Postoperative management

The surgical complication rate after cochlear implantation is estimated to be less than 5%. The most common problems are wound infection and wound breakdown. Rarely, extrusion of the device, facial nerve injury, bleeding, CSF leaks and meningitis can occur. Device-related complications include intracochlear damage, slippage of the array, breakage of the implant, and improper or inadequate insertion. Postoperative infection of the surgical site was treated by prolonged courses of antibiotics by Yu, et al. with excellent results. They suggest that a long course of antibiotics and limited I&D will treat the vast majority of wound infections without the need to remove the implant. Those patients that did not respond to this treatment protocol were often found to be immuno-compromised. Steenerson reported a 75% incidence of postoperative vertigo, but indicated that these patients did well after undergoing vestibular therapy. Other series do not show as high an incidence, nor the need for vestibular rehabilitation postoperatively. Stimulation of the facial or vestibular nerve by stray electrical current from electrodes outside or near the round window has also been reported. This is usually addressed by "turning off" the responsible electrodes and moving the electrical stimulation to electrodes located within the cochlea.

Recent reports of increased incidence of meningitis in cochlear implant recipients have prompted the CDC to recommend vaccination of implanted or soon to be implanted patients. Children less than 2 years old who have implants should receive pneumococcal conjugate vaccine (Prevnar). Children with implants 2 years and older who have completed the conjugate series should receive one dose of the pneumococcal poly-saccharide vaccine (Pneumovax 23 or Pnu-Imune 23). Children with implants between 24 and 59 months who have never received vaccination should receive two doses of pneumococcal conjugate vaccine two months apart and then one dose of pneumococcal polysaccharide vaccine at least two months later. Finally, persons age 5 years and older with cochlear implants should receive one dose of pneumococcal polysaccharide vaccine.

Although the incidence of device failure is very low, occasionally removal of the implant and reimplantation is necessary. These patients do surprisingly well. Alexiades, et al. showed that patients did as well or better after reimplantation (in the same ear) as with their first implant. Thus a history of implantation is not a contraindication to another cochlear implant. Long-term electrical stimulation from a cochlear implant has raised concern for damage to the auditory nerve. However, cochlear implants typically discharge less than one microcoulombs per square cm of electrode surface and long-term studies have shown no detrimental effects. In fact, studies following patients for up to 13 years show no decline in function. This finding is still true when the study population includes those that have been implanted multiple times. Research looking at cochlear implants under many environmental strains has shown them to be reliable and safe. Backous, et al. showed them to be stable when exposed to extreme barometric pressure changes (as experienced when scuba diving). MRI exposure should be avoided generally, but may be pursued when necessary.

Complications of cochlear implantation

Major complications include facial palsy, implant exposure due to flap loss and wound infection. Other complications include facial nerve stimulation, device failure, deterioration of hearing, tinnitus, temporary balance problems, numbness of scalp, loss of taste, electrode/device extrusion, CSF leak and meningitis.

Switch-on and mapping of cochlear implant

11

The switch-on and speech processor tuning is done 3 weeks after surgery. Mapping is done at periodic intervals till a stable map is achieved. Frequent mapping sessions are required and prolonged and intensive (re)habilitation after implantation is essential. Habilitation aims at improving receptive language skills and expressive skills. The habilitation program is started out based on baseline skills of the patient, periodical assessments of outcome needs to be done in terms of environmental sound, open set, closed set speech, speech discrimination and telephonic conversation. The recommended period for auditory verbal habilitation is 1 year.

Measuring level of performance

The outcomes of cochlear implantation are measured using the Category of Auditory Performance (CAP) and Speech Intelligibility Rating (SIR) scores, described by O'Donoghue et al., 1999. The extent of the auditory perception in terms of utility of auditory mechanisms to pursue day to day tasks from awareness of environmental sounds to making telephonic conversations and the ability to discriminate and understand speech with or without lip reading are assessed through CAP scores. SIR scores measure the outcome of cochlear implantation with respect to speech, measuring the intelligibility of speech and the quality, which might be recognizable by the listener. The overall outcomes need to be categorized accordingly, taking into account the number of months taken to achieve the necessary CAP and SIR scores.

Outcomes of cochlear implantation

The success of a CI program is directly dependent on its ability to address the issue of patient expectations and balance it with the outcomes. A multidisciplinary approach is required involving the ENT surgeon, audiologist, speech therapist, auditory verbal habilitationist, child psychologist and pediatrician. The patients and their family must also be highly motivated for the implant. Variables affecting the outcome of CI in children are the duration and etiology of deafness, age at onset of deafness, pre-implant amplification history, communication mode, age at implantation, type of speech processor used and duration of implant usage. In very young children, language acquisition is easier and hence the need for early implantation. Owing to the loss of neural plasticity in older pre-lingual deaf people, the response to implantation may not be optimal and extensive pre-op counseling regarding realistic expectations is vital. Factors influencing the overall outcomes are the transparency of the program, expertise of the team, patient motivation, family support and facilities for rehabilitation.

Although the perception of a successful implantation might vary from patient to patient, the primary goal of implantation has always been improved speech perception. Since implantation began, physicians have noted a wide range of outcomes. Some patients find little benefit after implantation and may even find the stimulation annoying. Others are able to function normally even without visual cues. Still others are able to listen to and enjoy music. Years of research has given us a better understanding of what variables might influence the results of implantation. The age of onset of deafness, as well as the length of time since the onset of hearing loss has both been shown to influence outcomes. Several studies have shown that patients who were pre-lingually deafened show the poorest outcome. Prelingually deaf children implanted before age 6 appear to be able to "catch up" to implanted postlingually deaf children within 2–5 years. These children, like their postlingual counterparts, are able to achieve open-set speech discrimination. Several studies have shown that implantation at an earlier age results in earlier achievement of open-set speech discrimination.

Govaerts, et al. showed that 90% of those implanted before age 2 were integrated into mainstream education whereas only 20–30% of those implanted after age 4 were ever integrated. These results are seen in children who are enrolled in aural/oral educational programs and who use oral language as their primary communication modality. The performance of implanted children is far better than those with equal hearing deficits who rely on vibrotactile devices or hearing aids. Generally, implantation of prelingually deaf adolescents and adults is significantly less successful, though results vary widely. Most authors now believe that the shorter the period of auditory deprivation, the faster and more complete will be the achievement of open-set speech discrimination. This has been shown to be true in the adult population, as well with children. Those patients who are implanted within a short time seem to retain the plasticity of the auditory system better than those who have been deaf for a period of years. Sharma, et al. compared children implanted after different periods of deafness. They showed that children with the shortest amount of time spent without auditory stimuli regained normal cortical responses more rapidly than all others. Specifically, those with 3.5 years of deafness or less showed age-appropriate P1 latencies (a marker of plasticity) after only 6 months of stimulation with a cochlear implant. The length of time required to reach age-appropriate latencies increased with increasing length of auditory deprivation. After age of 6 years, plasticity was greatly reduced.

Waltzman, et al. studied the long-term effects of cochlear implants in children. They followed the children after implantation for five to fifteen years and documented speech perception scores, device extrusion rates, and implant viability. They showed that implantation resulted in significant improvement of patient's speech perception and that this benefit remained stable (often improving) over the long-term. For the vast majority of the study group this resulted in assimilation into mainstream education. There was no significant incidence of device extrusion or migration and even when device failure necessitated reimplantation, long-term performance was not decreased. Recent studies looking at the economics of cochlear implants show cochlear implantation improves patient's quality of life and is cost-effective even in elderly patients (> 50 years old). Implantation results in significant benefit to the society as a whole, and to the individual. Unfortunately, cochlear implantation is more often a money-losing effort for everyone involved with implantation. Hospitals and physicians, as well as the other members of the rehabilitation team often find themselves without funding and support.

Difficult scenarios in cochlear implantation

With increasing experience in cochlear implantation, the indications for implant surgery have widened to include cochlear anomalies, syndromic associations and multiple handicapped individuals. Implantation is beneficial in such situations. However, the surgeon must anticipate challenges during implantation and also, the subsequent habilitation may be challenging.

Cochlear implantation in labyrinthitis ossificans

A common abnormality encountered is the ossified cochlea, mostly occurring as a post-meningitic sequelae, although other pathologies may predispose to ossification, including otosclerosis, chronic otitis media, ototoxicity, autoimmunity, trauma and others. This remains one of the significant surgical challenges for the otologist. It is diagnosed with a CT/MRI scan. Often the ossification is incomplete and if the surgeon drills forward along the basal coil for 4–5 mm the scala tympani will be identified. Care must be taken to avoid injury to the carotid artery which lies just anterior to the cochlea. In some cases of cochlear dysplasia CSF gushers have been encountered. This is managed by allowing the pressured fluid to drain off, and then proceeding with insertion as per routine. On confirmation of an obstructed basal turn, the proximal turn is drilled with a microdrill to a depth of 6–8 mm until an open lumen is discovered and the electrode array is inserted. In total ossification, a complete drill-out of the basal turn is required and the implanted array is seated in a trough that surrounds the modiolus. A double-array implant may be used with some electrodes into the basal turn and others into the second turn.

Cochlear implantation in Mondini's deformity/ large vestibular aqueduct syndrome

CSF leak during cochleostomy has to be sealed. A variety of techniques may be used to help control the flow of CSF including firm plugging of the cochleostomy using soft tissue coupled with reducing the flow of CSF by lumbar drainage and IV mannitol drip, if necessary. Such leaks may also be encountered in cases of enlarged vestibular aqueduct.

Auditory neuropathy/auditory dys-synchrony spectrum disorder (AN/ADSD)

Normal outer hair cell (OHC) function and dys-synchronous neural responses characterize this disorder. Patients will show a normal OAE with absent BERA waveforms, which is pathognomonic of this condition. Cochlear implants are a viable management option for patients with AN/ADSD and are beneficial in bypassing the desynchronous neural network, but the outcomes may be sub-optimal or guarded and the family needs to be counseled regarding the same.

Cochlear implantation in multi-handicapped individuals

11

Early diagnosis and rehabilitation of deafness and additional handicaps is crucial. An implant helps in the rehabilitation of deafness and other handicaps as well. However, patient selection criteria must be stringent. The decision to pursue implantation should be as fully informed as possible. Evaluation, surgical intervention, and post-implantation management of these patients can be challenging. Long-term intensive rehabilitation is essential after implantation. Jervell and Lange-Nielsen syndrome represents a rare cause of congenital hearing loss. Because of the potential for cardiac arrhythmias and sudden death, additional risks are involved in cochlear implantation. There is an early need for cochlear implantation in Usher's syndrome wherein the child is born deaf-blind and CI needs to be performed before the onset of complete blindness due to retinitis pigmentosa. Audtiory verbal habilitation is an immense task for these deaf-blind children and requires intense skill and motivation from the audiologist, therapist and parents.

Minimally invasive cochlear implantation

Due to improvements in cochlear implant technology, smaller and more powerful implantable cochlear implants have evolved which has enabled smaller external incisions, smaller skin flaps, shortened surgical time and faster healing. Current techniques in cochleostomy (Peep-hole Cochleostomy) and round window electrode insertion (soft insertion) have resulted in preservation of residual hearing. Unfortunately, peep-hole cochleostomy, sometimes called soft surgery, has occasionally led to mis-insertion of electrodes into the scala media and scala vestibuli because of lack of proper visualization and control.

Cochlear endoscopy

Cochlear endoscopy was first described by Balkany & colleagues (1990) who used flexible fiberoptic microendoscopes (0.7–1 mm diameter) (Fig. 11.9). Currently, the indications for cochlear endoscopy are limited and it is not recommended routinely during CI. The present indications are visualization of obstructed segments of the cochlea in labyrinthitis ossificans and the interior of the cochlea in cochlear dysplasia. Visualization of the interior of the cochlea

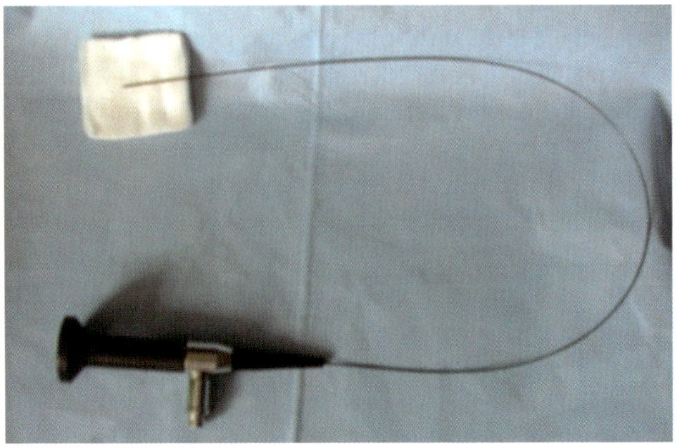

Fig. 11.9. Cochlear endoscope

will help in pre-insertion assessment as well as to verify proper insertion of the implant.

Perimodiolar and mid-scalar cochlear implantation

These implants are assumed to have a slightly enhanced speech perception. After the electrodes are inserted into the cochlea, the stylet is withdrawn and the electrodes come into a peri-modiolar/mid-scalar position. The electrode – neural interface seems to be minimal in this position and hence clarity of auditory inputs are much better.

Bilateral cochlear implantation

Bilateral CI has significant benefits which include improved speech perception in noisy environments and improved sound localization. Patients receive elimination of head-shadow effect and obtain significant benefits from summation effects (improvement in hearing threshold from redundant information presented to each ear) and squelch effects (improvement in hearing threshold from brainstem processing of inter-aural time and intensity differences). Speech perception in noise with bilateral implantation is significantly better than unilateral implantation and continues to improve even upto 24 months after implantation. Thus patients may be able to neurally integrate inputs from both implants to enhance speech perception over time. Further improvements in performance are to be expected with a greater understanding of the neural pathways and integration of binaural hearing along with improvements in implant programming and technology.

Electroacoustic stimulation (EAS)/ hybrid implants

One of the latest applications of implantable hearing technology combines electric and acoustic stimulation (EAS) into a hybrid device designed for individuals with binaural low-frequency hearing and severe-to-profound high-frequency hearing loss (Fig. 11.10).

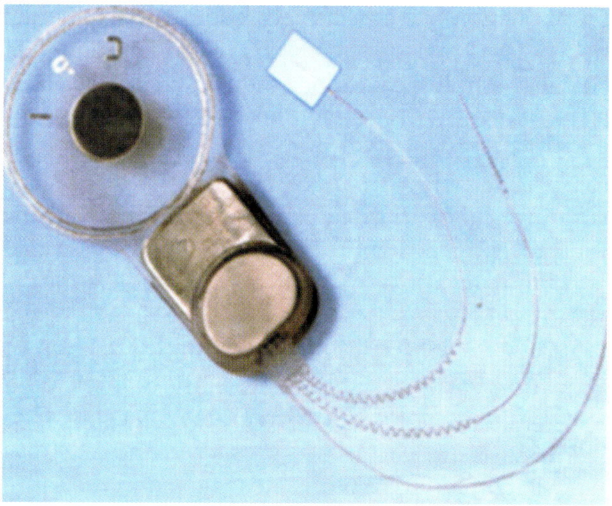

Fig. 11.10. CI double electrode array.

Indications for EAS

Currently, 15 million people worldwide fall into this group who would benefit from the hybrid hearing technology. Electroacoustic stimulation is the latest strategy conceptualized for residual hearing preservation in the implanted ear, in order to provide combined electrical stimulation and acoustic hearing for candidates with bilateral high frequency severe to profound sensorineural hearing loss. The addition of the electrical stimulation to such patients with existing residual low frequency hearing can provide clear speech recognition in background noise and better appreciation of musical notes.

The audiological candidacy criteria for EAS or hybrid technology vary somewhat across manufacturers. Low-frequency thresholds generally can range from 20 dB HL up to 60 dB HL through 750 Hz, and thresholds at 1000 Hz and above must generally exceed 60 to 70 dB HL. Preoperative speech perception criteria require that aided CNC monosyllabic word recognition score in the ear to be implanted cannot exceed 50%–60%. After surgery, the average low-frequency hearing loss ranges from 10 to 20 dB, depending on the electrode array and nature of the surgical technique. Some individuals, however, have a more significant loss of low-frequency acoustic hearing in the implanted ear ranging from > 20 dB to total loss of hearing.

Literature has shown that individuals with binaural high frequency hearing loss may not gain significant benefit from traditional hearing amplification. Possible reasons for the lack of amplification benefit is the presence of cochlear dead regions, which are more common with thresholds above 70 dB HL and the high levels required to make high-frequency speech audible may, in fact, degrade the signal. Although these individuals may not obtain much benefit from high-frequency amplification, their relatively good low-frequency hearing may disqualify them from conventional cochlear implant candidacy. As a result, individuals with good low-frequency hearing and severe-to-profound high-frequency hearing loss can experience significant difficulty in everyday communication, particularly in noisy backgrounds, where low-frequency information alone is not sufficient to allow high levels of speech understanding.

In 1999, Christoph Von Ilberg published the first article on cochlear implantation in a patient who still had considerable low frequency hearing. The low frequency hearing was preserved and a CI was used in combination with a hearing aid in the same ear. Results showed that acoustic stimulation of the low frequencies and added CI stimulation had a synergistic effect on outcomes which led to excellent speech perception, particularly in noise. In recent times, implant surgeons are employing soft surgical techniques which include a smaller cochleostomy or round window insertion performed gently with thinner electrode arrays and/or perimodiolar electrodes (atraumatic cochlear insertion) which contributes to hearing preservation with standard cochlear implants. The hybrid device uses a shortened cochlear implant electrode array that is inserted just 10 mm – 20 mm into the cochlea (versus 20 mm – 30 mm for a conventional implant), covering the basal 2/3rd of the cochlea. A successful surgical outcome allows for monaural electric stimulation of the basal cochlea for high-frequency information without damaging apical cochlear structures that transmit low-frequency acoustic information. This combination allows for the integration of electric and acoustic perception in the same ear.

Components of hybrid implant

The EAS system consists of two parts: a cochlear implant with a soft and flexible electrode array for preservation of residual low frequency hearing, and a speech processor which combines the cochlear implant component with conventional acoustic stimulation in one comfortable and compact device. EAS patients wear an in-the-ear (ITE) hearing aid in the implanted ear (which can amplify sound signals upto 43 dB acoustical gain) in combination with an external ear-level or body-worn speech processor or an integrated hearing aid/speech processor on the implanted side (Fig. 11.11).

The hybrid implant has a specialized microphone competent for parallel processing of sounds. The acoustic and electric digital sound processing components of the EAS processor receive sound signals from this single microphone. The parallel processing of these signals is performed separately and optimized for both acoustic stimulation (focusing on low frequency hearing) and cochlear implant stimulation (focusing on high frequency hearing). This microphone automatically adjusts to incoming sounds in order to capture all the vital cues necessary for understanding speech clearly without requiring special programming or the use

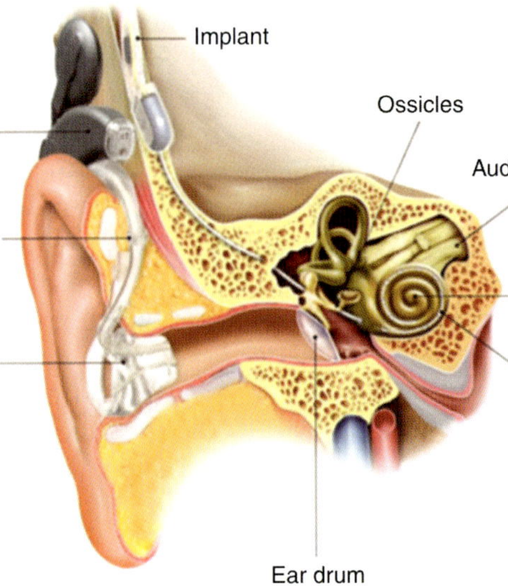

Fig. 11.11. The MedEl EAS system.

11

of a switch to shuffle between the two modes of hearing.

Benefits of hybrid hearing

Patients with a non-progressive, mild to moderate low frequency hearing loss combined with a profound hearing loss in high frequencies are ideal candidates for EAS. A recent study compared the speech perception performance for monosyllabic CNC word recognition for listeners using the EAS system. All the subjects had similar degrees of pre- and post-implant hearing loss, configurations, etiologies, and duration of deafness. Cochlear implant recipients without acoustic hearing served as the control group. Results proved that EAS recipients performed better than conventional, long-electrode cochlear implant recipients. Bimodal hearing yielded higher levels of performance than conventional unilateral cochlear implantees. Monosyllabic word recognition performance for hybrid recipients was comparable to standard unilateral implant recipients; however, hybrid patients using a hearing aid on the other ear have two acoustic-hearing ears, a condition that may provide real-world binaural benefits. Studies performed to assess the average speech understanding of monosyllables with EAS in comparison to results with hearing aid use, show that after one year of experience with the EAS system, the users achieved a speech score of 75%, which means, 3 out of 4 monosyllables in quiet were understood correctly.

Research efforts are underway presently redefining the EAS/hybrid hearing system, to determine the appropriate length of the array, number of intracochlear electrodes, mapping strategy, long-term stability of the residual hearing, spectral range for amplification and preoperative audiological and speech perception criteria, to provide a balance between maximizing post-operative performance, with minimal loss of low-frequency hearing. Plenty of data is emerging on the outcomes of EAS globally at present and the potential positive implications for preserving binaural residual hearing, has now been fully understood.

The Indian scenario

Difficulties in the Indian context have been mainly the prohibitive cost, the problems of introducing a radical technology in a developing country and logistic difficulties. The dilemma of balancing such an advanced technology, with the requirements of a developing country still largely remains. The hurdle begins right at the inception of the CI program, with problems in initiating a program due to limited resources and expertise (Surgeon/Audiologist/AVT unit) with open resistance to the concept of AV therapy.

Two successful models of the CI program have developed in India. The Chennai model echoes the international model wherein all wings of CI program such as surgery, audiology and AV therapy lie under one roof and the patient gets the surgery and habilitation at the same center. This model has the advantage of having more integration among the various professionals dealing with the patient. This concept of a self-sustaining, comprehensive CI program with surgery, audiology and auditory verbal therapy all under one roof was introduced in 1997 at Madras ENT Research Foundation (MERF), Chennai and has worked successfully since then. The Mumbai model, on the other hand, has independant units with the surgeon, audiologist and AV therapist acting as seperate entities. Here the surgeon passes over the patient to AV therapist after surgery, to take over the habilitation of the patient at his centre where the audiologist visits for switch-on and mapping as required. This Mumbai model to some extent dilutes the responsibility of the surgeon. The advantage of this model is that no major capital investment is necessary from any single center and seems to be preferred by most private clinics.

Unique challenges in Indian CI program

Certain individual challenges are unique to the Indian context. First is the distance between CI facilities or between the CI clinics and the patient's residence. This problem of distance has now been bridged by establishing satellite centres with telemedicine facility, for interaction with the parent clinic by video-conferencing and by developing habilitation packages for patients to train at home. Second is the problem faced in creating uniform habilitation facilities for a multilingual society. This multilingual barrier has proved to be a much bigger challenge than the distance issue, with a plethora of languages posing a unique set of challenges to our auditory verbal therapists. Speech material and other habilitation material have had to be developed in several Indian languages. Bearing in mind the extreme paucity of qualified and trained auditory verbal therapists, the task seems to be daunting. Thus the need of the hour is a "Lingual Map", which needs to be charted for uniform habilitation of various implantees, in their own mother-tongues with the child's parents themselves forming an active and integral part of AV therapy.

In India, it is estimated that there are 1 million potential implantees and the major problem remains the cost factor. The cost-utility ratio (cost per quality adjusted life year) of cochlear implants has been extensively studied here as elsewhere, and it is more than apparent that in relation to several other medical and surgical interventions, cochlear implantation is extremely cost effective and has significant quality-of-life-benefits. The overall cost of the basic implant in India, including surgery and post-implant habilitation (for one year) is approximately Rs 6 lakhs, and for the more advanced contour implant, the total cost will be Rs 10 lakhs. While the cost of the implant is decided by the manufacturer and is paid directly to them, the entire surgical and habilitation package for one year is in the range of Rs 100 thousand, which is extremely low as compared to other centres abroad. Although cost-effectiveness of the implant cannot be disputed, the real issue is in coming up with the total payment upfront. The cost of the implant, surgery and habilitation represents a lifetime saving of a Class-I Govt officer. As many parents are ready to part with their lifetime savings in the interest of their children, the responsibility of the surgeon becomes enormous with a virtually 0% error margin.

However, there have been promising developments in the area of funding. The Government funds implants for the Armed Forces and their families. Certain Government run industries and banks cover the cost of the implant and surgery for their employees and their dependants. Despite these developments, over 90% of the population is still not covered by any medical insurance or bank loans. To help these patients with raising of the necessary funds, some banks have come forward with special schemes with low interest, long-term loans and policies. The scenario is still very fluid and constantly changing in this regard. However, it is heartening to know that solutions are being worked out in this front at present.

To face all the above issues head on, the Cochlear Implant Group of India (CIGI) was started in 2003, bringing under its umbrella the various professionals like surgeons, audiologists and auditory-verbal therapists. This group has set for itself an ambitious agenda of voluntary self-regulation to ensure that uniform standards are maintained in all the various CI programs in India. The CIGI has brought out a Consensus document on various issues pertaining to cochlear implantation in India. It has initiated several new CI clinics of universal standard all over the country with comprehensive training of the surgeons, audiologists and auditory verbal therapists in the various aspects of this program. It has also taken upon itself the role of conducting workshops and training the professionals since 2003. This has worked out very well, with 20 individual teams of surgeons, audiologists and AV therapists participating in the hands-on training last year at Chennai.

The initial resistance to CI has been replaced by a frank desire on the part of most surgeons to get into the CI bandwagon. Paradoxically, this has created its own problem, with many CI clinics opening without the necessary infrastructure. CIGI, has therefore brought out a Consensus document on various issues pertaining to cochlear implantation in India, stating the minimum desirable and requisite facilities for initiating a CI program. It is the hope of CIGI that all CI companies will respect and support these norms without looking at the commercial angle alone, bearing in mind the long-term interest of patients. Cochlear implantation in a developing country like India has posed its own set of unique challenges. Despite these several hurdles, the Indian cochlear implant scenario is very much on the upward trail, with an exponential growth in the number of CI clinics and implants being done every year. The major hurdle for these clinics is to overcome the cost factor and habilitation difficulties in a multilingual society, while preserving the uniform international standards of CI programs around the world. The overall outcomes from several clinics around India have been largely gratifying, since they adhere to the international CI program norms well. It is vital for such clinics to actively interact and exchange their cumulative experiences for advancing the Indian CI program to the highest level. Only such a cohesive, comprehensive and integral team approach by all professionals can yield a useful and productive outcome. As cochlear implant surgery and technology continue to evolve, the future is towards fully implantable devices, improved speech coding strategies and cochlear hair cell and auditory nerve growth factors integrated within an implant. Such implants coming into the market at subsidized rates will aptly serve the needs of a large developing country like India.

Future directions in cochlear implantation

Auditory neural prosthesis has become highly successful in restoring normal hearing to profoundly deaf individuals. Partial insertion cochlear implantation has been proposed as treatment for those patients who have residual low-frequency hearing with high-frequency sensorineural hearing loss. Other implant strategies include brainstem implantation for those without an intact cochlear nerve. Good results have been reported. Bilateral cochlear implants are expected to help patients with clear sound localization, music appreciation and speech comprehension in noise. A new "minimally invasive" approach which allows for cochlear implantation through a small (5 cm) incision over the post-auricular area is on the vogue and initial results are satisfactory using this technique. Cochlear implant surgery and technology continue to evolve. In the future, fully implanted devices (like the TIKI prototype), improved speech coding strategies, cochlear hair cell and nerve growth factors used in conjunction with an implant may be available.

CONCLUSION

Cochlear implant is the most significant advancement of 21st century in the field of otology. Sensorineural hearing loss is one of the most common congenital anomalies which affect children worldwide and causing severe to profound degree of handicap, which is considered as social stigma in our society. Pre-operative diagnosis, patient counselling and postoperative speech therapy are important parts of cochlear implant surgery. It helps to restore hearing by integration of an external circuitry with peripheral apparatus and central circuitry of the brain; electronically it stimulates the cochlea/auditory nerve and higher auditory centres in the brain. This chapter is designed to know about indication, components, surgical techniques, habilitation/rehabilitation protocols and overall outcomes of cochlear implantation surgery.

SUGGESTED READING

1. Cochlear Implants. Textbook by Susan Waltzmann & Noel L. Cohen (Thieme Publishers, 2000).
2. Miyamoto, Richard and Kirk, Karen, Cochlear implants. In Bailey, Byron (ed). Head and Neck Surgery – Otolaryngology, 3rd edition. Philadelphia, Lippincott-Raven, 2001, pp. 1949–59.
3. Osberger MJ. Cochlear implantation in children under 2 years. Candidacy considerations. *Otolaryngol Head Neck Surg*, 1997; 117: 145–8.
4. Tyler RS, Dunn CC, Witt SA, et al. Update of bilateral cochlear implantation. Current Opinion. *Otolaryngol Head Neck Surg*, 2003; 11: 388–93.
5. Charles C, Santina D, Lustig LR. Surgically implantable hearing aids. Cummings Otolaryngology: Head and Neck Surgery, 2007, 4th edition, Vol. 4, pg 3579.
6. Kiefer J, Pok M, Adunka O, Stuerzebecher E, Baumgartner WD, and Schmidt M. Combined electric and acoustic stimulation of the auditory system: results of a clinical study. *Audiol Neuro-Otol*, 2005; 10: 134–44.
7. Kartush JM et al. Cochlear Implantation. Am Acad Otolaryngol Head & Neck Surg Foundation, Inc. Alexandria, VA, 1994.
8. Toh EH, Luxford WM. Cochlear and brainstem implantation. *Otolaryngol Clin North Am*, 2002; 35(2): 325–42.
9. Francis HW. Impact of coclear implants on the functional health status of older adults. *Laryngoscope*, 2002; 112 (8): 1482–8.
10. Sharma A, Dorman MF, Spahr A. A sensitive period for the development of the central auditory system in children with cochlear implants: Implication for age of implantation. *Ear & Hearing*, 2002; 23(6): 532–9.
11. O'Donoghue GM, Nikolopoulos TP. Minimal access surgery for pediatric cochlear implantation. *Otol Neurol*, 2002; 23(6): 891–4.
12. Govaerts P J, DeBeukelaer K, Deceulaer G, Yerman M, Somers T, Schatteman I, Offeciers FE. Outcome of cochlear implantation at different ages from 0 to 6 years. *Otol Nuerotol*, 2002; 23(6): 885–90.
13. Truy E, Ionescu E, Ceruse P, Gallego S. The binaural digisonic cochlear implant: surgical technique. *Otol Neurotol*, 2002; 23(5): 704–9.
14. Schramm D, Fitzpatrick E, Sequin C. Cochlear implantation for adolescents and adults with prelinguistic deafness. *Otol Neurotol*, 2002; 23(5): 698–703.
15. Sharma A, Dorman MF, Spahr AJ. Rapid development of cortical auditory evoked potentials after early cochlear implantation. *Neurol Report*, 2002; 13(10): 1365–8.

16. Backous DD, Dunford RG, Segel PM, Christnes C, Paul HNB. Effects of hyperbaric exposure on the integrity of the internal components of commercially available cochlear implant systems. *Otol Neurotol,* 2002; 23(4): 463–7.
17. Hassanzandeh S, Farhadi M, Daneshi A, Emamdjomeh H. The effects of age on auditory speech perception development in cochlear-implanted prelingually deaf children. *Otolaryngol Head Neck Surg,* 2002; 126(5): 524–7.
18. Waltzman S B, Cohen NL, Green J, Roland JD. Long-term effects of cochlear implants in children. *Otolaryngol Head Neck Surg,* 2002; 126(5): 505–11.
19. Gantz B J, Tyler RS, Rubinstein JT, Wolaver A, Lowderm M, Abbas P, et al. Binaural cochlear implants placed during the same operation. *Otol Neurotol,* 2002; 23(2):169–80.
20. Patel AK, Barkdul G, Doherty JK. Cochlear implantation in chronic suppurative otitis media. *Operative Technique Otolaryngol,* 2010; 21: 254–60.

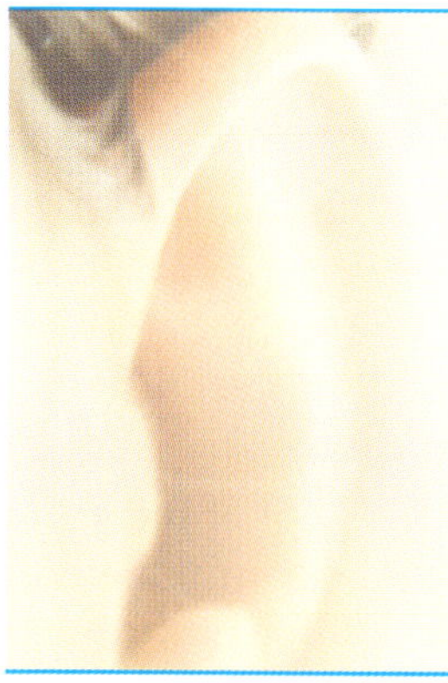

CHAPTER 12

Otoplasty

P.S. Bhandari

The external ear enjoys a special place in society all over the world. It is meant to be flaunted and adorned. Ear piercing is routine, with a range of jewellery pieces concentrating in enhancing its natural beauty. Persons with deformed ears have to limit their range of hairstyles. There is a definite need to reconstruct the deformed ear of both sexes (Figs. 12.1 and 12.2).

Total ear reconstruction is one of the most difficult problems faced by a plastic or ENT surgeon because of multiple stages of reconstruction, prolonged hospitalization and high cost. Multiple staged reconstructions make it prone to complication. Even a small complication at any stage can completely change the total outcome in ear reconstruction. It needs total dedication, long experience, artistic skill and high level of craftsmanship to carve out an ear framework out of costal cartilage. This is difficult to achieve. With the pioneering work of Tanzer, Brent, and others great advancements have been made in ear reconstruction.

Two basic raw materials which are required for ear reconstruction are:

1. Framework
2. Draping skin/cover

Framework

Quality framework made up of silastic and porous polyethylene (Mdpor. Porex, College Park) are available in the market. Cronin et al. used a commercially available silastic framework for ear reconstruction with good results. But its use has gone down tremendously because of high incidence of infection and extrusion. A polyethylene framework is a new material and has shown promising results. The porous polyethylene framework becomes rapidly vascularized with soft tissue in-growth and collagen deposition. But, long follow-up and more work is required to establish it as a viable alternative to costal cartilage for ear framework which is tissue of the choice for ear reconstruction. Although, in patient who have calcified rib cartilage or in patients with inadequate costal cartilage, porous polyethylene can be a viable alternative for ear framework.

Draping skin/cover

Cover to be used for framework depends upon the quality and quantity of skin available in the auricular region. If the skin in the auricular region is healthy, then it is the tissue of choice to be used as cover. If the skin is not available due to scarring then the temporoparietal facial flap is used to cover the framework.

The ear is approximately 85% grown by the age of 4 years so theoretically ear reconstruction can be started at the age of 4–5 years, but the author is of opinion that it should be deferred till the age of 10 years when sufficient costal cartilage is available for quality framework fabrication.

Ear reconstruction is done in four stages. In the first stage, ear framework is implanted in the auri-

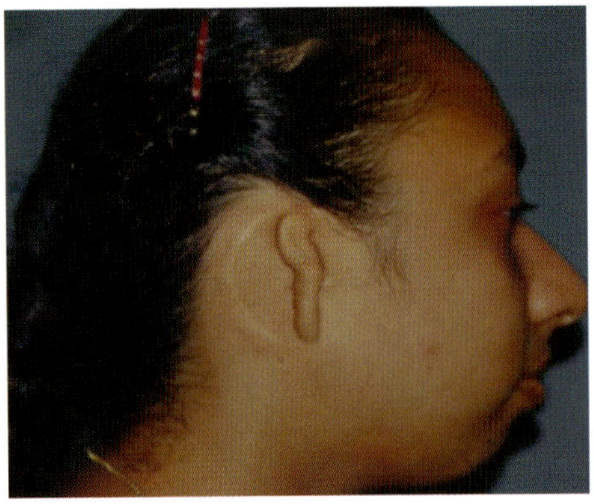

Fig. 12.1. Microtia preoperative.

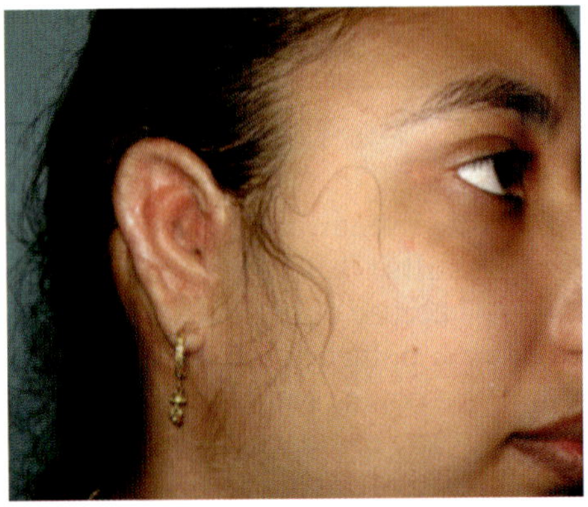

Fig. 12.2. Microtia postoperative.

cular region. In the second stage, congenitally displaced lobule is placed in alignment with reconstructed auricle. In the third stage, ear framework is elevated from the scalp. In the fourth stage, external auditory meatus and tragus is reconstructed.

Preoperative planning is extremely important and an essential step in ear reconstruction, where the following plan is formulated:

1. The size, shape, and site of the ear to be reconstructed.
2. The type of cover available for draping of the ear framework.

12

The size and shape of the ear to be reconstructed are decided with the help of a template made up of a plain radiographic film tracing of the normal ear. Two templates are made – one helps in cartilage framework fabrication and the other helps in deciding the size and direction of the ear.

The ear is reconstructed around the external auditory meatus if it is present. Otherwise, the location of the ear is decided with the help of following points:

1. External auditory meatus is placed just posterior and at the same level to that of the temporomandibular joint.
2. A point is marked at the angle of the mandible. A vertical line is drawn through this point. The ear is placed posterior to this line.
3. Distance between outer canthus of the eye and crus of the helix of the normal ear is measured. This distance is taken over to the deformed side and a point is marked for the crus helix of the ear to be reconstructed.
4. Upper margin of the ear is kept at the same level as that of the normal ear in unilateral deformity and to the level of the eyebrow in cases of bilateral deformity.

The orientation of the ear is decided by the direction of normal ear. In bilateral deformity of ear, it should be placed 15 to 20 degrees more vertical to the axis of nose.

Skin cover to be used for coverage of cartilage framework is decided by the condition, quantity and quality of skin available in and around the auricular region.

Surgical procedure

Stage I

Framework fabrication (Fig. 12.3)

A horizontal incision is made just above the costal margin. The synchondrotic portion of the sixth and seventh ribs is taken with an extra perichondrial dissection to obtain an unmarred specimen and is used to reconstruct the basal framework. Eighth rib is taken to reconstruct the helical margin. With the help of a template, cartilage fabrication is carried out.

Framework insertion

If the skin in the aurical region is normal, then a thin cutaneous pocket is created in the normal postauricular skin through a small incision at the middle of posterior margin of external meatus. The framework is introduced after securing absolute hemostasis. Skin is coapted to the framework with the help of a suction catheter. If the skin is in the auricular region is scarred then temporoparietal fascial flap based on superficial temporal artery and vein is raised. Fascia is turned down and is wrapped around the cartilage framework. The fascial flap is

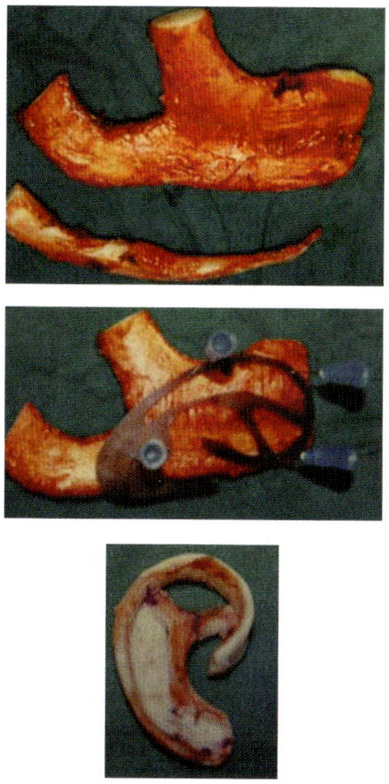

Fig. 12.3. Surgical steps.

co-opted to the cartilage with the help of a suction catheter and is covered by split-thickness skin graft.

In the postoperative period, suction drain is taken out on the third postoperative day and dressing is changed on the seventh postoperative day. During the postoperative period, the delicate contours of reconstructed ear are quite often masked as a result of prolonged edema, thick draping skin, larger then required temporoparietal fascial flap, organized hematoma, or inflammatory exudates. In most of the patient's edema subsides within 6 to 8 weeks of operation and ear contours begin to show through the skin.

Stage II

This involves recreating or reposition of the lobule. If lobule is present but out of alignment, it is merely realigned with the reconstructed ear. If reconstruction of lobule is required, several techniques have been described. Zenteno Alanis and Feldman described useful technique for lobule reconstruction. It is also possible to use cartilage to support the constructed lobule.

Stage III

In this stage, implanted cartilage is elevated from the scalp and thick split thickness skin graft is applied over the resulting raw area.

Stage IV

An incision is given along the margin of reconstructed concha and an anteriorly based flap is raised which is folded on itself to form the tragus and the resulting raw area is split skin grafted to create this external auditory meatus.

Total ear reconstruction is a difficult problem, but if the following points are heeded, success can be achieved in most cases:

1. Careful preoperative planning to decide size, site, direction of ear, and cover to be used for ear framework.
2. Use of autogenous costal cartilage for reconstruction of ear framework.
3. During framework fabrication, triangular fossa and scapha should be made as wide and as deep as possible to leave room for draping skin. Otherwise, the draping skin fills the grooves and masks the contours.
4. Helical and conchal augmentation by a cartilage strip should be done.
5. Skin pocket should be of adequate size. Otherwise, tight skin tents over the contours leaving a dead space for blood to collect, leading to masking of the contours.
6. While making a skin pocket, skin should be raised as thin as possible so that it drapes well over the contours of reconstructed ear. At the same time it should be thick enough to survive.
7. The temporoparietal fascial flap should be of optimum size, neither too small nor too large.
8. Absolute hemostasis should be achieved.
9. Antiseptic and aseptic precautions should be taken.
10. No bolster suture should be used for coaptation of skin temporoparietal fascial flap.
11. Triamcinolone acetonide injection should be used in case of masking contours.
12. Take care to avoid exposure of cartilage while raising it from the scalp in stage III

If one can achieve an ear that does not attract attention from people, success has been achieved.

CONCLUSION

Otoplasty is a challenging job for otorhino laryngologists. The basic material used for ear reconstruction is a framework of cartilage and draping of skin. Usually this procedure is carried out in many stages and better otoplasty requires lot of patience. If one can achieve an ear that does not attract the attention from people, the success has been achieved.

SUGGESTED READING

1. Brent B. The correction of microtia with autogenous cartilage grafts: I. The classic deformity. *Plast Reconstr Surg*, 1980; 66: 1–12.
2. Brent B. Auricular repair with autogenous rib cartilage grafts. Two decades of experience with 600 cases. *Plast Reconstr Surg*, 1992; 90: 355–374.
3. Brent B. Reconstruction of auricle. *In:* McCarthy JG, editor. Plastic Surgery, Vol. 3. Philadelphia: W.B. Saunders Co. 1990: 2094.
4. Brent B. Byrd HS. Secondary ear reconstruction with cartilage graft covered by axial random and free flaps of temporoparietal fascia. *Plast Reconstr Surg*, 1983; 72: 141–152.
5. Nagata S. A new method of total reconstruction of the auricle for microtia. *Plast Reconstr Surg*, 1993; 92: 187–201.
6. Bhandari PS. Total ear reconstruction in post-burn deformity. *Burns*, 1998; 24: 661–70.
7. Bhandari PS. Use of triamcinolone acetonide injection in ear reconstruction. *Ann Plast Surg*, 2000; 45: 458–61.
8. Bhandari PS. Total ear reconstruction in post-burn deformity. *Clin Plast Surg*, 2002; 213–20.

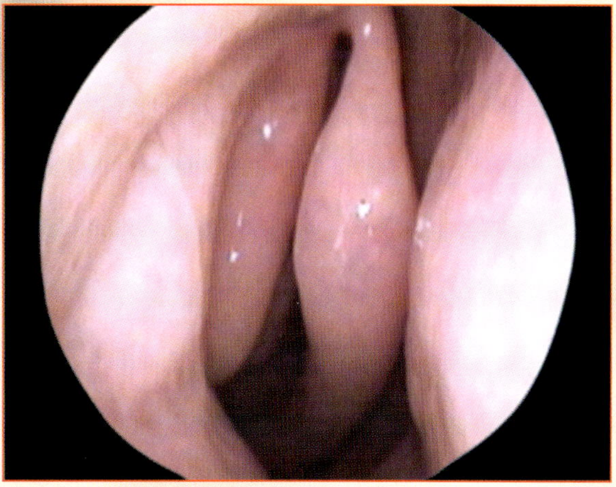

SECTION 3

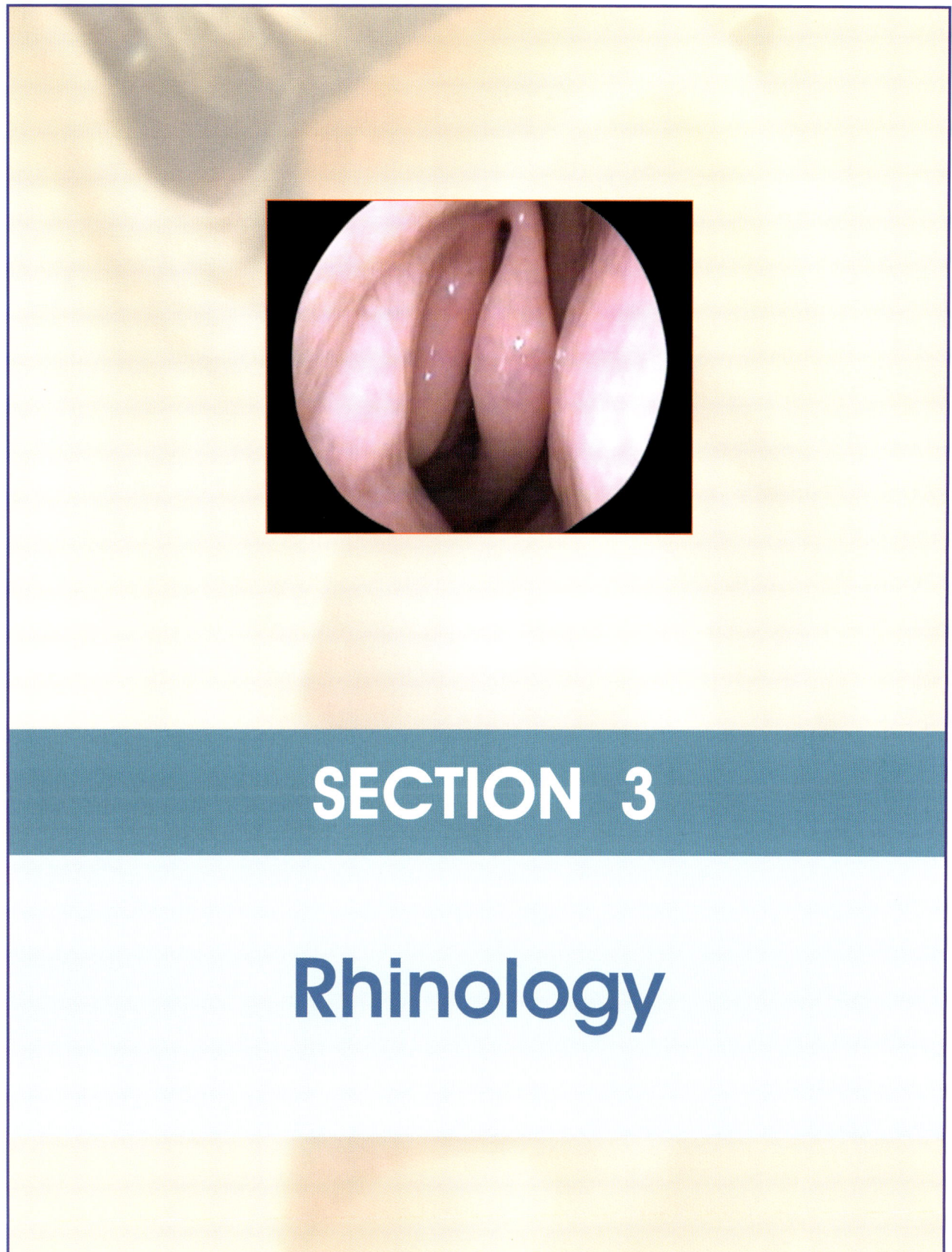

Rhinology

CHAPTER 13

Nasal Mucociliary Clearance in Health and Diseases

Jyoti Yadav

Mucociliary clearance is an important physiological defence mechanism of the upper as well as lower respiratory tract. The respiratory passage is lined by pseudostratified ciliated columnar epithelium resting on basement membrane with numerous goblet cells beneath which lies continuous layer of mucous and serous glands secreting mucus which bathe the cilia and microvilli. Cilia beat in metachronous fashion at a frequency of 10–15 beats/second to propel the mucus at a speed of 0.25–0.75 cm/minute.

The mucociliary system of the airway forms a highly efficient defence mechanism that protects the lungs against inhaled particles including living organisms like bacteria, viruses, fungi, mycoplasma and chemical irritants. The vital part of this system is an adequate quantity of mucus with appropriate rhinological quality and adequately functioning cilia, which allow the continuous exchange of covering fluid layer and removal of engulfed particles. The mucociliary system is regarded as the means of purification at tracheobronchial level, but at the nasal level it acquires more value as it is directly involved in filtration and air conditioning functions. Nose is an easily accessible organ, so in many centers the measurement of nasal mucociliary clearance (NMC) has been used as a screening procedure for congenital abnormalities that would alter mucociliary clearance in the nose and lungs. Any disturbance in number and movement of cilia and mucus production leads to an altered NMC as in adenotonsillar hypertrophy, which causes stagnation of secretions and secondary infection. A permanently deranged mucociliary mechanism predisposes to chronic sinusitis and chronic obstructive lung diseases. The abnormalities of mucociliary transport mechanism may occur as a result of abnormal function of cilia or unusual characteristics of mucus. Variation in the nature of mucus or in anatomic and physiologic integrity of cilia may be a result of disease, drug or environmental influences, like oxygen deprivation, proteolytic enzyme action, bacterial toxins, noxious gases, chemicals and metals. Numerous factors affect mucociliary clearance. They are moisture, temperature, pH, smoke, atmospheric pollutants, radiations, drugs like steroids, adrenaline, atropine and diseases like deviated nasal septum, nasal polyps, Young's syndrome and adenoid hypertrophy. The values of NMC have been reported in different parts of world with wide variation depending upon various geographical, physiological and pathological conditions.

STRUCTURE

Nasal mucosa

Human nasal cavity is lined by three types of epithelia which are squamous, respiratory and olfactory. Squamous lies in anterior part of nose and is without cilia. Within 1 cm of nostrils, a transitional epithelium is present that precedes the respiratory epithelium. The olfactory epithelium is found in the posterosuperior part of nasal cavity. Respiratory epithelium is the major lining of nose and possesses mucociliary system. This epithelium is composed of ciliated and nonciliated columnar, goblet and basal cells. Respiratory epithelium is continuous with lower respiratory tract.

Cilia

They are motile hair-like appendages extending from surface of epithelial cells and contain an axoneme which is a bundle of microtubules arranged as nine outer doublets and a central pair. The axoneme is surrounded by a specialized extension of cell membrane and ciliary membrane. It is assembled in a fixed pattern at the cell surface, above the basal bodies. A doublet microtubule is composed of two subfibers 'A' and 'B'. Subfiber 'A' has inner and outer dynein arms with ATPase activity. Adjacent doublets are connected by nexin lines and radial spokes connect the microtubule with central pair. Sliding movements of microtubules generate movement of cilium. The dyenin arms on subfiber 'A' of one doublet walk along subfiber 'B' of an adjacent doublet as ATP is hydrolysed. The active sliding of outer doublets relative to one another generates curvature, and the force between adjacent doublets is generated by dynein cross bridges. The radial spokes resist the sliding motion, which is converted into local bending. Nexin is highly extensible protein which keeps adjacent doublets together during sliding. The length and width of cilia is between 5–10 µm and 0.1–0.3 µm respectively. The number of cilia per cell is approximately 200 with a density of 6–8 cilia/µm. The beating of cilium has three phases, an effective stroke, during which the cilium is extended maximally, the rest phase in which it is parallel to the cell surface and the recovery stroke. Cilia beat in close coordination in a metachronal wave by adjusting their frequency and phase of beating in response to neighbouring cilia.

The ciliary beat frequency is regulated by several factors, like temperature, intracellular calcium and cAMP levels and by extracellular ATP. The optimum range of temperature for ciliary activity is 28–35°C. Extracellular ATP increases the intracellular calcium ion level in cell which increases ciliary beat frequency. Mechanostimulation by foreign particles or mucus on cilia increases ciliary beat frequency. Dual regulation of ciliary beat frequency is beneficial for mucus transport, because mechanical stimulation would provide local control to elevate beat frequency in the immediate vicinity of mucus load, whereas neurohormonal stimulation regulates the general level of ciliary activity throughout the airways.

NASAL SECRETIONS

The mucus layer which covers the respiratory epithelium is divided into two layers, i.e., periciliary layer and a more gellous upper layer. Periciliary layer has low viscosity fluid with thickness slightly less than the length of an extended cilium and it is probably formed by epithelial cell exudates. Periciliary layer is covered by more viscous upper layer of about 0.5–5 µm deep, which is secreted by goblet cells. It contains mucins which are glycoproteins and form 80% of its dry weight. Mucus is viscoelastic liquid and has 2% glycoproteins, 1% immunoglobulins, 1% lysozyme and lactoferrin, 1% inorganic salts and 95% water. Mucus is expelled from the goblet cells as highly condensed granules by exocytosis and undergoes massive swelling to form a viscoelastic gel that is transportable by cilia. The viscous properties enable mucus to efficiently accept the energy transfer from cilia, while its elastic properties enable it to relax sufficiently to be propelled. If mucus composition remains balanced, a gel layer persists on the surface. Hyposecretion of mucus usually brings about changes in mucus to make the sol layer more viscous and impedes ciliary function.

MUCOCILIARY CLEARANCE

Mucociliary system helps in removing foreign substances and particles from nasal cavity and prevents them from reaching the lower airways. This system has been described as a "conveyer belt" in which ciliated cells provide the driving force, and mucus performs as a sticky fluiditic belt that collects and disposes of foreign particles. Efficiency of mucociliary system depends on physiological control of ciliated cells and rheological properties of mucus blanket. Metachronal coordination of cilia maintains a continous forward thrust on mucus. The presence of several metachronal waves under a blanket of mucus spreads the propulsive movement so that the whole blanket moves as a unit.

The efficiency of nasal mucociliary system depends on three factors, that is, the amount of ciliary input which is determined by length and density of cilia and their beating frequency; the amount of mucus and depth of periciliary layer; and the viscoelastic properties of mucus. Changes in any of these parameters impair mucociliary clearance system.

NORMAL VALUES

Various investigators have reported different nasal mucus transport rate, wide range being 4.2–10.8 mm/minute in healthy individuals. Passali et al. reported the normal values of nasal mucociliary clearance time in healthy children as 9.96 minutes. The mean value of NMC time in India at Nagpur and Rohtak are reported to be 7.1 and 7.5 respectively.

MUCOCILIARY TRANSPORT MEASUREMENT METHODS

There are several methods to evaluate efficiency of nasomucociliary clearance which include direct observation of dyes or particles deposited on nasal mucosa, use of radioactive microdroplets, single radioactively tagged resin particle and radiopaque Teflon disks monitored by external device. The study of mucociliary transport and clearance in vivo is divided into two categories. The first one is determination of total nasal clearance of a deposited dose, by measuring clearance of a radiolabelled solution from nasal cavity. The clearance of radioactivity from nasal cavity is measured with a gamma camera. In second category, those methods are included which determine the mucus flow rate or mucociliary transport time is measured by speed of radiolabelled markers placed in nasal mucosa and the transport of particle is followed by a gamma camera. The main drawback of this method is administration of radioactive material to volunteers. Radioactive Teflon disks mixed with bismuth trioxide as an alternative were administered nasally and detected by roentgenography. Another most simple and inexpensive method of estimating mucus flow in vivo is by using dyes as markers. Particles or drops coloured by a strong dye or other coloured substance, like edicol orange, indigo carmine or charcoal are placed into anterior part of nasal cavity. The time for the dye to appear in the pharyngeal cavity is measured by monitoring its appearance in pharyngeal cavity. Drawback of this method is that constant monitoring is required which is inconvenient for the volunteer.

Anderson et al. described a very simple, noninvasive, easily reproducible and economical method consisting of depositing a particle of saccharin on the nasal mucosa and observing the time when the subject reported the first taste of sweetness. A 1.5 mm diameter particle of saccharin is placed 1 cm behind the anterior end of inferior turbinate on the floor of nasal cavity and the time required to perceive a sweet taste by the subject is noted. Subjects are asked to refrain from any nasal manipulation. The test is performed on both sides of nasal cavity with an interval of one hour and the average value of NMC is to be recorded. The disadvantage of saccharin test method is that threshold for sweet taste varies from individual to individual. Secondly, performing multiple saccharin tests in a short period of time is impossible because sweet taste requires approximately four hours disappearing completely. So, to overcome the disadvantages of both these methods, a combination of a dye and a saccharin method has been used by several researchers. In modified saccharin test three molar aqueous sodium saccharin solutions (1 μl) are applied with a wiretrol capillary on inferior concha instead of saccharin particles. The outcome of mucociliary transport rate studies depends on whether the tracer is insoluble (like particles, inert dyes and Teflon disks) or soluble (like saccharin dye solutions). Insoluble particles will be transported by mucus layer. While soluble markers dissolve in both mucus and periciliary layer and their transport rate reflect the transport rate of both the layers.

FACTORS AFFECTING NASAL MUCOCILIARY CLEARANCE

Several factors which affect nasal mucociliary clearance time are described below.

Age

Little is known about the effects of aging on nasal mucociliary clearance. Subjects older than 40 years age had significantly slower ciliary beat frequency, and longer NMC time than their younger counterparts and that is why elderly persons have more frequent occurrence of respiratory infections. While others found the mucociliary transport to be independent of age and sex. Sakakura et al. found NMC 14.6 ± 9.8 minute in age group of 18–39 years; 11.5 ± 5.7 minute in age group of 40–59 years and 120 minutes or more in age of 60–100 years. Yadav et al. observed significant increase in NMC time in 6th and 7th decades, which was more marked in 7th decade and this may be the one of the reasons for increased susceptibility of elderly to sinusitis, chronic bronchitis, deep lung infections and increased incidence of pneumonia. Svartengren also found that long-term clearance from small airways decreases with age.

Tonicity

Hower studied the effect of tonicity of saline nasal douching solutions on mucociliary clearance in order to ascertain whether hypertonicity conferred any advantage which was found to improve mucociliary clearance with solutions of 5% tonicity. The effect is probably brought about by changes in mucus rheology. Andrew et al. observed that hypertonic saline nasal irrigation improves mucociliary transit time of saccharin, while buffered normal saline had no such effect.

pH

The best pH for ciliary activity is 7–8. The cilia beat above pH 6.4 and will function in slightly alkaline fluids of pH 8.5 for long periods. If pH is reduced to 6.4 or less, the ciliary activity is arrested. A rise in pH is better tolerated. In systemic disease patients like diabetes, the NMC and oral pH values were significantly different as compared to healthy subjects.

Temperature

The optimum temperature for ciliary activity is 28–33°C. The normal human nasal temperature has been recorded as about 32°C. The fall in temperature decreases the frequency of ciliary motion. Below 18°C the frequency slows down, stopping completely between 12 to 7°C. At 40°C, ciliary activity slows down and at 43°C it stops completely. If these temperature extremes last for a short period of time, then this cessation of ciliary activity is reversible.

13

Exercise

For years physicians have observed a high incidence of upper respiratory tract infections after strenuous exercise. Mucosal surfaces represent a first line of defence against infections; pollutants or organisms entrapped in respiratory secretions are cleared by mucociliary transport. Muns observed impairment of NMC upto several days after strenuous exercise, which might be partially caused by abnormally functioning cilia.

Dry oxygen inhalation and humidity

Nakamura did not find any adverse effect of inhalation of dry oxygen on NMC. A reduction in the amount of secretion or a loss of humidity at the mucosal surface will tend to reduce the sol layer, bringing the gel layer into close contact with the cilia thus impeding their action. The addition of a few drops of saline may rehydrate the mucus and restore normal mucociliary transport.

Drying, viscosity and elasticity

Adequate moisture is essential for maintenance of integrity and normal function of cilia. Drying of slight degree causes cessation of ciliary activity and prompt moistening restores normal activity. Absence of mucus removes protective action of lysozymes.

According to Tremble, smoky atmosphere also interfere with ciliary action by causing drying in the persons residing in overheated and underhumid rooms. For efficient ciliary action, a balanced film of moisture and mucus of suitable viscosity is essential. While Atsuta found no significant correlation between NMC and elasticity, a change in viscosity of mucus, by an alteration in composition of secretion, produces a thicker gel layer impeding its passage through sinus ostia causing mucus retention.

Composition of tissue fluids

For efficient nourishment of cilia bearing cells, various ions must be present in correct proportions. According to Lillie sodium alone caused slowing and ultimately cessation of movement, while potassium allowed the action to continue but ammonium led to partial paralysis. While Gray found that proper concentration of potassium is essential for functioning of cilia which contract permanently in higher concentration. Magnesium has little effect, whereas hydrogen ions affect cilia adversely.

Atmospheric pollutants

The three major gaseous pollutants sulphur dioxide, nitrous oxide and ozone along with inorganic particles like sulphide and nitrate salts exert an irritating effect on respiratory mucosa and adversely affect mucociliary activity.

Johnson et al. found that NMC time is prolonged in women using biomass fuel and peak expiratory flow rate is reduced significantly in them. NMC function is significantly impaired in workers who have been exposed to wood dust in the furniture industry for more than 10 years.

Inflammation

When inflamed, the mucosa of sinuses swells rapidly. When bacterial or viral infection is present then not only the mucosal cells are affected but the entire mucosal surface may be partially destroyed or paralysed and thus unable to provide its mucociliary clearance function.

Drugs

The observed effects of intranasal administration of various drugs on NMC are described here. Cocaine solution of 2.5% is almost harmless if applied for shorter periods but continuous application for one hour stops ciliary activity; its 5% solution causes arrest of ciliary activity in 2–3 minutes; while its 10% solution produces such effect immediately. Local anaesthetics like lidocaine 5%, procaine 5% and tetracaine 0.1% have similar action. Adrenaline 1 : 1,000 causes reversible inhibition of ciliated cells when they are exposed to it for 20 minutes. Acetylcholine causes increase in rate of ciliary beating. Atropine causes reduction in secretion of nose, depressing ciliary activity. Ether and chloroform even in higher concentration in the inspired air have no effect on ciliary activity. However, both of these on direct application cause immediate paralysis. Antiseptics, except those of silver compounds in 2.5–5% strength, are also harmful. Topical antibiotics such as penicillins or streptomycin slightly stimulate the mucociliary movement. Bromhexine used as mucolytic agent in chronic sinusitis has a stimulatory effect.

Antihistamines slow down the action of cilia. High concentration of α_1-agonist, phenylephrine decrease ciliary beat frequency, whereas lower doses increase it in vivo. Propranolol (β-antagonist) decreases ciliary beat frequency in a dose-dependent fashion. Following one week's therapy with corticosteroids, the rate of saccharin clearance is reduced which is secondary to a change in ciliary beat frequency. Oxymetazoline and 3% sodium chloride solution are found more effective in mucociliary clearance. Hypertonic saline inhibits NMC which is reversible when replaced with isotonic solution. With hypotonic saline, the ciliary movement ceases permanently. Isotonic solutions are harmless or rather useful when used in sprays. Nasal continous positive airway pressure does not significantly affect mucus transport in vitro but it can acutely increase NMC.

Smoking

NMC is a biomarker of nasal mucus function. In vitro studies have shown that cigarette smoke is a potent inhibitor of ciliary transport activity. Persons smoking bidi or unfiltered cigarettes had significant depression of ciliary activity. The clearance was prolonged as the number of cigarettes smoked and the duration of smoking increased. It was greater among those who gave a history of nasal exhalation of inhaled smoke. The mechanism of effects of smoke on NMC is that the cigarette smoke consists of gaseous and particulate phases. Gaseous phase is water soluble and is trapped mainly in the upper respiratory tract which is responsible for acute effects of smoke. The particulate phase settles down deeper and has role in pathogenesis of chronic disorders. Ciliated cells are damaged by smoking leading to metaplasia and dysplasia.

Proenca et al. found that in smokers although the mucociliary clearance immediately after smoking is similar to non-smokers, eight hours after smoking it is reduced, and this reduction is closely related to the smoking habits. Ercy et al. found in a smoking cessation programme contributed to improvement in mucociliary clearance among smokers from the 15th day after cessation of smoking, and these beneficial effects persisted for 180 days. Side stream tobacco smoke exposure acutely alters human nasal mucociliary clearance.

Nasal cycle

A significant difference in NMC is found in congested and decongested phases of nasal cycle but nasal mucociliary clearance time in diseased states did not show significant differences in transport between two phases of nasal cycle.

Naomi et al. found that mucociliary clearance is impaired in acutely ill patients with no airway manipulation and correlates with simple markers of underlying disease severity. Mucociliary dysfunction may help to explain the increased susceptibility of hospital acquired respiratory infection in critically ill patients.

Common cold

In common cold patients, there is loss of cilia in first week but they recover within three weeks. It had been observed in patients of sinusitis that the mucociliary transit time was found prolonged as compared to normal control group.

Lower respiratory tract diseases

Significant prolongation of NMC is found in lower respiratory tract diseases. Coughing acts as defence mechanism of lung when mucociliary clearance system is defective. Awotedu and others observed abnormal mucociliary clearance in patients of asthma and bronchiectasis which is due to combination of mucus abnormality and ciliary malfunction. Andersen et al. did not find any alteration in NMC with the duration of disease in bronchiectasis, implying that per se duration of illness is of no consequence and prolonged NMC was present from the very beginning and is possibly responsible for causation of disease, since a positive correlation exists between nasal mucociliary and pulmonary clearance. Singh et al. and Yadav et al. also observed significantly prolonged NMC time in patients of diseases of lower respiratory tract like bronchiectasis, chronic bronchitis and bronchial asthma. No relationship of NMC with duration of disease was observed. Some authors even observed an impaired mucociliary transport in patients who have been hospitalized in intensive care units and had developed pneumonia and retention of secretions. In patients of lower respiratory tract diseases, the defective mucociliary clearance can be due to abnormalities in its ciliary or mucus components or a combination of both. The mucoid sputum obtained from bronchiectasis patients is found to have high viscosity and for ideal mucociliary clearance, mucus should have high elasticity and low viscosity. According to Currie et al. the impaired mucociliary clearance in these patients is due to high viscosity of respiratory secretions. Waite et al. observed abnormalities of nasal cilia under the electron microscope in these patients. Ramos et al. observed that pulmonary rehabilitation can acutely increase nasal mucociliary clearance in COPD patients that may have clinical implications.

Adenoiditis

It is a common problem in children consequent to recurrent viral or bacterial upper respiratory tract infection leading to hypertrophy of nasopharyngeal lymphoid tissue. The catarrhal child is invariably having adenoidal hypertrophy. Yadav et al. and Ranga et al. observed significant impairment in NMC in patients of adenoiditis and adenotonsillar hypertrophy. After adenotonsillectomy, NMC is restored to normal. Yadav et al. also found impaired NMC even in healthy children of 4–11 years age which was due to subclinical adenoiditis. However, clearance returned to normal level at the time of puberty which coincides with adenoid involution.

Rhinitis

Schuhl found a significant difference in NMC between allergic and non-allergic rhinitis which is due to changes in rheology of nasal mucosa as a consequence of underlying inflammatory process in rhinitis. A unilateral nasal challenge accelerates the mucociliary transport system bilaterally in the nose of subjects with hypersensitivity such as allergic rhinitis. Maurizi et al. studied ciliary ultrastructure and NMC in chronic and allergic rhinitis. All the patients had an increased mucociliary time and a reduced velocity regardless to the pathology. Different ultrastructural alterations observed include both central and peripheral microtubules alterations, absence of dynein arms, absence of radial spokes, ciliary membrane alterations, compound cilia, disorientation of central tubules. According to them mucociliary clearance determination represents the only method to evaluate, even if in an indirect fashion, the percentage of ciliary abnormalities, as no direct quantitative method has been described and ciliary ultrastructural alterations can be of diagnostic value only if associated with mucociliary clearance time and velocity determination. We observed lesser clearance time in perennial allergic rhinitis which may be to cope up with excessive secretions.

Chronic rhinosinusitis

It decreases ciliary beat frequency and factors accounting for it are amount of ciliated cells, orientation of cilia, epithelial metaplasia and secretions. Purulent sputum in sinusitis contains factors like serine proteases and this enzyme is probably a product released by the host phagocytic defenses and impairs ciliary activity. In human, nasal epithelium with or without inflammation, no definite difference was seen. After rinsing the infected mucus, the ciliary movement rapidly recovers. Mucus may protect cilia against bacteria. Disorientation and loss of cilia is likely to have a role in pathogenesis of rhinosinusitis.

Radiation

Irradiation causes decreased mucociliary clearance in animal models. Patients who receive radiotherapy had no clearance of saccharin from nasal cavity at a minimum of 20 minutes. These patients had higher prevalence of nasal congestion, poor drainage and facial pain after radiation therapy. Stringer et al. observed that radiation therapy to nasal cavity causes decrease in NMC and this alteration should be considered while selecting therapy for malignancies in nasal area. Surico et al. observed the effects of radiotherapy of head in children over nasal mucociliary function. They found that irradiation of head in children impairs mucociliary function even permanently which may predispose children to upper respiratory tract infections. Careful monitoring of such patients should be done to detect the clinical effects of functional changes as early as possible and to prevent evolution to chronic diseases.

Boushy et al. reported changes at autopsy due to irradiation in the lung parenchyma and trachea in patients of bronchogenic carcinoma and they observed fibrosis of tracheal epithelium and decreased number of goblet cells. Irradiation decreases ciliary beat frequency by affecting ciliated epithelium and decreasing the number of mucus-secreting glands. Singh et al. also observed significant increase in NMC time after radiotherapy in patients of head and neck carcinoma. The increase in NMC time was higher in patients with carcinoma of tonsil, nasopharynx and palate where the nasal cavity came under irradiation field.

Cystic fibrosis

McShane et al. observed that abnormalities appeared in cystic fibrosis in adults with the symptoms of chronic sinus disease, suggesting a secondary rather than primary phenomenon. Studies to explore this mechanism in distal more sparsely ciliated airways could aid an understanding of pathogenesis and the development of new treatments.

FUNCTIONAL ENDOSCOPIC SINUS SURGERY

This minimal invasive surgery is based on restoration of physiology. In chronic maxillary sinusitis previously Caldwell-Luc's operation with inferior meatus antrostomy was done which was not found to be effective as cilia still beat in the direction of natural osteum. In FESS middle meatus antrostomy is done which restores mucociliary clearance and hence not only good aeration but mucociliary clearance is also restored with good results in sinusitis.

CONCLUSION

Mucociliary clearance is an important physiological defence mechanism of respiratory tract. Two main components of NMC are cilia and mucus of proper rheological quality. It depends on age, pH, temperature, viscosity, elasticity, pollutants, inflammation and nasal cycle. It may be affected by various diseases of nose, paranasal sinuses and lower respiratory tract. It may also get affected by smoking, radiation, certain systemic diseases like diabetes.

SUGGESTED READINGS

1. Petruson B, Hansan HA, Karlsson G. Structural and functional aspects of cells in the nasal mucociliary system. *Arch Otolaryngol*, 1984; 110: 576–81.
2. Procter D, Wagner H. Clearance of particles from the nose. *Arch Environ Health*, 1965; 11: 366–71.
3. Postic WP. Assessment and treatment of adeno-tonsillar hypertrophy in children. *Am J Otolaryngol*, 1992; 13: 259–64.
4. Currie DC, Pavia D, Agnew JE, Lopez-Vidriero MT, Diamond PD, Cola PJ et al. Impaired tracheobronchial clearance in bronchiectasis. *Thorax*, 1987; 42: 126–30.
5. Toremalm NG. Aerodynamic and mucociliary function of upper airways. *Eur J Respir Dis*, 1985; 66: 54–6.
6. Davis RJ. The assessment of nasal mucociliary clearance and the effects of drugs. *Respir Med*, 1994; 88: 89–101.
7. Golhar S, Arora MML. The effect of cryodestruction of vidian nasal branches on nasal mucus flow in vaso-motor rhinitis. *Indian J Otolaryngol*, 1981; 97: 12–4.
8. Toss M. Goblet cells and glands in the nose and para-nasal sinuses. *In:* The Nose, edited by D Procter and I Anderson, Amsterdam: Elsevier Biomedical Press 1982: 99–144.
9. Sleigh MA. Some aspects of the comparative physiology of cilia. *Am Rev Respir Dis*, 1966; 93: 16–31.
10. Wanner A. State of the art. Clinical aspects of muco-ciliary transport. *Am Rev Respir Dis*, 1977; 116: 73–121.

11. Yergin B, Saketkhoo K, Michaelson E, Serafini S, Kovitz K, Sackner M. A roentgenographic method for measuring nasal mucus velocity. *J Appl Physiol*, 1978; 44: 964–8.
12. Passali D, Bianchini Ciampoli M. Normal values of mucociliary transport time in young subjects. *Int J Pediatr Otorhinolaryngol*, 1985; 9(2): 151–6.
13. Wig U, Jindal NK, Goel H, Chawla RK, Yadav SPS. Nasal mucus clearance in nasal and paranasal sinus disorders. *Indian J Chest Dis Allied Sci*, 1988; 30: 177–80.
14. Anderson I, Camner P, Jensen PL, Philipson K, Proctor DF. A comparison of nasal and tracheobronchial clearance. *Arch Environ Health*, 1974; 29: 290–3.
15. Anderson I, Lundquist G, Jensen PL, Philipson K, Proctor DF. Nasal clearance in monozygotic twins. *Am Rev Respir Dis*, 1974; 110: 301–5.
16. Ho JC, Chan KN, Hu WH, Lam WK, Zheng L, Tipoe GL, et al. The effect of aging on nasal mucociliary clearance beat frequency and ultrastructure of respiratory cilia. *Am J Respir Crit Care Med*, 2001; 163(4): 983–8.
17. Sakakura Y, Ukai K, Majima Y, Hurai S, Harada T, Miyoshi Y. Nasal mucociliary clearance under various conditions. *Acta Otolaryngol*, 1983; 96: 167–73.
18. Yadav J, Ranga RK, Singh J. Effect of aging on nasal mucociliary clearance. *Clin Rhinol*, 2011; 4(1): 1–3.
19. Svartengren M, Falk R, Philipson K. Long term clearance from small airways decreases with age. *Eur Respir J*, 2005; 26: 609–15.
20. Hower JJ, Dowley AC, Condon L, EL-Jassar P, Sood S. The effect of hypertonicity on nasal mucociliary clearance. *Clin Otolaryngol*, 2000; 25: 558–60.
21. Talbot AR, Herr TM, Parsow DS. Mucociliary clearance and buffered hypertonic saline solution. *Laryngoscope*, 2009; 107: 500–3.
22. Negus VE. The action of cilia and the effect of drugs on their activity. *J Laryngol Otol*, 1934; 49: 571–85.
23. Selimoglu MA, Selimoglu E, Kurt A. Nasal mucociliary clearance and nasal and oral pH in patients with insulin dependent diabetes. *Ear Nose Throat J*, 1999; 78: 585–90.
24. Muns G, Singer P, Wolf F, Rubinstein I. Impaired nasal mucociliary clearance in long distance runners. *Int J Sports Med*, 1995; 16: 209–13.
25. Tremble GE. Clinical observation on the movement of nasal cilia: An experimental study. *Laryngoscope*, 1948; 58: 206–24.
26. Atsuta S, Majma Y. Nasal mucociliary clearance of chronic sinusitis in relation to rheological properties of nasal mucus. *Ann Otol Rhinolaryngol*, 1998; 107: 47–51.
27. Lillie RS. The relation of ions to contractile processes. *Am J Physiol*, 1934; 112: 468–76.
28. Cralley LV. The effect of irritant gases upon the rate of ciliary activity. *J Industrial Hygiene Toxicol*, 1942; 24: 193–8.
29. Priscilla J, Padmavathi R, Ghosh S, Paul P, Ramadoss S, Balakrishnan K, Thanasekaraan V, Subhashini AS. Evaluation of mucociliary clearance among women using biomass and clean fuel in a periurban area of Chennai: A preliminary study. *Lung India*, 2011; 28: 30–3.
30. Black A, Evans JC, Hadfield EH, Macbeth RG, Morgan A, Walsh M. Impairment of nasal mucociliary clearance in woodworkers in the furniture industry. *Br J Indust Med*, 1974; 31: 10–17.
31. Bang FB, Bang BG, Foard MA. Responses of upper respiratory mucosa to drugs and viral infections. *Am Rev Respir Dis*, 1966; 93: 142–9.
32. Ewart G. The effect of two topical anaesthetic drugs on the mucus flow on respiratory tract. *Ann Otol Rhinol Laryngol*, 1967; 76: 359–67.
33. Greenwood G, Pittenger RE, Constant GA, Ivy AC. Effect of zephiran chloride, tyrothricin, penicillin and streptomycin on ciliary action. *Arch Otolaryngol*, 1946; 43: 623–28.
34. Goel H, Jindal NK, Wig U, Chawla RK, Yadav SPS. Effect of bromhexine on nasal mucus clearance in chronic maxillary sinusitis. *Indian J Chest Dis Allied Sci*, 1989; 31: 33–6.
35. Naul S, Ozturk O, Korkmaz M, Tutkua A, Batman C. The effect of topical agents of fluticasone propionate, oxymetazoline and 3% and 9% sodium chloride solution on mucociliary clearance in the therapy of acute bacterial rhinosinusitis in vivo. *Laryngoscope*, 2009; 122: 320–5.
36. De Oliveira LR, AlbertiniYagi CS, Flgueirdo AC, Sadiva PH, Lorenzi-Fiho G. Short term effect of nCPAA on nasal mucociliary clearance and mucus transportability in healthy subjects. *Respir Med*, 2006; 100: 183–5.
37. Kensler GJ, Battista SP. Components of cigarette smoke with ciliary depressant activity. *New Engl J Med*, 1963; 269: 1161–6.
38. Singh I, Mehta M, Singh J, Yadav J. Nasal mucus clearance in chronic smokers. *Indian J Chest Dis Allied Sci*, 1994; 36: 133–6.
39. Auarback O, Hammond EC, Garfinkel L. Changes in bronchial epithelium in relation to cigarette smoking. *New Engl J Med*, 1979; 300: 381–6.
40. Cipulo Ramos EM, De Toledo AC, Xavier RF, Fosco LC, Vieira RP, Ramos D, Jardim JR. Revesibility of impaired nasal mucociliary clearance in smokers following a smoking cessation programme. *Respirology*, 2011; 16(5): 849–55.
41. Bascom R, Kesavanathan J, Fitgerald TK, Cheng KH, Swift DL. Sidestream tobacco smoke exposure acutely alters human nasal mucociliary clearance. *Environ Health Perspectives*, 1995; 103: 1026–30.
42. Littlejohu MC, Steinberg CM, Hokamson JA, Quiun FB, Bailey B. The relationship between the nasal cycle and mucociliary clearance. *Laryngoscope*, 1991; 102: 117–20.

43. Nakagawa NK, Franchini ML, Driusso P, De Oliveira LR, Saldiva PHN, Lorenzi-Filbo G. Mucociliary clearance is impaired in acutely ill patients. *Chest*, 2005; 128: 2772–7.
44. Mahakit P, Pumhirun P. A preliminary study of nasal mucociliary clearance in smokers, sinusitis and allergic rhinitis patients. *Asian Pac J Allergy Immunol*, 1995; 13: 119–21.
45. Rutland J, Cole PJ. Nasal mucociliary clearance and ciliary beat frequency in cystic fibrosis compared with sinusitis and bronchiectasis. *Thorax*, 1981; 36: 654–8.
46. Awotedu AA, Babalola OO, Lawani EO, Hart PD. Abnormal mucociliary action in asthma and bronchiectasis. *African J Medicine Medical Sci*, 1990; 19: 153–6.
47. Singh I, Yadav J, Singh R, Raj B. Nasal mucociliary clearance in diseases of lower respiratory tract. *Lung India*, 1998; 16: 159–61.
48. Yadav J, Verma A, Gupta KB. Nasal mucociliary clearance in bronchial asthma. *Indian J Allergy Asthma Immunol*, 2005; 19: 21–3.
49. Yadav J, Ranga RK, Singh J. Nasal mucociliary clearance in adenoiditis. *Indian J Physiol All Sci*, 1999; 80: 896–8.
50. Ranga RK, Singh J, Gera A, Yadav J. Nasal mucociliary clearance in adenotonsillar hypertrophy. *Indian J Peditr*, 2000; 67: 651–2.
51. Yadav J, Ranga RK, Singh J, Gathwala G. Nasal mucociliary clearance in healthy children in a tropical country. *Int J Pediatr Otorhinolaryngol*, 2001; 57: 21–4.
52. Schuhl JF. Nasal mucociliary clearance in perennial rhinitis. *J Investig Allergol Clin Immunol*, 1995; 5: 333–6.
53. Maurizi M, Ottaviani F, Paludetti G, Almadoni G, Zappone C. Adenoid hypertrophy and nasal mucociliary clearance in children. A morphological and functional study. *Int J Pediatr Otorhinolaryngol*, 1984; 8: 31–41.
54. Yadav J, Verma A, Singh J. Nasal mucociliary clearance in patients of perennial allergic rhinitis. *Indian J Allergy Asthma Immunol*, 2003; 17: 89–91.
55. Sykes DA, Wilson R, Greenstone M, Currie DC, Steinfort C, Cole PJ. Deleterious effects of purulent sputum solution on human ciliary function in vitro: at least two factors identified. *Thorax*, 1987; 42: 256–61.
56. Stringer SP, Stiles W, Slattery WH 3rd, Krumerman J, Parsons JT, Mendenhall WM, et al. Nasal mucociliary clearance after radiation therapy. *Laryngoscope*, 1995; 105: 380–2.
57. Surico G, Muggeo P, Mappa L, Muggeo V, Conti V, Lucarelli A et al. Impairment of nasal mucociliary clearance after radiotherapy for childhood head cancer. *Head Neck*, 2001; 23(6): 461–6.
58. Boushy SF, Helgason AH, North LB. The effects of radiation on the lung and bronchial tree. *Am J Roentgenol*, 1970; 108: 284–92.
59. Singh I, Jakhar KK, Das BP, Yadav J. The effect of irradiation on mucociliary clearance. *Indian J Chest Dis Allied Sci*, 1995; 37: 115–8.
60. McShane D, Davies JC, Wodehouse T, Bush A, Geddes D, Alton EW. Normal nasal mucociliary clearance in cystic fibrosis children: Evidence against a CFTRL-related defect. *Eur Respir J*, 2004; 24: 95–100.

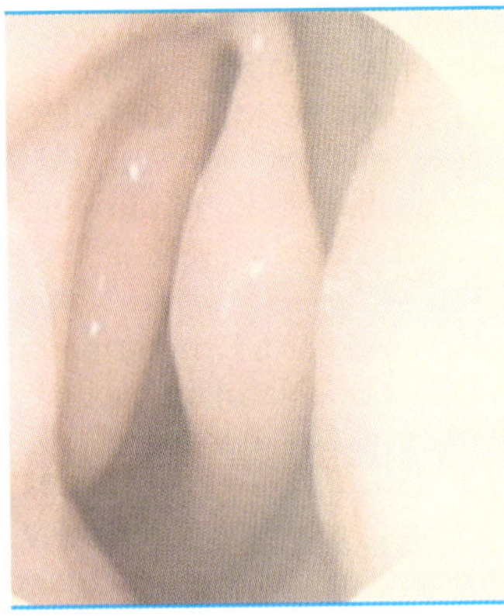

CHAPTER 14

Rhinosinusitis

Rijuneeta, Grace Budhiraja

Rhinosinusitis is on the rise in developed as well as developing countries. Its incidence is increasing globally among patients of all ages. It affects 14% of U.S. population annually.

Most of the clinicians still think that allergy is the cause of rhinosinusitis than infection. The latest etiology is thought to be fungal in origin. It is appropriate to use the term "Rhinosinusitis" as rhinitis precedes sinusitis.

VIRAL RHINOSINUSITIS

It is a common but self-limiting disease. It usually lasts for 3–10 days and improves with due course of time except few which change to other type of rhinosinusitis. The pathophysiology starts with stage of infection followed by stimulation of multiple inflammatory pathways, inflammatory mediators and parasympathetic stimulation leading to engorgement of vessels (Figs. 14.1A & B).

This leads to sneezing, pain and cough reflexes. Two hundred species of virus are known to cause rhinosinusitis. Common viruses are: Rhinovirus, Influenza, Parainfluenza, Corona and Respiratory syncytial virus. Hamory et al. could prove viral etiology only in 16 percent of cases. The pure viral stage of the disease is soon contaminated by the following common bacterias such as *Moraxella*, *Pneumococcus*, *Streptococcus* A, etc.

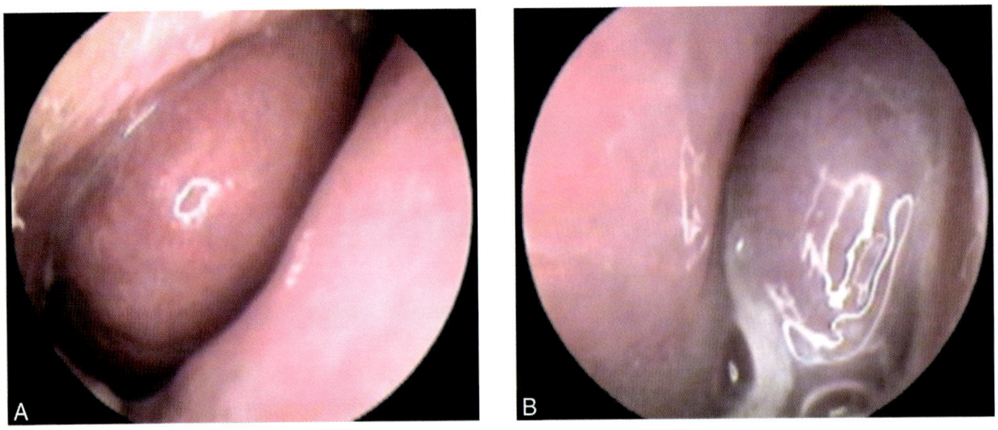

Fig. 14.1A & B. Endoscopic view of acute viral rhinosinusitis.

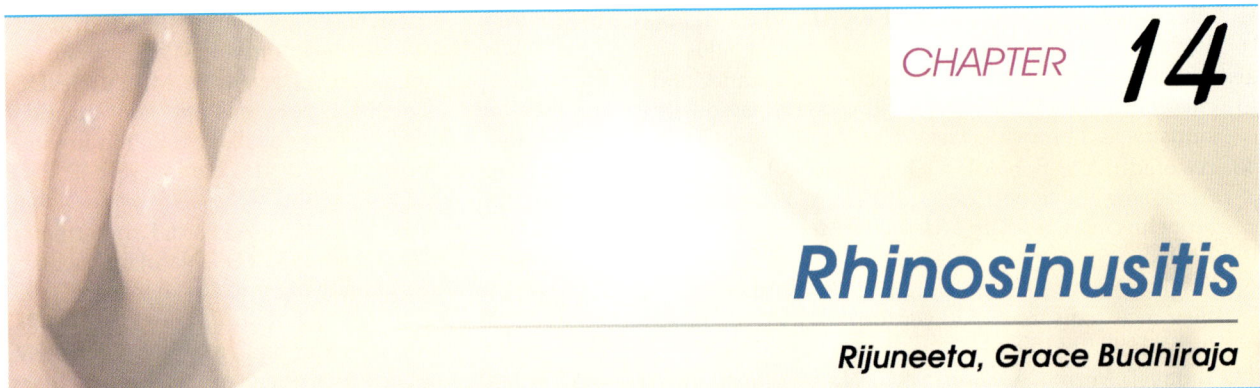

BACTERIAL RHINOSINUSITIS

It is usually multifactorial. Various causes are infection, allergy, environmental factors, local anatomical changes, metabolic disorders, mucosal abnormalities and trauma. The following are the routes for infection to reach sinuses in order of frequency: Rhinogenic (commonest), Dentogenic and Iatrogenic (including trauma). The following mechanisms like part of commensal population, sneezing/coughing and nose blowing (by creating differential pressure) and obstruction of sinus ostium (by reducing oxygen tension/increase in lactic acid concentration, which favour bacterial growth) have been identified. The usual organisms responsible for the causation of chronic bacterial rhinosinusitis are as follows: *Streptococcus milleri, Haemophilus influenzae, Streptococcus pneumoniae, Staphylococcus aureus* (coagulase negative and positive) and anaerobic (need to be considered). Lanza and Kennedy defined rhinosinusitis as "the condition manifested by an inflammatory response involving the following; the mucus membrane (possibly including the neuroepithelium) of the nasal cavity and paranasal sinuses, fluids within these cavities, and/or underlying bone. Rhinosinusitis has been classified as: Acute: lasting for 4 weeks, Subacute: 4–12 weeks, Recurrent acute: 4 episodes/year each episode lasting 7–10 days with no intervening symptoms and Chronic: 12 weeks. Acute sinusitis is defined as sinus inflammation of acute onset with duration of symptoms for more than seven days but less than four weeks or less than 12 weeks, which are completely resolved after medical therapy leaving no significant residual mucosal damage (judged on clinical basis only). The most prominent presenting symptoms in acute sinusitis are facial pain, congestion, purulent discharge, anosmia, hyposmia and fever. It is rapid in onset. On examination, the mucosa is congested and swollen. Mucopurulent discharge may be noted in the middle meatus (Figs. 14.2A & B).

The presence of purulent discharge is enough to arrive at clinical diagnosis. Chronic rhinosinusitis is defined as persistent inflammation of nose and paranasal sinuses with mild grade symptoms and signs for the duration of more than 12 weeks. These persistent inflammatory changes are seen on CT imaging or endoscopy, four weeks after starting the appropriate medical therapy, without patient having suffered from an intervening acute infection, a definition that presupposes that every patient undergoes CT scan. The symptoms and findings are similar to acute rhinosinusitis. The findings are also same as that of acute with the exception that the presence of nasal polyposis is considered as a sign of chronicity.

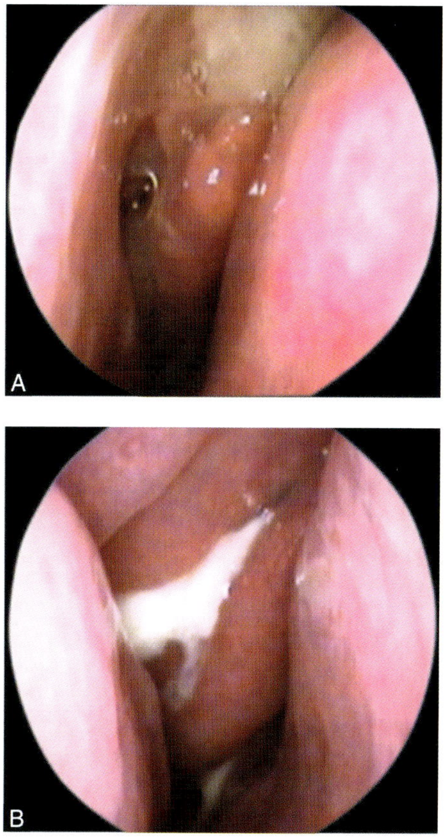

Fig. 14.2A & B. Endoscopic view of bacterial sinusitis.

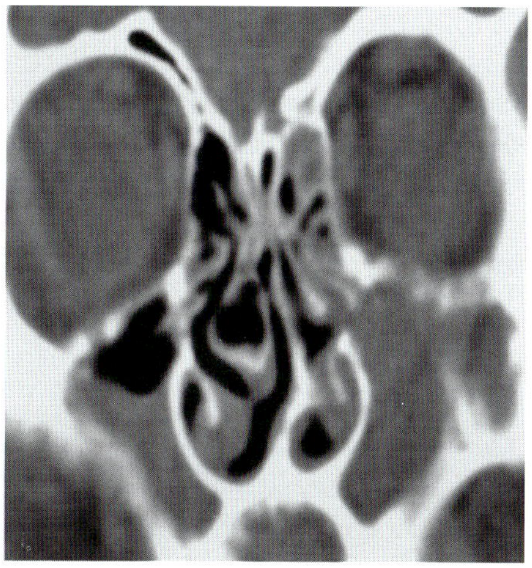

Fig. 14.3. Coronal CT showing DNS, concha bullosa and polyps in sinuses.

It is rarely seen as a result of acute infection. The nasal mucosa is hyperemic. *Streptococcus viridans, Streptococcus pneumoniae, Haemophilus influenzae* and *Haemophilus parainfluenzae* are common causative organisms. Recurrent acute sinusitis is defined as one to four episodes (at least one documented by clinician) of acute rhinosinusitis treated with antibiotics in the past year. It should be separated by a symptoms-free interval of antibiotics of eight weeks, and either an imaging study (CT, MRI, or plain radiographs) showing rhinosinusitis, or evidence of rhinosinusitis on nasal endoscopy during one of the episodes. Acute exacerbation on chronic rhinosinusitis is defined as episode of acute inflammation on chronic pathology with worsening of existing symptoms or appearance of new symptoms. There is a complete resolution of acute (but not chronic) symptoms in between the episodes.

FUNGAL RHINOSINUSITIS

The diagnosis of fungal rhinosinusitis is very challenging though methods of investigations are improving. Lately fungal rhinosinusitis has also been included in the list of indications for functional endoscopic sinus surgery. Fungal rhinosinusitis was initially reported in 1791 by Plaignaud. *Aspergillus* was identified as a causative organism for rhinosinusitis in 1983 by Mackenzie. Its incidence is on the increase over the last two decades. This increase in frequency has been attributed to increase in immune suppressed patients, improvement in diagnosis and rise in predisposing factors like diabetes, AIDS, prolonged administration of steroids, post-transplant patients, children with leukaemia, prolonged granulocytosis and prolonged hospitalization. *Aspergillus* (80%) is the most common causative organism. The other species are *Mucor* and *Candida. Aspergillus fumigatus* is more common in Europe and North America whereas in Middle East (Sudan) *Aspergillus flavus* takes the upper hand.

Classification

It has been classified as following:

Invasive disease

Types of invasive disease include:

1. Acute invasive (fulminant) fungal rhinosinusitis.
2. Granulomatous invasive fungal rhinosinusitis.
3. Chronic invasive fungal rhinosinusitis.

Non-invasive disease

Types of non-invasive disease include:

1. Saprophytic fungal infestation.
2. Aspergilloma (Fungal ball).
3. Eosinophil related fungal rhinosinusitis including allergic fungal rhinosinusitis (AFRS).

INVASIVE FORM

Sinonasal region is rarely the site of primary pathology in invasive fungal infections. It usually involves other areas such as maxillary and ethmoid sinuses. It is seen both in immunocompetent as well as immunocompromised patients. Early symptoms of invasive fungal rhinosinusitis include nasal obstruction, rhinorrhea, facial hematoma and epistaxis. Common symptoms are retroorbital and sinus pain, fever, orbital swelling and nasal congestion. Complications usually occur as a result of local invasion. They include involvement of internal carotid artery, ophthalmic artery occlusion, cavernous sinus thrombosis, intracerebral extension of infection.

Aspergillus is the most common causative organism of chronic invasive fungal rhinosinusitis. It is a saprophyte found in soil, dust and decaying organic matter. All species of *Aspergillus*, e.g., *flavus, fumigatus* and *niger* can be pathogenic in man. The pathophysiology is speculative and is thought to be combination of both type I (IgE) and type III (immune complex) immunologic reactions.

Acute fulminant, rhinocerebral mucormycosis, invasive aspergillus rhinosinusitis

This clinical condition was first described by McGill et al. It is a rare clinical entity. The primary etiologic agent belongs to the Mucoraceae family (Morpeth et al.). The most common organism is *Aspergillus* closely followed by *Mucor*, and *Candida*. Rapidity of the diseased process is entirely dependent on the immunocompetence of the host. The outstanding histopathological features are fungal vascular invasion with vascular thrombosis and tissue infarction; centrifugally spreading necrotizing reaction with minimal cellular infilterate, often have a necrotic nasal ulcer. This condition commonly manifests with fever, facial pain and swelling, nasal obstruction, and rhinorrhoea (McGill et al. & Kavangh et al.) If the infection progresses into orbit then patient may present with visual symptoms and

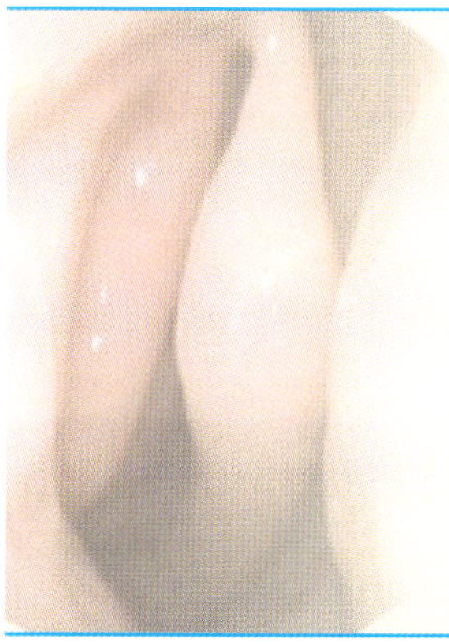

CHAPTER 16

Management of Epistaxis

R.K. Ranga, S.P.S. Yadav

Epistaxis (Greek word meaning nose bleed) is one of the most common complaints in all age groups, which have prevalence of 10–20%. Anterior epistaxis is more common in children and young adults while posterior nasal bleed is mostly seen in older patients with arteriosclerosis or hypertension. It is more common during hot dry climates with low humidity. Most of the episodes of epistaxis do not affect the hemodynamics but sometimes may cause great anxiety not only to the patient but to their relatives also. There is tendency for the bleeding to stop by itself or may be controlled with home remedies. However, massive bleeding sometimes proves fatal. There are different modalities of treatment. Home remedies like pinching of nose or pouring cold water on the face and head may stop epistaxis and the patient may not need any further treatment. In majority of cases the cause of epistaxis is not identifiable which is termed as idiopathic.

Hippocrates commented that holding pressure on the nose helped to abate the bleeding. Others tried writing magical words on the forehead with the patient's own blood, having the patient sniff and own fried blood into their nose, and wear red colour amulets. Carl Michel (1871), James Little (1871) and Wilheim Kiesselbach were first to identify the nasal septem's anterior plexus as a source of nasal bleeding. Pilz was the first to surgically treat epistaxis with ligation of the common carotid artery in 1869. This work was followed by Seiffert ligating the internal maxillary artery via maxillary sinus in 1928. Henry Goodyear performed the first anterior ethmoid artery ligation for the treatment of epistaxis. The medical fraternity's understanding of epistaxis has increased dramatically. However, treatment, though somewhat modified over the years, has continued to include techniques first noted several thousand years ago.

ANATOMY AND PHYSIOLOGY

For its role of humidifying and warming inspired air, the nasal mucosa has a rich blood supply derived from both the internal and external carotid systems, with extensive anastomoses between these blood vessels. The external carotid artery is the main contributor to the blood supply of the nasal mucosa by its eight branches; the facial artery and the maxillary artery are the main sources of blood to the nose. The facial artery (external maxillary artery) is less significant than the internal maxillary artery. It gives rise to the superior labial artery, which enters the nose just lateral to the nasal spine. It sends two branches to the nose: the septal branch to the anterior nasal septum and floor and the alar branch to the nasal ala. The most significant contribution from the external carotid is the internal maxillary artery. Several terminal branches of the internal maxillary artery exist in its third, or pterygopalatine, portion. As the artery enters the pterygopalatine fossa it gives off (among others) the sphenopalatine and greater palatine arteries.

The sphenopalatine artery enters the nasal cavity through the sphenopalatine foramen located at the posterior limit of the middle turbinate. It gives off the posterior septal branch which courses over the nasal roof underneath the sphenoid bone to supply the septum inferiorly and anteriorly, as well as the posterior lateral nasal branch which supplies the turbinates and meati (as well as the ethmoid and maxillary sinuses). The greater palatine artery can originate from the internal maxillary, sphenopalatine, or descending palatine arteries. It descends through the pterygopalatine canal, to emerge from the greater palatine foramen as the greater palatine artery. It then courses anteriorly in close contact with the alveolar ridge where it makes an upward turn, passing through the incisive foramen to supply the anterior, inferior nasal septum.

The internal carotid artery has no contributing branches in the neck. It passes through the petrous portion of the temporal bone and turns sharply, running near the lateral surface of the sphenoid bone. It runs close to the cavernous sinus and pierces the dura lateral to the anterior clinoid process. This is where it gives off its first intracranial branch, the ophthalmic artery, which enters the superior orbital fissure and gives off (among others) the posterior and anterior ethmoid arteries. The posterior ethmoid artery branches off the ophthalmic artery shortly after it enters the orbit. It passes medially to exit the orbit through the posterior ethmoid foramen, located 3 to 7 mm anterior to the optic nerve. It travels through the posterior ethmoid air cells, enters the anterior cranial fossa, and penetrates the cribiform plate to reach the nose. This artery supplies primarily the superior turbinate and a corresponding area of the septum. The anterior ethmoid artery, which is the larger of the two, branches off from the ophthalmic artery anterior to the posterior ethmoid artery and exits the orbit through the anterior ethmoid foramen, located about 10 mm anterior to the posterior ethmoid foramen. It travels through the anterior ethmoid air cells, enters the anterior cranial fossa, and enters the nose through the open nasal slit (a space between the crista galli and the cribiform plate). It nourishes the anterior superior septum and lateral walls.

Several areas within the nose are associated with a high frequency of epistaxis. The first is located along the anterior caudal septum where the sphenopalatine, greater palatine, anterior ethmoid, and superior labial arteries anastomose. This is the area that is known as Kiesselbach's plexus or Little's area. It is estimated that approximately 80% to 90% of all epistaxis occurs in this area, especially in children and young adults. The site associated most frequently with posterior epistaxis is known as Woodruff's plexus and is located where the sphenopalatine artery enters the nasal cavity through the sphenopalatine foramen at the posterior limit of the middle turbinate.

SITE

Various sites of nasal bleeding like Kiesselbach's plexus (Little's area) which is situated at the anterior inferior part of nasal septum and 90% of anterior bleeding occurs from this site. Other sites are inferior turbinate and nasal floor, Woodruff's plexus, middle turbinate, middle meatus, bilateral septum in bleeding diathesis, nasopharynx and sinus cavities.

ETIOLOGY OF EPISTAXIS

The etiology of epistaxis is not always straight forward, however, trauma is the most common cause of epistaxis which may be blunt trauma or digital trauma (nose picking), the latter is most common cause in children. In elderly patients hypertension induced arteriosclerotic vessels, which lie under the delicate mucosa are unable to retract and clot easily when get damaged and cause bleeding. Fear and anxiety due to bleeding and the pain associated with epistaxis management may further elevate the blood pressure causing a vicious cycle. Multiple causes of epistaxis can be divided into two broad categories: local and systemic.

There can also be epistaxis with trauma to the sinuses, orbits, middle ear, and base of skull (if the trauma involves the anterior sphenoid sinus wall causing laceration of the posterior septal branch of the sphenopalatine artery). Chronic irritation in nose causes crusting and excoriation with formation of friable granulation tissue that bleeds easily on further nose picking. Surgical procedures of the nose and sinuses such as rhinoplasty, septoplasty, turbinoplasty and endoscopic sinus surgery as well as orbital floor procedures can cause epistaxis usually from the mucosal incisions, but less frequently as a result of complications such as transection of vessels and septal perforations. Barotrauma sustained from flying or scuba diving can cause hemorrhage within the paranasal sinus cavities with subsequent epistaxis. Anatomical or

Table 16.1. Common causes of epistaxis

Local	
Inflammatory	Rhinosinusitis, nasal polyposis, chronic infections like TB, syphilis, rhinoscleroma
Trauma	Nose picking, iatrogenic facial trauma, foreign body in nose, surgery
Idiopathic	Little's area, Woodruff's plexus
Neoplastic	Benign, e.g., angiofibroma, inverted papilloma Malignant, e.g., squamous cells carcinoma, olfactory neuroblastoma, melanoma
Drugs/ inhalants	Cocaine, tobacco, heroin, wood-dust, cannabis, etc.
Miscellaneous	Wegener's granulomatosis, midline granuloma
Systemic	
Coagulation disorders	Haemophila, specific factor deficiency
Thrombo-cytopenia	Bone marrow aplasia, hypersplenism, DIC
Platelet dysfunction	von Willebrand's disease, leukemia, uraemia, bypass surgery
Drugs	Aspirin, anticoagulants, immunosuppression, alcohol, chloramphenicol, chemotherapy
Miscellaneous	Liver failure, hypothyroidism, vitamin K deficiency

structural deformities are another local etiology of epistaxis. Septal spurs and deviations involving the cartilaginous or bony septum can cause epistaxis by interrupting the normal airflow pattern inside the nasal cavity. Eddy currents are produced that dry the adjacent nasal mucosa and cause crusting with subsequent epistaxis. Bleeding just posterior to a septal deformity may be difficult to arrest thus requiring septoplasty. Septal perforations secondary to various etiologies can cause epistaxis. Granulation and crusting occur on the margins of the perforations which bleed easily. Inflammatory conditions usually manifest as congestion and blood streaked mucus, but can also develop frank epistaxis. Various local inflammatory reactions can alter the normal mucosa, causing dryness and crusting, which allows introduction of bacteria and subsequent formation of granulation tissue.

Increased vascularity and greater friability of the vessels are characteristic of inflamed tissue. Such conditions causing local inflammation include upper respiratory infection, allergic rhinitis, sinusitis, nasal polyposis, environmental irritants, and toxic chemicals. Patients with recurrent epistaxis may have fibrinolytically active bacteria in the nasal cavity that produce streptokinase and staphylokinase. Nasal foreign bodies, usually lodged in children and mentally retarded individuals, should be suspected with unilateral foul discharge. Foreign bodies that cause bleeding usually have sharp edges, irritating chemical properties, and/or porosity. Bleeding occurs from the inflamed mucosa and granulation tissue around the foreign body. Intranasal parasites, including leeches, can lodge in the nose or nasopharynx and cause bleeding. Benign and malignant tumours in the nasal cavities, nasopharynx, and sinuses can present with epistaxis. They cause bleeding indirectly from erosion into normal sinonasal structures or directly from tumours of high vascularity. Bleeding is usually unilateral and can be intermittent or constant.

Tumours like nasal hemangioma, hemangiopericytoma, papilloma, squamous cell carcinoma, adenoid cystic carcinoma, adenocarcinoma, and melanoma are the common causes of epistaxis. Juvenile nasal angiofibroma should be considered when a male adolescent presents with nasal obstruction, epistaxis, and a nasal or nasopharyngeal mass. Aneurysms of the extradural or cavernous sinus portion of the internal carotid artery can cause life-threatening epistaxis. Often a history of cranial surgery or head trauma with sudden onset of unilateral blindness and cranial nerve deficits such as anosmia and involvement of cranial nerves II–VI. Due to the inaccessibility of this area, bleeding from this is usually treated with arterial embolization.

The second major category of disorders causing epistaxis is the systemic factors. These factors usually cause repetitive episodes of epistaxis because of their effect on the vessels either directly or indirectly. Hypertension and atherosclerotic changes are associated with epistaxis, especially posterior nosebleeds in the older patient. Posterior epistaxis was often referred to in the past as "cardiovascular epistaxis" due to its association with hypertension. Accumulation of atheromatous material in the blood vessels and replacement of the muscular tunica media of the arteries by fibrous tissue decrease the hemostatic capabilities of the arteries. Although no scientific studies have shown any significant differences in the prevalence of nosebleeds between patients with or without hypertension, the treatment of epistaxis should include measurement of blood pressure and treatment if needed.

Any condition that impairs or decreases clotting factors and/or platelets can cause epistaxis that is difficult to control. Blood dyscrasias are usually seen in the alcoholic patient or in the patient with a debilitating systemic disease, immunodeficiency, or a lymphoproliferative disorder. Thrombocytopenia is defined as < 100,000 platelets/mm^3, but no spontaneous bleeding occurs until < 40,000. There can be spontaneous mucous membrane bleeding at 10–20,000. The thrombocytopenia can be due to decreased production caused by cytotoxic agents, aplastic anemia, malignancies, etc. or an increased destruction caused by prosthetic heart valves, DIC, sickle cell crisis, TTP, ITP, drugs, hypersplenism, etc. Platelet dysfunction occurs when there is sufficient quantity of platelets but they do not function properly. The most common cause is the use of aspirin and other NSAIDs which impair platelet function by inhibiting cyclooxygenase which is associated with thromboxane production from arachadonic acid. This biochemical pathway is important for platelet aggregation. Systemic disorders such as uremia and liver failure, as well as vitamin deficiencies also predispose to platelet dysfunction causing epistaxis. Clotting factor abnormalities should be suspected if there is a history of easy bruising, prolonged bleeding, and/or family history of the former. Primary coagulopathies include factor VIII deficiency (hemophilia A), factor IX deficiency (hemophilia B or Christmas disease), factor XI, and von Willebrand's disease. Deficiencies of fibrinogen, prothrombin, factors V, X, VII, and XII are extremely rare.

Secondary coagulopathies such as liver disease and vitamin deficiencies can cause bleeding due to diminished synthesis of clotting factors or exacerbate epistaxis. Drugs can affect the clotting mechanism such as coumadin which antagonizes the action of vitamin K and heparin which inactivates thrombin via anti-thrombin III. Systemic illnesses such as DIC can consume clotting factors. Hereditary hemorrhagic telangiectasia also known as Osler-Weber-Rendu disease is the most common disease of vascular structure. It is autosomal dominant disease. However, its overall incidence is low.

The pathologic condition is the lack of contractile elements in the vessel walls which makes it difficult to stop the epistaxis spontaneously. The telangiectasias are composed of dilated venules and capillaries or small AV malformations that can be found in the skin and mucosal surface of the aerodigestive and genitourinary tracts, although they can occur anywhere on the body. The telangiectasias bleed in response to minor trauma. The most common symptom is recurrent, spontaneous epistaxis that begins with puberty and worsens with age. These patients often require hundreds of blood transfusions. Tests of clotting factors and platelet function are usually normal. Treatment is difficult and usually unsuccessful. Alcohol abuse can predispose to epistaxis by decreased clotting factor synthesis, bone marrow suppression, platelet inhibition, and vitamin deficiencies. Systemic toxic substances such as heavy metals and infectious diseases such as typhoid fever, nasal diphtheria, whooping cough, scarlet fever, rheumatic fever, and leprosy. Cardiovascular conditions such as congestive heart failure, mitral stenosis, and coarctation of the aorta can predispose to epistaxis because of increased systemic vascular resistance that is translated back to the nasal mucosa.

MANAGEMENT

In the management of epistaxis three treatment are required like assessment of patient, non-surgical and surgical.

Assessment of patient (Fig. 16.1)

It includes a history-taking regarding excess alcohol intake, chronic pulmonary diseases, bleeding tendencies, hypertension and cardiovascular diseases which can cause epistaxis or can increases morbidity or mortality in compromised patients. History of trauma, site of bleed, recurrent attacks of sinus infection, sinonasal surgery or any drug intake (aspirin, anticoagulants) is obtained. Initially during the physical examination, the adequacy of the airway and circulating blood volume should be assessed. A general physical examination should be performed with particular attention to the skin and mucous membranes for vascular lesions. Thorough examination of the nasal cavity should then be performed in order to locate the site of bleeding as well as possible septal deviations or mucosal and structural abnormalities within. During the

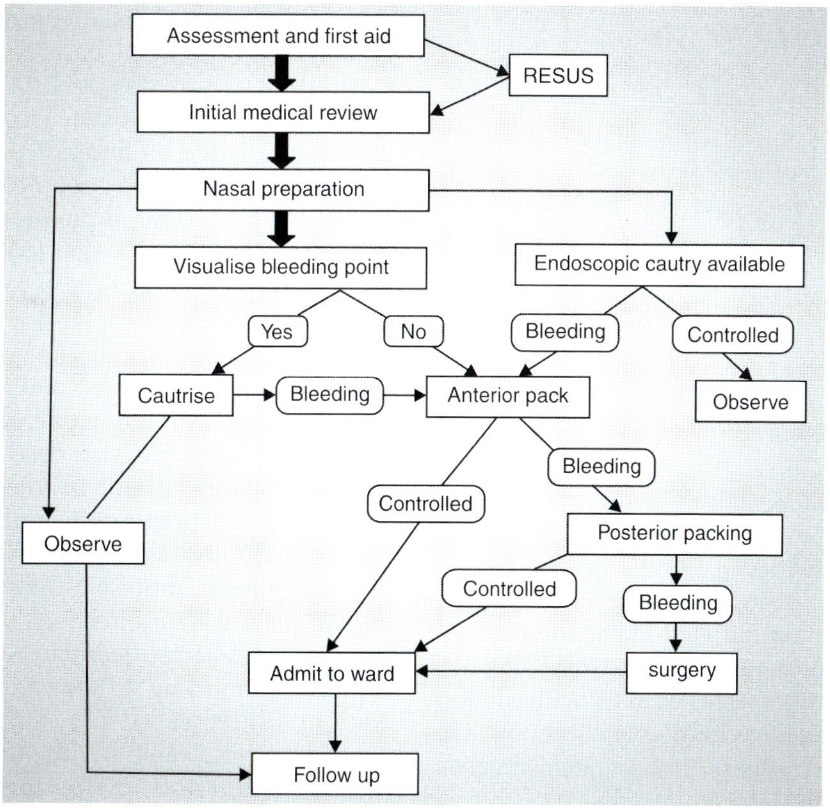

Fig. 16.1. Epistaxis management protocol.

examination particular attention should be paid to assure both physician and patient comfort.

Assess blood loss, monitor blood pressure and pulse rate. All patients with bilateral anterior nasal packing or posterior nasal packing should be admitted, intravenous fluid line maintained and oxygen should be given. High risks patients (elderly, debilitated, alcoholics with liver diseases) and unstable patients need constant monitoring. Bed rest with head elevation is advised. Humidification of room along with low flow oxygen by face mask for patients with posterior packing. Broad-spectrum antibiotics with adequate hydration. Complete blood count and management of hypertension if existing. Fresh blood (cross matched) transfusion if required. Vitamin supplement like C, K and calcium are also required for haemostasis.

Non-surgical treatment

Traditionally, patients are initially managed with topical vasoconstrictors, packing or cauterisation. Most of time these methods can stop bleeding upto 80–90% cases. Topical treatments include epinephrine, pseudoephedrine, xylocaine with adrenaline and cocaine. Nasal packing is used for placement of constant pressure on nasal mucosa. Mostly material used in packing is ribbon gauze with soframycin ointment and merocel and sometimes can be supplement with thrombin, oxycellulose or fibrin. The three locations of packing are anterior, posterior and anterior/posterior. These should be kept inside at least for 3–5 days to allow vessels to develop a mature thrombus. The main advantages of such a packing are simple, easy to perform and does not require any inpatient monitoring, but few disadvantages like nasal obstruction, sinusitis, risks of pressure necrosis of nasal mucosa, hypoxia, bacteremia, epiphoria, toxic shock syndrome and otitis media.

Merocel packing

It is a polyvinyl alcohol derivative (PVA), which is highly advanced biocompatible synthetic material (Fig. 16.2). It is produced by a chemical reaction resulting in cross-linked polyvinyl alcohol with a completely open cell structure. The final PVA sponge material has 100% open pores in its structure with no dead-end pockets to hold residues.

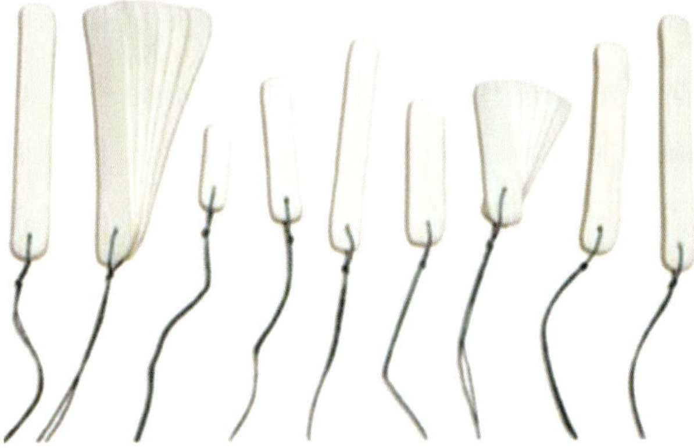

Fig. 16.2. Different size of merocel packs.

The structure, along with the sponge's unique reticulated form, makes it both absorbent and hydrophilic. The merocel material is exceptionally strong and durable, yet soft and comfortable when hydrated. It is gamma-radiated, distinctive micro-state 100% open pores, pore formers. It is very easy to use by just cleaning the nasal cavity with suction and insert in to nasal cavity (Fig. 16.3). Long size merocel pack covers the nasopharyngeal mucosa and stops the posterior bleeding also.

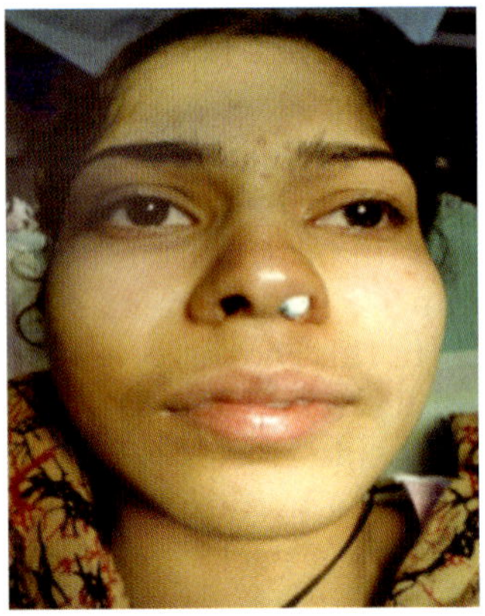

Fig. 16.3. Merocel pack in situ in left nasal cavity.

Posterior packing

A posterior pack should be placed if a posterior nosebleed continues despite a properly placed anterior pack. The standard posterior pack is made up of finely rolled gauze or lamb's wool tied in the centre with two long pieces and one short piece of umbilical tape or 0-silk ties. The patient needs to be given sedation and adequate anesthesia prior to placing the pack. A small red rubber catheter is passed through the each bleeding nostril and brought out from the mouth. The two long ties are then secured to the distal end of the catheter and pulled back through the nasal cavity as the catheter is withdrawn from the nose until the pack is secure in nasopharynx or choana. Traction on the ties is maintained while an anterior pack is placed. The ties are then fastened over a dental roll in front of the nostril by placing a piece of plastic tube. The small suture previously tied to the pack is used to retrieve the pack at the time of removal in 4–7 days.

All patients with posterior packs should be admitted to the hospital. The elderly and patients with cardiopulmonary or blood gas changes should be admitted to an intensive care unit for close monitoring. These patients need to be observed for changes brought about by the abnormalities in respiratory function: hypoventilation, hypoxemia, cardiac arrhythmias, and possible cardiac arrest. Broad-spectrum antibiotics to counteract possible middle ear and sinus infections as well as aspiration pneumonia and septicemia are needed. Oxygen supplementation by 40% oxygen via facemask to counteract decreased pO_2 and increased pCO_2 which occurs in patients with posterior nasal packs. Mild sedation and analgesia needs to be used judiciously so as not to cause significant respiratory depression. The patient should be kept on intravenous fluid therapy as well as monitored with pulse oximetry, electrocardiography, blood gases, and serial hematocrits.

Balloon therapy

This relies on either direct pressure or more commonly, the accumulation of blood within the nasal cavity leading to tamponade. There are several types of inflatable balloon packs which are commercially available and designed especially for epistaxis management. Advantages of inflatable balloon packs include easily inserted, less traumatic to the patient, and allows a partial nasal airway. Disadvantages include less effective than a standard pack since the pressure applied to the nose is not equal and some balloons are inflated with water whereas some need to be inflated with air.

Foley catheter

A Foley catheter size 12–16 French is placed along the floor of the nose until visualized in the nasopharynx. The balloon is then inflated with 3–4 ml of water or air and the catheter is retracted anteriorly to wedge the balloon snugly onto the posterior choana. After this nasal cavity is then packed anteriorly with ribbon gauze or a nasal sponge anterior pack, then balloon is held firmly in place with an umbilical clamp at the anterior nares or the catheter is secured with a piece of tubing slid tightly against the anterior pack either by artery forceps or by suture. It is important in these cases to protect the columella and ala nasi with a soft dressing; otherwise it is susceptible to pressure necrosis. To avoid this 2–3 cm of endotracheal tube is slid over the catheter and kept out before inserting in the nose. This tube will be just at the anterior nasal packing and clamp will lie just anterior to it. Other complications include posterior displacement of the balloon with potential airway compromise, deflation in situ (which is more likely to occur with air inflation) and rupture of the balloon which, when it contains water, could result in aspiration. Recent evidence suggests that balloon rupture is more likely with the use of paraffin paste. It is important to note that the Foley's catheter is, in fact, not licensed for nasal use.

Brighton balloon

This is specifically manufactured for the treatment of epistaxis. It has a postnasal balloon and a mobile anterior balloon that is independently inflated. Other specialised balloons include the Simpson plug and the Epistat nasal catheter (Figs. 16.4 and 16.5).

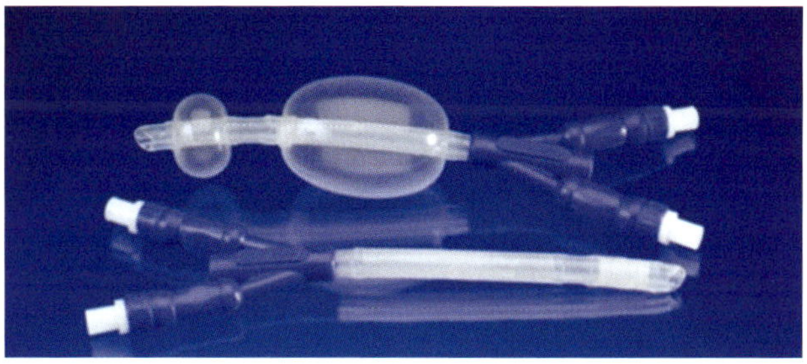

Fig. 16.4. Epistat nasal catheter.

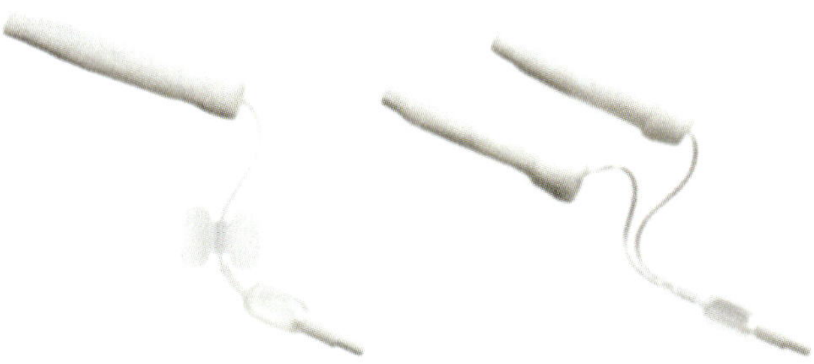

Fig. 16.5. Nasal tamponade with carboximethylcellulose fabric for unilateral or bilateral nostril.

Cauterisation of bleeder

Once the active or inactive bleeding site is identified, chemical or electrical cautery can be used to attempt to arrest the bleeding. Silver nitrate/trichloroacetic acid should be applied to the bleeding site for at least 30 seconds. The excess acids should be removed from the nose to prevent it from spreading and injuring healthy nasal mucosa. Beware of performing overly aggressive cautery on both sides of the nasal septum as cartilage exposure or septal perforations can occur. Since actively bleeding vessel is almost impossible to cauterize using silver nitrate, coagulation electrocautery (Fig. 16.6) with suction bovie may be the next choice. It provides a greater depth of penetration, so it is more likely to cause exposure of either cartilage or septal perforation. Since coagulation electrocautery is more painful than using silver nitrate, the patient may need injection with local anesthetic. Antibiotic ointment should be applied to the cauterized area until it is healed. Even posterior bleeding sites can be treated with chemical or electrical cautery after visualization with a rigid or flexible endoscope. This has been found to lessen the distress and morbidity associated with nasal packing and the need for more extensive surgical procedures.

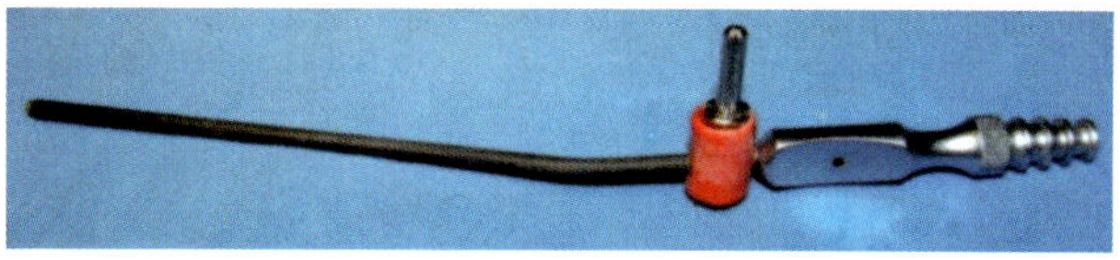

Fig. 16.6. Coagulation electrocautery with suction bovie.

Surgical treatment

Any non-surgical treatment that fails to stop bleeding then surgical intervention or embolisation is next step to control bleeding. In such conditions before doing surgical intervention patient should be haemodynamically stable. Most cases of surgical intervention require general anesthesia, although in frail elderly patient, local anesthesia with sedation can be used. Surgical intervention option can be transmaxillary internal maxillary artery ligation, transoral internal maxillary artery ligation, anterior/posterior ethmoid ligation, external carotid ligation, endoscopic sphenopalatine artery ligation and septoplasty. For patients with hereditary hemorrhagic telangiectasia septodermoplasty, laser, and nasal closure are surgical options.

Transantral internal maxillary artery ligation

Transantral internal maxillary artery ligation is treatment of choice for recalcitrant epistaxis which is performed under general anesthesia. This procedure is performed via a Caldwell-Luc approach through maxillary sinus in which posterior sinus wall is carefully removed and the pterygopalatine fossa contents exposed. Dissection should perform under the operating microscope which allows the surgeon to ligate the distal branches of the internal maxillary artery (sphenopalatine and posterior nasal) under direct vision. There is a 10–15% technical failure rate. Complications (25–30%) include pain in teeth, damage to teeth, damage to sphenopalatine ganglion or vidian nerve, damage to infraorbital nerve, oroantral fistula, and sinusitis.

Transoral internal maxillary artery ligation

The transoral approach is reserved for patients with hypoplastic maxillary sinus and is generally less effective as the ligation is more proximal to the bleeding. An intraoral approach to the maxillary artery provides access to the first and second parts of the artery between the ramus of the mandible and the temporalis muscle. The posterior portion of the maxilla is exposed through a posterior gingivobuccal incision beginning at the second molar. Blunt dissection is then performed with the finger and the buccal fat is dissected or retracted. After the temporalis muscle is split and partially dissected, the internal maxillary artery is visualized at the base of the wound or brought out into the field by a nerve hook then clipped and divided. The advantages of this procedure include its feasibility in children and comminuted fractures of the maxilla. Disadvantages include – the site of ligation is more proximal than the transantral approach with a greater chance of failure due to collateral circulation, frequently results in trismus that may take up to 3 months to resolve due to the manipulation of the temporalis muscle, and can result in damage to the infraorbital nerve.

Anterior/posterior ethmoid artery ligation

This is reserved for patients with superior bleeding or in conjunction with internal maxillary artery ligation for patients with an unknown bleeding site. The approach is made via a Lynch incision and the periorbita is carefully dissected free from the medial orbital wall. The anterior ethmoid artery is located about 14–18 mm posteriorly to this. If the posterior ethmoid artery has to be ligated, it is located 10–12 mm posterior to the anterior ethmoid artery. Care must be taken in this area since the optic nerve is only 4–6 mm posterior to the posterior ethmoid artery. Once identified, the arteries are ligated and divided. The effectiveness of this procedure is not always known, but complications include stroke, blindness, ophthalmoplegia, and epiphora.

External carotid artery ligation

External carotid artery ligation is performed through an incision made in the neck along the anterior border of the sternocleidomastoid muscle at the level of upper border of thyroid cartilage. After two branches of the external carotid artery are identified to avoid ligation of the internal carotid artery, the external carotid artery is ligated. When doing the ligation care must be taken to avoid injury to the vagus, the superior laryngeal nerve, the hypoglossal nerve, the sympathetic chain, or the mandibular branch of the facial nerve. This technique is simple and the anatomy is familiar to most otolaryngologists. The disadvantages of this procedure are that it is less effective than other ligations due to greater collateral blood flow.

Endoscopic coagulation of sphenopalatine artery for posterior epistaxis

The use of endoscopes has revolutionised many nasal surgeries including the management of epistaxis. Posterior epistaxis can be successfully treated with endoscopic coagulation of sphenopalatine artery with successful results and minimal complication. This procedure is carried out either unilaterally or bilaterally. These cases present with profuse posterior epistaxis that persists or recurs despite conservative measures. The nasal cavity is packed with cottonoids soaked in 4% xylocaine with oxymetazoline 0.1%. Hypotensive anesthesia is used to reduce bleeding so as to maintain a clear surgical field. Endoscope is used to examine nasal cavity and an incision is made in the posterior part of middle meatus, posterior to the maxillary ostea around 1 cm anterior to the posterior end of middle turbinate. The mucoperichondrial flap is raised posteriorly until the sphenopalatine artery and its branches are identified. These vessels are coagulated with electrical diathermy. Surgicel is inserted to the area and merocel pack is placed for 24 hours. The submucoperiosteal dissection reduces bleeding, shortens operating time and allows relatively easy identification of sphenopalatine artery. This allows direct positive control over the major vessel supplying the posterior nasal cavity. The length of hospitalization is reduced to just two days post-operatively.

Angiography and embolisation

When neither non-surgical or surgical intervention controls the epistaxis or epistaxis is due to congenital arteriovenous malformation, aberrant arterial vessels, nasal tumours, facial trauma and intractile cases of posterior epistaxis, then embolisation is required. Selective angiography can be used as a diagnostic as well as a therapeutic tool to control epistaxis. After the anatomy is defined and the bleeding site is identified, the bleeding site is embolized with polyvinyl alcohol, Gel-foam particles or coiled springs. This procedure can embolize vessels close to the bleeding site therefore minimizing collaterals. It is effective only when the bleeding rate is > 0.5 ml/min. Success rate is about 90%, with a complication rate of 0.1%. Disadvantages are that only external carotid artery or branches can be embolized and severe complications such as hemiplegia, facial paralysis, and skin necrosis can occur.

Septoplasty

It should be performed in cases where the bony nasal spur is prominent and causes the epistaxis.

Hereditary hemorrhagic telangiectasia

This is also known as Osler-Weber-Rendu disease which is an autosomal dominant fibrovascular dysplasia. Septodermoplasty is used most often in patients with such hemorrhagic disorder. After telangiectatic anterior nasal mucosa is removed from the anterior half of the septum, floor of the nose and lateral wall, a spilt thickness skin graft is placed. Cutaneous, myocutaneous, or microvascular free flaps can also be used in place of the skin graft. There have also been good experimental results from the use of autografts of cultured epithelial sheets derived from the patients buccal mucosa. Patients will get recurrence of epistaxis due to ingrowth of telangiectasia into the grafts or flaps, but the severity and frequency of bleeding is significantly reduced. The neodymium-yttrium-garnet (Nd-YAG) laser or argon laser has been used to photocoagulate epistaxis lesions, especially in those with hereditary hemorrhagic telangiectasia. Retreatment is usually necessary, but the severity and frequency of bleeding is generally improved. Topical estrogen combined with argon plasma coagulation is known to induce metaplasia of nasal mucosa to thick layers of keratinizing squamous epithelium.

CONCLUSION

Epistaxis is a common otorhinolaryngological emergency encountered in our practice, which is caused by various etiological factors like inflammatory, traumatic, neoplastic, coagulopathies, drug-induced and idiopathic. It may be minor which resolves spontaneously or so severe that proves fatal. Traditional methods of management of anterior and posterior epistaxis are nasal packing, which is associated with marked discomfort and several complications. In recent times merocel nasal packing avoiding complication of traditional nasal packing is more potent in controlling epistaxis. Posterior epistaxis is controlled by anterioposterior nasal packing, nasal balloon tamponades and arterial ligation. However, endoscopic cauterization of bleeder is more effective method. In hereditary hemorrhagic telangiectasia septodermoplasty, laser, and topical estrogen is beneficial. Any mechanical deviation of nasal septum with spur which causes epistaxis, septoplasty is helpful in controlling epistaxis.

SUGGESTED READING

1. Pope LER, Hobbs CGL. Epistaxis: An update on current management. *Postgrad Med J*, 2005; 81: 309–14.
2. Barlow DW. Effectiveness of surgical management of epistaxis at a tertiary care center. *Laryngoscope*, 1997; 107: 21–4.
3. Kucik CJ, Clienney T. Management of epistaxis. *Am Fam Physician*, 2005; 71: 305–11.
4. Shin EJ, Murr AH. Managing epistaxis. *Current Opinion in Otolaryngol Head Neck Surg*, 2000; 8: 37–42.
5. Prepageran N, Krishnan G. Endoscopic coagulation of sphenopalatine artery for posterior epistaxis. *Singapore Med J*, 2003; 44: 123–5.
6. Pringle MB, Beasley P, Brightwell AP. The use of merocel nasal packs in the treatment of epistaxis. *J Laryngol Otol*, 2007; 110: 543–6.
7. Stankiewicz, James A. Nasal endoscopy and control of epistaxis. *Current Opinion in Otolaryngol Head Neck Surg*, 2004; 12: 43–5.

8. Srinivasan V, Sherman W, O'Sullivan G. Surgical management of intractable epistaxis: Audit of results. *J Laryngol Otol*, 2000; 114: 697–700.
9. Sadick H, Gotte K, Riedel F, Hormann K. Topical estrogen combined with argon plasma coagulation in the management of epistaxis in hereditary hemorrhagic telangiectasia. *Ann Otol Rhinol Laryngol*, 2002; 111: 222–7.
10. Mohammed ME. Therapeutic embolisation in treatment in intractable epistaxis. *Arch Otolaryngol Head Neck Surg*, 1995; 121: 65–9.
11. Quinn F. Epistaxis pearls from the internet. *UTMB-Otolaryngology website*, 1997.
12. Paul J, Kanotra SP, Kanotra S. Endoscopic management of posterior epistaxis. *Indian J Otolaryngol Head Neck Surg*, 2011; 63(2): 141–4.

CHAPTER 17

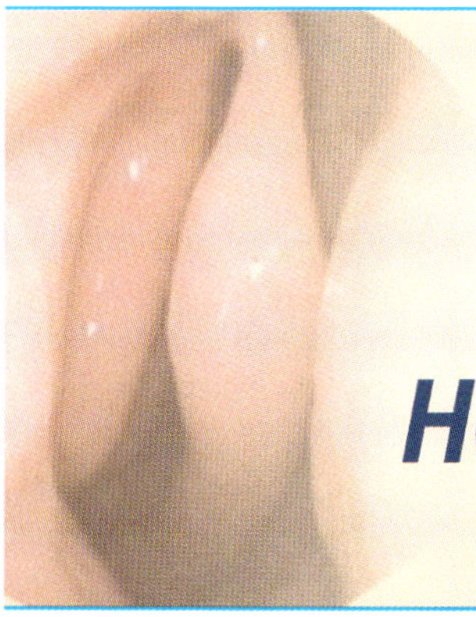

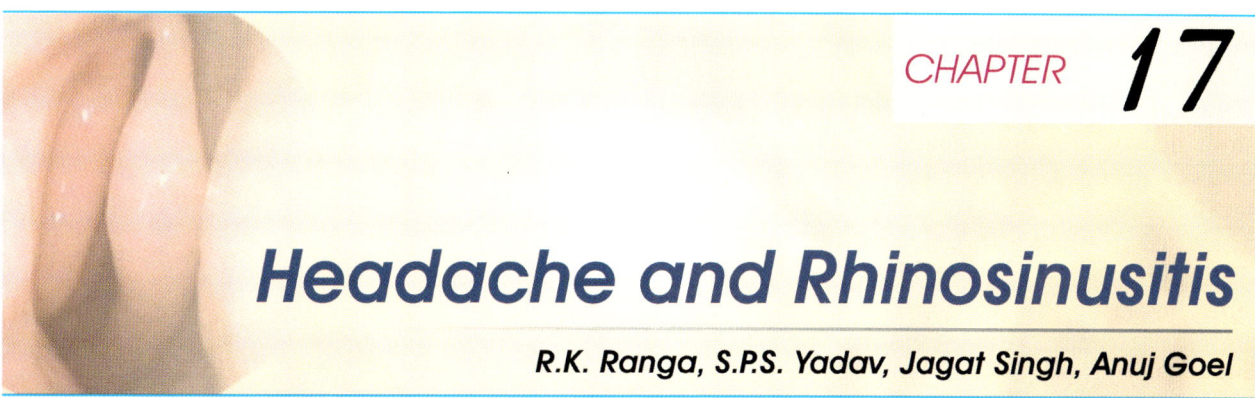

Headache and Rhinosinusitis

R.K. Ranga, S.P.S. Yadav, Jagat Singh, Anuj Goel

Headache is nearly a universal human experience and its lifetime incidence is estimated to be at least 90%. Otolaryngologist frequently deals with the symptoms of headache and the patient often believes the headache is sinus related. Sinus headache is an extremely common clinical entity experienced by millions of people throughout the world. Although sinus headache is commonly diagnosed and seem to be widely recognized by medical practitioners. Therefore, otolaryngologists must have thorough understanding of headache and how the symptomatology may or may not relate to the sinuses.

Typically sinus headache refers to episodes of pain over the sinus area of the face or around the eyes, which is often associated with nasal congestion, rhinorrhoea, facial pressure, lacrimation, nausea and sensory sensitivity. The onset of sinus headache is often related to changes in weather. Like other common primary headache disorders, the sinus headache is to a large extent self-diagnosed and self-treated with wide range of highly promoted over-the-counter remedies. The effectiveness of these products is generally unknown, although recent studies suggest that high degree of dissatisfaction with self-treatment exists, and several headache specialists have publicly expressed concern that overuse of these products can complicate an underlying headache disorder such as migraine. Sinus headache is frequently misdiagnosed and subsequently ineffectively treated.

Historical review

There are many etiological concepts of sinus headache origin hypothesis proposed more than five decades ago. Review of literature concludes that etiologic concepts of sinus headache is due to creation of negative pressure in the occluded sinus cavity as the air is absorbed by the tissue. This was proposed by McBride in 1891. Greenfeild Sluder also discussed the role of the trigeminal system in generation of nasal symptom and medical intervention with sphenopalatine ganglion blocks.

Harold Wolff proposed the vascular theory of migraine in 1948. He described an experiment in which he stimulated various portion of the nasal cavities and sinus passages. In an experiment catheters were inserted into oroantral fistulous tract secondary to dental extraction. Both positive and negative pressures were applied to induce pain. Moderate pain was induced at 50 mmHg positive pressure and 250 mmHg negative pressure. Wolf found that pain could be elicited from much lower pressure applied in the area of the osteum that connects the maxillary sinus with nasal passage. McAuliffe and colleagues challenged the earlier hypothesis of negative pressure in the occluded sinus cavities. They hypothesized that there are likely more anatomic areas of pain generation.

Presently sinus headache is supposed to be a secondary headache associated with sinonasal pathology. Nasal headache caused by structural abnormalities is considered an unproven clinical entity. Such headache is rarely anything more than misdiagnosed migraine. Low and Willet reported that correction of sinonasal pathology improves the symptoms of headache postoperativly. Therefore, sinus headache is not a single entity but a heterogeneous group of headaches that share location of headache but have diverse causes. Neurophysician and otorhinolaryngologist might consult on different subsets of patients with the complaint of sinus headache.

Site of pain (Figs. 17.1, 17.2 and 17.3)

Pain from sinonasal diseases can be present in many areas of the face and referred to a distant area of the head or neck region. On percussion the sinuses in cases of sinusitis reveal inexact and often misleading information. As tension headache can cause tenderness of facial muscle and scalp, percussion of the forehead may elicit pain misleading to the possibility of frontal sinusitis.

Pain over the forehead may be a frontal or ethmoid sinus pathology or muscle contraction tension headache.

Sometimes multiple sinuses involvement makes the pain and symptoms confusing. These cause pain in several locations and this facial pain may confuse the practitioner.

History-taking in headache is important to sort out the etiology of facial pain and pressure. It is important to know the location of the pain, the nature of pain (pulsating, steady, squeezing, lancinating-like, sharp, dull, mild, and moderate and severe) as well as the duration and frequency of headache. Many patients have more than one kind of headache. It is important to know how many kinds of headaches are present, what makes the headache better or worse and whether associated symptoms such as aura, nausea, vomiting, photophobia and phonophobia. It is also very important to know about associated sinonasal symptoms such as nasal obstruction, nasal discharge and alteration in taste/smell.

Causes of sinonasal headache

There are many causes of alteration of sinonasal physiological function. Acute rhinosinusitis of

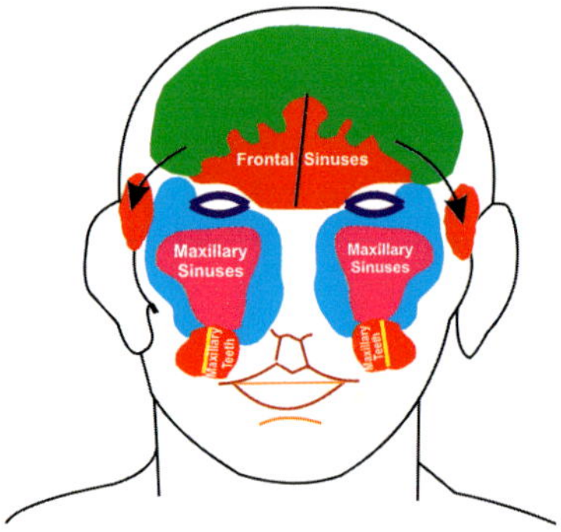

Fig. 17.1. Pain over maxillary sinus may be located over the maxillary sinus or radiate to canine teeth and into temporal region

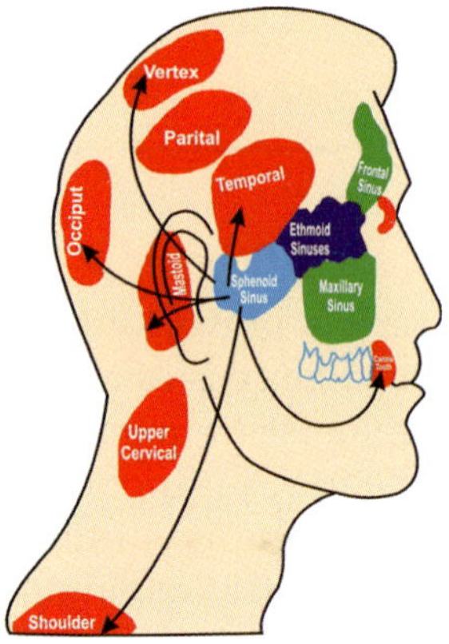

Fig. 17.2. Ethmoid sinusitis can produce pain most often in the medial canthal area, but also pain can extend into parietal and temporal areas and into the upper cervical area.

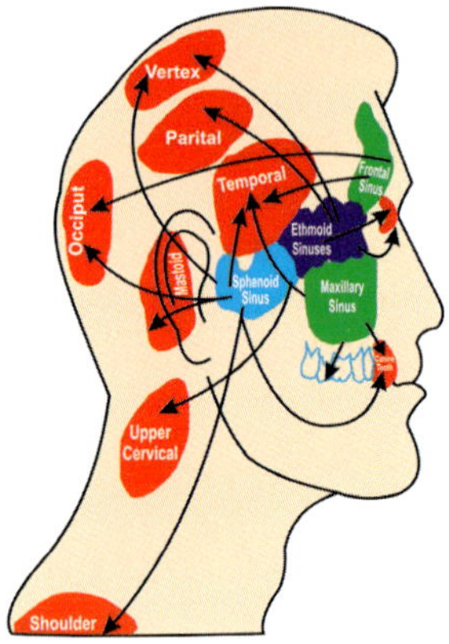

Fig. 17.3. Sphenoid sinusitis will generally produce a retro-orbital headache, but it can extend to the temporal region, vertex, occiput and even into the shoulder and canine teeth.

maxillary, frontal, ethmoid and sphenoid can cause sinus headache. Pathologically the osteomeatal complex can be blocked by polyps, altered pattern of pneumotisation of middle turbinate, uncinate process, agar nasai cell, ethmoid sinus and frontal sinus and inflammatory process in the mucous membrane of this area. A paradoxically bent middle turbinate may be asymptomatic, but it can cause pressure over the mucosa of middle meatus and that can cause pain in various areas. Septal deviation is also a common cause of sinus headache (Figs. 17.4, 17.5 and 17.6).

Concha bullosa either unilateral or bilateral can cause the pressure over the part of middle meatus area and headache (Fig. 17.7). Minimal pathology may cause edema in osteomeatal complex which results from air pollutants, nasal congestion or allergies. Abnormalities of uncinate process also cause obstruction in the anterior osteometal complex (Fig. 17.8). The pain from these areas is referred to the zygomaticotemporal nerve in the temporal region.

Pathological process may occur in the posterior osteometal complex (sphenoethmoid recess) caused by abnormalities of superior turbinate such as concha bullosa, edema or polyposis. Various clinical features leading to diagnosis of sinusitis are depicted in Table 17.1.

Diagnosis is made when two or more major factors are present or one major and two minor factors are present and there is purulence on examination.

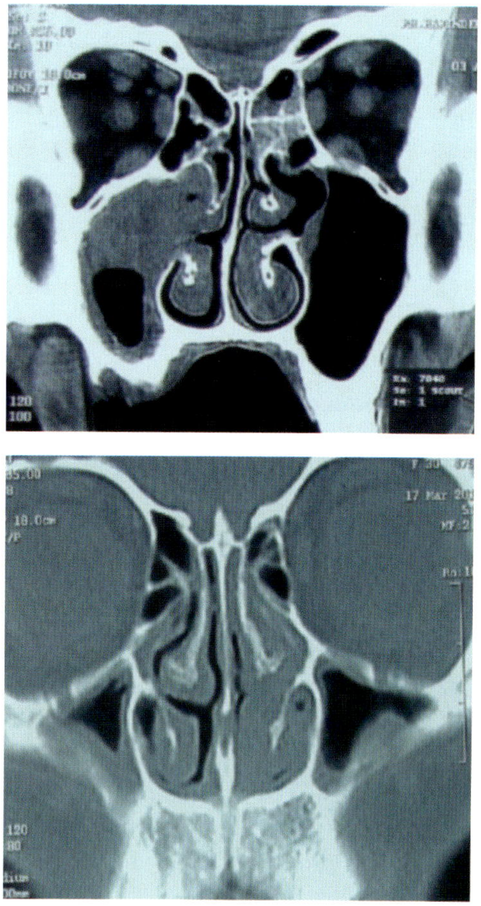

Fig. 17.4. Coronal CT views showing blocked osteomeatal complex.

Biochemical basis

The biological basis of pain is not totally understood. But there are certain irritants, infections, thermal changes that cause the release of substance P and other mediators which are still to be discovered. Substance P causes an orthodromic impulse that travels to the cerebral cortex and causes sensation of both primary and referred pain. There is also an antidromic impulse that travels from cerebral cortex

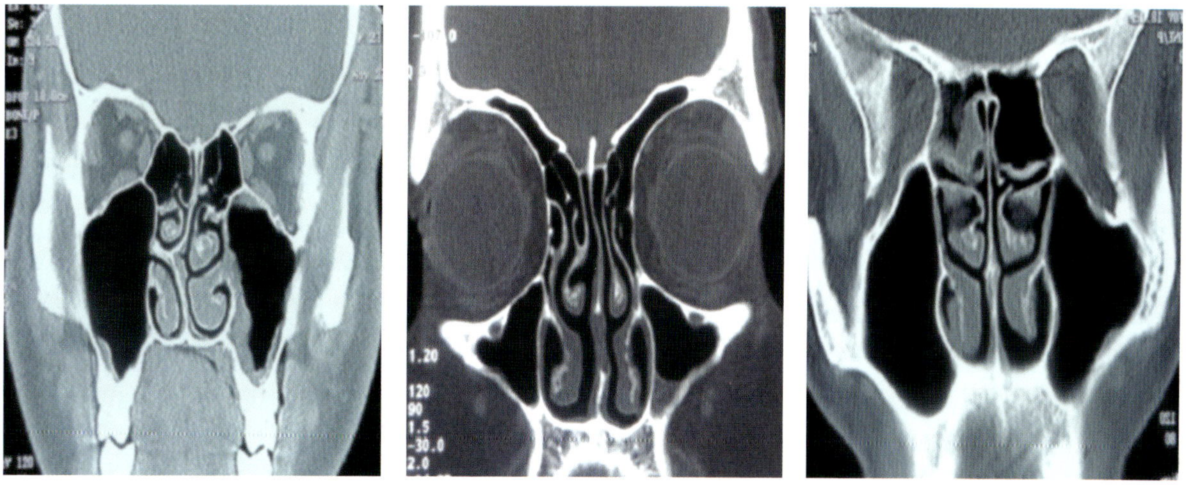

Fig. 17.5. Coronal CT views showing septal deviation, unilateral and bilateral paradoxical middle turbinate.

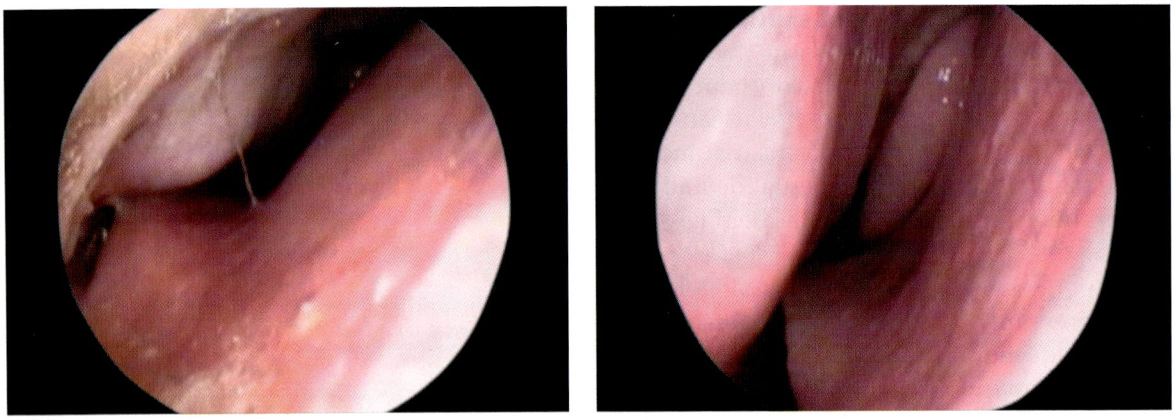

Fig. 17.6. Endoscopic views showing sharp septal deviation.

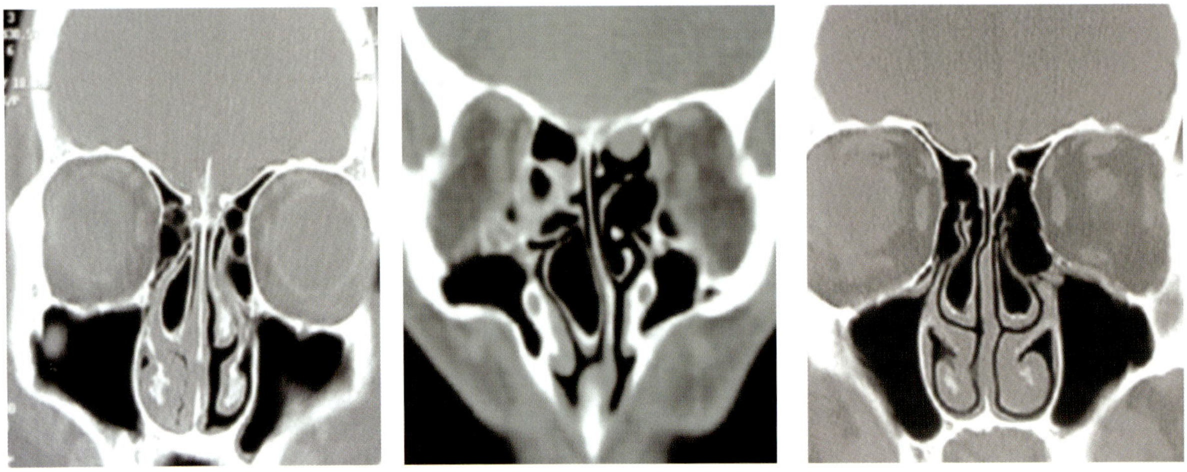

Fig. 17.7. Coronal CT scans PNS showing small and large unilateral and bilateral concha bullosa.

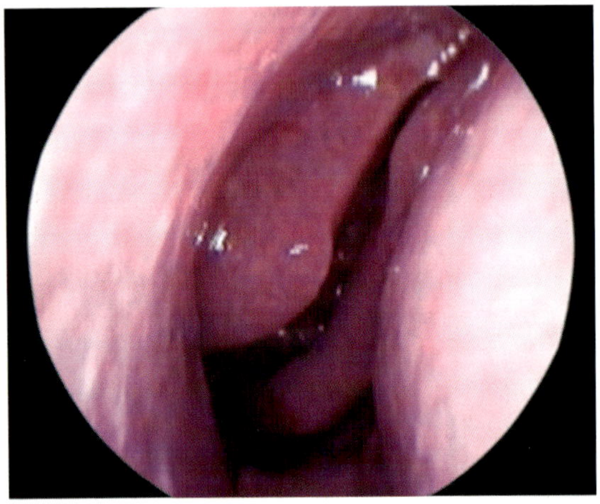

Fig. 17.8. Endoscopic view showing enlarged uncinate process.

Table 17.1. Sinusitis guidelines definition and diagnosis

Major factors	*Minor factors*
Nasal congestion/fullness	Cough
Nasal obstruction/blockage	Ear pressure/fullness
Nasal purulence/drainage	Fatigue
Facial pressure/pain	Halitosis
Hyposmia/anosmia	Headache
Fever	Maxillary dental pain

to nasal mucosa. This process causes the congestion and hypersecretion of nasal mucus which causes increase in mucosal mechanical pressure and contact. If there is already some degree of a compromised sinus outflow because of an anatomical abnormality, the problem is compounded and pain is worsened. This causes increased release of substance P and subsequent increase in nasal congestion and hypersecretion, resulting in a vicious cycle. We always make an attempt to break this cycle with decongestants, mucolytes, antibiotics, steroids or surgery.

Diagnosis of sinus headache

Sinus headache is defined by International Headache Society (I.H.S.) diagnostic criteria in the setting of an infection. Process requires verification through imaging and confirmation by response to appropriate antibiotics. IHS Nomenclature Committee concludes that headache is not recognized as symptom of chronic sinusitis unless there is a superimposed acute infection. The diagnostic criteria for headache were revised in 2003, but the nasal and ocular symptoms were again conspicuously absent in the diagnostic definition of migraine. Essentially, sinus headache remains a headache secondary to inflammatory pathologic conditions, although there is a statement in the new criteria that sinus headache is often confused with migraine.

Diagnostic criteria for rhinosinusitis were defined in the ENT literature by Lanza and Kennedy in 1997. In this diagnostic scheme rhinosinusitis is subdivided into acute, recurrent acute, subacute, chronic and acute exacerbations of chronic. Headache in absence of other diagnostic criteria was not considered diagnostic of sinusitis.

Plain X-rays have a poor specificity and sensitivity in diagnosis of sinus headache. However, computed tomography (CT) visualizes all anatomical landmarks of nose and paranasal sinuses. Both sections – axial and coronal – are necessary for assessment. MRI have limited role in diagnosis of sinus headache.

Rigid endoscopy

In routine diagnostic endoscopy visualize all three passes in the nose.

- First endoscopy pass visualizes the septum, inferior meatus, Eustachian tube opening and nasolacrimal duct opening.
- 2nd pass: Middle turbinate, uncinate process, hiatus semilunaris and septum should be visualized.
- 3rd pass: Sphenoethmoidal recess area and olfactory area are visualized.

Previous theories implicating contact point as a cause of facial pain have been discredited, as they are found frequently in an asymptomatic population as in those with pain and these patients often respond to low dose amytriptyline.

Sinus headache is a secondary headache but we have to differentiate from primary headache like migraine and tension type headaches.

Headache attributed to rhinosinusitis by the international classification of headache disorders

A. Frontal headache accompanied by pain in one or more regions of the face, ears or teeth and fulfilling criteria C and D.

B. Clinical, nasal endoscopic, CT and/or MRI imaging and/or laboratory evidence of acute-on-chronic rhinosinusitis (1, 2).

C. Headache and facial pain develops simultaneously with onset or acute exacerbation of rhinosinusitis.

D. Headache and/or facial pain resolves within 7 days after remission or successful treatment of acute-on-chronic rhinosinusitis.

Note:

1. Clinical evidence may include purulence in the nasal cavity, nasal obstruction, hyposmia/anosmia and/or fever.
2. Chronic sinusitis is not validated as a cause of headache or facial pain unless relapsing in to an acute stage.

Migraine headache

Migraine headaches are recurring with periods free of pain. There are two types of migraine: migraine with aura (classical) and migraine without aura (common). Migraine headaches are typically moderate to severe in intensity, unilateral, palasitle, and lasting for several hours. It is usually associated with nausea, vomiting, photophobia, phonophobia and irritability. During the attack time the sufferer will usually have pale facies, mostly likes dark and quiet environment.

There are numerous triggers to bring on migraine headache. These include stress, fatigue, over-sleeping, fasting or missing a meal, vasoactive substances in food (e.g., nitrates in processed meats), caffeine, alcohol, menses, change in barometric pressure and changes in altitudes. Such headaches often occur on weekends, when there is a change in typical sleep pattern, eating and activity schedules.

Most migraine headaches occur in young adults and women, who account three times more than men. Many women have such episodes of headache few days before the menstrual cycle. There is a positive family history for migraine in over 70% of patients. The onset is generally during adolescence and migraine headaches tend to diminish by the fifth or sixth decade of life.

Tension-type headache

It is also known as muscle contraction headache which is most common. It is a combination of neurogenic, vascular and muscle contraction. The headache is usually a bandlike pain with pressure in forehead, temples, over the top of head, or down the neck and in the shoulders. It is described as a pressure or tightness. It is most often of moderate intensity, but not disabling and can persist more than half a month. The discomfort worsens as the day progresses and rarely worsens with activity. Tension headaches are more of workweek headache versus migraine of weekend type headache. They are triggered by stress, anxiety, drug habituation, cervical spondylitis, temporomandubular joint disorders and some occupational situation. Most of the patients complain of pain in forehead and are referred to otorhinolaryngologist assuming it to be a sinus headache.

Cluster headache

It is not as common as migraine or tension headache. The patient is awakened in early hours, often walking around in distress, with the pain lasting 30 minutes to 2 hours. Nausea is absent but frequently there is rhinorrhoea, unilateral nasal obstruction, lacrimation and sometimes conjunctival infection. It is common in males between 20–40 years of age. It may be precipitated by alcohol, cold temperature, or excitement. Myosis or facial flushing may be seen. It typically presents with a severe, unilateral, stabbing or burning pain, which may be frontal, temporal, and ocular, over the cheek or even in maxillary teeth. Patients will often surmise that they have a sinus infection rather than cluster headache because of the associated nasal stiffness and periorbital pain. Like other headaches, the history points to cluster rather than sinus headache.

MANAGEMENT

In case of sinus headache caused by nasal sinus disorder, the site of obstruction is frequently much more important than the extent of the disease, and minor obstruction can cause great deal of pain. There may be a concentration of sensory nerve fibers around the ostia of sinuses. It would result in small lesions and obstruction in anterior or posterior osteomeatal complex to produce a great deal of pain, pressure and pansinusitis. For treatment of sinus headache correct the pathological causes of sinonasal ailment either by correction of mechanical obstruction like DNS or functional endoscopic sinus surgery. Allergic condition treated with newer antihistaminic, antifungal agents and intranasal corticosteroids.

Migraine treatment

A simple analgesic provides effective relief from migraine. Absorption is impaired by gastric stasis during migraine; this may be helped by the addition of an antiemetic and large dose of aspirin. First line treatments for migraine include the use of β-blockers and tricyclic antidepressants such as amytriptyline. These medications exert their effects via multiple pathways both within and outside that of the central nervous system.

Table 17.2. Comparison of diagnostic symptoms for migraine and tension-type headache

Migraine without aura	*Episodic tension-type headache*
History of >5 lifetime attacks lasting 4 to 72 hours	History of >10 lifetime attacks lasting 30 minutes to 7 days
Headache characterized by at least 2 of the following 4:	Headache characterized by at least 2 of the following 4:
Moderate to severe pain	Mild to moderate pain
Unilateral	Bilateral
Throbbing quality	Pressure
Aggravated by activity	Not aggravated by activity
Associated features	Associated features
Nausea and/or vomiting	No nausea and/or vomiting
Photophobia and phonophobia	No photophobia and phonophobia
No evidence of underlying cause	No evidence of underlying disease

17

Non-steroidal antiinflammatory drugs such as paracetamol are also helpful and drug of choice in some patients. Triptans are more effective than simple analgesics. Triptans can be given in dose sumatriptan 50/100 mg, naratriptan 2.5 mg, zolmitriptan 2.5/5 mg, rizatriptan 10 mg and almotriptan 12.5 mg. Triptans are relatively safe drugs; concern about cardiac toxicity has only rarely been realized in clinical practice. However, triptan should never be used in those with or at risk of cardiac ischemia.

Prophylaxis of migraine

The prevention of migraine with daily drug treatment should be considered only after acute treatment has been optimized, however, over-medication should be avoided, lifestyle modification tried and episodes are recorded for 1–3 months. Most agents often provide partial benefit only, which may take 1–5 months to achieve optimal effects. Commonly used drugs are as follows: amitriptyline 5–10 mg, flunarizine 5–10 mg, propranolol 20–40 mg, valproate 500 mg, methysergide 1 mg and pizotifen 0.5 mg.

Patient must be informed that occurrence after starting prophylaxis does not mean treatment failure. Comorbid disease, such as depression or insomnia, may suggest amitriptyline as intial choice, hypertension indicates a beta-blocker. It is unusual to offer prophylaxis for less than two attacks a month. Treatment should be titrated first for tolerability then for efficacy. After 6 months of effective treatment, phased withdrawal should be considered.

CONCLUSION

Sinonasal headache is a common ailment encountered in otorhinolaryngological practice with many varied causes like infection, neoplasm, septal deviation and malpneumotisation of sinuses which affect the osteomeatal complex physiology. It can be confused with headache of other kinds such as migraine, tension and cluster. When headache is the only symptom, it probably is not of sinus origin. The correct diagnosis can usually be reached by history, physical examination, diagnostic endoscopy and radiological imaging. Treat the cause of headache then headache will subsides spontaneously. Effective treatment is rewarding to the patient's productivity and quality of life are greatly improved.

SUGGESTED READING

1. Topics on otorhinolaryngology, head and neck surgery edited by Swift A (CBS Publisher 2009).
2. Phillips J, Longridge N, Mallinson A, Robinson G. View and perspectives: Migraine and vertigo: A marriage of convenience? *J Head Face Pain*, 2010; 50; 25–8.
3. Sinus surgery: endoscopic and microscopic approaches. Edited by Levine HL & Clemente MP (Thieme Publisher 2005).
4. Cady RK, Schreiber CP. Sinus headache or migraine? Considerations in making a differential diagnosis. *Neurology*, 2002; 58(9): 10–14.
5. Perry BF, Login IS and Kountakis SE. Nonrhinogenic headache in a tertiary rhinology practice. *Otolaryngol Head Neck Surg*, 2004; 130: 449–52.
6. Daudia AT and Jones NS. Facial migraine in a rhinological setting. *Clin Otolaryngol All Sc*, 2002; 27: 521–5.
7. Spierings EL. Migraine mechanism and management. *Otolaryngol Clin N Am*, 2003; 36: 1063–78.
8. Cady RK and Schreiber CP. Sinus headache: a clinical conundrum. *Otolaryngologic Clin N Am*, 2004; 37: 267–88.
9. Jones NS. Sinus headaches: avoiding over- and mis-diagnosis. *Expert Rev Neurother*, 2009; 9(4): 439–44.
10. Aaseth K, Grande RB, Kvaerner K, Lundqvist C and Russell MB. Chronic rhinosinusitis gives a ninefold increased risks of chronic headache. The Akershus study of chronic headache. *Cephalagia: An Int J Headache*, 2010; 30(2): 152–60.

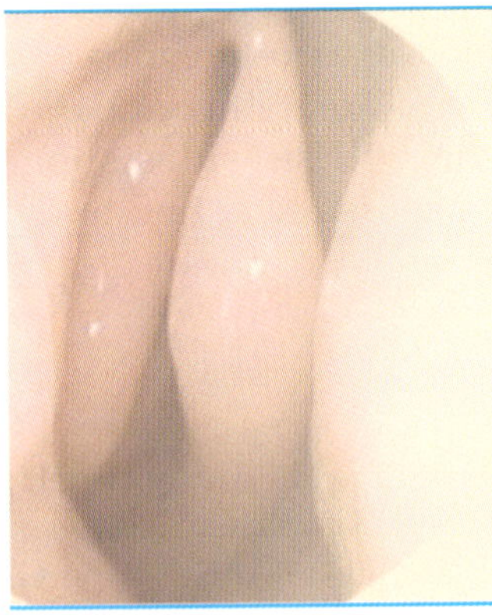

CHAPTER 18

Crooked Nose

Brajendra Baser, Shenal Kothari

Nose has a major impact on the overall appearance of the face as it occupies central position in midface. Crooked nose is typically characterized by external deformity with underlying septal defect (Fig. 18.1). Crooked nose deformity is because of both bony and cartilaginous defects. The forces applied on septum by the surrounding bones and skin determines its shape and therefore to achieve proper correction of septum these forces need to be corrected at the same time. Surgical aim for crooked nose is to provide a nose which looks good and breathe well.

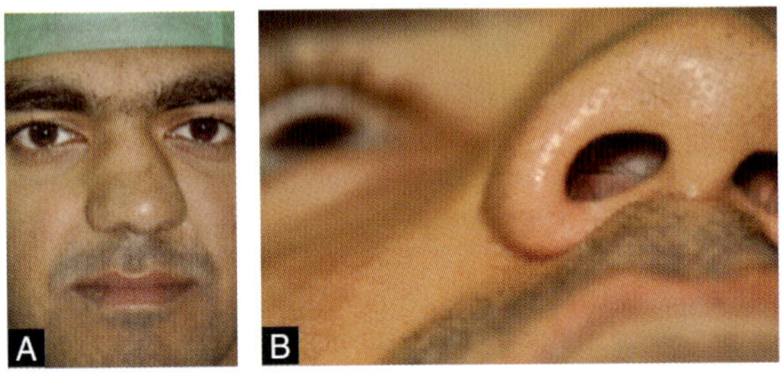

Fig. 18.1. Patient with crooked nose with deviation of septum which is completely blocking the right nostril. **A.** Front view; **B.** Basal view.

Etiology

Although the correction of deviated nose is considered as a difficult task and only experienced surgeons comprehend the precision required for this kind of rhinoplasty. It calls for meticulous analysis of the problem and surgical technique

1. **Traumatic (common):** Nasal trauma in adults is usually easily treatable because there is no preexisting soft tissue or skeletal deformity. Neglected or partially treated nasal fractures may produce progressive nasal changes because of scarring and contracture and therefore require greater attention.

   Childhood trauma is a different situation, as damaged septal cartilage may regenerate incompletely or grow on one side only. The deformed cartilage exerts force on soft tissues, bone and skin leading to asymmetrical cartilaginous and bony vault.
2. **Diseases of nose:** Autoimmune, connective tissue diseases and neoplasm may cause resorption of supporting structures leading to collapse of nasal valves and crooked nose deformity.
3. Post-surgical.
4. Congenital.

Classification

Crooked nose can be subdivided into three groups:

1. Deviated nose – dorsum deviated to one side of facial midline.
2. Asymmetric – straight but irregular dorsum.
3. True Crooked nose – 'c' or 's' shaped dorsum.

Chief presentation

- External deformity

- Nasal obstruction
- Recurrent rhinitis
- Epistaxis
- Psychological problems

Examination

The nose is analyzed in relation to entire face. Detailed facial analysis is useful in diagnosing structural nasal pathology. Facial aesthetic units (vertically divided into 5 equal parts and horizontally into 3 equal parts) are evaluated separately and in conjunction with nasal dorsum, nasal tip, side walls, nasal alae, columella and soft tissue triangle.

Assessment of skin condition is an important factor. It is important as it has a bearing on the anticipated tissue reaction, wound healing and surgical outcome. Thick skinned should be shown realistic picture. Similarly connective tissue type becomes significant. It affects skin wrinkling, tissue tension, elasticity and mobility of skin.

Determine the nature of deviation. Weather it is a true deviation or it is because of unilateral collapse of cartilage. Pseudo-deviation should also be ruled out.

Analysis of nasal tip is a must for determining the desired surgical approach. The concept of equilateral rhomboid of nasal tip must be kept in mind for all rhinoplasties.

Palpation of nose is done for bony irregularities. It allows for preoperative planning of osteotomies and wedge resection.

Watch for collapsing ala during inspiration. This is because of external valve collapse and is seen in patients who had undergone aggressive reduction rhinoplasty.

Evaluation of septal relationship to turbinates is necessary as compensatory turbinate hypertrophy may lead to nasal obstruction. The internal nasal valve is formed by junction of quadrangular cartilage, anterior end of inferior turbinate and floor of nose. This valve should be between 10 and 15 degrees. If the valve is less than 10 degree it produces sense of nasal obstruction. Positive Cottle's test is indicative of internal nasal valve collapse.

A complete internal nasal examination repeated with the aid of topical decongestant and nasal endoscopy allows better visualization of posterior and dorsal septum.

Photographic documentation is important in diagnosis and planning surgery. Postoperative photographs serve to document immediate outcome and function as a historical record to follow surgical changes. The photographs are taken in following standard views viz. frontal, right and left lateral, oblique and basal. The possible outcome is discussed with patient using preoperative photographs.

SURGERY

Aufricht rightly stated, "Where the septum goes, there goes the nose". Therefore septal correction should always be included in the surgical plan.

Principles

1. Majority of crooked nose require extensive septal reconstruction.
2. All deviated structures must be mobilized and positioned.
3. Osteotomies to be planned precisely.
4. Preservation of septal supports while carrying out septal correction.
5. Septal mucoperichondrium attachments to be maintained.

Steps

General anesthesia combined with local infiltration of lignocaine adrenaline solution.

Exposure

Open rhinoplasty approach is preferred as it gives a complete view of asymmetry. The septum is completely exposed. Care should be taken to avoid perforation of mucoperichondrial flap.

Mobilization of deviated structures

Any bony or cartilaginous deviation from midline should be mobilized and replaced in correct midline position. Osteotomies are done for deviated nasal bone. Incised wounds give better healing, hence all osteotomies should be as clean cut and smooth as possible. For this it is important that the osteotome is sharpened and optimally grounded and preferably a 2 mm osteotome is used. This will also help in reducing post-op consequences like hematoma, ecchymosed or lid edema. Due importance should be given to the cartilaginous framework. Displaced cartilage is freed from septum fixed in its anatomical position maintaining

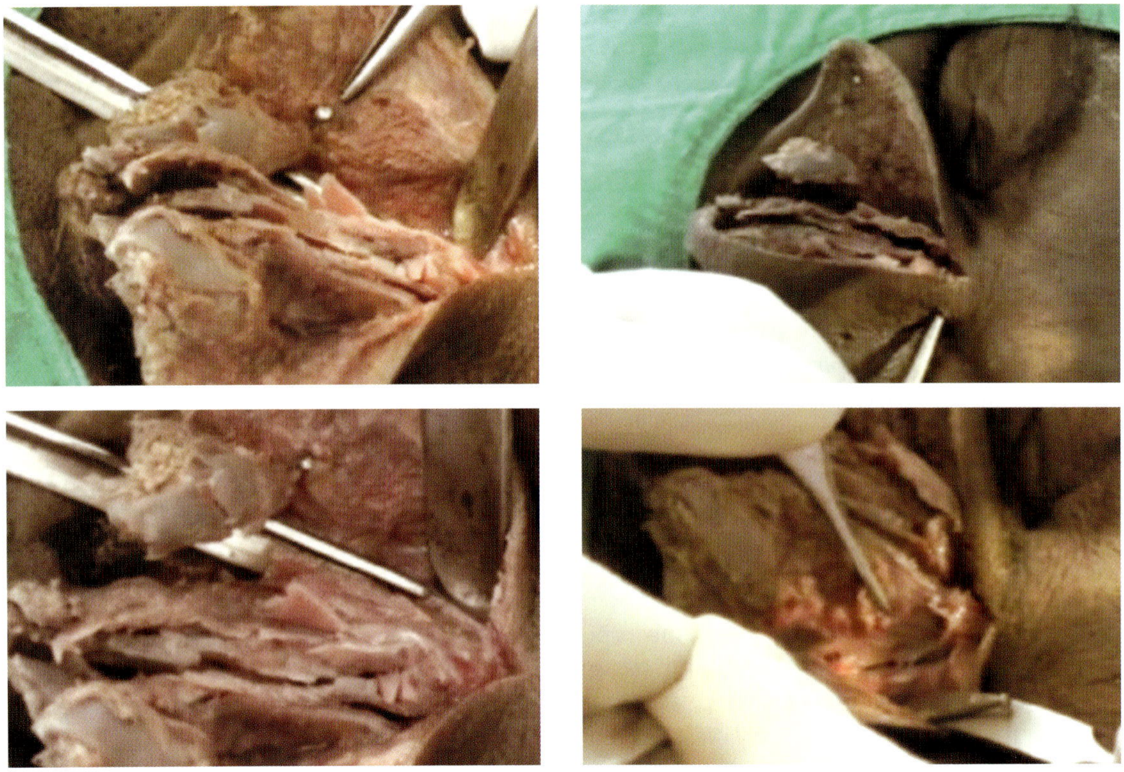

Fig. 18.2. Lateral osteotomy. Osteotomy done from (**A**) low to (**B**) high; Incisions (**C**) for external osteotomy; (**D**) Osteotomy line.

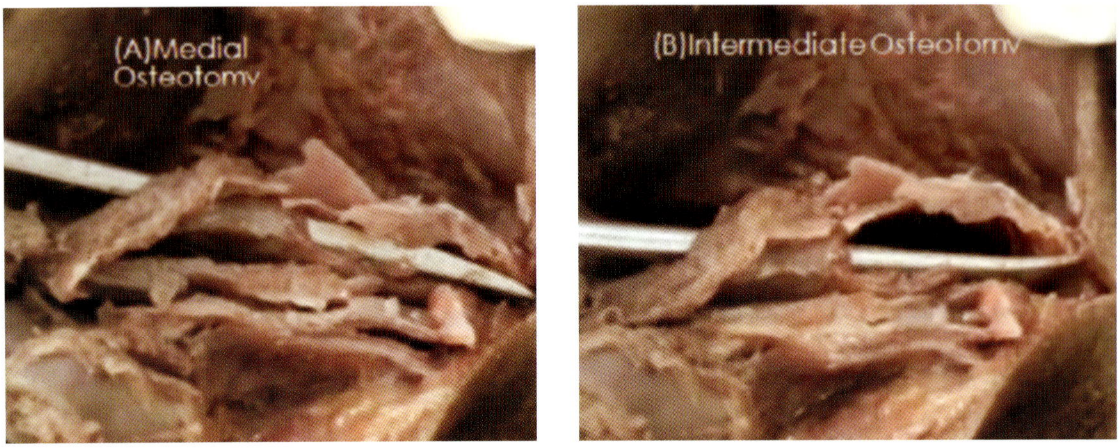

Fig. 18.3. A. Medial osteotomy; **B.** Intermediate osteotomy.

symmetry and position of upper and lower lateral cartilages. This can be achieved by trimming them or using spreader graft and positioning sutures (Figs. 18.2 and 18.3).

Septal reconstruction

The septum is completely delivered out, straightened and reshaped into L shape and replaced in its place. This cartilage is fixed in its position by suturing it with surrounding periosteum or by making drill hole in the nasal spine (Fig. 18.4). This can be further supplemented with internal septal splints, suture splints or autologous ethmoidal splint.

Caudal septal deviation is managed by adequate mobilization, excision of excess cartilage with suture fixation (Fig. 18.5).

At times rasping may be required on the deviated side or a little augmentation be considered on the concavity of the deviation.

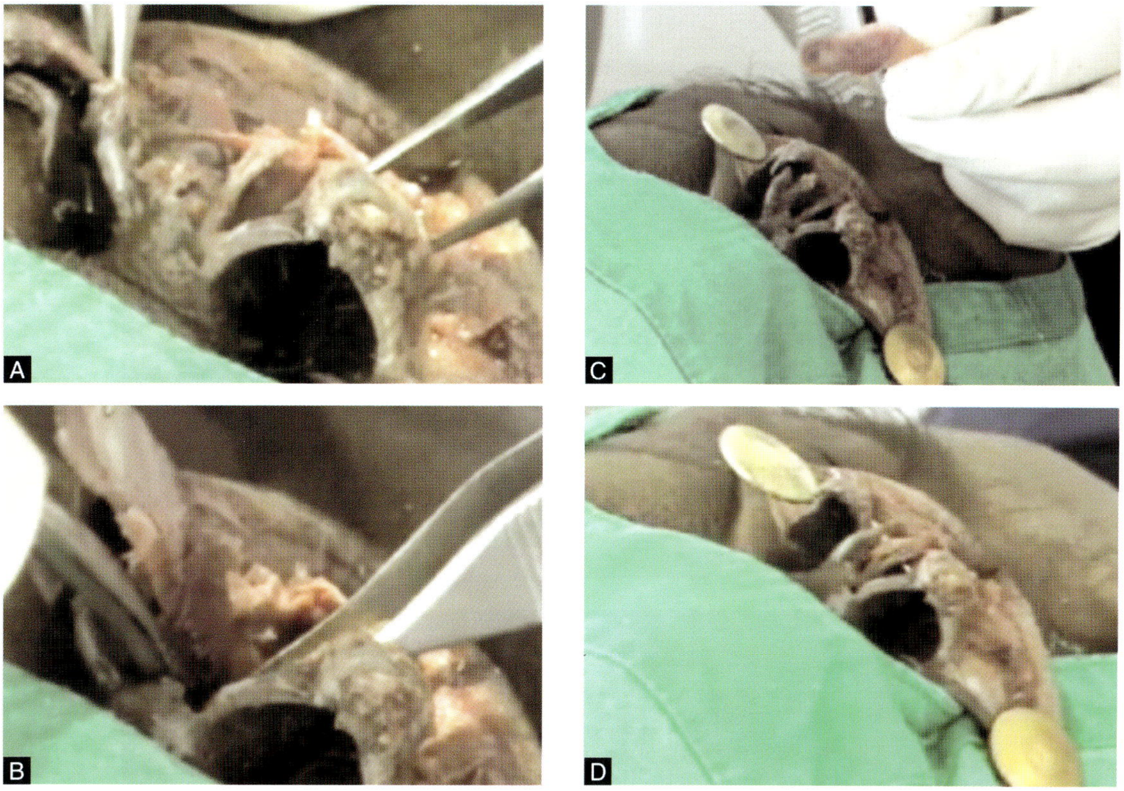

Fig. 18.4. A. Exposure of septum; **B.** Removal of the entire septum; **C.** Excised septum; **D.** Positioned septum between the alar cartilages.

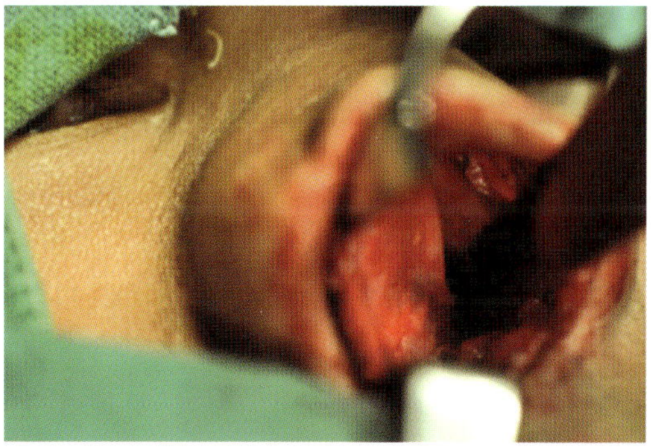

Fig. 18.5. Septal cartilage being removed.

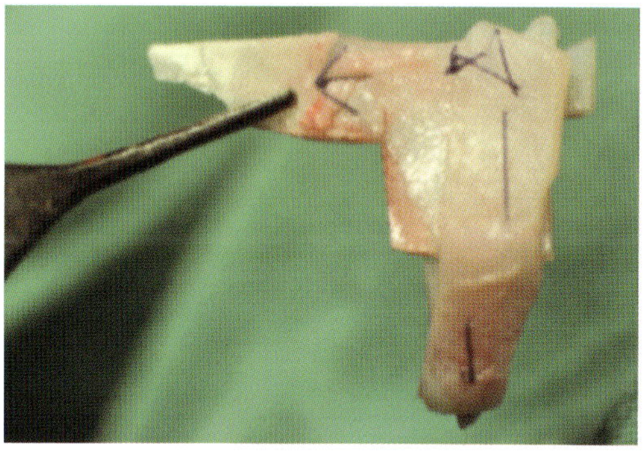

Fig. 18.6. L-shaped cartilagenous dorsal support.

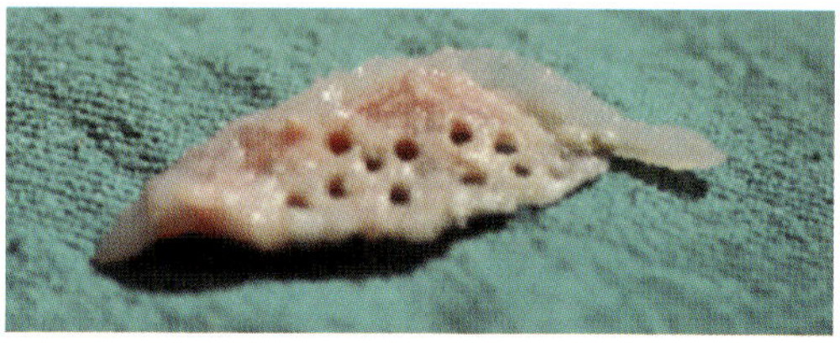

Fig. 18.7. Perforated bony septal support for dorsum.

Dorsal onlay grafts

Defects in dorsum and midline vault can be filled with sliced cartilage (Fig. 18.6) or dorsal bony support (Fig. 18.7). Large septal spreader grafts are used to support middle and lower nose which also serve in improving internal nasal valve functioning.

The nose is packed for 24 hours and external cast applied for two weeks.

Postoperatively facial swelling is unavoidable. It results from tissue handling and therefore the procedure should be as atraumatic as possible. An overly aggressive approach may be disastrous, it can lead to long-term contractures or distortions and disparity between the two sides.

PREOPERATIVE AND POSTOPERATIVE IMAGES OF SOME PATIENTS

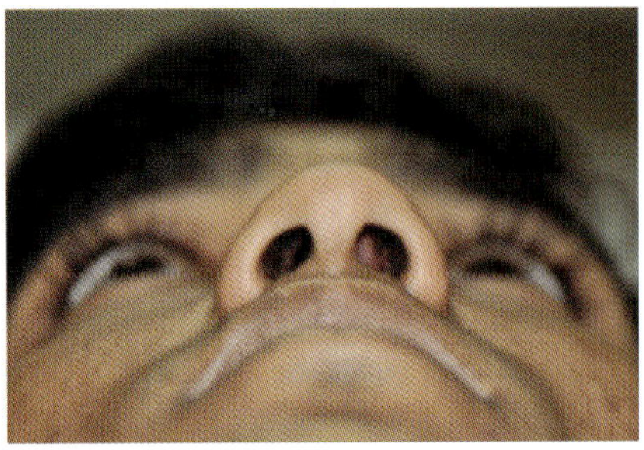
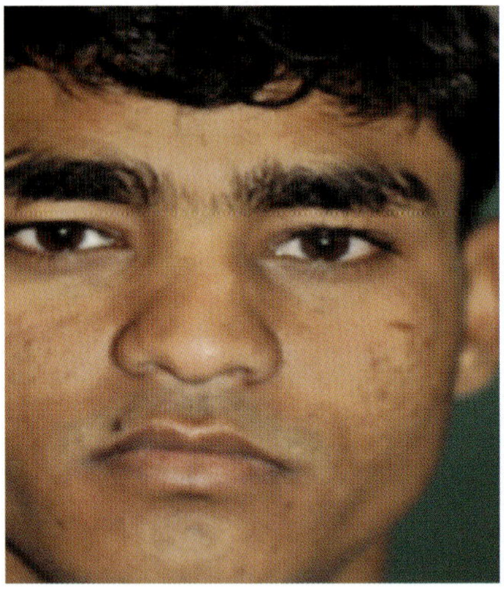

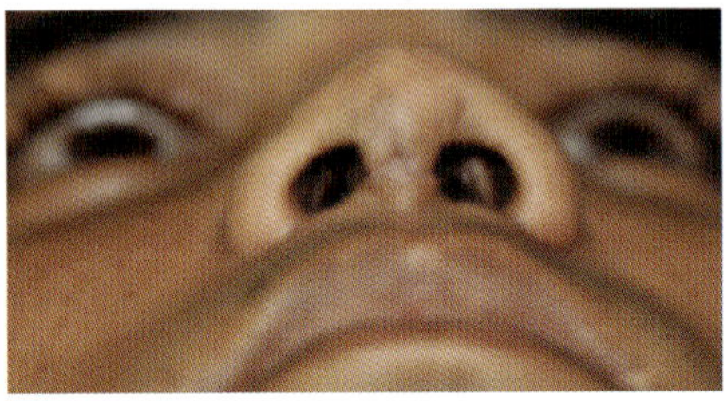
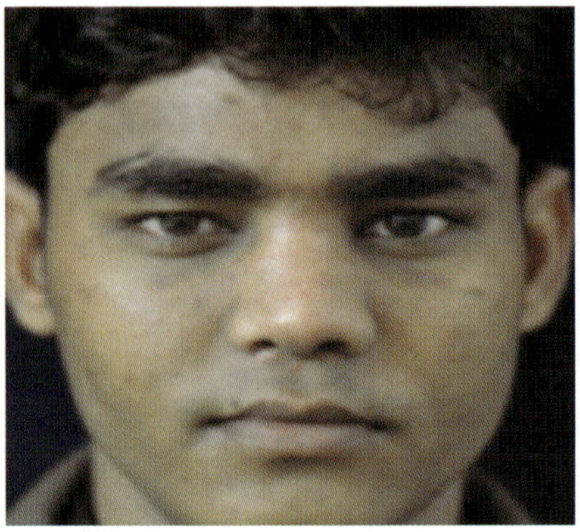

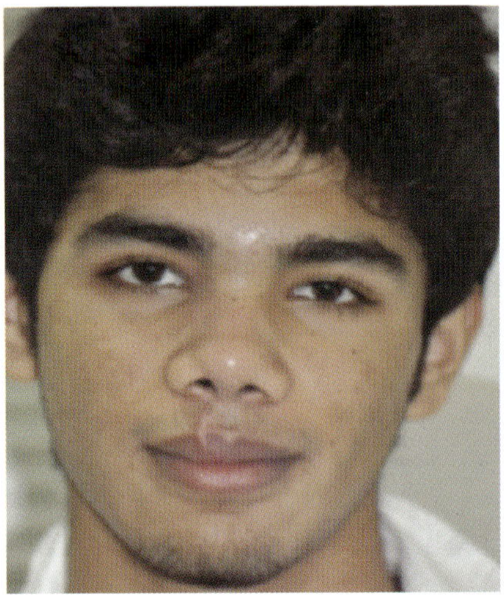
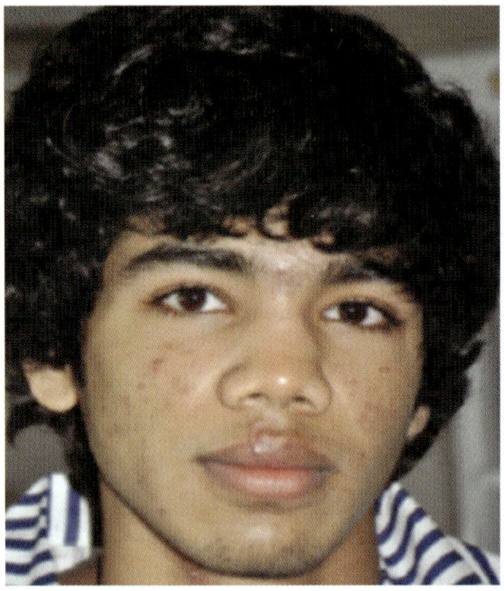

Crooked nose with DNS

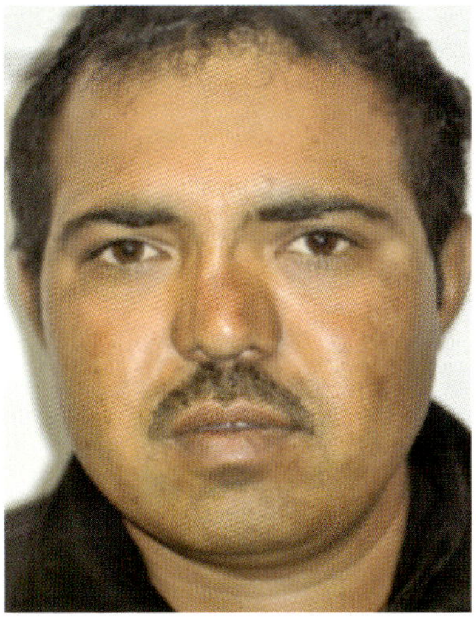
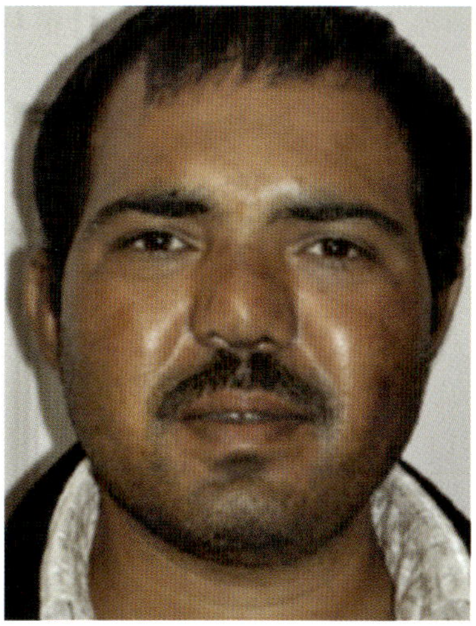

After two revisions

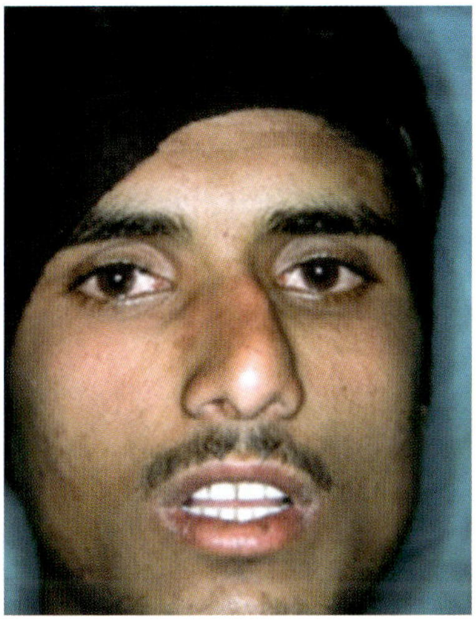

Before

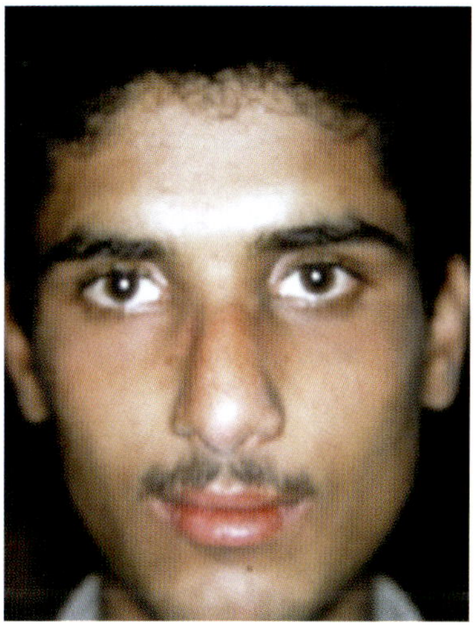

After

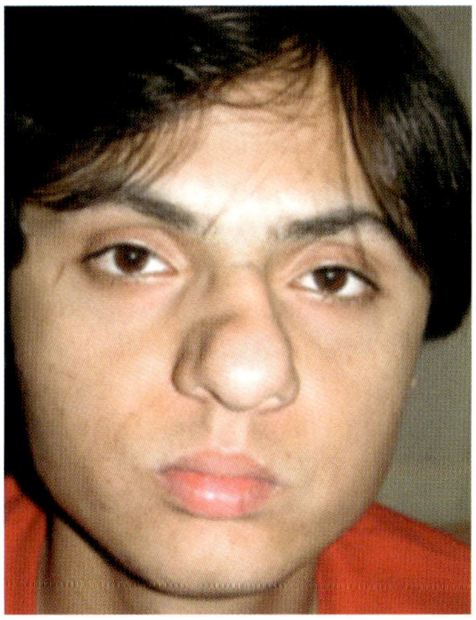

Before

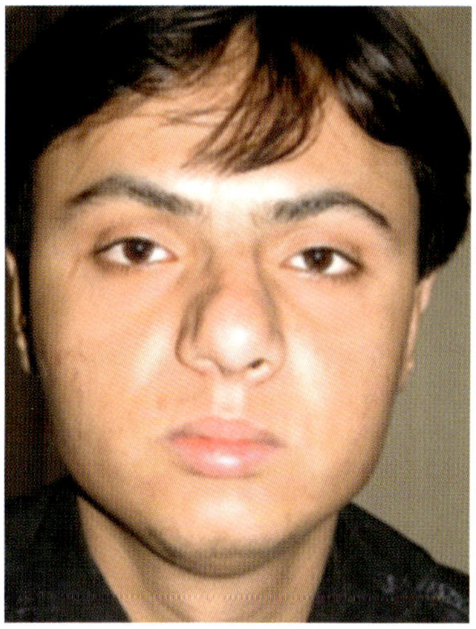

After

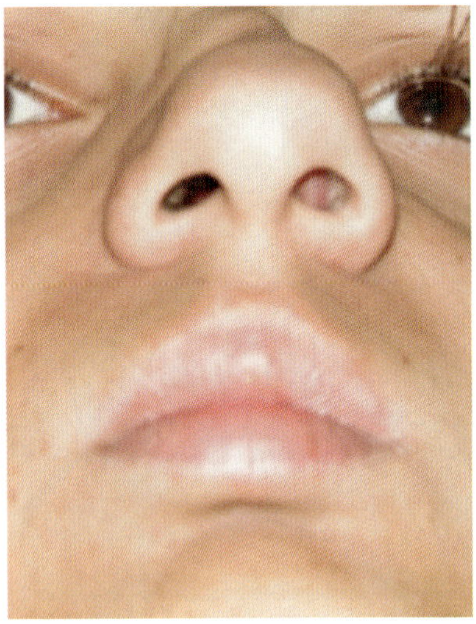

Before

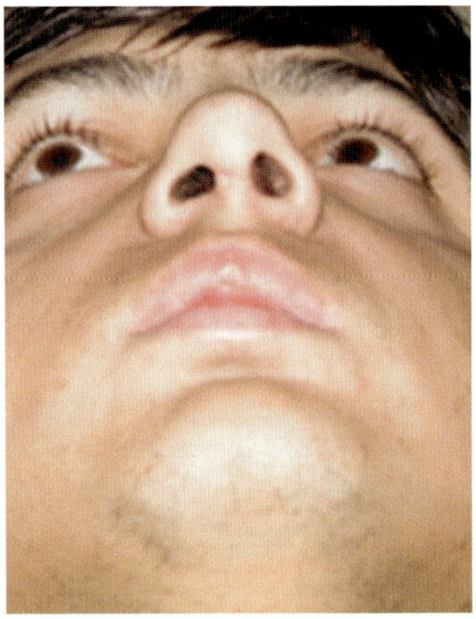

After

CONCLUSION

Preoperative patient evaluation and counseling forms the most essential part of cosmetic surgery.

It is true that minor defects meticulously corrected are not as well appreciated as gross defects converted to a less severe deformity. Therefore it is important to be realistic and make the patient understand as to what can be or cannot be achieved postoperatively.

In routine, few basic principles should be kept in mind to treat crooked nose. These are:

- Dorsum of nose – height (reduction/ augmentation) and smooth contour.
- Osteotomy – as per the requirement single/ multiple.
- Septum – resection, correction, harvest graft material, use of spreader graft or autologous ethmoid splint.
- Restoration of tip support when required.

Above all every rhinoplastic surgeon should be able to realize the associated complications and treat them.

18

FURTHER READING

1. Watzinger F, Wutzl A, Wanschitz F, Ewers R, Turhani D, Seemann R. Biodegradable polymer membrane used as septal splint. *Int J Oral Maxillofac Surg*, 2008; 37: 473–7.
2. Gurlek A, Ersoz-Ozturk A, Celik M, Firat C, Aslan S, Aydogan H. Correction of the crooked nose using custom-made high-density porous polyethylene extended spreader grafts. *Aesthetic Plast Surg*, 2006; 30: 141–9.
3. Baser. B. Aesthetic and Functional Rhinoplasty, 2nd edition, 2004.
4. Achauer BM, VanderKam VM, Celikoz B, Jacobson DG. Augmentation of facial soft-tissue defects with Alloderm dermal graft. *Ann Plast Surg*, 1998; 41: 503–7.
5. Fanous N. Unilateral osteotomies for external bony deviation of the nose. *Plast Reconstr Surg*, 1997; 100: 115–23.
6. Gunter J. Management of the deviated Nose. The importance of septal reconstruction. Clin Plat Surg, 1988; 15: 43–55.
7. Holt GR. Garner EI, Mc Larey D. Postoperative Sequelae and complications of rhinoplasty. *Otolaryngol Clin North Am*, 1987; 20: 853–76.
8. Wright MR, Management of patient Dissatisfaction with results of Cosmetic procedures. *Arh Otolaryngol Head Neck Surg*, 1980; 106: 466–71.
9. Bernstein L. Surgical anatomy in rhinoplasty. *Otolaryngol Clin North Am*, 1975; 8: 549–558.
10. Aufright G. Rhinoplasty and Face. Plast Reconstr Surg, 1969; 43: 219.

CHAPTER 19

Endoscopic Excision of Angiofibroma: Operative Techniques and Applied Anatomy

Brajendra Baser, Shenal Kothari, Anshul Vijay

Various approaches for excision of JNA range from wide midfacial degloving to minimally invasive endoscopic excision. All the open techniques have the disadvantage of prolonged and cosmetically unacceptable morbidity (delayed facial growth in children, deformities or massive bleeding). While endoscopic excision has an inherent advantage of avoiding facial scars and providing magnified panoramic view under direct vision, thus it allows better tumour delineation and dissection from adjacent tissues.

The property of juvenile nasopharyngeal angiofibroma to grow along the tissue planes following a path of least resistance can be put to a great advantage when working with a endoscope as it allows better identification of the interface between the tumour and rest of the structures. Therefore, complete dissection and detachment followed by excision is possible endoscopically without damage to child's developing facial skeleton. In this way it takes care of the growth of the face and maintains cosmoses. The duration of surgery and hospitalisation both are reduced, also there is better control of bleeding.

Hence, endoscopic excision is the first line of treatment even for extensive tumours reaching the optic chiasma or the middle cranial fossa. Better understanding of the endoscopic anatomy and availability of angled scopes allows wide exposure of surgical field and therefore aids in total tumour removal.

Pre-surgical study of each individual case helps to decide the most appropriate surgical plan. However, embolisation is essential in every case as it controls the intra-op and post-op bleeding. The vessels that need to be embolised are internal maxillary artery, ascending pharyngeal artery, sphenopalatine artery and descending pharyngeal artery depending upon which is the feeder vessel. Embolisation also helps to reduce the tumour volume. All these effects in turn assist in giving a less bloody operative field and therefore avoid recurrence and/or residual tumour. Polyvinyl crystals or crushed gelfoam are used for embolisation. This is done 24–36 hours prior to surgery by Seldinger technique from the right femoral artery. Embolisation is usually uneventful and alleviates need for blood transfusion.

APPLIED ANATOMY

Pterygopalatine fossa is a pyramid-shaped space bounded anteriorly by maxillary sinus, posteriorly by pterygoid process and anteromedially by palatine bone (Fig. 19.1).

It contains fat, pterygopalatine ganglion, maxillary nerve, nerve of pterygoid canal and maxillary artery.

The fossa is important clinically because of its communications with vital structures as shown in Fig. 19.2.

The pterygopalatine canal connects the pterygopalatine fossa with the hard palate via the

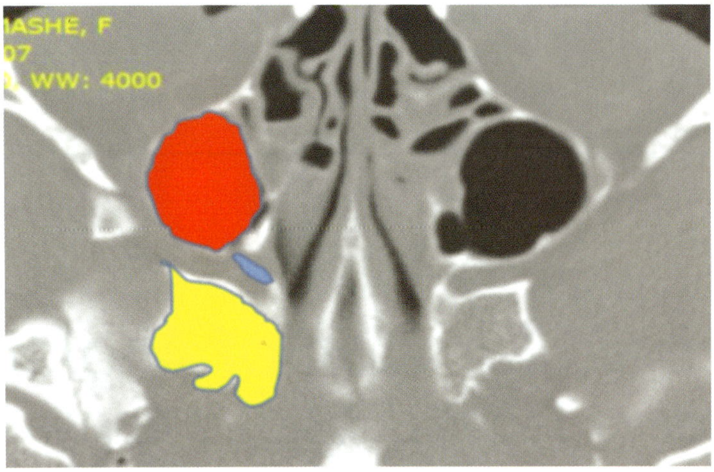

Fig. 19.1. Walls of pterygopalatine fossa maxillary sinus (red), pterygoid process (yellow), and palatine bone (blue).

greater (anteriorly placed, single) and lesser (posteriorly placed, may be more than two) palatine canals opening into their respective foramina on the hard palate and containing respective neurovascular bundle (Fig. 19.3). In this way these channels allow the tumour to reach the hard palate.

The sphenopalatine foramen opens into the nasal cavity on either side. This opening allows growth of angiofibroma into the nasal cavities and postnasal space (Fig. 19.4). Sometimes tumour may grow posterosuperiorly towards foramen lacerum and foramen ovale to enter the middle cranial fossa. It contains the sphenopalatine vessels and nasopalatine and superior nasal nerve.

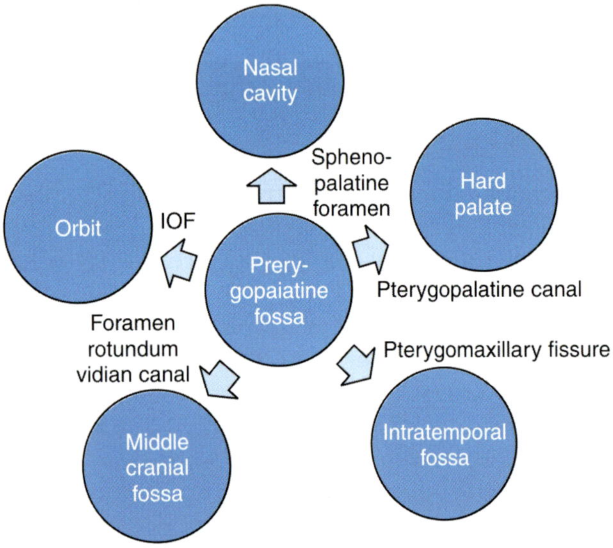

Fig. 19.2A. Communications of pterygopalatine fossa.

Inferior orbital fissure is the route leading from pterygopalatine fossa to the orbit. It is through this channel that the tumours spread into the orbital fossa. It contains the inferior orbital and zygomatic branch of V-2 nerve, inferior orbital vessels and inferior ophthalmic vein. The pterygomaxillary fissure connects the pterygopalatine fossa to infratemporal fossa (Fig. 19.5).

The two foramina that communicate the pterygopalatine fossa with the middle cranial fossa

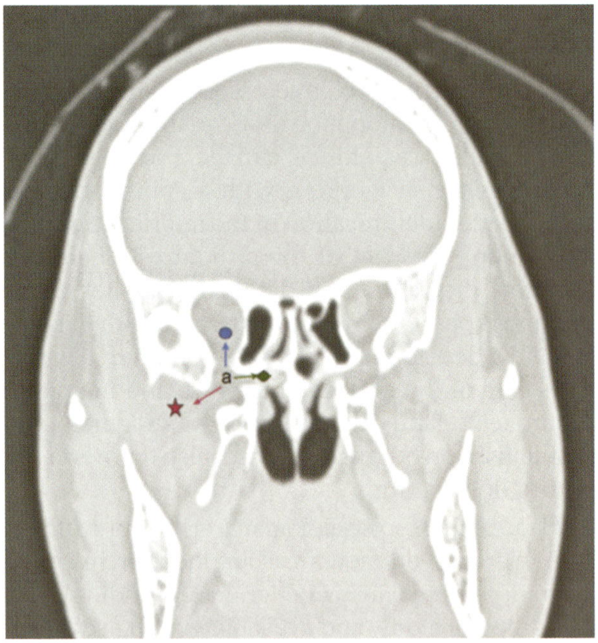

Fig. 19.2B. Communications of pterygopalatine fossa. Orbit – inferior orbital fissure (blue circle); infratemporal fossa – pterygomaxillary fissue (red star); and nasal cavity – sphenopalatine foramen (green diamond).

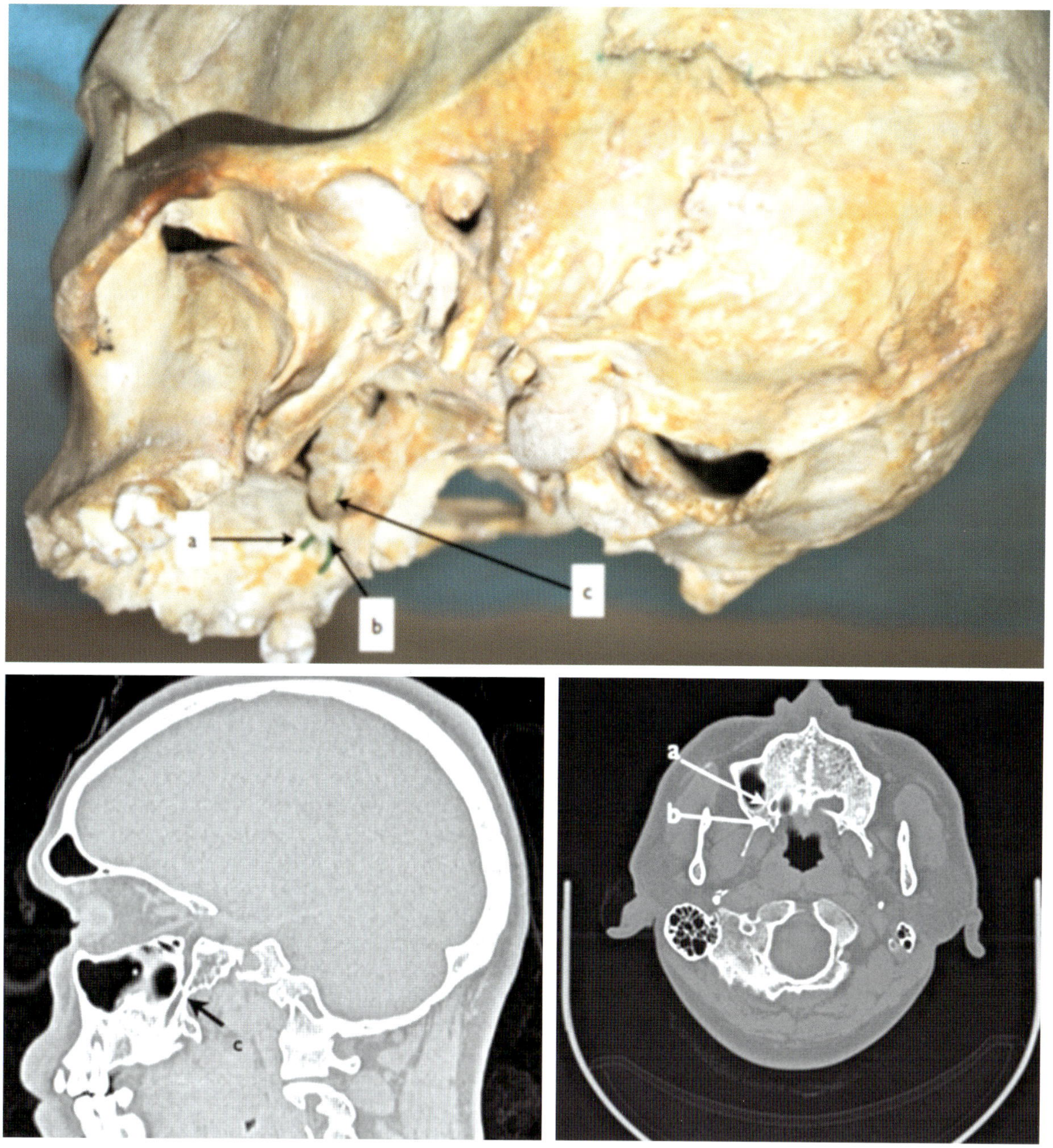

Fig. 19.3. a – Greater palatine foramen; b – Lesser palatine foramen; and c – Pterygopalatine canal.

are the foramen rotundum and the pterygoid canal (transmits nerve and artery of pterygoid canal, also called Vidian canal, leads into the foramen lacerum). Foramen rotundum (transmits maxillary nerve) is not seen at the norma basalis and can be identified on superior surface. It opens into the pterygopalatine fossa on its posterior wall (Fig. 19.6).

Mode of spread of juvenile nasopharyngeal angiofibroma is anteriorly into the nasal cavity and paranasal sinuses, laterally to the infratemporal fossa through pterygomaxillary fissure or orbit through inferior orbital fissure, superiorly into the sphenoid (and then through its posterior wall progressing to cavernous sinus or pituitary optochiasm), posterosuperiorly into the middle cranial fossa or medially into nasopharynx and then contralateral extension (Fig. 19.7).

Surgical plan is tailored as per each individual case after assessing the tumour size and its extensions. All cases are done under GA with patient

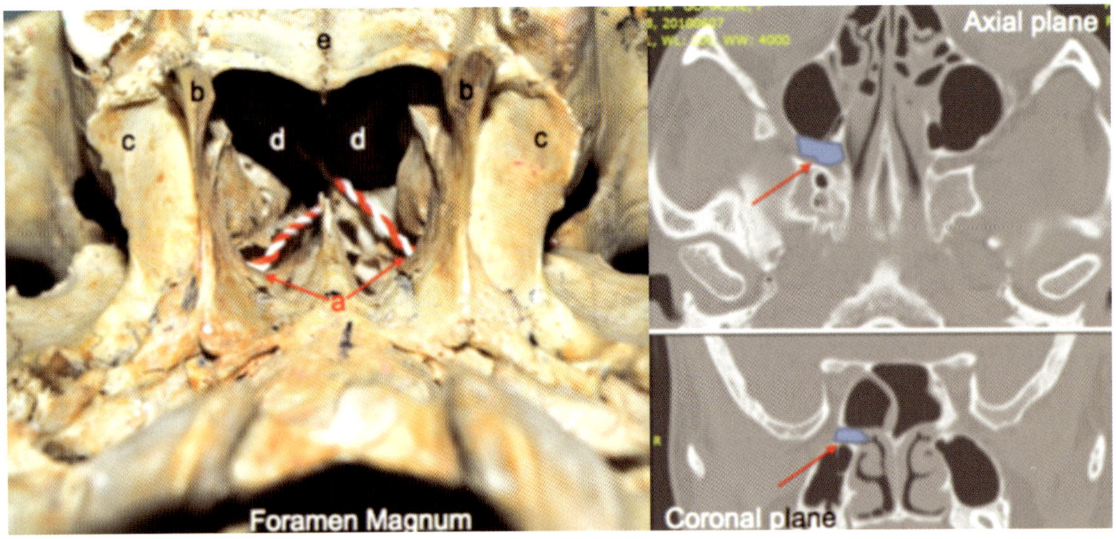

Fig. 19.4. d – Communication with nasal cavities; a – Through sphenopalatine foramen; b – Medial pterygoid plate; c – Lateral pterygoid plate; and e – Hard palate.

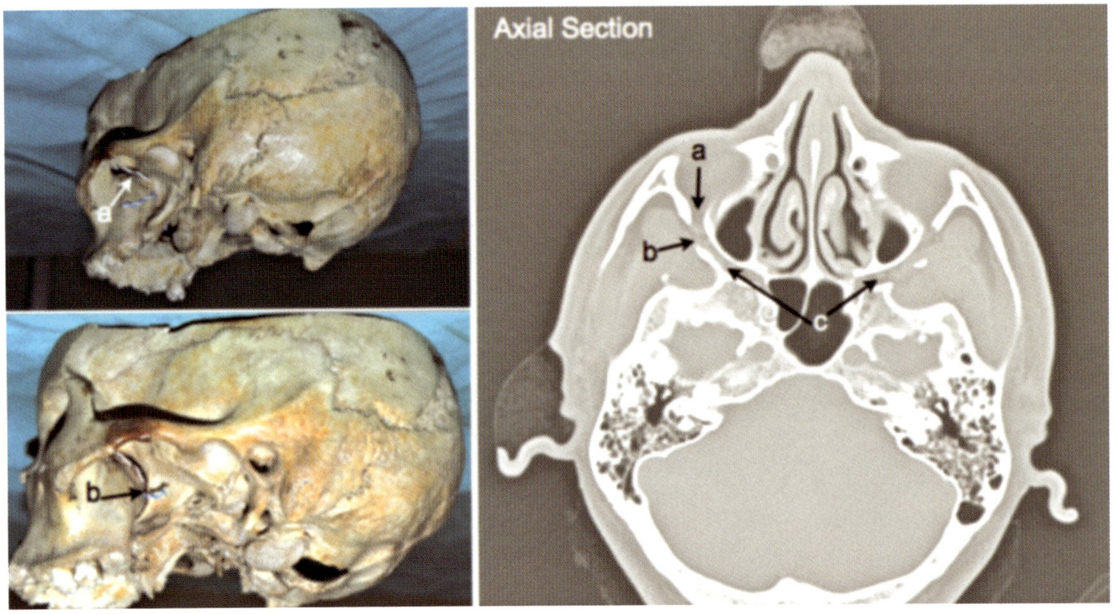

Fig. 19.5. a – Inferior orbital fissure; b – Pterygomaxillary fissue; c – Pterygopalatine fossa.

19

in semisitting position. After standard painting and drapping, 200–250 ml of tumescent solution is injected all around the tumour, on the septum, the middle and inferior turbinates and into the tumour under direct vision using a zero degree sinoscope. The tumescent solution is prepared from 500 ml saline, 25 ml 2% plain lignocaine, 5 ml sodabicarb and 1 ml adrenaline (Fig. 19.8).

Adequate surgical exposure of the operative field and adequate area for instrumentation is the key to successful endoscopic excision of JNA. Instruments used are standard FESS set along with 0, 30 and 45 degree sinoscopes. Haemostasis is better achieved with the availability of cautery (both monopolar and bipolar, Ligassure and harmonic). Microdebrider aids to the clean haemostatic tissue removal. Plester's elevator and tonsillar dissector are other very useful instruments for blunt dissection during traction.

Although it is believed that more advanced tumours reaching the infratemporal fossa and intracranial fossa must be managed with a combined

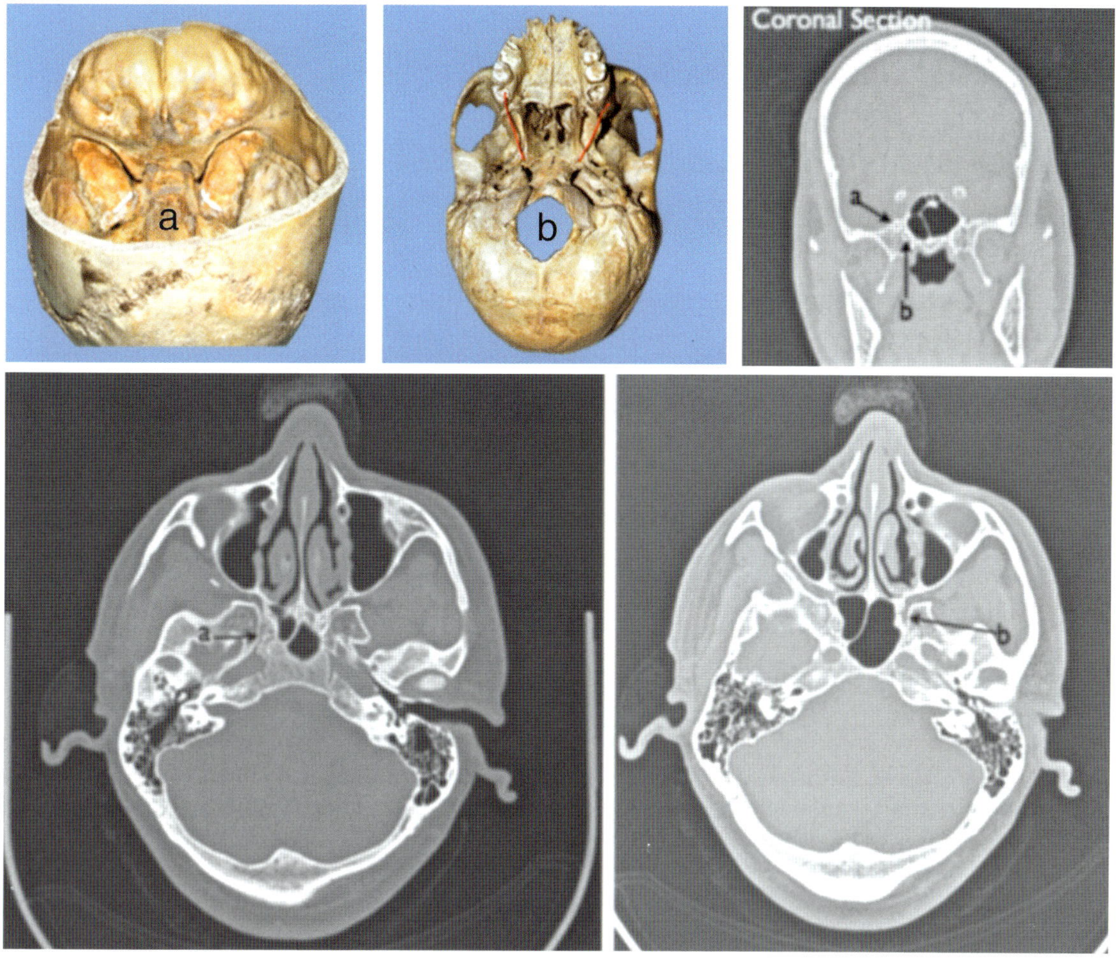

Fig. 19.6. Foramen rotundum (a) and pterygoid canal (b) allow middle cranial fossa extension of tumour.

approach, the endoscopic technique described below can dissect, detach and excise most extensive tumours also.

STEPS

1. Tumour assessment

Pre-op tumour assessment is done from the radiological studies with and without contrast and also from the angiography during embolisation. Intra-op nasal endoscopy assists in co-relation of the pre-op study. This knowledge of tumour extent and its extensions is essential for the best surgical outcome. Septal attachments of tumour if any should be clearly understood (Fig. 19.9).

2. Creation of working space

(a) Create septal window

Periosteal flaps are raised in the posterior part of the septum (Fig. 19.10 A–D) which was infiltrated previously. The septum along with adjoining cartilaginous portion is excised. The mucoperiosteal left is removed by microdebrider. In this way a septal window is created to be used as a port for instrumentation by the assistant allowing a two surgeon–two nostril approach. The size of the window should be big enough to allow instrumentation (Fig. 19.11).

(b) Resection of turbinates

The inferior turbinate is cauterised just below the hillock using a bipolar cautery to provide haemostasis. This is then cut with turbinectomy scissors and removed with forceps. Similarly the middle turbinectomy is performed (Fig. 19.12 A, B).

3. Uncinectomy

Uncinectomy is done followed by infundibulotomy. The anterior and posterior fontanelle are removed using a microdebrider. The bony part of the medial

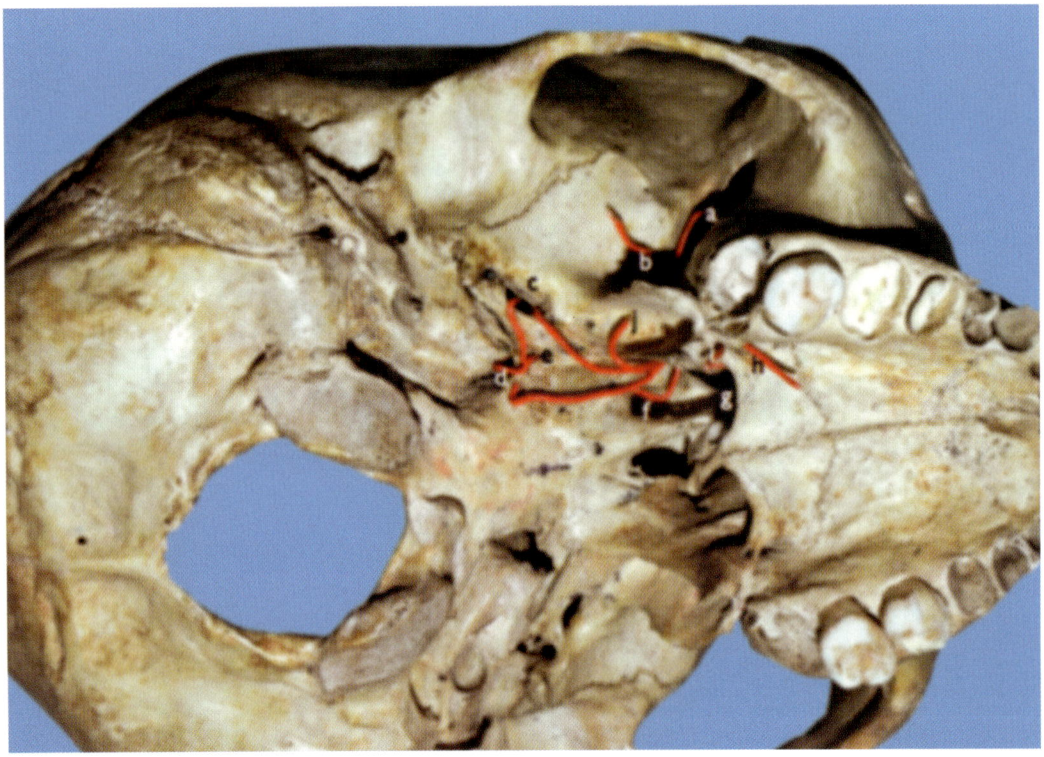

Fig. 19.7. Spread of angiofibroma towards — a – orbit, b – infratemporal fossa, c – foramen ovale, d – foramen lacerum, e – Vidian canal, f – sphenoid opening, g – sphenopalatine foramen, h – greater palatine foramen, i – lesser palatine foramen, and h – interpterygoid space.

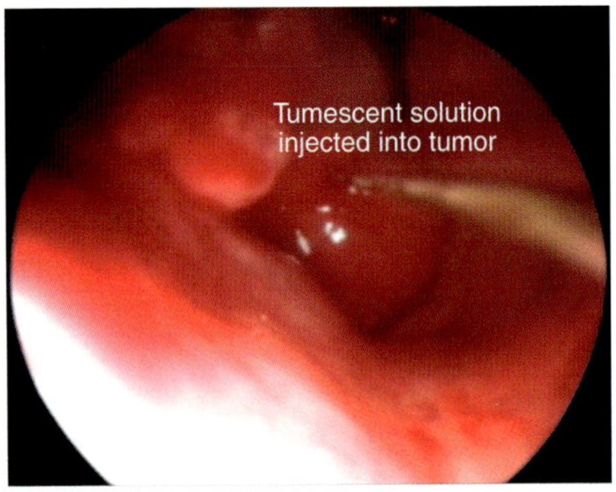

Fig. 19.8. Tumescent solution injected into tumour with a 26 gauge spinal needle.

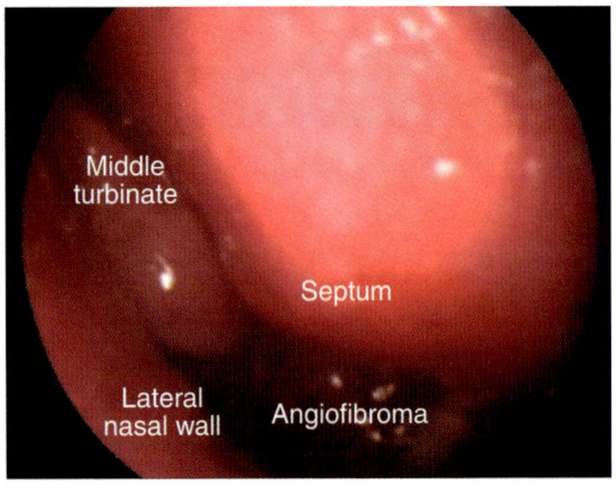

Fig. 19.9. Assessment of the tumour.

19

wall are then punched out with Kerrison's punch. In this way entire maxillary wall is removed and a direct view into the maxillary sinus is possible.

4. Creation of antral window

The pterygopalatine fossa lies posterior to posterior maxillary wall and therefore this wall has to be removed to reach the tumour. An antral window (Fig. 19.14 A, B) is made to visualise the posterior wall and then remove it from medial to lateral direction with punches (Fig. 19.14 C). This is done by introducing the scope through the antral window and instruments are worked through the nasal cavities. During this manoeuvre care is taken to identify the internal maxillary artery in the pterygopalatine fat (Fig. 19.14 D) which is then sealed with bipolar cautery to further enhance haemostasis.

An easy identification of tumour, fat and internal maxillary artery is possible only through the precise endoscopic view. Also, it allows view of infratemporal fossa far laterally specially with angled scopes (Fig. 19.14 E).

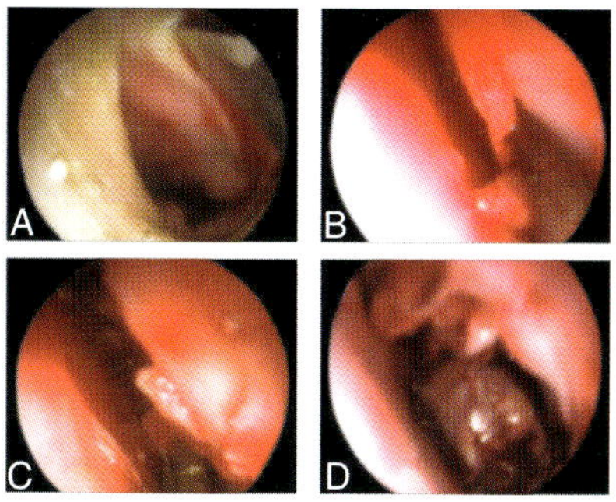

Fig. 19.10. A. Incision in the posterior portion of septum. **B.** Elevation of mucoperiosteal flaps. **C.** Removal of bony septum. **D.** Creation of desired septal window.

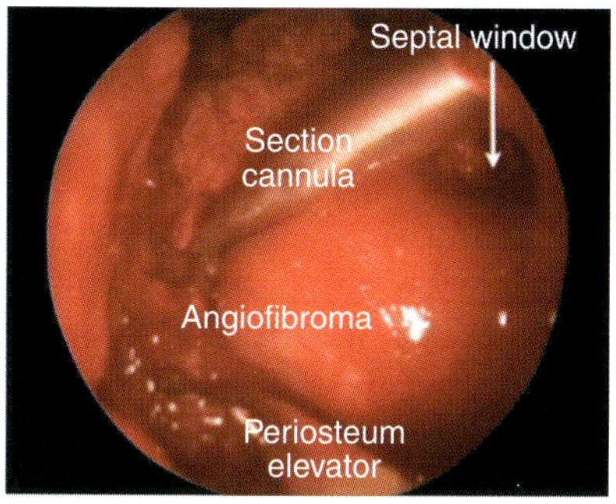

Fig. 19.11. Intrumentation through two windows allows better handling.

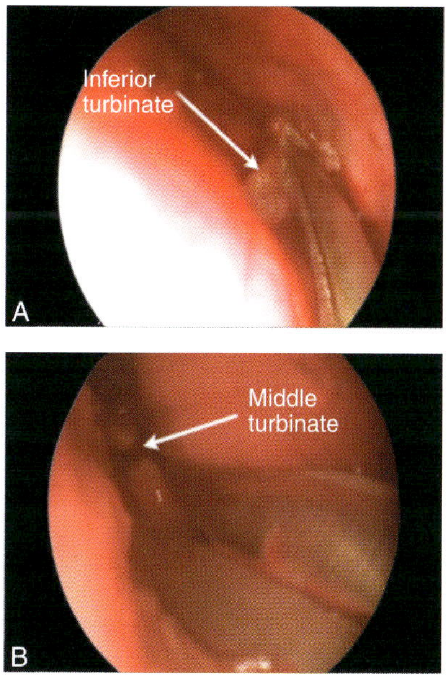

Fig. 19.12. A. Resection of the inferior turbinate. **B.** Resection of the middle turbinate.

5. Removal of the intracranial tumour extensions

The dissection is further continued superiorly maintaining constant progressive traction in a downward direction and detaching the tumour

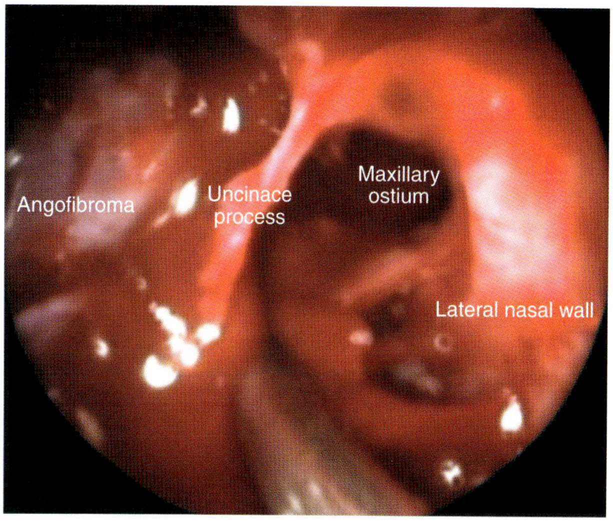

Fig. 19.13. Uncinectomy and infundibulotomy.

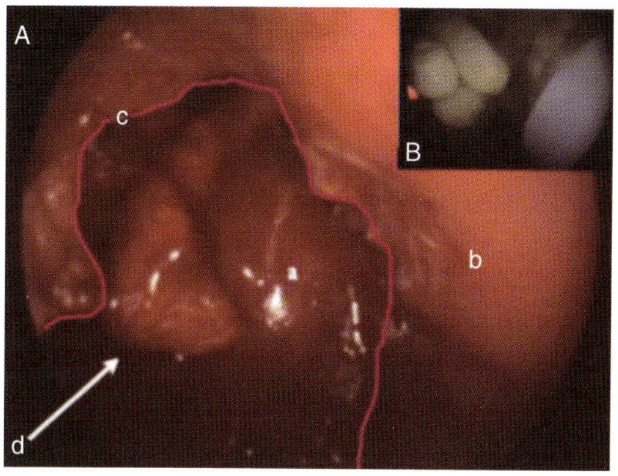

Fig. 19.14A. a – Angiofibroma; b – Lateral nasal wall; c – Outline of widened maxillary ostium opening at the lateral nasal wall; and d – Direct visualisation of the most lateral aspect of posterior maxillary wall and pterygopalatine fossa. **B.** Endoscope introduced through antral cannula.

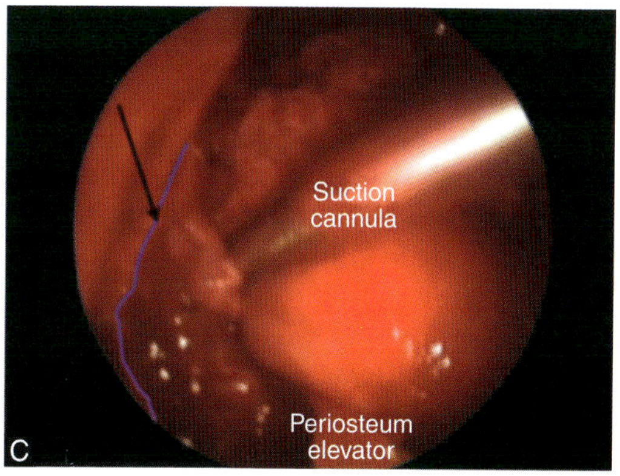

Fig. 19.14C. Angiofibroma excised under transantral endoscopic control. Lateral end of posterior maxillary wall outlined by arrow.

19

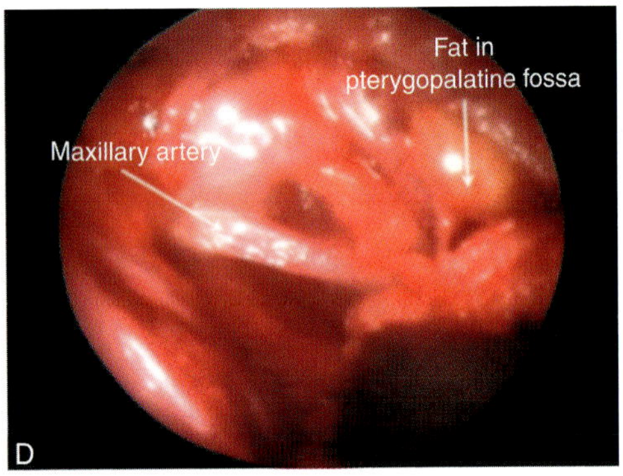

Fig. 19.14D. Maxillary artery and fat occupying the pterygopalatine fossa.

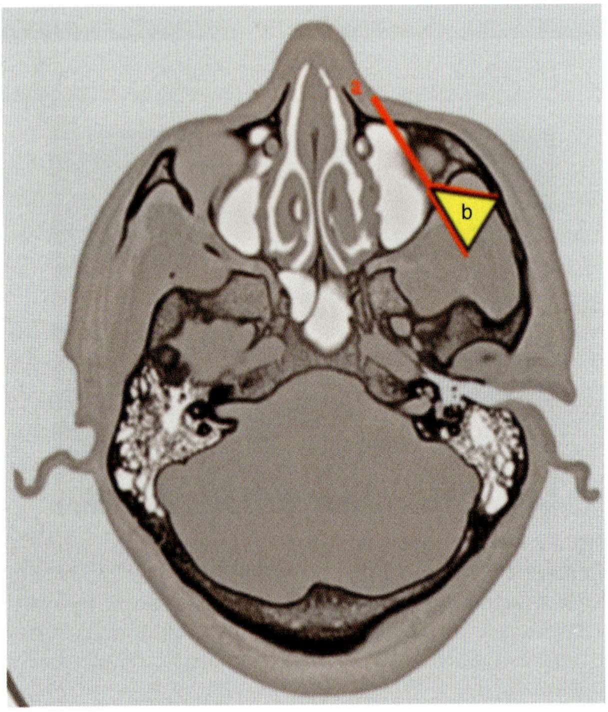

Fig. 19.14E. Transantral window used as extra port for instrumentation. a – Endoscope reaching pterygopalatine fossa through the transantral window; and b – Area illuminated as per the angulation of the scope.

from the inferior orbital fissure and the foramen ovale and foramen rotundum and then proceeding towards the middle cranial fossa extension which may at times show bony erosion but the dura mater is intact in most cases. Complete removal is confirmed by assuring a smooth surface of the dissected portion (Fig. 19.15).

6. Dealing with the infratemporal extension

Once the intracranial extension is dissected, the dissection is carried to the infratemporal fossa. The

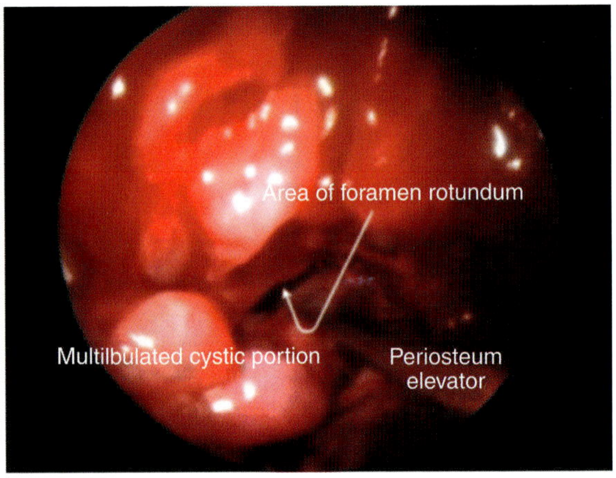

Fig. 19.15. Intracranial multilobulated cystic extension of tumour pulled out down and medially from the area of foramen rotundum.

bone at the junction of the anterolateral and posterior maxillary wall is punched out. This allows access and direct visualisation of the infratemporal region. Continuing with blunt dissection with elevator and applying continuous traction away from the tumour helps to dissect out the complete lateral extension. Once detached from all the surrounding structures the tumour can be removed.

Excision of contralateral extension when present is done in two ways, either it is removed en-bloc with the main tumour or it may be dealt with after removing the main tumour mass. However, bilateral juvenile nasopharyngeal angiofibroma are of uncommon occurrence.

At times the angiofibroma is attached to the septum, septal mucosa is cauterised all around the attachment area with bipolar as much as accessible.

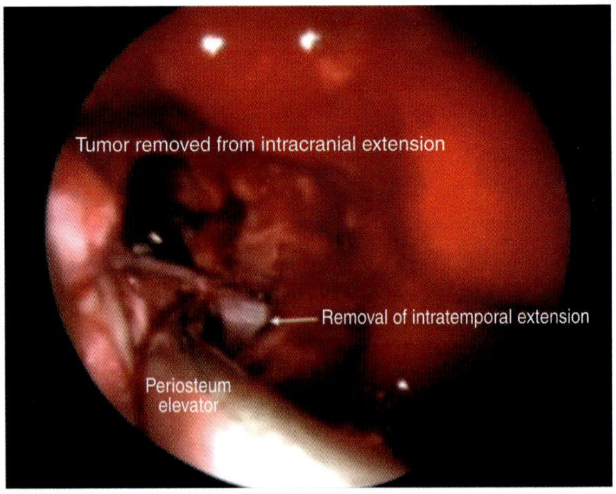

Fig. 19.16. Dissection of the infratemporal fossa after clearing the posterior wall of maxilla.

This is done to control bleeding from posterior ethmoid artery supplying this part of the nose. This part of the septum is then excised along with the angiofibroma. With the control of bleeding the chances of complete clearance increase and recurrence is minimised.

Cases with angiofibroma reaching the interpterygoid space require removal of the medial pterygoid plate. An extended removal of medial maxillary wall further posteriorly with Kerrison's punch helps to remove medial pterygoid plate and access the interpterygoid space carefully salvaging the greater and lesser palatine vessels and nerves.

Once the tumour is out, the bleeding spontaneously reduces. It is now possible to inspect the cavity endoscopically, and a note of bleeding or residual mass if any can be made and managed accordingly. Also, the excised mass is inspected for any breach over its surface which may help in deciding if any portion is left behind. Another method that can help in ascertaining complete tumour removal is comparing the size of the removed mass with that as revealed radiologically. With huge angiofibromas reaching to the shenoid roof, optic chiasma can be identified (Fig. 19.17).

The operated cavity is covered with surgicel followed by gel foam packing and merocel introduced on either side. Anterior nasal packing is done, posterior pack is not required routinely. Again the oral cavity is inspected for haemostasis. Blood transfusion is routinely not required with endoscopic approach.

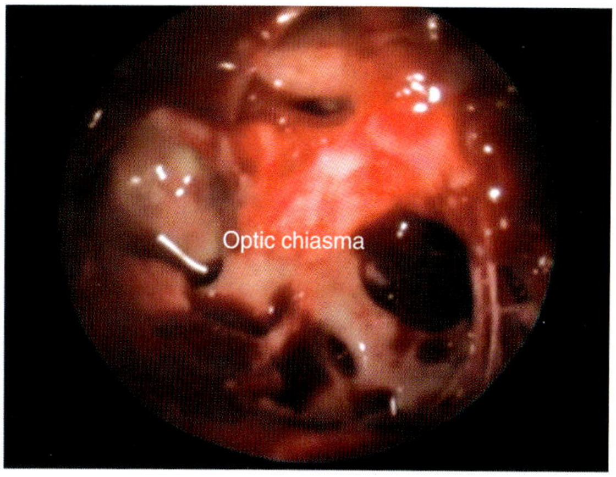

Fig. 19.17. Optic chiasma seen after complete angiofibroma excision and bleeding stops.

Endoscopy has inherent advantage of low morbidity, better aesthetically, panoramic-magnified-direct visualisation of the nasal cavity and skull base which gives good surgical control. Post-op inspection is easier and more complete endoscopically (Fig. 19.18).

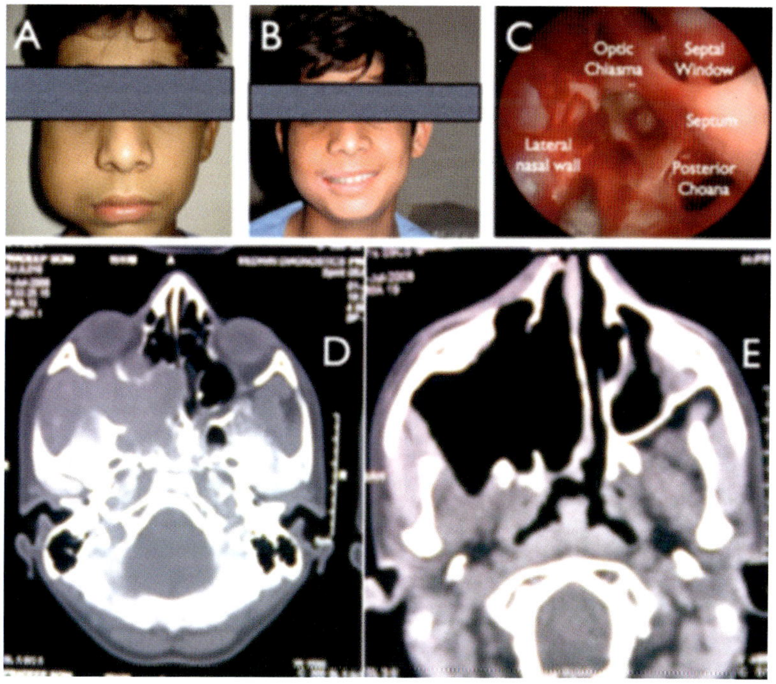

Fig. 19.18A. Pre-op appearance. **B.** Post-op cosmesis maintained. **C.** Endoscopic image 2 years post-op. **D.** Pre-op CT scan. **E.** Post-op CT scan.

CONCLUSION

To conclude, endoscopic approach is minimally invasive and has the inherent advantage of early rehabilitation and few complications. The knowledge of endoscopic anatomy helps to reach paratubal area, sphenoid sinus, orbital apex, optic nerve, clivus, hypophysis, cavernous sinus, foramen lacerum, foramen ovale, foramen rotundum. Postoperatively it allows serial easy follow-ups of sinonasal cavity, crusts removal and irrigation.

It avoids incision on face with minimal destruction of the facial bones and hence does not affect facial growth. Other definite advantages are decreased blood loss and hosptalisation. All the follow-ups are possible under local anaesthesia with ease of defining anatomical structures and removal of any asymptomatic masses if present. Morbid conditions like infraorbital neuralgia, facial disfigurement, epiphora, nasal tip deformity, plating, osteotomies, maxillomandibular fixation etc. can be avoided.

Use of high illumination, magnification and panoramic view provided by endoscope with a two nostril–two surgeon approach as described above definitely decreases the morbidity in patients with advanced Juvenile Nasopharyngeal Angiofibromas.

SUGGESTED READING

1. Fisch U. Infratemporal approach for epipharyngeal tumours. *Laryngoscope*, 1983; 93: 36–44.
2. Batsakis JG. Tumours of the Head and Neck: Clinical and Pathological Considerations. 2nd ed. Baltimore: Williams & Wilkins; 1979: 296–300.
3. Radowski D, McGill T, Healy GB, et al. Changes in staging and treatment. *Arch Otolaryngol Head Neck Surg*, 1996; 122: 122–9.
4. Onerci TM, Yucel OT, Ogretmenoglu O. Endoscopic surgery in treatment of juvenile nasopharyngeal angiofibroma. *Int J Pediatr Otorhinolaryngol*, 2003; 67: 1219–25.
5. Mojitaba MA, Seyed-Hadyi SA, Nasrin Y, et al. Endoscopic excision of juvenile nasopharyngeal angiofibroma: Complications and outcomes. *Otolaryngol Head Neck Surg*, 2010; 31: 343–349.
6. Tandon DA, Bahadur TS, Kacker SK, et al. Nasopharyngeal angiofibroma: a nine year experience. *J Laryngol Otol*, 1988; 105: 547–52.
7. Kamel RH. Transnasal endoscopic surgery in juvenile nasopharyngeal angiofibroma. *J Laryngol Otol*, 1996; 110: 962 8.
8. Ernesto P, Vittorio S, Giorgio F, et al. Endoscopic treatment of benign tumours of the nose and paranasal sinuses. *Otolaryngol Head Neck Surg*, 2004; 131: 180–6.
9. Gilles R, Patrice TBH, Patrick F, et al. Exclusive endoscopic removal of juvenile nasopharyngeal angiofibroma: Trends and limits. *Acta Otolaryngol Head Neck Surg*, 2002; 128: 928–35.
10. Nicolai P, Berlucchi M, Tomenzoli D, et al. Endoscopic surgery for juvenile angiofibroma: When and how. *Laryngoscope*, 2003; 113: 775–82.
11. Naraghi M, Kashfi A. Endoscopic resection of nasopharyngeal angiofibromas by combined transnasal and transoral routes. *Am J Otolaryngol*, 2003; 24: 149–54.
12. Wormald PJ, Van Hasselt A. Endoscopic removal of juvenile angiofibromas. *Otolaryngol Head Neck Surg*, 2003; 129: 684–91.
13. Iannetti G, Belli E, De Ponte F, et al. The surgical approaches to nasopharyngeal angiofibroma. *J Craniomaxillofac Surg*, 1994; 22: 311–16.
14. Jorissen M, Eloy P, Rombaux P, et al. Endoscopic sinus surgery for juvenile nasopharyngeal angiofibroma. *Acta Otorhinolaryngol Belg*, 2000; 54: 201–19.
15. Scholtz AW, Appenroth E, Kammen-Jolly K, et al. Juvenile nasopharyngeal angiofibroma: Management and therapy. *Laryngoscope*, 2001; 111: 681–7.
16. Lim IR, Pang YT, Soh K. Juvenile angiofibroma: Case report and the role of endoscopic resection. *Singapore Med J*, 2002; 43: 208–10.
17. Eloy P, Watelet JB, Hatert AS, et al. Endonasal endoscopic resection of juvenile nasopharyngeal angiofibromas. *Rhinology*, 2007; 45: 24–30.
18. Mann WJ, Jecker P, Amedee RG. Juvenile angiofibromas: Changing surgical concept over the last 20 years. *Laryngoscope*, 2004; 114: 291–3.
19. Yadav SPS, Singh I, Chand R, Sachdeva OP. Nasopharyngeal angiofibroma. *J Otolaryngol*, 2002; 31: 346–8.

CHAPTER 20

Endoscopic Dacryocystorhinostomy

Nishi Gupta

Endoscopes have revolutionized the way we look at the pathologies of nose and orbit these days. Like any other new procedure the acceptance of endoscopic procedure was low initially. But its high success rate with much less morbidity has enhanced the popularity of this procedure. Endoscopic DCR aims at communicating the lacrimal sac with the nasal cavity bypassing the obstructed nasolacrimal duct. There is increased awareness amongst patients and surgeons about endoscopic DCR and it has become the treatment of choice for chronic dacryocystitis. There is still a lot of limitation in finding the complete cure of epiphora. The limitation lies in cases with associated canalicular block.

Endoscopic DCR is a simple surgery in hands of an expert sinus endoscopic surgeon. The sac lies quite anterior, with favourable anatomy the procedure is easy and the results are excellent. This technique of endoscopic DCR was first devised by West more than a century ago. Owing to the lack of good instruments the technique did not gain momentum until the advent of endoscopes with camera and monitor unit.

Endoscopic dacryocystorhinostomy offers an alternative to conventional technique for the patients who want to avoid a scar on the face. It is a safe, fast and effective method to relieve an obstruction distal to the common cannaliculus. It is a procedure of choice in patients with history of chronic dacryocystitis, lacrimal abscess, mucocele, dacryolithiasis and failed external DCR.

PREOPERATIVE EVALUATION

Clinical features

Watering from eye is the most important symptom in patients presenting with dacryocystitis. Watering is mostly unilateral but it can be bilateral. In children with congenital dacryocystitis the nasolacrimal duct block is generally bilateral.

Watering from the affected eye in some patients can be profuse with blurring of vision due to the formation of a film over the cornea. It interferes with vision and needs to be corrected. If not corrected infection occurs in the stagnated secretions and the sac gets filled with purulent discharge. This thick discharge keeps getting regurgitated when the sac is full and makes the patient very uncomfortable. The eyelashes are sticky due to thick discharge. Skin lying over the sac gets infected in some cases leading to reddish inflamed look. Some people present with bulge in the medial canthal area.

Examination

Examination starts from the lids and punctum (Figs. 8.1 and 8.2).

Age of the patient is an important criterion. Laxity of lids in old age can lead to lacrimal pump failure and epiphora. Lid laxity is rare in young adults and children unless there is paralysis of the facial nerve leading to the loss of blinking reflex.

Absence or malformation of punctum can also lead to epiphora (Fig. 20.3).

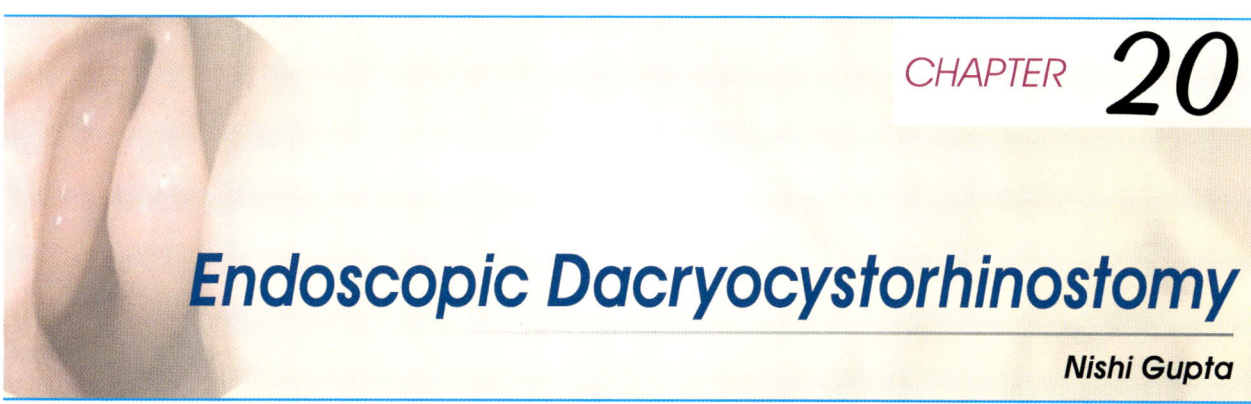

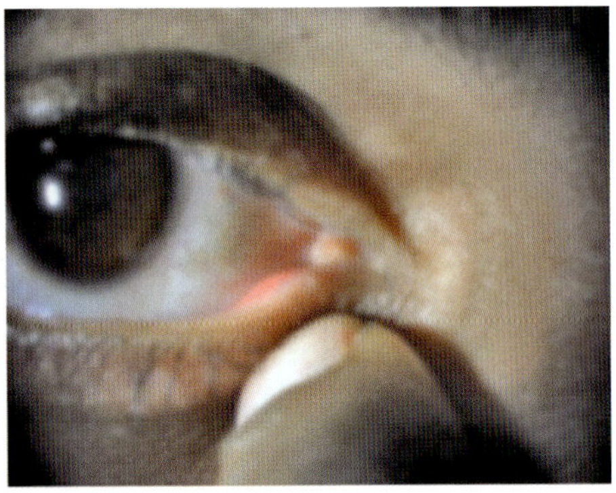

Fig. 20.1. Examination of lower punctum.

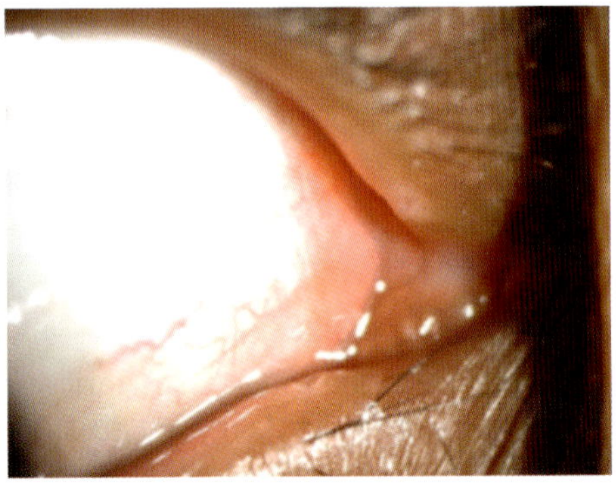

Fig. 20.2. Examination of both puncta.

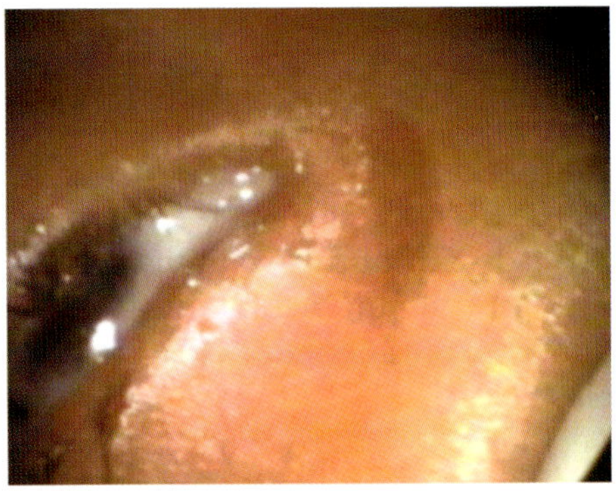

Fig. 20.3. Purulent epiphora filling the eye.

The single most important diagnostic criterion for detecting the obstruction in the nasolacrimal duct is ROPLAS test. ROPLAS is regurgitation of PUS on pressure over the lacrimal sac area (Fig. 20.4). An index finger is used to put pressure just below the medial canthal area.

In adults if ROPLAS is not positive, syringing with irrigation of the lacrimal system is performed to find the site of block.

The approach to a child with epiphora is quite different from that of an adult. In children it is not possible to carry out syringing to find the exact site

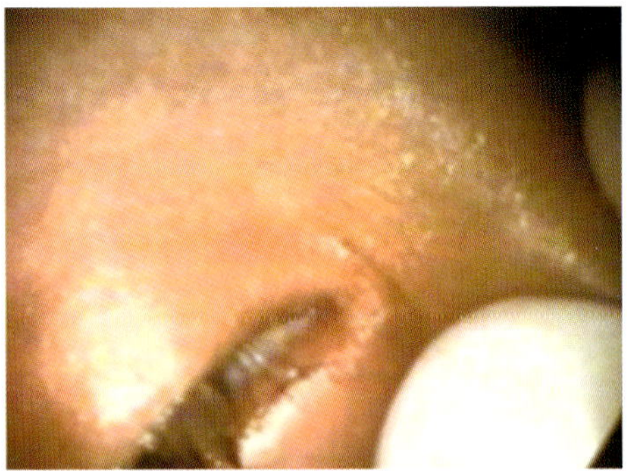

Fig. 20.4. ROPLAS test positive a definite indication for DCR.

of block. In such cases few drops of dye are instilled into the eye and dye disappearance from the eye is noted. If the dye disappears, it indicates a patent system. If the dye does not disappear it indicates a blocked system.

Role of nasal endoscopy

- Nasal endoscopy may not be required in cases where nasal cavity is roomy and the lateral wall along the root of MT is visible clearly. In children it is not possible to do nasal endoscopy without anaesthesia. Thus clinical judgement forms the basis of selection of cases for surgery. In cases requiring a revision surgery, it is mandatory to carry out the nasal endoscopy, as it helps in better planning.
- In cases where the landmarks are not clear on anterior rhinoscopy, nasal endoscopy is a must. It is done for examination of the nose and also to rule out any pathology. The most important finding is the high posterior deviation of the septum that requires septoplasty. Prior planning is a must as it involves two surgeries rather than one. If not corrected, the septal deviation may make it very difficult to negotiate the endoscope and even if we can reach there, the area over the lacrimal sac remains obscured. To prevent messing up in the area with mucosal laceration due to less space it is important to correct the septal deviation. Sometimes it may be possible to inject xylocaine adrenaline that helps in shrinking the septal mucosa moving the deviated portion of the septum away from the lateral wall. It must be remembered at this point that the surgeon gets adequate space to work at the time of surgery if the deviation is not severe. If not so, the surgical correction (limited endoscopic septoplasty) should be done. Otherwise the septal mucosa that

was shrunken during surgery will come back to its normal position to maintain the deviation and may block the rhinostomy. The chances of synechia formation also increase in such cases.

- Middle turbinate may be hypertrophied with a concha bullosa and thus needs to be resected in order to facilitate access to the lacrimal sac area. On the other hand, middle turbinate is the important landmark that guides the surgeon about the location of the lacrimal sac. Absence of middle turbinate may not only confuse the surgeon about the location of the sac but can also lead to serious complications.
- Role of nasal endoscopy is crucial in cases with history of previous surgery, e.g., a failed DCR or functional endoscopic sinus surgery for nasal polyps. One may find the landmarks completely absent. If preoperative evaluation is proper it is easy to explain the prognosis to the patient.
- Nasal endoscopy in revision cases may also reveal presence of synechiae making the revision very difficult. These synechiae if present are released in the same sitting.
- The endoscopic finding may give us an idea about the likely cause of failure of the previous surgery.

Upper vs. lower punctum

Since 70% of secretions from the lacrimal gland are drained through the lower canaliculi and 30% from the upper canaliculi, it is important to keep the lower canaliculi functional. It is, therefore, better if the syringing is done through the upper punctum during preoperative and postoperative assessment rather that lower punctum, though with experience we have seen that it makes no difference in expert hands whether lower or the upper canaliculi is used. Complications may occur in hands of less skilled people and also in cases of transcanalicular laser DCR. Canalicular scarring carries a bad prognosis and should be avoided at any cost.

Steps of probing and syringing

Canalicular direction is peculiar and needs to be understood well (Fig. 20.5).

4% xylocaine with 1: 100000 adrenaline drops are instilled into the eye.

- Position and appearance of the lower punctum is examined by retracting the lid.
- Punctum is dilated with punctal dilator. The dilator is rotated between the thumb and the index finger for easy insertion.

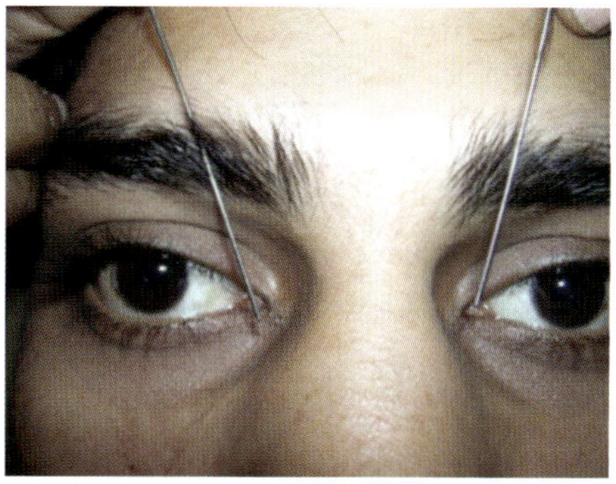

Fig. 20.5. Direction of canaliculi as shown in probes.

- The cannula is then inserted vertically 1–2 mm (Fig. 20.6), and the lid is stretched with finger, the cannula is turned horizontly to 90° to make it parallel to the canaliculus (Fig. 20.7). Progressively thicker dilators can be used if more dilatation is required.

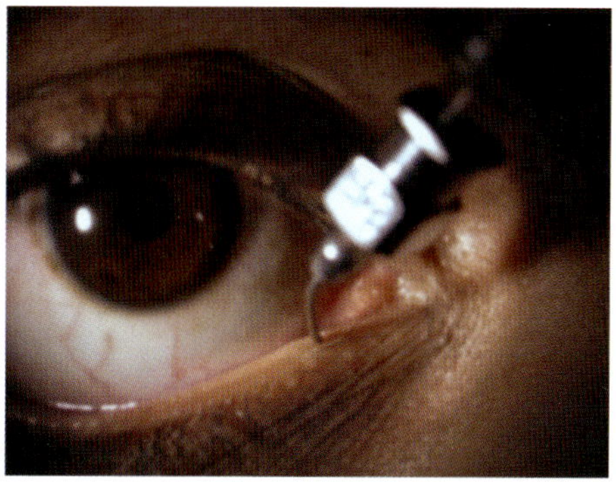

Fig. 20.6. Vertical insertion of lacrimal canula.

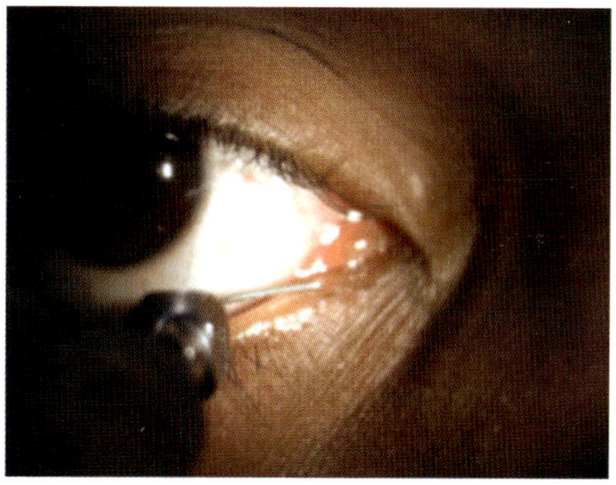

Fig. 20.7. Canula inserted horizontally.

- A small size (no. 1 or 2) Bowman's probe is passed through the punctum using the same technique as that of the dilator. The probe is directed vertically downwards, turned to 90° and is pushed gently.

20

- The canaliculus is maintained in stretched position during this process (Fig. 20.8). If the steps are not followed, the probe strikes against a fold of mucosa and not only gives a false positive result showing a blocked system but also produces a false passage if force is exerted (Fig. 20.9).

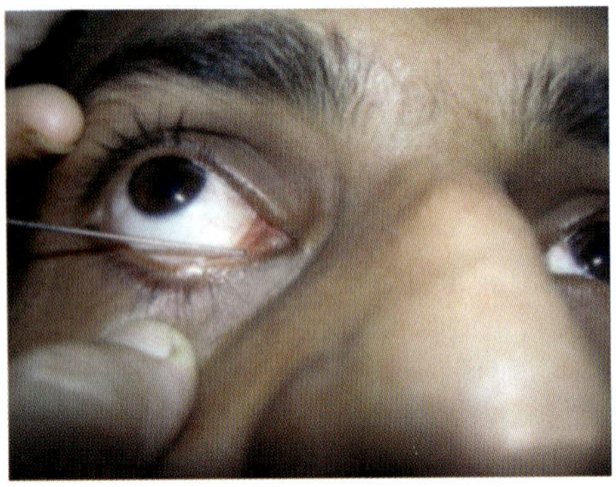

Fig. 20.8. Correct technique of probing.

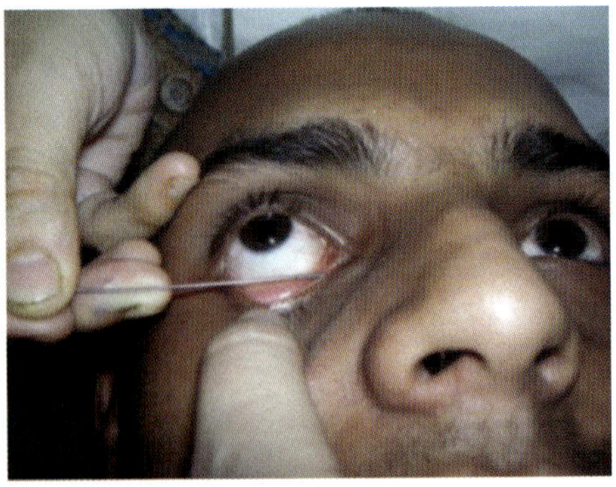

Fig. 20.9. Incorrect technique of probing.

- Presence of soft block indicates a canalicular block while the presence of hard block is indicative of NLD block.

The steps of syringing are same as that of probing. The canula is inserted in the same way as the Bowman's probe. The tip of the canula is than tilted horizontally and the saline is pushed to check the level of block.

Syringing results

- Free flow of fluid into nose on syringing and irrigation indicates a patent nasolacrimal duct system.
- Regurgitation of fluid through the opposite punctum indicates a blocked nasolacrimal duct.
- Regurgitation through both the puncta may indicate a blocked common canalliculi as well as it could be a blocked nasolacrimal duct. To differentiate the two it is easy if the regurgitation fluid is mixed with purulent discharge. It indicates a common canalicular block.

For further differentiation probing is done to find any soft block if present.

Investigations

- Probing and syringing remain the mainstay of diagnosis, but for more information CT scan can be done. It gives us an idea of the surrounding structures in the nose in relation to the sac.
- CT DCG is again very informative in failed cases and in trauma leading to entrapment of the sac.

Flowchart indicating operation decision-making based on sac syringing

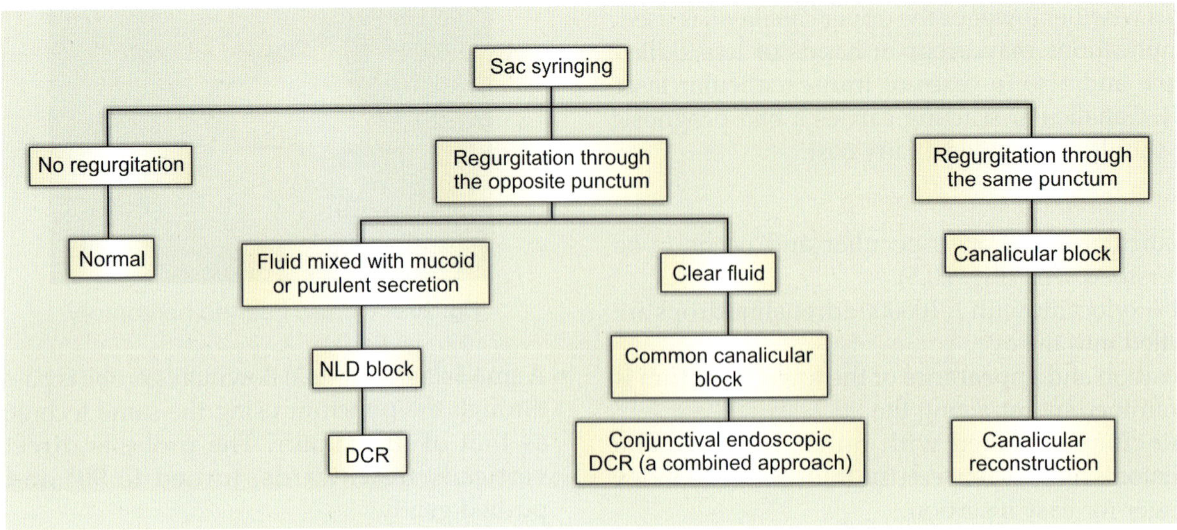

- MRI can be done to rule out diverticula of the lacrimal sac.
- Lacrimal scintillography can provide additional information about the pumping mechanism of the lacrimal pathway.

Preoperative preparation

Discussion with the patient about the procedure should be done. More time needs to be devoted to the patients with previous failed surgery or those with guarded prognosis. In cases of partial canalicular block need of intubation should be discussed. Informed consent should be obtained from the patient, explaining that an endoscopic cleaning may be required in the event of recurrence of symptoms.

Premedication

Premedication in the form of intramuscular fortwin 30 mg and phenargan 25 mg is given. It is used only for patients to be operated under local anaesthesia. We do most of our operations under general anaesthesia. Old-age patients who are thin built are operated under local anaesthesia. Those with medical conditions making them unfit for anaesthesia are also operated under local anaesthesia with premedication. Premedication should be administered at least 30–45 minutes prior to surgery for better analgesia.

Packing of nose

Nose is packed with sofrol packs having one end attached to a silk thread. The thread is tied to one end of each pack for its easy retrieval. The sofrol packs are made up of soft cloth and avoid damage to the nasal mucosa. In adults adrenaline packs can be used in a concentration of one in 20,000 and in children a concentration of 1 in 40,000 can be used safely.

Local anaesthesia

Technique of local anaesthesia

- External block (Fig. 20.10) is given using 0.25% bupivacaine and 2% xylocaine solution. The site of block is at the infraorbital margin at the junction of medial third with the lateral third, palpating the bony margin all the time. Another block is given in the intratrochlear area and around the suptraorbital rim medially.
- Internal block (Fig. 20.11) is given in the nose on the lateral wall of the nose and middle turbinate.

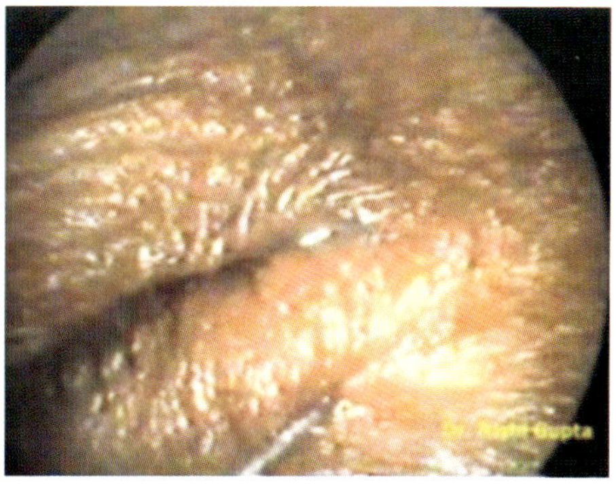

Fig. 20.10. External block in a case operated under local anaesthesia.

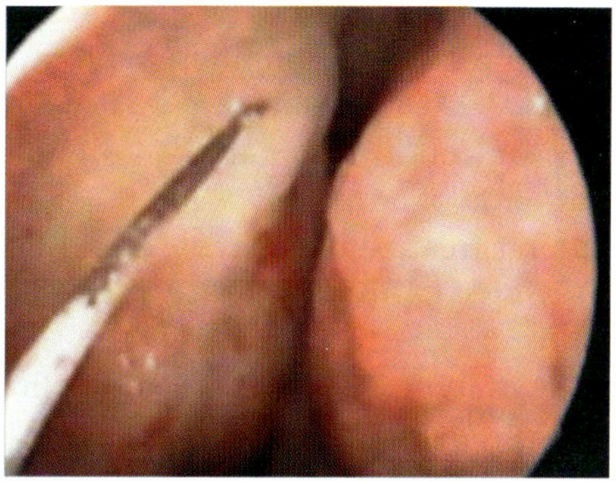

Fig. 20.11. Internal block on lateral wall of nose.

Advantages of local anaesthesia

- The procedure is quick as the bleeding is less.
- Cost to the patient is less.
- Patients unfit for anaesthesia can be safely operated under local anaesthesia. Operating these medically unfit elderly patients under local anaesthesia is a boon as these patients have associated cataract. Cataract surgery cannot be performed without a patent nasolacrimal duct. This is due to the fact that regurgitation of infected secretions from the sac in the eye can cause endophthalmitis. Regurgitation is due to blocked NLD. Endophthalmitis is a dreaded complication, fearing which an ophthalmologist does not go for surgery in such cases. Restoring the patency of lacrimal sac cases by doing a DCR is necessary in such cases.

Limitations of local anaesthesia

- Adequate anaelgesia is difficult to obtain by infiltration in cases with acute inflammation of the sac or lacrimal sac abscess.
- Patients with hypertension may have a rise in blood pressure during surgery. It may not be possible to achieve a hypotensive field.

- In well-built or obese middle-aged females surgery during local anaesthesia may be difficult.
- Surgeon needs to be well versed with the technique of local anaesthesia with particular block sites to be infiltrated. Inadequate infiltration may force the surgeon to abandon the surgery.

Preoperative preparation of the nasal mucosa

Adequate hemostasis is very important for good results. Therefore, a concentrated solution of xylocaine adrenaline is used. Concentration of adrenaline used is different in different cases. Concentration of adrenaline to be used depends on following factors:

- In children readymade solution of 2% xylocaine with 1 : 2,00,000 adrenaline can be used.
- Elderly patients also cannot tolerate high concentration of adrenaline.
- Patients on treatment for hypertension, cardiac disease, etc. cannot tolerate high doses of adrenaline.
- Any known hypersensitivity to adrenaline.

We use adrenaline in a concentration of 1 : 80,000 in healthy adults. Surgeon needs to have a good repo with the anaesthetist in such cases. In most of the cases the blood pressure shoots up with higher doses, but it is not uncommon to find a reflex bradycardia in patients with concentrated solution of xylocaine and adrenaline.

Technique of preparing solutions in different concentration of adrenaline

Adrenaline ampoule is available as 1 in 1000 adrenaline.

20 cc of saline/20 cc of lignocaine is mixed to 1 ml of adrenaline leading to a final composition of 1 : 20,000 solution.

- 1 ml of adrenaline = 1 : 1000 units
- 100 ml of lignocaine/saline (added to 1 ml of adrenaline) = 1 : 100,000
- 80 ml of lignocaine (added to 1 ml of adrenaline) = 1 : 80,000
- 40 ml of lignocaine (added to 1 ml of adrenaline) = 1 : 40,000

If the requirement is of 50 ml of lignocaine in a concentration of 1 : 100,000 of adrenaline, add 50 ml of lignocaine to half cc of adrenaline solution to make it 1 : 100,000.

If 25 ml of lignocaine has to be prepared in a concentration of 1 : 100,000, then add 25 ml of lignocaine to one-fourth ml of adrenaline to make it 1 : 100,000.

General anaesthesia

Advantages of general anaesthesia

- It is possible to have better control over the operative field under GA.
- No external block is required and thus there is no side effect of local infiltration.
- Patients with hard bone and difficult anatomy require drilling that can be done comfortably under GA.
- Revision cases are time-consuming making the patients uncomfortable under local anaesthesia.
- It is possible to have a good hypotensive field under general anaesthesia.

Disadvantages of general anaesthesia

- Risk of GA lies with every case and more with patients with systemic diseases.
- Cost of GA incurred to the patient is more than local anaesthesia.

Surgical technique

The landmark for finding the lacrimal sac is the ridge formed by the frontal process of maxilla and the root of the middle turbinate on the lateral nasal wall (Fig. 20.12). High posterior deviation of the septum obscures the landmarks as it is difficult to negotiate the endoscope beyond the deviated portion. In such cases limited endoscopic septoplasty is done to remove the deviated portion of the septum.

The surgical technique thus involves two procedures:

1. Endoscopic septoplasty.
2. Opening the lacrimal sac.

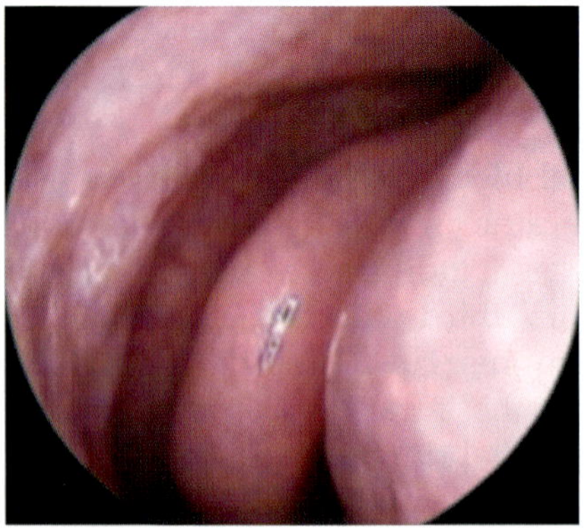

Fig. 20.12. Endoscopic view of lacrimal sac landmark.

Endoscopic septoplasty

Endoscopic septoplasty obviates the need of conventional septoplasty involving complete lifting up of the flaps in such cases.

- An incision over the deviated portion of the nasal septum is given with the help of a 15 no. blade.
- Once the incision is complete the mucosal flap is lifted using Freer's elevator.
- The flap is retracted by the assistant using a blunt instrument. This is the limitation of endoscopic septoplasty as the two hands of the surgeon are busy and an assistant is required.
- Deviated portion of the septum is incised and removed. This creates adequate space for negotiation of endoscope.

Opening the lacrimal sac

Landmark for identifying the lacrimal sac is the lateral wall of the nose anterior to the uncinate process, i.e., the ridge formed by the frontal process of maxilla and the root of the middle turbinate. In more than 75% of cases the upper limit of the sac lies above the anterior attachment of the middle turbinate (Fig. 20.13). So the incision should extend a little higher to the upper limit of the anterior attachment of the middle turbinate. This helps in complete exposure of the sac.

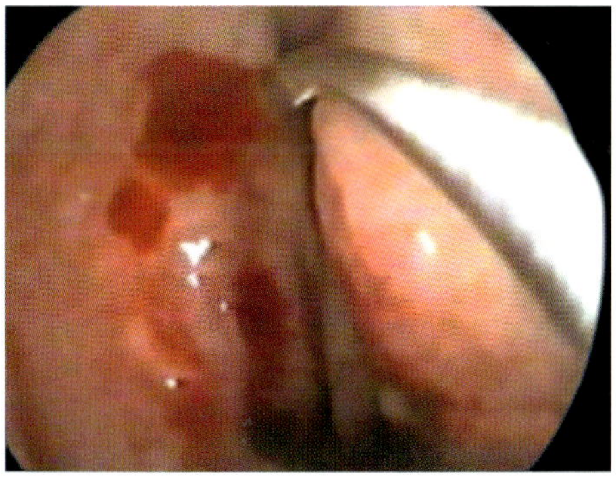

Fig. 20.13. Incision marked by sickle knife.

This landmark on the lateral wall is infiltrated using a long curved 26 no. needle. Points injected on the lateral wall are: the frontal process of maxilla and over the lateral wall of nose just above the upper end of inferior turbinate. Adequate hemostasis is achieved by waiting for 10 minutes after the infiltration.

The mucosa overlying the bone of the ascending process of the maxilla is thin, spillage occurs if one tries to inject while the needle is hitting the bone. In order to avoid spillage withdraw the needle a little bit after it hits the bone and inject the drug to notice the fullness and blanching.

Clear concept about the location of sac is enough to reach the sac without difficulty in all the cases, right from the beginning of the learning curve.

A beginner may still use a rigid fibre-optic light probe if available. This 20 gauge light cable may be inserted either through the lower or the upper punctum. The upper canaliculus is preferred as it allows the light to pass straight into the sac. The light within the nasal cavity is seen using 0° Hopkin's endoscope with the endoscopic illumination at the lowest setting. This allows for accurate identification of the intranasal position of the sac. The sac is found just anterior to the head of middle turbinate but may be obstructed with intervening ethmoid cells.

The transillumination in the nose lies just behind the ridge formed by the frontal process of maxilla and the root of the middle turbinate. The position of NLD can be observed as a vertical ridge just anterior and inferior to the middle turbinate. In most of the cases, the whole process can be completed with a zero degree endoscope alone. However, sometimes 30° scope is required in cases with difficult anatomy such as merging of anterior lacrimal crest with the lateral wall with no ledge of bone marked clearly. One has to tilt the 0° endoscope to visualize the whole of the sac area in such cases.

The incision (Fig. 20.14) starts on the lateral wall 1 to 1.5 cm anterior to the uncinate process. A horizontal incision then starts from the upper end of the vertical incision and similarly another horizontal incision starts medially from the lower end of the vertical incision, making a U-shaped incision with its base resting inferiorly.

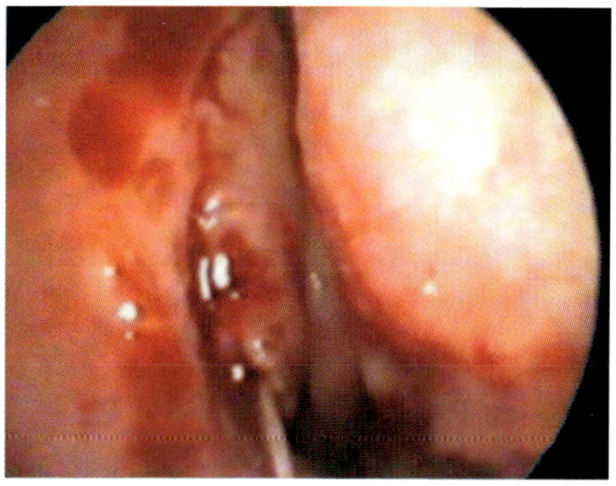

Fig. 20.14. Complete incision on lateral wall of nose.

Various modifications of the incision are possible, e.g., it can start from a horizontal incision at the upper part that starts from the medial to lateral on the lateral wall and then turns vertically down to join another horizontal incision and then finally a U shape incision with its base resting inferiorly.

Once the incision is complete the overlying mucosa is separated with the help of a periosteal elevator. This mucosal flap is preserved for lining the exposed bone at the end of the surgery. It helps in better healing of the osteum and prevents adhesions and contracture of the rhinostomy made. Sometimes it may not be possible to make those clear flaps and difficult and narrow nasal cavity makes visualization difficult. If necessary, the flap can be sacrificed in such cases.

Ledge of bone is seen exposed after the mucosal flap is lifted. Kerrison's punch is used to remove the bone starting from the lower border of the ledge and the removal is continued up gradually (Fig. 20.15). The sac starts getting visible after few punches. Pressure is applied over the medial canthal area to notice the bulge of the sac into the nose. The sac lies between the lacrimal bone and the frontal process of maxilla. While in some cases (more so in children) the lacrimal bone is thin and can be perforated with the help of a blunt dissector but the window needs to be widened using a bone punch.

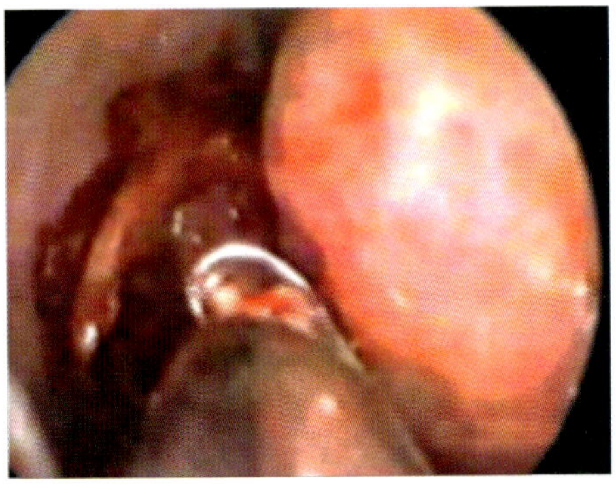

Fig. 20.15. Kerrison's punch used to remove the edge of bone.

20

Complete exposure of the sac is the key to success. It is tempting to note the sac bulging into the nose after few punches. Temptation of opening the sac with a nick in its wall should be resisted at this stage. This may otherwise lead to an incomplete surgery where sac will start pouring pus once the incision is given and it will make further dissection difficult. The sac therefore must be exposed all along its longitudinal axis where fundus of the sac should also be exposed. This upper limit can be identified by probing of the lower canaliculi to make sure that it lies horizontally and there is no blind sac part covering its tip. Sac should be dissected upto this level at least and in some cases even higher than this. The sac's upper border is seen curving laterally. Drill may be required in some cases to remove this bone higher up (Fig. 20.16). This is due to the fact that the bone may be hard in the upper part and it is difficult to remove with bone punch. Sometimes it is difficult to engage the Kerrison's punch in this area due to variable anatomy. Use of curved bone punch is not able to transmit the same force at the tip that is possible with the straight Kerrison's punch. Use of drill is mandatory in such cases, however, if the surgeon is not comfortable with the drilling into the nose he could use chisel and hammer.

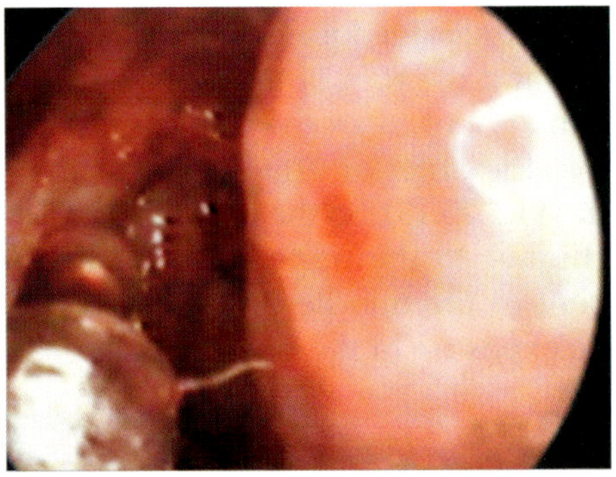

Fig. 20.16. Drill used to remove the bone.

Drilling helps in smooth cutting of the bone and exposes the sac at the fundus. One should be cautious to cover the shaft of the burr with a plastic sheath to avoid damage to the nasal vestibule. The accepted size of the osteum is 12 to 15 mm. We believe it is the site of the osteum that is important not the size in endoscopic DCR. The opening made higher remains patent for a long time. The size of opening in external DCR is very important, because the surgeon needs adequate flaps to suture it with the nasal mucosa.

Following instruments can be used for making a bony window:

- **Hajek's bone punch.** It is an instrument that is used in external DCR. It is a short and stout punch, works excellent for hard bone that may not be possible to remove with Kerrison's punch. This punch, due to its short length, is able to exert more pressure over its tip.

- **Kerrison's punch.** It is a specially designed punch for endoscopic sinus surgery. It is the most important instrument for opening the lacrimal sac as well.
- **Drill with straight or angled handpiece.** Otologic drill machine can be used for drilling in the nose. Microdebrider with special long burrs for DCR surgery can also be used.
- **Chisel and hammer.** These can be used as an alternate option at a site where Kerrrison punch fails. The advanatages are fast removal of bone, as the big chunks can be removed and also its ability to remove hard bone. It can however be dangerous as the fracture line can extend upto base of skull causing CSF leak. Therefore controlled pressure should be applied for bone removal in this area.
- **Laser cutting of bone.** This is used only because it is available for other surgeries and thus can add the advantage of the facility being present.

Once the bone is removed, the periosteum is incised and the sac is approached. Thin-walled sac is identified. There are various ways by which we can identify and confirm the sac.

- Pressure is applied on the medial canthal area to note the movement of the sac into the nose.
- Tenting of the sac is noted into the nose by passing a probe into the canaliculi that enters the sac causing its tenting into the nose.
- The sac is pushed into the nose and an incision is given over it with the help of a sickle knife. Thick pus coming out of the sac is sucked out (Fig. 20.17). The incision is enlarged and the medial wall of the sac is removed using bone punch.

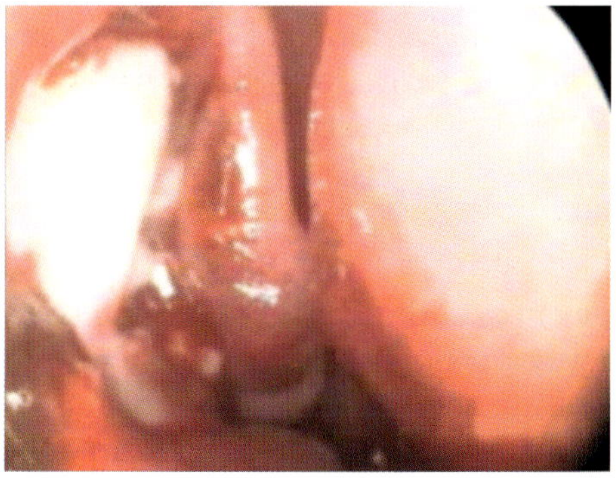

Fig. 20.17. Thick pus coming out of the sac.

- Lumen of the sac is examined, syringing with irrigation is done with dilute betadine solution to check its free flow into the nose. Syringing helps in detecting canalicular block if present. Sometimes even though the sac is completely opened and the common canalicular opening can be seen, it may not be patent due to partial or complete canalicular block.

If there is resistance to the flow of fluid into the nose after the sac is opened it suggests either

(i) the sac remnant is left, or
(ii) adequate bone removal has not been done, or
(iii) there is presence of canalicular block.

Procedure of silicone stenting
(Figs. 8.18, 8.19 and 8.20)

The preferred choice is bicanalicular silicone stent. It comes with metallic guard at its two ends. One metallic guard is passed through the lower punctum and the other through the upper punctum and the two ends are brought out into the nose and tied over a silk thread that helps in easy retrieval of the stent. The metallic ends are cut and the two ends of the tube are tied in the nose. The tube should not be too tight or else it will cause slitting of the canaliculi. Loose silicone stent tends to prolapse into the medial canthal area causing irritation and watering (Fig.

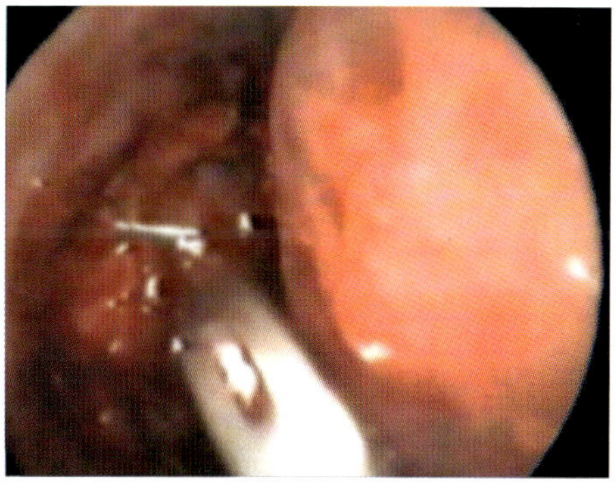

Fig. 20.18. Metallic guard of silicone coming out of nose.

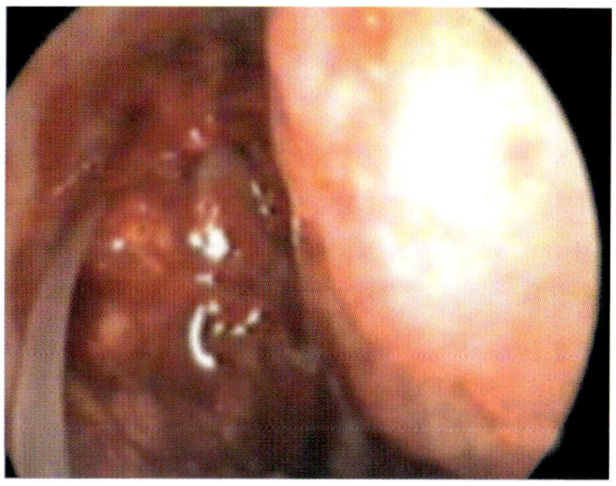

Fig. 20.19. Silicone stent view coming out of nose.

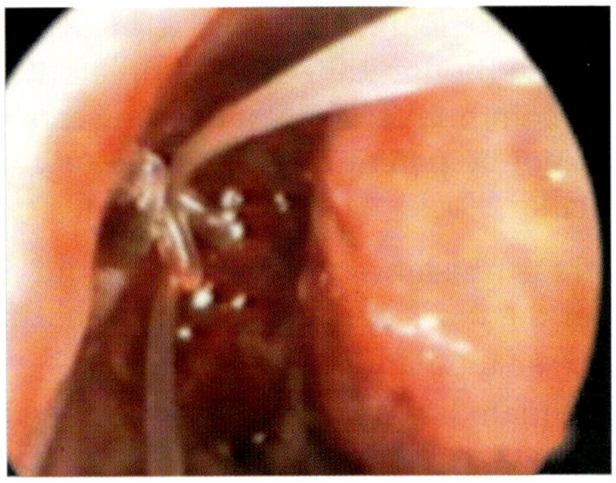

Fig. 20.20. Silicone stent tied in the nose.

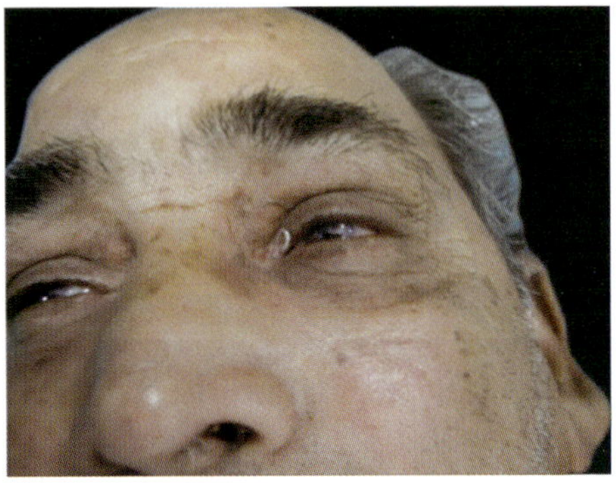

Fig. 20.21. Complication of stent prolapsing out of the eye.

20.21). Silicone tube is seen as a loop in the medial canthal area. The optimal time for keeping the tube in place is 6 weeks, but the duration differs in various conditions and in some with intractable epiphora and common canalicular block, it is kept for 6 months to one year.

Difficulties during endoscopic DCR

- Anatomical variations are a challenge in endoscopic DCR. While some cases can be finished in ten minutes, others take more than an hour.
- Sometimes bone is extremely thick making its removal difficult. It is advisable to use drill in such cases to remove the bone completely. Use of drill makes the procedure lengthy and technically more difficult.
- One has to be careful to avoid contact of the drill with the endoscope as this may damage the optical axis of the endoscope.
- If the sac is small and contracted it can be challenging for the surgeon.
- Vestibular skin may get damaged with the shaft of the rotating burr. The shaft of the burr is covered with a plastic sheath which can be made out of the intravenous intubation set.

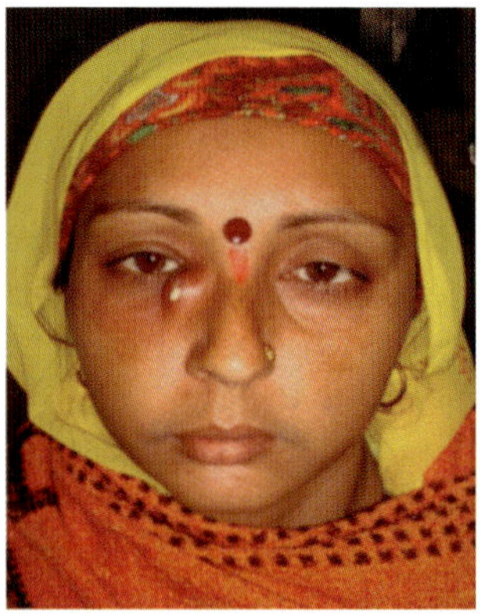

Fig. 20.22. Lacrimal sac abscess right side.

- There may be difficulty in locating the sac, especially in revision cases. The landmarks are destroyed and the tissue scarring makes identification difficult. In such cases light cable is very helpful. This light cable is passed through the lower canaliculi and the illumination in the nose is noted to locate the sac.
- There might be inadequate space to work. Ledge of bone on the lateral wall may not be well demarcated. This short length of the ridge is due to higher attachment of the upper end of the inferior turbinate.
- Hypertensive patient with hypertrophied and vascular mucosa may bleed more than normal.
- Stenotic puncta may be not only difficult to locate, but can also cause persistent symptoms after surgery. May be due to inability of the tears to flow through this narrow punctum into the lacrimal sac. Such cases are managed with dilatation and stenting of pathway. If the punctum is too narrow to be identified, a microscope is used for easy identification.
- High posterior deviation of the septum may pose a temporary threat and is solved by limited endoscopic septoplasty.

How to improve the success rate in endoscopic DCR

Case selection is the key to success. During ENT residency one is not trained enough to do syringing and assessing the site of block and thus relies on the other surgeon. It is good to have an ophthalmic colleague with you, but it is advisable to do the syringing yourself. Since it is the only diagnostic method we use along with probing wherever required. It is essential to judge it preoperatively to avoid surprises on the table.

One should be well versed with the technique of probing and syringing. It helps in detecting a soft block indicating a common cannalicular or an isolated canalicular block. Thus syringing by itself is the most important part of analysis. If the common canalicular obstruction is present, a bicanalicular stent can be passed through the block after endoscopic opening of the sac. This is to treat any canalicular block if present.

Site of the rhinostomy should be higher up. Its position can be decided with the help of probe introduced into the lower canaliculus. Once the sac is opened intranasal, the surgeon should pass the probe through the lower canaliculus to judge the direction of probe. The direction should be horizontal with no tilting downward of the probe required to enter the nose. The probe through the lower canaliculus should be passed horizontally and this probe should be visible in the nose in the same direction. If a block is felt at the tip of the probe at this level despite a complete opening of the sac, it means that there is a remnant of the sac that is still not opened. Higher dissection is required in such cases. An otologic drill or a microdebrider with a special burr can be used to remove the bone higher up. Bony window needs to be widened so that the sac can be opened all along its long axis. Long-term results are good in such cases.

Most of the endoscopic DCR in the hands of less skilled surgeons fail because of the remnant of the sac left behind.

Synechia formation is another reason of failure. In most of the cases the middle turbinate adhesion with the lateral wall is seen. It can be avoided by preserving the mucosal flap and raw bone can be covered with these flaps. This is the nasal mucosal flap which was earlier sacrificed. With the passage of time it was realized that this flap preservation leads to the better epithelization. It also tends to avoid closure of the rhinostomy as seen in some cases.

Postoperative management

Packing of the nose

- Packing of the nose should be done cautiously as it contributes to the success of the procedure. In patients where flap preservation is not possible for various reasons, sinus pack is placed over the rhinostomy. Tip of the sinus pack is trimmed and kept towards the lumen of the sac. It helps in keeping the lumen patent and prevents synechiae formation. The mucosal tags around the osteum epithelize well with the surrounding mucosa in a week's time. It helps in maintaining long-term patency by avoiding contracture at the primary site. This pack is removed after 7 days, as during this time complete epithelisation of the mucosa occurs.
- In cases where flaps are preserved, it is better to pack the nose with gel foam. This is to avoid disturbing the flaps till healing occur and thus gel foam is left in the nasal cavity for 2–3 weeks. This pack is supported with Vaseline guaze that is removed after 48 hours.
- Use of sinus pack in children is not advocated because sinus pack fits snugly and gradually swells with absorption of secretions. Sometimes considerable force has to be exerted to pull out the pack that can be painful in children. Children are thus packed with Vaseline guaze packs. In children, results of DCR are otherwise also excellent and the risk of adhesions is less. Bone is thin and can be removed easily, thus less raw area is created.
- Sofratulae or glycerine packs are removed after 48–72 hours.
- Sinus pack should not be placed in cases with bicanalicular silicone stenting. Though other surgeons may have varied opinion on this, our apprehension is that if the stent or its silicone thread gets entangled in the sinus pack, its removal can cause complication. There could be damage to the puncta or canaliculi with the pull over the stent or there could be an accidental extrusion of the silicone stent.
- Systemic antibiotics, systemic decongestants, analgesics and serratiopeptidase are given as per requirement.
- Decongestant nose drops are given in post-operative patients.
- Syringing is done on day 1, day 7, after one month and then after 3 months.

Advantages and disadvantages of endoscopic DCR

Advantages

- The associated nasal pathology can be corrected in the same sitting.
- There is no scar, thus morbidity is less. Though in external DCR also scar may not be visible after

few weeks. But it is not uncommon to find patients with hypertrophied scar in the medial canthal area and if the pathology is bilateral, scars in the most prominent part of the face gives an ugly look to the patient.

- There is no injury to the adjacent medial canthal structures. Thus, it is more physiological as the medial palpebral ligament is preserved. The normal pumping mechanism of orbicularis muscle over the canaliculi is maintained.
- Bilateral surgeries can be performed in the same sitting only in endoscopic approach to lacrimal sac. This is not possible via external route.
- Revision surgery should always be done endoscopically. As there is no visible cut, it does not look like a revision surgery to the patient.
- Endoscpic approach to lacrimal abscess obviates the need of an incision and drainage prior to DCR. Unlike external DCR where an incision and drainage of the sac is required, in endoscopic DCR the abscess can be drained into the nose with a dacryocystorhinostomy in the same sitting. It therefore saves the patient of two surgeries and helps in saving time and money both. Two sittings are required in external DCR because the skin over the abscess is fragile and it is not possible to suture the skin flaps in this condition.
- There is no error in osteum location like seen in external DCR.
- There is no error in bone removal
- Common canalicular obstruction is a limitation with both external and endonasal DCR. It is better as it is less mutilating surgery by adopting an endonasal approach followed by stenting of the lacrimal pathway.
- Scarring at the rhinostomy site can cause blockage of the osteum. Follow up of the patient with persistant epiphora is easy as the mucosal overgrowth can be removed endoscopically.
- Difficult tube removal can be managed by endoscopic control.
- Intervening ethmoid cells can be removed in the same sitting
- An enlarged middle turbinate poses threat to external DCR, as it is blind surgery and enlarged turbinate can get damaged leading to bleeding.
- Deviated nasal septum can be corrected in the same sitting.

Disadvantages

It is difficult to think about the disadvantage of endoscopic DCR. One could put it the other way by saying there is no extra advantage of endoscopic DCR over external DCR in certain case. These cases are, e.g., lacrimal sac fistula with chronic dacryocystitis. Fistulectomy is must in all the cases except children. It therefore does need an external incision and a dacryocystorhinostomy can be done through the same incision. Endoscopic DCR with fistulectomy by an external incision is done in such cases, but there is no added advantage of endoscopic DCR over external DCR in such cases.

Size of rhinostomy was an issue earlier at the time of advent of endosciopic DCR. But it is possible to make as large a window as required by endoscopic DCR. The procedure involves opening the sac all along its longitudinal axis. Thus the size of the window is as big as the size of the sac. This also therefore is not a disadvantage.

The only theoretical disadvantage is that it is not possible to suture the flaps of the lacrimal sac with the nasal mucosa in endoscopic DCR. It was therefore thought to compromise the results by an early closure of the rhinostomy. Studies by many authors and our own experience have proved that the success rate of endoscopic DCR is at par with the external DCR. It is therefore not mandatory to suture the flaps for better results.

Results of endoscopic DCR

A successful DCR case will not only be patent to syringing but endoscopic documentation of the rhinostomy is also important. Workers use various techniques of documenting results. Most important is to have a patent rhinostomy. One can however record pre and postoperative clinical pictures of patients with lacrimal sac mucocele presenting as a bulge below the medial canthal area (Fig. 20.22).

Transcanalicular laser DCR

Transcanalicular laser DCR is gaining popularity amongst eye surgeons and is technically an easy procedure. 20 guaze diode laser fibres is passed through the lower punctum into the canaliculi and the lacrimal sac and laser is fired. Once the sac is opened, pus can be seen coming out of the sac into the nose. The ostium is widened and syringing is done with dilute betadine solution.

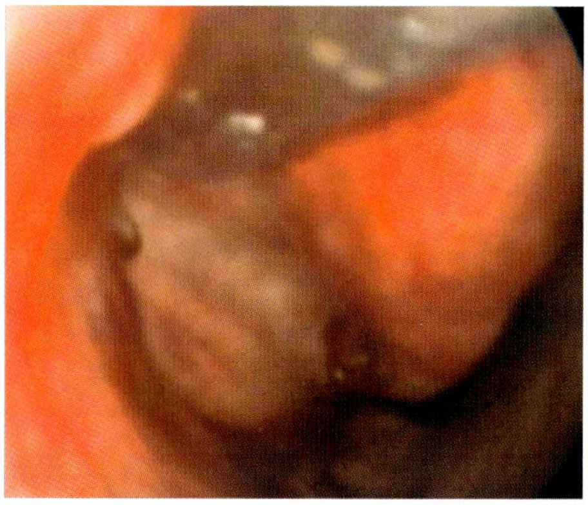

Fig. 20.23. Stenting of congenital dacryocystitis

Word of caution

If the laser is fired while the cannula is still in the canaliculi it may lead to permanent scarring and stenosis of the canaliculi leading to epiphora.

Outcome

The results of transcanalicular DCR are not very encouraging as only a small size window can be made. The window is located more inferiorly and tends to close faster.

Management of paediatric epiphora

Good clinical judgement is required for treating the paediatric epiphora. The challenge lies in finding:

1. The right age for intervention.
2. Available management option for treating epiphora in children.
3. Stage at which an intervention should be planned.
4. How to diagnose the site of obstruction in children as syringing is not possible in them, thus the diagnosis is based on history and clinical examination.
5. When to seek help from an ophthalmology colleague.

To decide the age for intervention

By intervention here we mean probing and syringing in congenital NLD obstruction. There are various schools of thought about the timings. This is based on the fact that the nasolacrimal duct that is blocked in some children since birth and opens up as the child reaches six months of age. Probing and syringing therefore should be avoided before six months. Early probing should be considered in cases where purulent discharge causes embarrassment and disability to the child.

Available management option for treating epiphora in children

- Probing and syringing of the nasolacrimal duct.
- Stenting of nasolacrimal duct using a bicanalicular silicone stent (Fig. 20.23).
- Endoscopic DCR.
- Stenting of NLD a latest concept in treatment of congenital dacryocystitis.

When is an endoscopic DCR indicated in children?

- Theoretically endoscopic DCR in children is not recommended before 3 years.
- Practically, congenital lacrimal abscess with fistula should be operated immediately.
- If the age is more than three years with ROPLAS (regurgitation of pus on pressure over the lacrimal sac) the child should be operated.

CONCLUSION

Nasolacrimal duct anatomy has close relationship to lateral wall of nose. Nasolacrimal system blockage is caused by chronic dacrycystitis, lacrimal abscess, mucocele, dacryolithiasis and failed external DCR. Endoscopic DCR is safe, quick, less traumatic, minimal blood loss and last but not the least avoids external scar, more so in lacrimal abscess which can be done in a single stage. It has high success rate in primary and secondary cases, with few complications. Deviated nasal septal and paranasal sinus pathology can be corrected at the same sitting.

SUGGESTED READING

1. Arruga H. Ocular surgery. McGraw Hill Book Co. Inc. 4th edition, 1956.
2. Austen DP. Lacrimal dilatation and syringing. *Optometric News*, 1–7.
3. Blaylock WK, Moore CA, Linberg JV. Anterior ethmoid anatomy facilitates dacryocystorhinostomy. *Arch Ophthalmol*, 1990; 108; 1774–7.
4. Kong YT, Kim TI, Kong BW. A report of 131 cases of endoscopic laser lacrimal surgery. *Ophthalmolo*, 1994; 101: 1793-1800.
5. Stormo LPS, Gipson J. Endocanalicular laser assisted dacryocystorhinostomy: an anatomical study. *Arch Ophthalmol*, 1992; 110: 1488–90.
6. Linberg JV, Anderson RL, Bumsted RM, Barrers R. Study of intranasal osteum in external dacryocystorhinostomy. *Arch Ophthalmol*, 1982; 100: 1758–62.

7. Mickelson SA, Kim DK, Stein IM. Endoscopic laser assisted dacryocystorhinostomy. *Am J Otolaryngol,* 1997; 18: 107–11.
8. Michalos P, Pearlman SJ, Avila EN, Newton JL. Hemispherical tip contact Nd:Yag translacrimal-nasal dacryocystorhinostomy. *Ocular Surg News,* 1995; 13: 40.
9. Pearlman SJ, Michalos P, Leib ML, Moazed KT. Translacrimal transnasal laser assisted dacryocystorhinostomy. *Laryngoscope,* 1997; 107: 1362–5.
10. Silkiss RZ, THC: YAG nasolacrimal duct recanalization. *Ophthalmic Surg,* 1993; 24: 772–4.
11. Woog JG, Metson R, Puliafito CA. Holium Yag endonasal laser dacrycystorhinostomy. *Am J Ophthalmol,* 1993; 116: 1–10.
12. Ranga RK, Advin, Yadav SPS. Endo- DCR: Is it an end of the road for external DCR? *J Indian Med Assoc,* 2008; 106: 228–31.

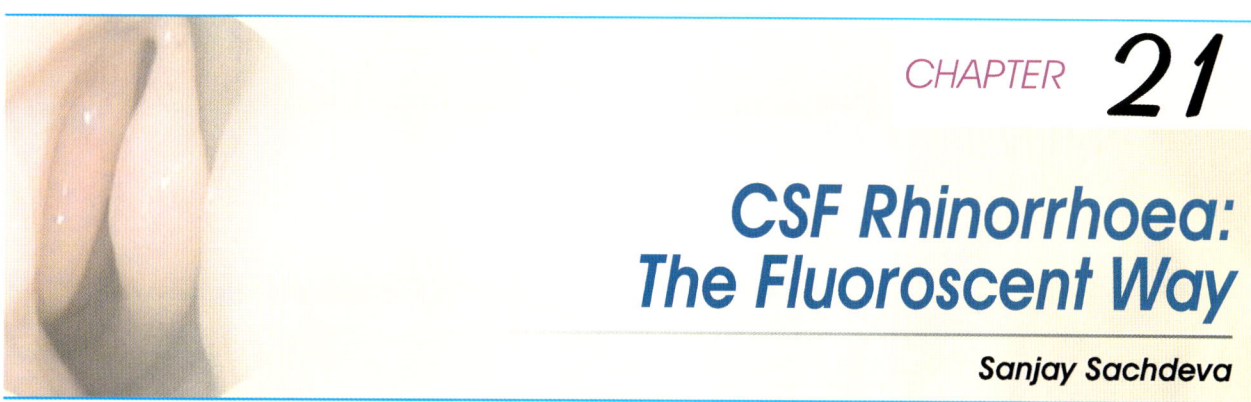

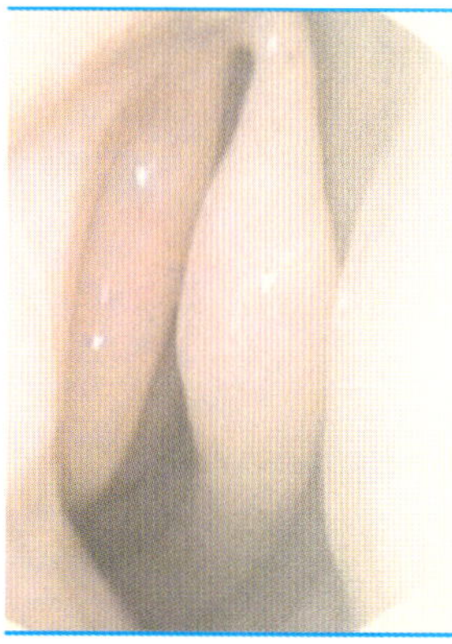

CHAPTER 21

CSF Rhinorrhoea: The Fluoroscent Way

Sanjay Sachdeva

Cerebrospinal fluid (CSF) leak occurs when there is an osseous as well as dural defect at the skull base, with direct communication of the subarachnoid space to the extracranial space, usually via nose or a paranasal sinus. Dura provides a waterproof seal that prevents spinal fluid from escaping. CSF leaks occur when there is a breakdown of this barrier. Greater proportion of CSF leaks resolve spontaneously. CSF leak persisting for more than 7–10 days causes significant risk of developing meningitis and brain abscess. So, persistent CSF leak is potentially lethal and surgical treatment is often required.

Cerebrospinal fluid (CSF) rhinorrhoea was first described by Galen in 200 BC. St. Clair Thompson reported the first series of patients with spontaneous leakage in 1889. Many attempts to correct CSF leak were done in the 20th century, although the first well-succeeded surgical approach was attributed to Dandy in 1926, when he sutured the fascia lata over dural defect, on the posterior wall of the frontal sinus, by intracranial route. In 1964, Vrabec and Hallberg described endonasal approach to repair CSF leak in the cribriform lamina.

The advancement in radiology and endoscopic nasal surgery has provided ways to solve this potentially dangerous condition. The surgical management of CSF leak has changed significantly after the introduction of functional endoscopic sinus surgery (FESS) in the management of sinusitis. It is currently accepted that endoscopic intranasal management of CSF rhinorrhoea is the preferred method of surgical repair, with higher success rates and less morbidity than intracranial surgical repair in selected cases. Laboratory tests for confirming the presence of the CSF in nasal fluid can yield false positive results and radiological evaluation has never been foolproof when it comes to small leaks and multiple leaks. CT/MR cisternogram can localize the direct defect in 85% cases while intrathecal fluorescein injection aided localization. Endoscopic repair of CSF rhinorrhoea has success rate of 92%. Endoscopic repair of CSF rhinorrhoea requires composite graft and fibrin glue.

Types

- Traumatic
- Iatrogenic
- Spontaneous

TRAUMATIC

CSF rhinorrhoea commonly occurs following head trauma (frontobasal skull fractures), as a result of intracranial surgery, or destructive lesions. Frontal bone anterior table is strong enough to withstand certain amount of pressure, but once this is fractured, concertina effect is transmitted to the ethmoid labyrinth and cribriform plate, in particular, both being extremely fragile. Cribriform plate is perforated by olfactory fibres, making it still weaker. Moreover, dura and arachnoid are closely adherent to cribriform plate. Hence any trauma is likely to tear them leading to a CSF leak.

Physical examination of nose reveals clear fluid stream on position testing, Valsalva manoeuvre or compressing both jugular veins (Queckenstedt-Stookey test). Halo sign is also diagnostic of CSF leaks (Fig. 21.1). Ooze or bleed, if it is mixed with CSF, may not clot, which becomes an important sign during surgery.

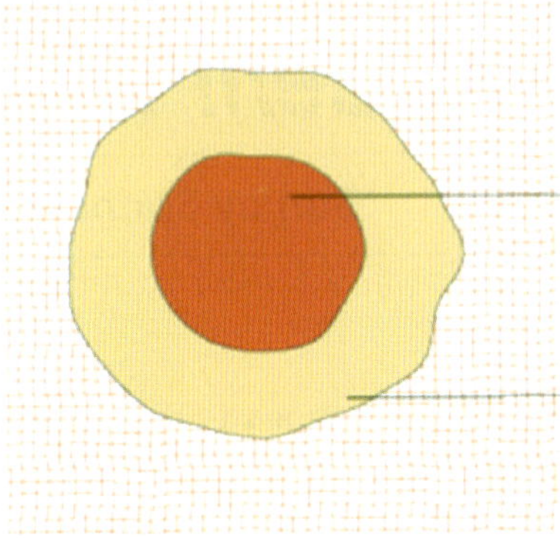

Fig. 21.1. Halo sign showing red (blood) and clear CSF.

Sudden negative pressure created around the leak, either by suction or otherwise, may lead to air being sucked inside the opening. If air goes inside the CSF compartment and does not come out because of ball valve effect, tension pneumoencephalus results. Patient would complain of increasing headache if patient is conscious. This can be diagnosed by plain radiology or CT scan of the head.

Such condition would require immediate surgical intervention. If the leak is small and intermittent it may be wise to let it heal spontaneously, which might take 3 to 4 weeks. Infections in the nose have to be avoided all times at all cost.

Indications of immediate action in traumatic CSF leak

1. Large continuous leak with skull base bony defect of more than 2 cm.
2. Tension pneumoencephalus.
3. Multiple sites of injury and leak as seen by CT scan (Fig. 21.2).

We are likely to miss one or two if endoscopic approach is used.

If traumatic leak persists for more than 4 weeks, then chances of self-healing are remote and this would need endoscopic repair.

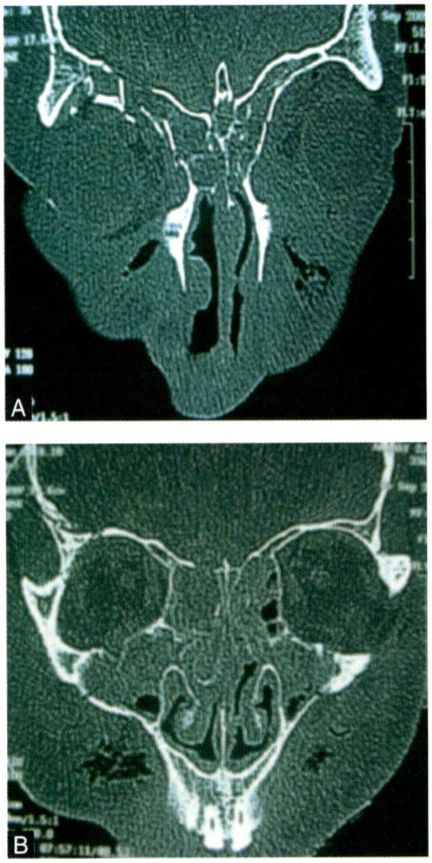

Fig. 21.2 A & B. CT scan showing multiple leak sites.

IATROGENIC LEAK

Diagnosing CSF rhinorrhoea during active leak is the best time for repair. So, a great deal of suspicion is required at the time of surgery. Any surgeon is capable of opening the dura, but experience would ensure that it is diagnosed and repaired in time. One must be aware that one has gone beyond the confines of nose and sinuses well in time so that damage is negligible and remediable. It may be difficult to recognize CSF in a pool of blood, but as mentioned earlier a strong suspicion is the key to diagnosis. Clear fluid washing away blood may be seen if leak is copious, blood collected from the site does not clot as it is mixed with CSF (Fig. 21.3). Fluid collected from the site if kept on the blotting paper leaves two fluids with different consistencies which move at different rates on the blotting paper, making what is known as target sign. Jugular pressure or Valsalva done by the anaesthetist increases the flow of leak from the suspected site. A black hole may be appreciated as the opening of the dura and arachnoid against white background of the bone and

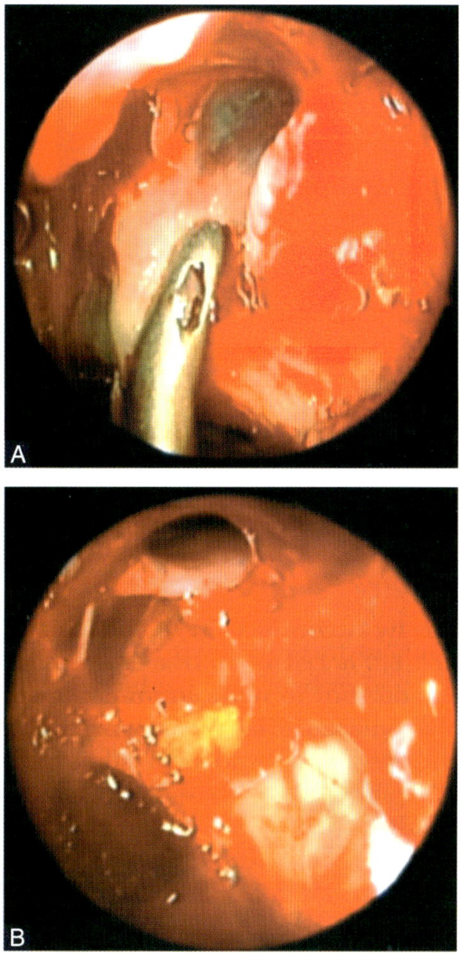

Fig. 21.3 A & B. Endoscopic view of CSF leak.

pink-red of the nasal mucosa. Pulsations of intracranial tissues can be visualized quite easily and CSF leak may come out in a pulsatile manner.

Best time to repair is at the time of trauma during surgery. The leak is identified and sealed with muscle or fat. Middle turbinate forms a good material to scaffold the fat or fascia in the dural hole.

SPONTANEOUS LEAK

Patient with spontaneous leak may not give a history of old trauma (Fig. 21.4). This may be intermittent and recurrent. Obvious causes of non-traumatic CSF rhinorrhoea, such as congenital malformations or tumors and/or nothing in the history or at surgery consistent with a traumatic or iatrogenic origin. The leaks may have periods of remission, but since CSF does not have precursors of self-healing like fibrinogen, platelets, etc. They are known to persist unless closed surgically.

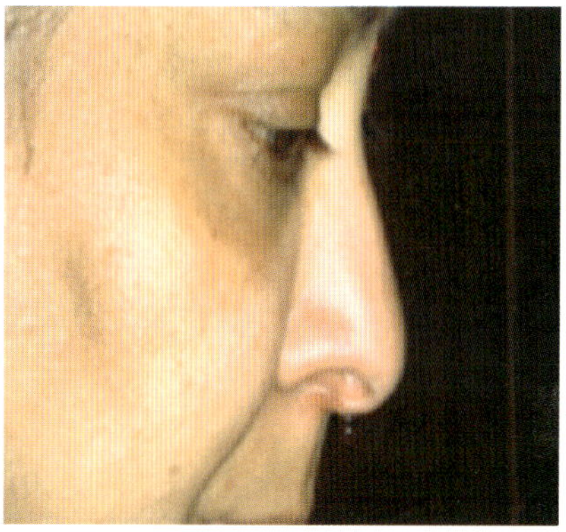

Fig. 21.4. Spontaneous leak.

Meningitis being an inflammatory process may heal at the end of the process.

They are commonly seen in menopausal and perimenopausal age because of osteoporosis. The pulsations of vessels at the skull base, both anterior or posterior ethmoidal artery, may thin down already thin skull base. These areas, in clinical practice, are certainly the commonest sites where spontaneous leaks are found.

If leak is present intermittently and is missed with MRI, CT cysternography (Fig. 21.5), though an invasive procedure, may be able to pick it up.

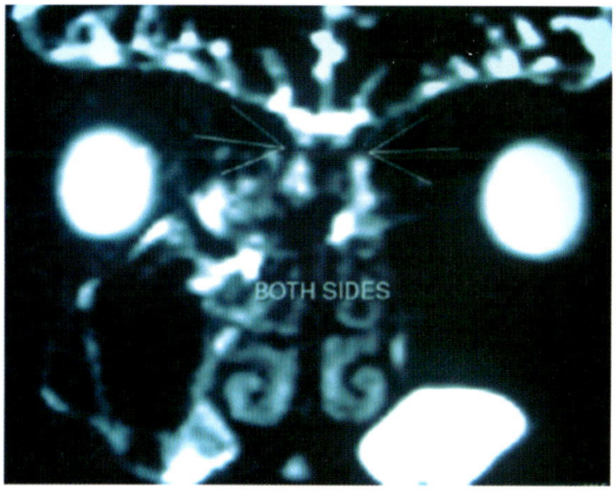

Fig. 21.5. MRI cysternography showing the CSF leak.

Most of these repairs are advised to be done endoscopically, unless the leak is in frontal sinus, where combined approach is required.

Ophthalmic consultation is taken to rule out papilloedema to rule out raised intracranial tension.

Fluorescein injected into CSF compartment may be a good tool to diagnose even small leaks.

Once leak is identified and a fair estimate of its size has been made, the plan is to close it immediately with either local flap of nasal mucosa or using fascia, fat and muscle from the thigh or temporal region. The opening needs to be plugged first to stop active leak, lest no assembly will stay in actively leaking situation. This can be achieved by plugging muscle or fat. In all these situations the skull base is devoided of its mucosal lining. After the bone is made bare and opening in dura and arachnoid identified by using Blue filter. The fluorescein that escapes the opening is seen as brilliant fluoroscent in a dark background (Fig. 21.6).

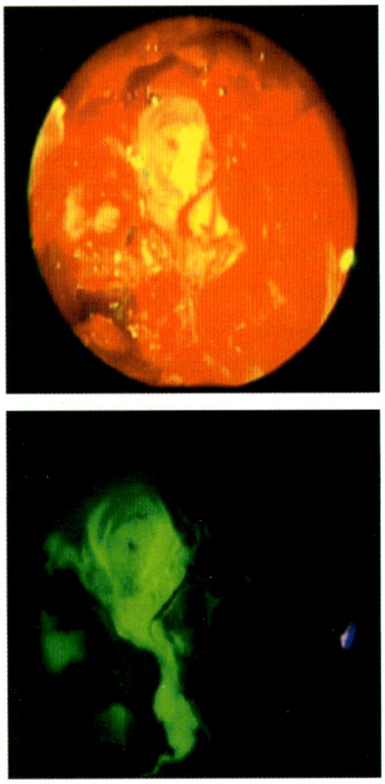

Fig. 21.6. Endoscopic view of leak after flourescein.

Endoscopic technique

After achieving good anesthesia, the middle turbinate is utilised to support this antigravity assembly with good results as the support is by local structure with inherent nasal mucosa. It has to be assured that no nasal mucosa gets submerged or assembly does not occlude frontal or sphenoid sinus. The same precaution is taken when fibrin glue is used to strengthen the assembly. At this point of time, Blue filter has justification, since it ensures results of repair in terms of absence of fluoroscent at the site of surgery (Fig. 21.7).

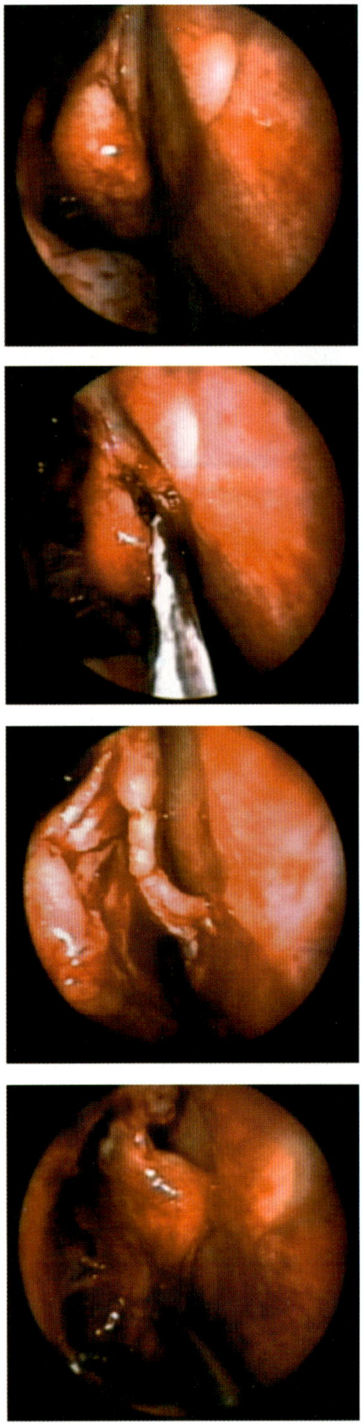

Fig. 21.7. Endoscopic views of rotating middle turbinate to support the leak. Graft material used at bared area.

In very small leaks cauterising the edges may stop the leak. This has to be done with caution as excessive use of cautery can increase the size of the leak. Nasal cavity needs to be packed well to keep the assembly of fascia, fat, muscle or flap in place.

Packs are kept for 5 days with adequate antibiotic cover. Patient is advised to take adequate rest, avoid blowing nose, lifting of weights, constipation and crowded places where there is chance of picking up a respiratory infection.

Postoperative care and follow up is must to help facilitate the healing process and closely monitor for CSF leakage. Repaired site takes 4–6 weeks to achieve complete healing.

The value of broad spectrum antibiotic prophylaxis in patients with CSF leakage is debatable. The question of the use of prophylactic antibiotics in patients with CSF rhinorrhoea stems from the reasonable assumption that a communication between a sterile environment (intracranial vault) and a nonsterile environment (sinonasal cavity) will ultimately result in infection of the sterile compartment.

The use of prophylactic antibiotics in patients incurring skull base injuries during endoscopic sinus surgery has not been studied in a randomized controlled fashion. However, administering antibiotics in this setting is reasonable because the skull base injury occurred during surgery for chronic inflammatory/infectious sinusitis and implantation of bacteria into the sterile compartment may have occurred.

CONCLUSION

A cerebrospinal fluid rhinorrhoea (CSF leak) occurs when there is a fistula between the dura and the skull base and discharge of CSF from the nose. It may be traumatic, iatrogenic and spontaneous. Large leaks are diagnosed by CT/MRI, however, small leaks can be seen on fluorescein technique. Transcranial procedures are associated with a higher complication rate than extracranial procedures. Endonasal endoscopic approach can be preferred for the closure of uncomplicated CSF fistula, located at the anterior or posterior ethmoid roof and in the sphenoid sinus, due to its minimal postoperative morbidity.

SUGGESTED READING

1. Bhalodiya NH, Joseph ST. Cerebrospinal fluid rhinorrhoea: Endoscopic repair based on a combined diagnostic approach. *Indian J Otolaryngol Head Neck Surg*, 2009; 61: 120–6.
2. Wax MK, Ramadan HH, Ortiz O, Wetmore SJ. Contemporary management of cerebrospinal fluid rhinorrhoea. *Otolaryngol Head Neck Surg*, 1997; 116: 442–9.
3. Schick B, Ibing R, Brors D, Draf W. Long-term study of endonasal duraplasty and review of the literature. *Ann Otol Rhinol Laryngol*, 2001; 110: 142–7.
4. Paul P, Upadhay K. Endoscopic endonasal repair of traumatic CSF rhinorrhoea. *Indian J Neurotrauma*, 2010; 7: 67–70.
5. Lanza DC, O'Brien DA, Kennedy DW. Endoscopic repair of cerebrospinal fluid fistulae and encephaloceles. *Laryngoscope*, 1996; 106: 1119–25.
6. Lloyd KM, DelGaudio JM, Hudgins PA. Imaging of skull base cerebrospinal fluid leaks in adults. *Radiology*, 2008; 248: 725–36.

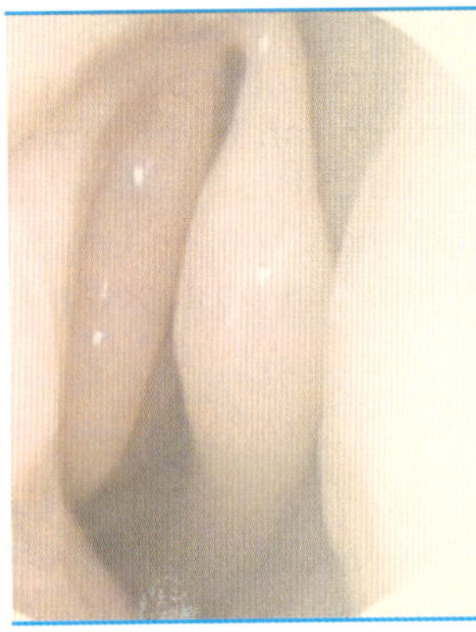

CHAPTER 22

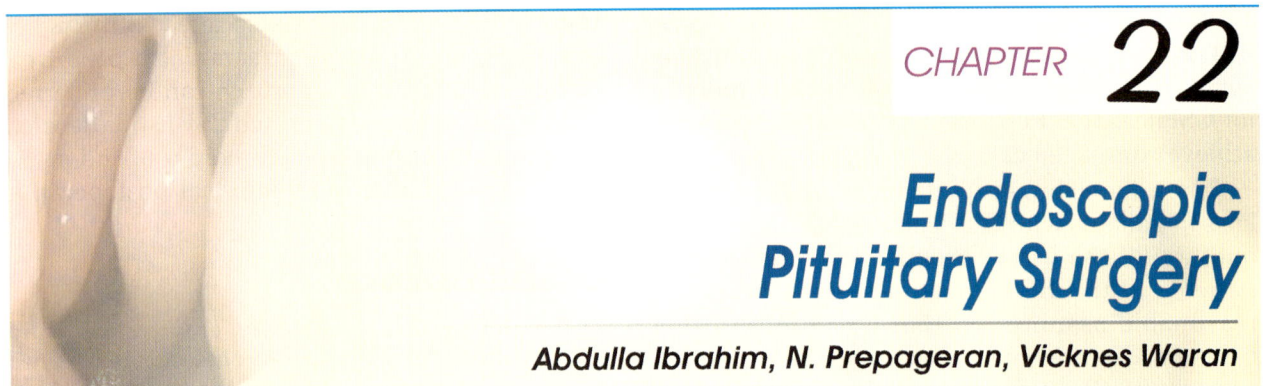

Endoscopic Pituitary Surgery

Abdulla Ibrahim, N. Prepageran, Vicknes Waran

This chapter is intended to describe the endoscopic approach to pituitary surgery highlighting the necessary steps of the procedure.

Surgeons have started routinely using a purely endoscopic technique to remove pituitary tumours. The endoscope has revolutionized the surgical treatment of pituitary tumours whereby allowing:

- Direct visualization and removal of tumour in otherwise difficult to reach areas. Prior to this breakthrough, most pituitary tumour surgeries were done in part "blindly".
- Unsurpassed illumination, magnification, and optical resolution of the surgical field.
- The use of two hands to perform precise movements in a four handed technique.

By operating through the natural pathway of the nose and nasal sinuses, this surgery can be performed without a visible scar on the face or scalp. There is less morbidity compared to traditional craniofacial surgery. Patients can often be discharged the day after surgery.

Background

Ten to fifteen percent of all intracranial neoplasms are the slow-growing pituitary adenomas which produce symptoms either by expansile forces when enlarged or metabolic dysfunction secondary to hormonal disorder. Diagnosis is best carried out by radiology and hormonal studies. Management can be medical, surgical or radiotherapy.

Surgical anatomy and embryology

The anterior lobe (adenohypophysis) of the gland develops from an evagination of ectodermal cells of the oropharynx known as Rathke's pouch and it is eventually pinched off from the oral cavity and becomes separated by the sphenoid bone of the skull (Figs. 22.1 and 22.2).

The posterior lobe (neurohypophysis) develops from neural crest cells as a downward evagination of the floor of the third ventricle of the brain.

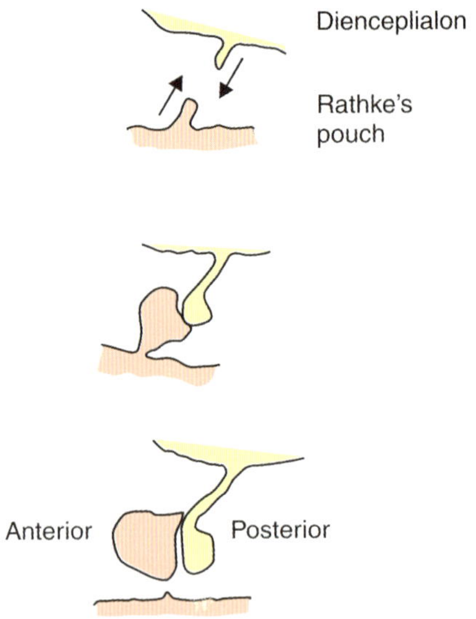

Fig. 22.1. Development of the pituitary gland. (*Courtesy:* med.mun.ca)

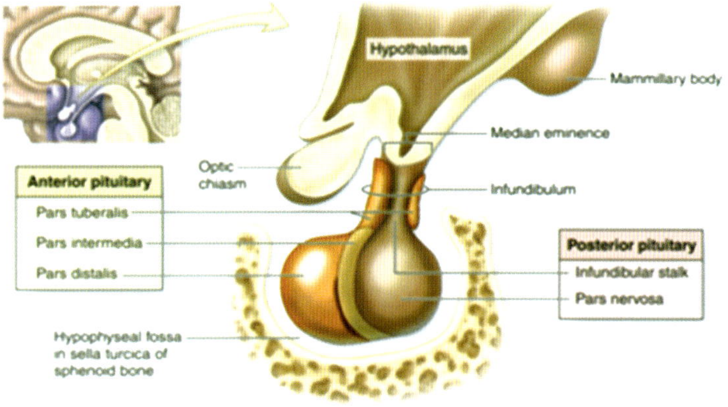

Fig. 22.2. Final position of the pituitary gland. (*Courtesy:* McGraw Hill Companies)

In the adult the gland weighs 500–900 mg and measures about 15 × 10 × 16 mm.

Surgical relationships

The pituitary gland is related to four surgically important structures (Fig. 22.3):

1. Optic chiasm, 9–14 mm superior to the pituitary gland and anterior to the pituitary stalk.
2. The cavernous sinuses situated in the middle cranial fossa on either side of the pituitary gland.

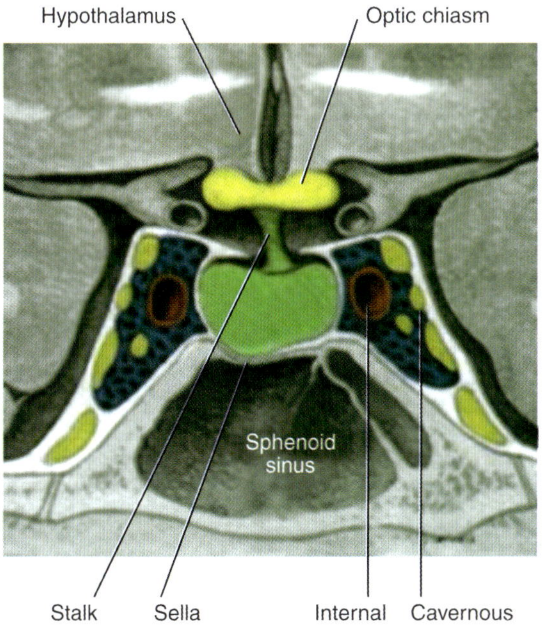

Fig. 22.3. Relationship of the pituitary gland to the various important structures. (*Courtesy:* Mayfield Clinic)

3. Intercavernous sinuses – The right and left cavernous sinuses communicate via intercavernous sinuses that pass anterior and posterior to the infundibulum (stalk) of the pituitary gland.
4. The hypothalamus which is situated superior to the optic tract and connects to the gland by the pituitary stalk.

Blood supply

The superior hypophyseal and inferior hypophyseal arteries (branches of internal carotid artery) and their respective transverse anastomosis supply the pituitary gland. Note please, that the anterior pituitary is not supplied directly (Fig. 22.4).

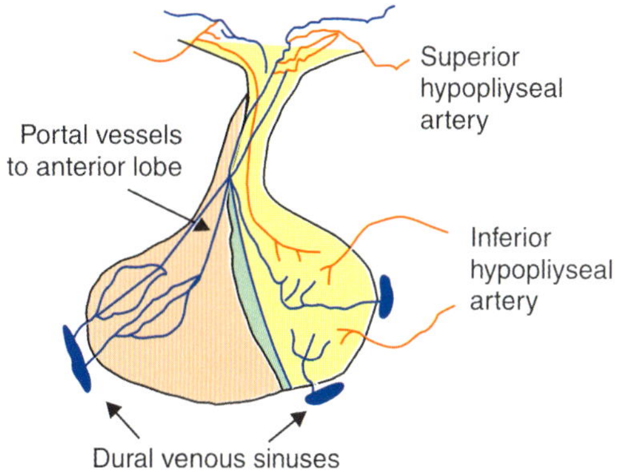

Fig. 22.4. Blood supply to the pituitary gland. (*Courtesy:* med.mun.ca)

Physiology

The pituitary gland is the master gland of the body because it controls most of the body's endocrine functions by means of the hypothalamic-pituitary

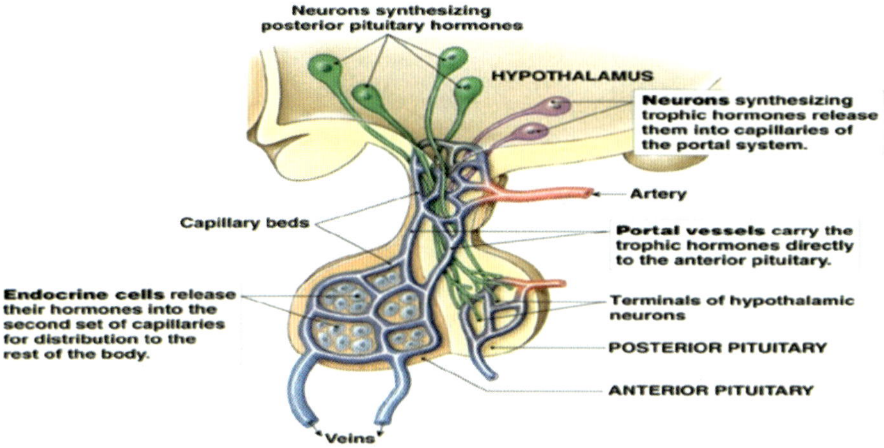

Fig. 22.5. Mode of production and transport of the pituitary hormones. (*Courtesy:* Pearsonsedu)

axis. It secretes various hormones required to maintain normal metabolic and cellular functions within the body (Fig. 22.5).

The anterior lobe of the pituitary gland secretes 6 hormones: thyroid-stimulating hormone (TSH), previously adrenocorticotropic hormone (ACTH), follicle-stimulating hormone (FSH), leuteinizing hormone (LH), growth hormone (GH), and prolactin (PRL).

The posterior pituitary gland secretes vasopressin and oxytocin (Fig. 22.6).

Pathology

Pituitary adenomas are almost always benign with no malignant potential. In general, pituitary lesions can be subdivided into nonsecretory and secretory tumours of the pituitary gland, other intrasellar tumours, and parasellar tumours. Functioning pituitary adenomas can be clinically classified by means of the hormone they secrete. Furthermore, pituitary adenomas can be differentiated by measuring the size of the tumour (Figs. 22.7 and 22.8).

- Microadenomas are defined as intrasellar adenomas as large as 1 cm in diameter without sellar enlargement and have little effect on the visual system or on the function of the gland.
- Macroadenomas measure more than 1 cm in diameter and cause sellar enlargement and pressure symptoms. They cause symptoms of

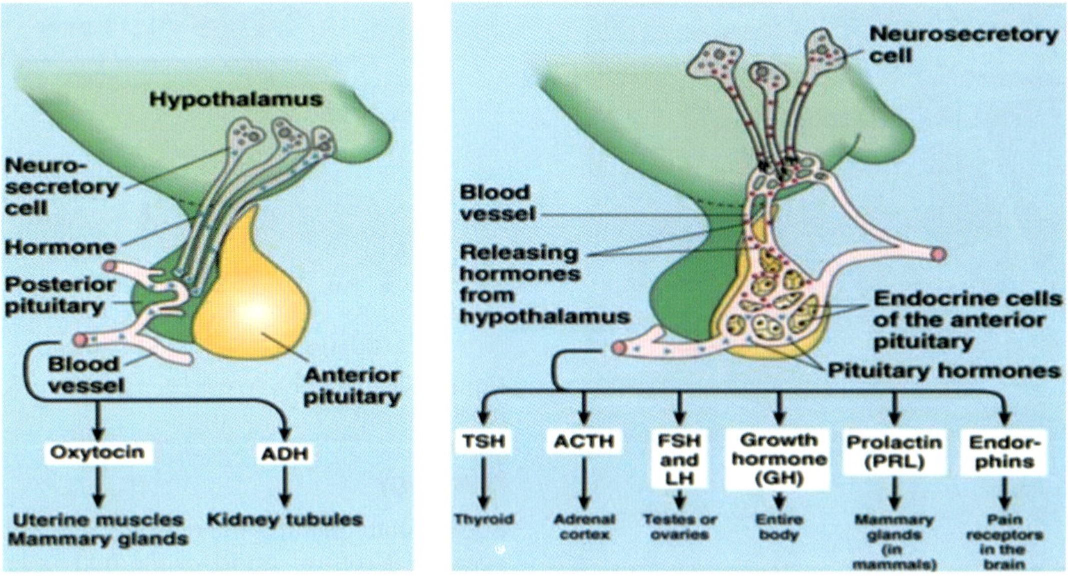

Fig. 22.6. Various endocrine role of pituitary gland. (*Courtesy:* Addison Wesley Longman)

22

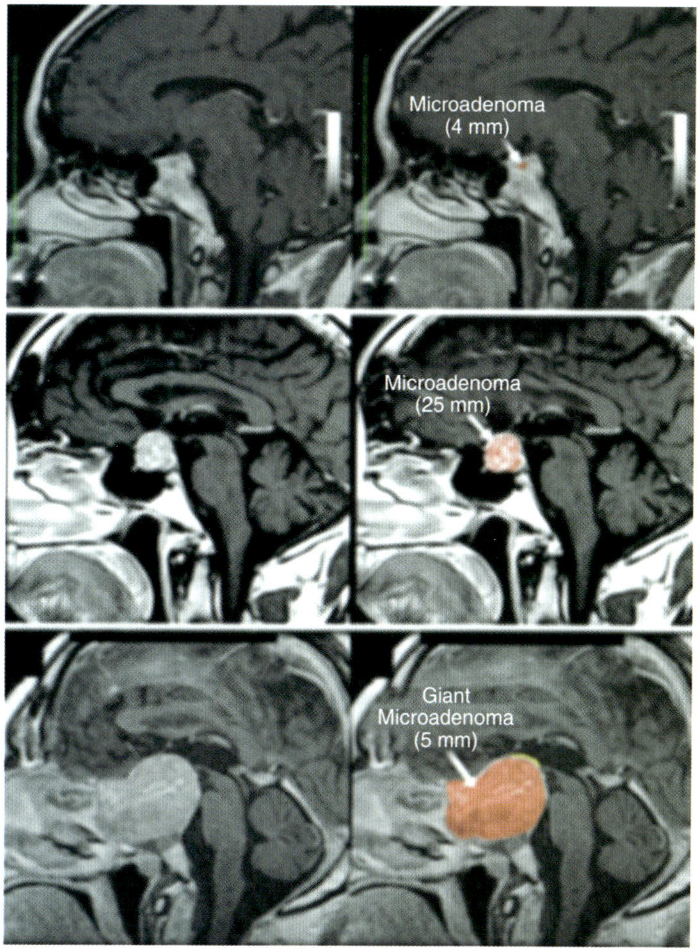

Fig. 22.7. Sagittal views: MRI images from three different patients with pituitary adenomas. The images on the right side have colorized to better show the tumour in red. The upper pair of images demonstrates how a small microadenoma can be difficult to detect. The middle and lower panels show how larger pituitary adenomas can grow upward toward the brain, and sometimes additionally into the nasal cavity. (*Courtesy:* neurosurgery.ucla.edu)

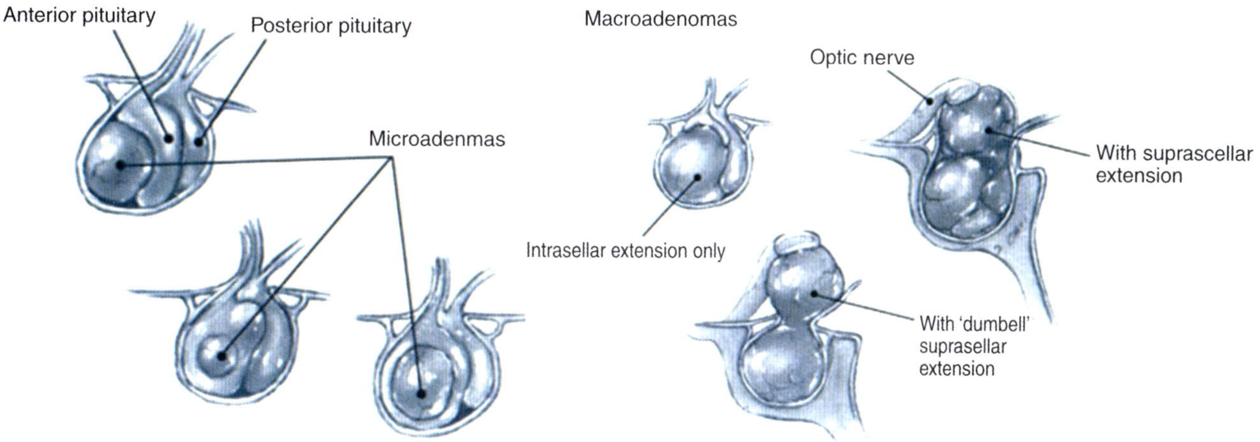

Fig. 22.8. Various presentations and growth patterns of both pituitary microadenomas and macroadenomas (*Courtesy:* An Atlas of Skull Base Surgery)

mass effect (e.g., headache). Macroadenomas include nonsecreting adenomas, PRL-secreting (chromophobe) adenomas, GH-secreting (acidophil) adenomas, ACTH-secreting (basophil) adenomas, and FSH- or TSH-secreting adenomas.

Pathophysiology

Pituitary adenomas exhibit pathology via the following mechanisms:

Pressure symptoms via tumour enlargement resulting in headache, nausea and vomiting. Superior growing tumours can impinge on the optic chiasm resulting in bitemporal hemianopia. Other cranial nerves in the cavernous sinus can also be involved with lateral extension.

Endocrine via hypo- or hypersecretion occurs.

The most common functioning pituitary adenomas are Prolactinomas. Excess production of prolactin by these tumours can cause amenorrhea, galactorrhoea and infertility.

Pituitary adenomas that produce excess adenocorticotrophic hormone cause Cushing's disease.

Excess secretion of growth hormone produces gigantism in children which primarily affects the active growth plates and acromegaly in adults wherein the soft tissues of the body such as the hands, face, tongue and lips are affected.

Thyroid stimulating hormone (TSH) producing adenomas are rare and can give rise to goitre or thyroid hyperfunction.

Pituitary dysfunction occurs when the enlarged adenoma compresses the normal surrounding functional pituitary tissue.

Frequency

Pituitary tumours represent 10–15% of all intracranial tumours, with an annual incidence of 0.2–2.8 cases per 100,000 persons. Incidental pituitary tumours are found in approximately 10% of autopsies. About 25–30% pituitary adenomas are nonfunctioning, 25% produce PRL, 20% produce GH, and 10% produce ACTH.

Mortality/morbidity

The mortality rate related to pituitary tumours is low. Advances in both medical and surgical therapies and the availability of hormone replacement have contributed to successful management.

- Morbidity related to macroadenomas is associated with expansion of the tumour into the optic tracts and the cranial nerves adjacent to the cavernous sinus and may include permanent visual loss, ophthalmoplegia, and other neurologic complications. Some tumours recur after radiation therapy and surgery. Pituitary apoplexy is rare complication of pituitary tumours caused by sudden bleeding into the tumour or infarction of the pituitary gland. Headache of sudden and severe onset is the main symptom, associated with visual disturbances or ocular palsy. Signs of meningeal irritation or altered consciousness may be present. Secondary adrenal failure due to ACTH deficiency may be life threatening.
- In rare cases, a pituitary adenoma may invade the orbit with devastating consequences to the integrity of the globe and ocular. Therefore, early recognition of this complication is of the utmost importance to begin appropriate treatment to minimize ocular and orbital damage.
- Surgery by means of the transsphenoidal approach is considered the technique of choice when pituitary surgery is indicated. Surgery has the advantage of rapidly lowering hormone levels. For microadenomas, the cure rate is greater than 50%. Tumours larger than 1 cm can recur and may require additional treatment. Infection, cerebrospinal leakage, vascular injury, double vision, visual loss, and pituitary deficiency are rare postoperative complications.
- A false aneurysm of the cavernous carotid artery and a carotid cavernous fistula have been reported as complications after trans-sphenoidal surgery.

Sex

In general, autopsy series show equal distributions of pituitary tumours between men and women.

- Corticotrophin-secreting tumours are an exception. These tumours occur mainly in women, with a female-to-male ratio of 4 : 1.
- In general, pituitary adenomas are diagnosed more frequently in women of childbearing age than in men probably because of the association of these tumours with menstrual irregularities. Amenorrhea is common in women with macroadenomas; this finding suggests a pituitary lesion.

Age

Tumours affect individuals of all ages, but the incidence increases with age, peaking between the third and sixth decades. Pituitary gigantism is very rare in the pediatrics age group; however, it is extremely rare in a child that is less than 3 years of age.

Diagnosis

Pituitary tumours are diagnosed using clinical and radiological tools.

Endocrinologists usually diagnose **secreting** tumours whereas the ophthalmologists diagnose the **non-secreting** tumours since they produce visual defects in the absence of any systemic signs.

The two most important radiological tools used to diagnose pituitary tumours are:

- MRI with contrast, it is useful to (a) confirm the presence or absence of tumour (b) delineate the exact size and extension of the adenoma (c) to assess vascular relationships to the tumour (d) to detect invasion of the surrounding structures (e) to localize microadenomas and differentiate it from surrounding normal pituitary gland, and (f) post-therapy to detect residual or recurrent tumour.
- CT scan of the paranasal sinuses is obligatory before any endoscopic surgery as it serves as a "road map" for the surgeon. CT scan is required (a) to find out other anatomical variations that may obstruct the sphenoid sinus ostium (b) to know the extent of sphenoid sinus pneumatisation (c) to look for variations in the attachments of the intra- and intersphenoid septae in particular to the carotid artery (d) to know the size of the sella, and (e) to ascertain sellar erosion and extent of tumour extension into the sphenoid sinus.

MANAGEMENT

All patients should have a thorough physical examination including nasal and sinus examination and an evaluation of cranial nerve function. For pituitary adenomas, visual compromise may occur when the tumour extends above the plane of the diaphragma sellae. Assessment of visual acuity, visual fields, and ocular motility should be routine, with emphasis on detailed examinations in patients with macroadenomas and suprasellar extension. In general, cranial nerves II, III, IV, and VI are not affected until significant parasellar tumour extension occurs. However, acutely expanding or developing lesions, such as haemorrhage within an existing adenoma or infarction (pituitary apoplexy), may also induce palsies of cranial nerves III, IV, and VI and may present as a surgical emergency.

Medical therapy

It can be considered for the following type of tumours:

- Prolactinomas are treated best with Bromocriptine. Orally active. First line therapy for prolactinomas. Normalizes serum prolactin (~ 95%) and shrinks tumours (~ 95%).
- Acromegaly can be treated with Octreotide, which reduces GH concentrations (~ 80%) and shrinks tumours (~ 30%).

Radiotherapy

Growth in nonfunctioning pituitary adenomas can be effectively controlled with fractionated radiotherapy. Growth is arrested in 70–90% tumours with radiation doses of 45 Gy given in 1.8 Gy fractions. The risk of optic neuropathy and visual loss is 1%. Approximately 50% of the patients develop hypopituitarism and require replacement hormone therapy. The combination of surgery and radiation therapy appears to improve the control of disease progression.

Surgery

Historical perspective

The first attempts to use the endoscope in sellar region surgery date back to 1963 when the French neurosurgeon Gerard Guiot proposed using endoscopy to supplement the transsphenoid transseptal approach to microsurgical exploration of the sellar cavity. More recently, the introduction of the endoscopic endonasal approach has offered a less-invasive alternative to access the pituitary gland, providing superior intraoperative imaging by virtue of angled lenses that allow panoramic views of the regional anatomy. This has allowed for more thorough tumour resection and fewer surgical complications having rendered the fully endoscopic endonasal approach the "gold standard" in pituitary surgery. Most patients are able to go home the day after surgery.

Surgical indications

1. Pituitary apoplexy.
2. Progressive mass effect from a large macroadenoma or other sellar mass.
3. Hyperfunctioning pituitary adenomas.
4. Failure of previous therapy.
5. Tissue diagnosis.

Surgical contraindications

All are relative and absolute only if medical co-morbidities pose as an anesthetic risk.

SURGICAL STEPS

The steps are divided into 3 stages: nasal, sphenoid and sella.

The surgery is carried out under general anesthesia in collaboration with the neurosurgeon and a neurosurgical anesthetic protocol.

Positioning

The patient is positioned in a semi-recumbent position (approximately 20° head up) with the head placed on a horseshoe headrest. The head is slightly extended (this enables the skull base to be in direct vision and perpendicular to the surgeon) and slightly rotated towards the surgeon who is on the right side of the patient. The nurse with the instrument trolley stands at the top of the patient's head. The C-arm if used is placed in the axial plane of the patient's head. The monitor with the camera and light source (on the trolley) is on the top left side of the patient's head, opposite the surgeon. The assistant stands to the right/opposite of the surgeon depending on the requirements of the procedure.

TIP: Extending the head is vital in endoscopic surgery of the frontal sinus, skull base (CSF leak repair) and sphenoid sinus surgery. If not, the surgeon will be operating with an "upward" view instead of a direct view that an extended head provides.

22

Preparation

The periumbilical region is aseptically cleansed with betadine (in anticipation for harvesting fat if need be) and the face cleansed with sterile normal saline/water.

The head is draped completely keeping the nose exposed only.

Nasal stage

Diagnostic endoscopy and decongestion

The 0° endoscope is used to inspect both nasal cavities. The side with the greater working room is chosen to commence surgery if the tumour is enlarged equally. If the tumour is predominantly on one side, the opposite nostril is chosen as after removal of posterior septum, this provides a direct route to the tumour and its lateral extension.

Prior to beginning the dissection, the endonasal anatomy is identified, including the middle and inferior turbinates, the choana, and, most importantly, the superior turbinates and sphenoid ostia to assist in orientation (Fig. 22.9).

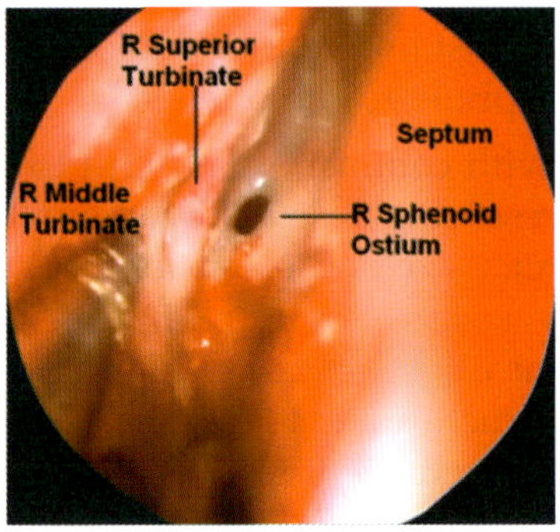

Fig. 22.9. Diagnostic endoscopy

Ribbon gauze soaked in 1 : 1000 epinephrine are packed in the spenoethmoidal recess bilaterally and in the space between the middle turbinate and septum on the side chosen for dissection to assist in the gentle lateralization without fracturing of the middle turbinate (Fig. 22.10).

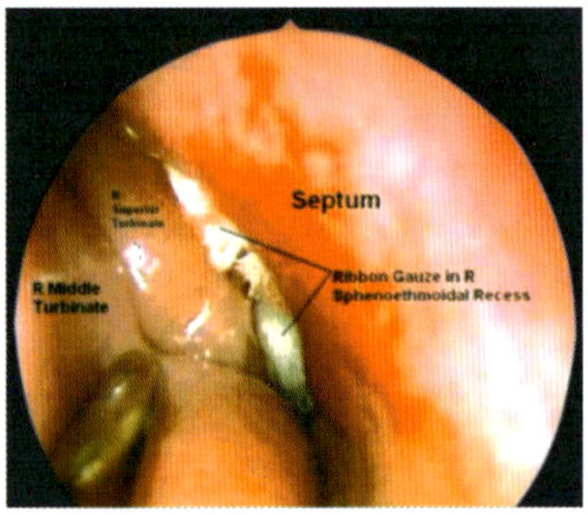

Fig. 22.10. Nasal packing.

Then using a 25-gauge 1.5-inch or spinal needle the anterior portion of the septum is injected submucosally with 0.2% bupivicaine with 1 : 200,000 epinephrine and the blanching is visualized tracking posteriorly (Fig. 22.11).

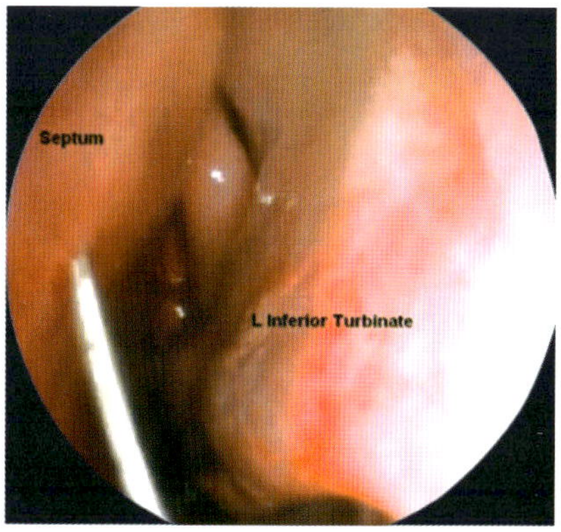

Fig. 22.11. Injecting the septum.

In the event of a concha bullosa or deviated septum obstructing access these are excised accordingly (Fig. 22.11).

HINT: Gentle packing will prevent mucosal trauma and bleeding that might interfere with visualization. Packing should be carried out under direct endoscopic vision to minimize trauma.

Raising a vascular pedicled nasoseptal flap (Hadad-Bassagasteguy flap (HBF))

As a standard protocol for transsphenoidal surgery we raise a nasoseptal flap routinely in anticipation of reconstructing cranial base defects to promote rapid and complete healing if the need arises thus avoiding complications caused by persistent communication between the cranial cavity and the sinonasal tract.

Two parallel incisions are carried out along the sagittal plane of the septum, one over the maxillary crest and the other 1 to 2 cm below the most superior aspect of the septum (this preserves the olfactory epithelium). These incisions are joined anteriorly by a vertical incision (posterior to the Killians' incision site). Elevation starts anteriorly with a Cottle dissector and is carried posteriorly to the anterior wall (rostrum) of the sphenoid sinus, below the sphenoid ostia, making sure that the flaps' postero-lateral neurovascular pedicle is preserved. Elevation of the flap is completed leaving it pedicled on the posterior septal neurovascular bundle. Once completely elevated, the flap is parked into the naso-pharynx until the sella phase of the surgery is concluded. During surgery, it is important to be careful with bone removal lateral to the pterygoid canal so that the vascular pedicle is not injured (Figs. 22.12, 22.13 and 22.14).

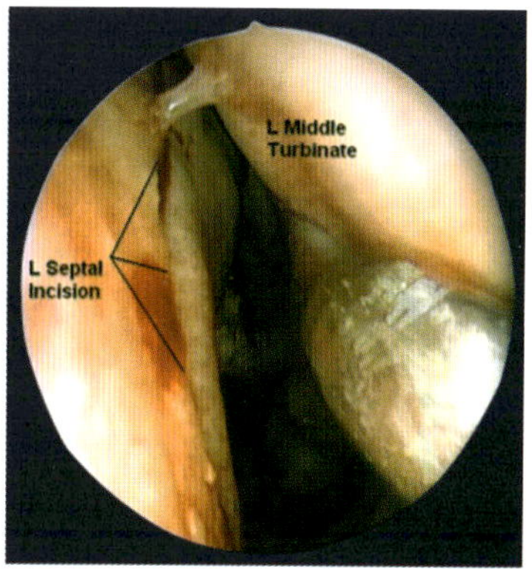

Fig. 22.12. Incising the mucoperichondrium.

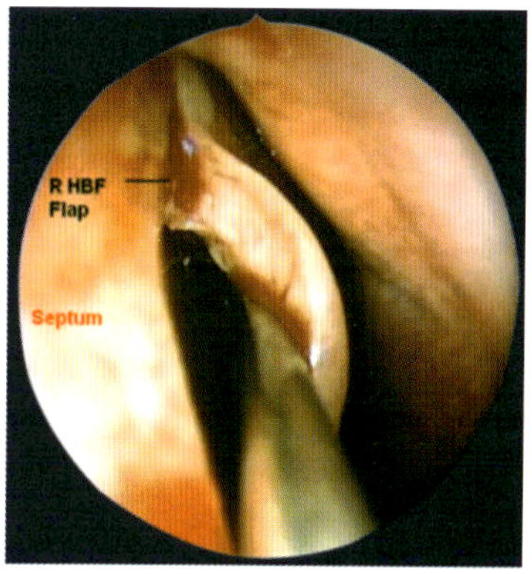

Fig. 22.13. Raising the HBF.

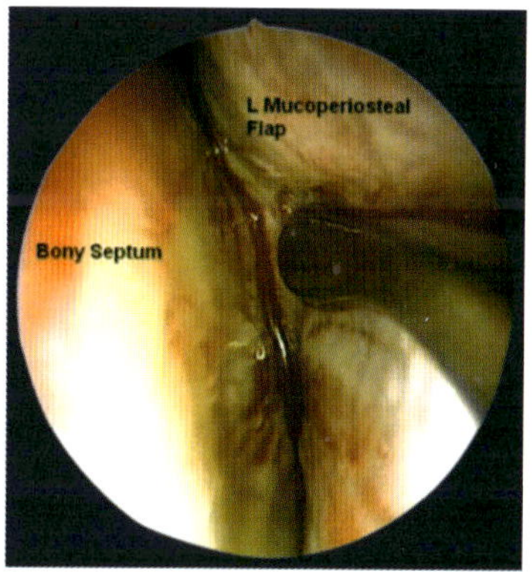

Fig. 22.14. Submucoperichondrial view of the HBF.

Locating the sphenoid sinus ostium

The perpendicular plate is dislocated from the septal cartilage and excised using a true-cut forceps until the sphenoid rostrum is exposed (Figs. 22.15, 22.16 and 22.17).

Using a monopolar diathermy the mucosa on the anterior sphenoid wall and rostrum is dissected laterally bilaterally to expose the anterior wall of the sphenoid (Fig. 22.18).

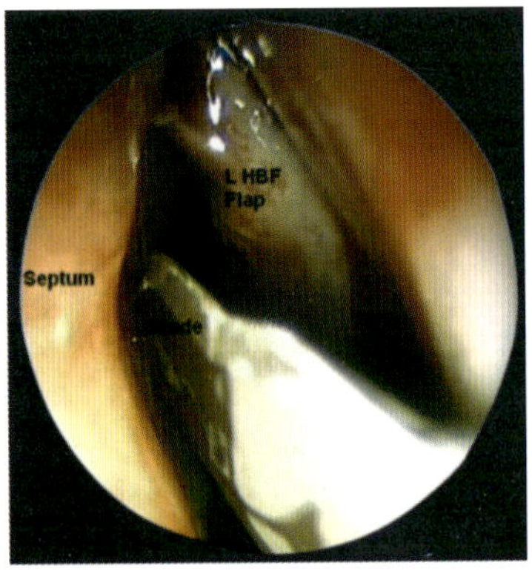

Fig. 22.15. Incising septal chondrium.

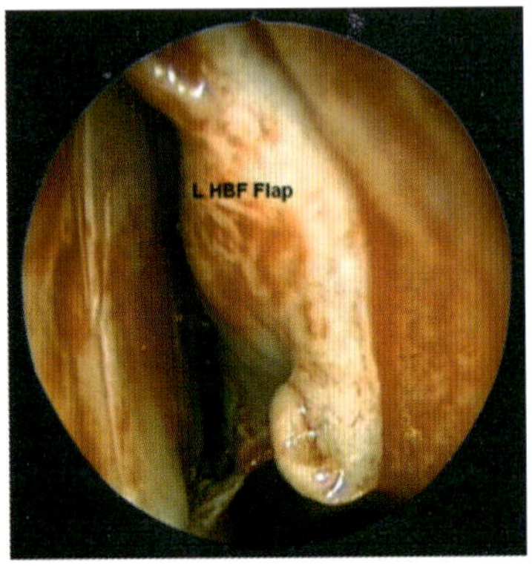

Fig. 22.16. Chondrotomy incision marks.

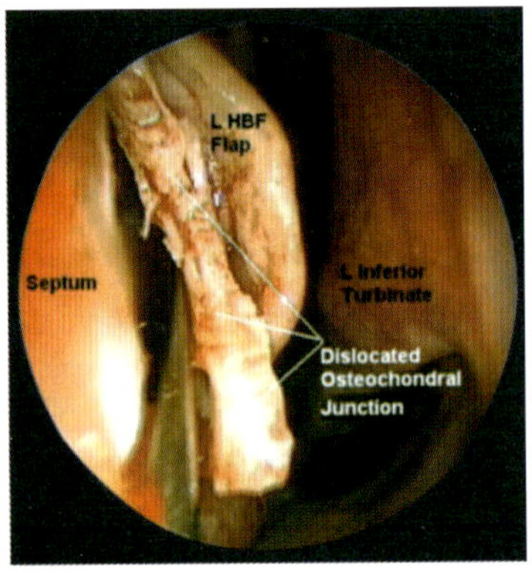

Fig. 22.17. Dislocated septal osteochondral junction.

The sphenoid sinus ostium may be seen bilaterally on the superior half of the diamond-shaped anterior wall of the sphenoid (Fig. 22.19).

TIPS: The procedure above can be carried out via cold instruments or a microdebrider depending on what is available in the center and surgeon's comfort level. In a four-handed technique, the posterior septum and their associated bilateral mucoperiosteums to facilitate use of endoscope on

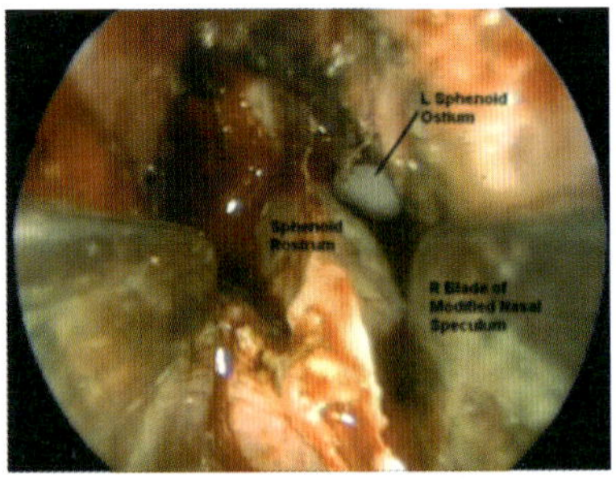

Fig. 22.18. Transseptal view of anterior wall of sphenoid sinus.

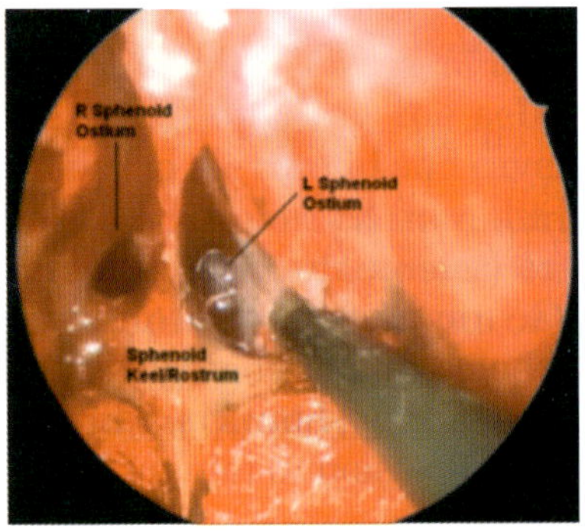

Fig. 22.19. Diathermy dissecting the mucosa of the sphenoid ostia.

one side and the use of an additional two instruments via the opposite nostril.

Sphenoid stage

Widening the sphenoidotomy

Prior to proceeding to this stage, the position of the sphenoid sinus is confirmed with an image intensifier (II) (Fig. 22.20).

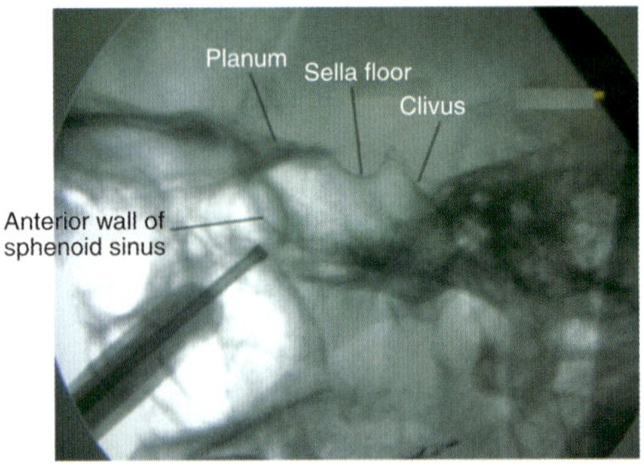

Fig. 22.20. Intraoperative II view of the position of anterior wall of sphenoid sinus.

A 2 mm downward Kerrison punch is used to widen the ostium inferiorly bilaterally whilst aiming towards the midline. Similarly the superior portion

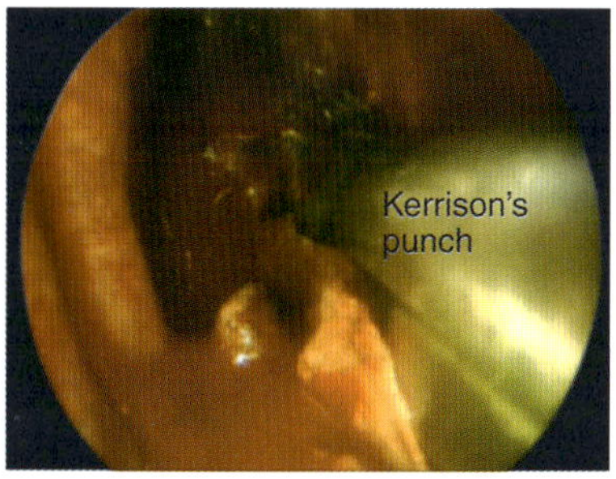

Fig. 22.21. Sphenoid ostium widening with Kerrison's punch.

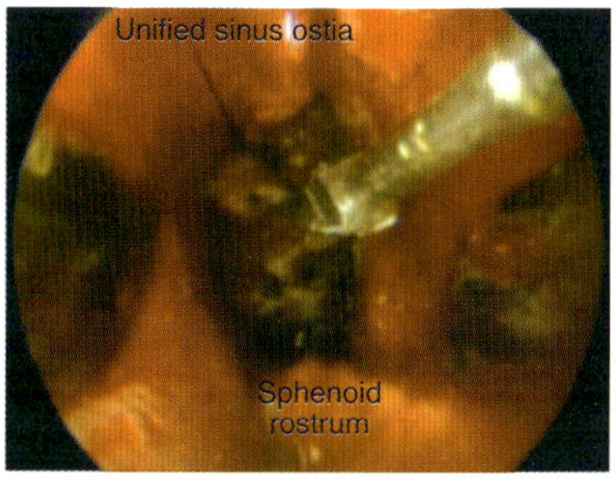

Fig. 22.22. Drilling the sphenoid rostrum.

of the sphenoid wall is punched out to delineate the margin of the planum sphenoidale (Fig. 22.21).

The rostrum of the sphenoid is drilled out to expose the clivus thus marking the inferior limit (Fig. 22.22).

Adequate sphenoidotomy includes visualization of the roof of the tuberculum sella superiorly, the bulge of the optic nerves at 10.00 and 2.00 O'clock, the area of the cavernous sinuses at 3.00 and 9.00 O'clock, the carotid bulge at 5.00 and 7.00 O'clock and the clivus interiorly (Fig. 22.23).

TIP: Cauterising the anteroinferior mucosa overlying the sphenoid wall will reduce bleeding.

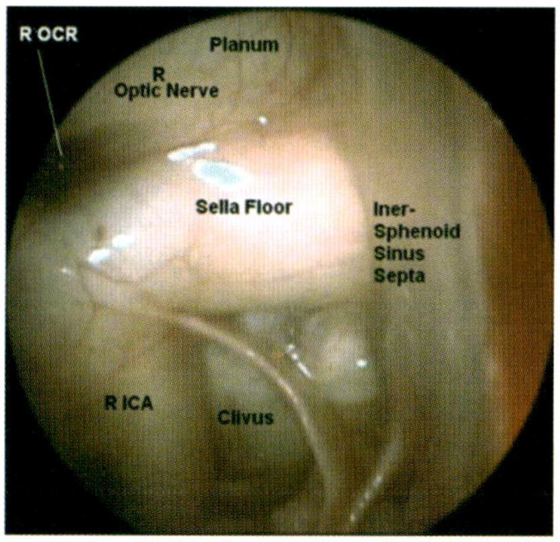

Fig. 22.23. Intrasphenoidal view of contents.

Sellar stage

There are two options to proceed from this stage:

- The four hand technique where the ENT surgeon holds the endoscope and suction through one nostril and the neurosurgeon operates through the other nostril with two free hands.
- The other technique is the introduction of a modified Killian nasal speculum (Uni Port) into the nostril and held open and positioned in place by a Fukushima retractor system (Fig. 22.24).

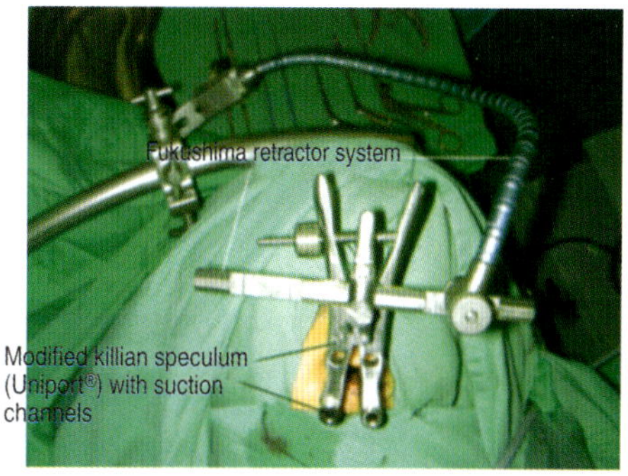

Fig. 22.24. Placement of uniport with Fukushima retractor system.

The decision as to the choice of procedure depends on what the neurosurgeon is comfortable with; it cannot be over emphasized to be familiar with different approaches so as to be able to work with different neurosurgeons.

The other option is to excise the contralateral posterior septal mucoperichondrium + osteum if a four-handed technique is used depending on the comfort level of surgeon.

Exposing the anterior sellar wall

Any intersphenoid septum obstructing the view of the sella is carefully removed using a true-cut forceps in order to expose the anterior wall of the sella noting that occasionally the septum may terminate on the carotid artery (in 32–40% of patients) (Fig. 22.25).

The mucosa over the sella is diathermied in the midline using a mono-polar and carefully dissected bilaterally to expose the sella bone.

HINT: Only remove septa obstructing access to the anterior sella wall. Diathermy of the mucosa overlying the sella will abort any unnecessary bleeding from the mucosa and reduce morbidity to the procedure.

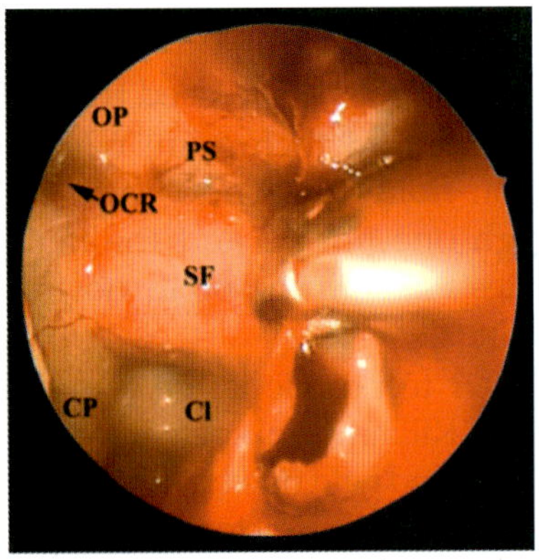

Fig. 22.25. Excising the intersphenoidal sinus septa.

Opening the anterior wall of the sella

The position of the sella may be confirmed using the C-arm in case of microadenomas or if any doubt exists about the position of the sella (Fig. 22.26).

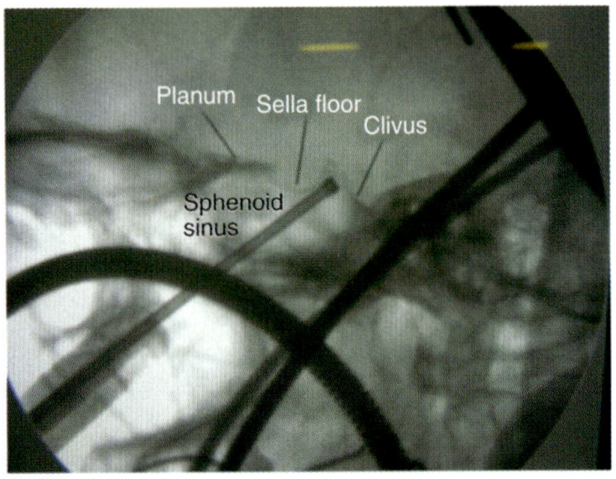

Fig. 22.26. View of the position of sella.

The sella can be opened in many different ways:

1. If the tumour has eroded or thinned out part of the bone then it is quite easy to use the smallest Kerrison punch to remove loose bone to expose the dura.
2. If the bone is firm and does not break easily with the pressure of the punch, then an osteotome may be used to make a window in the sella which can then be enlarged using punches (Fig. 22.27).
3. The third option is to use a drill to thin the bone prior to opening it.

The amount of exposure depends on the size of the sella and tumour extension and is as follows:

Superiorly the tuberculum sella, inferiorly the floor and the cavernous sinus and carotid artery laterally. In cases of microadenoma, a small opening localized to the tumour is enough.

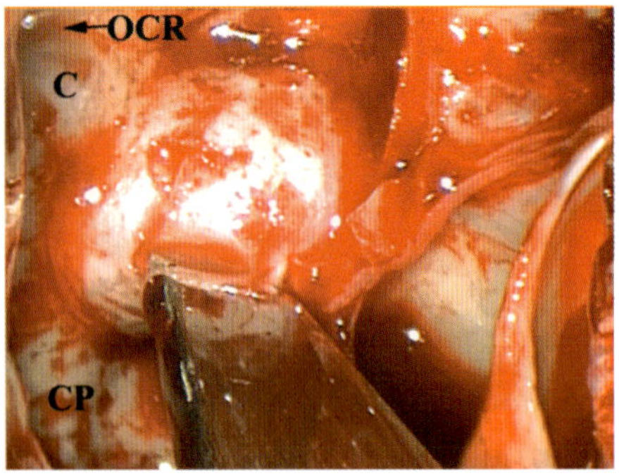

Fig. 22.27. Osteotomy of the sella.

HINT: It is extremely important to be aware of the midline when opening the sella to avoid accidental injury to the carotid and cavernous area. The midline can be confirmed from the base of the sphenoid inferiorly (rostrum-vomer) or remaining anterior sphenoid wall-septum attachment superiorly. It is also possible to stay between the optic nerves and the carotid bulges. It is best to start with opening or widening sellas which are eroded with tumour (or) have very thin bone prior to using an osteotome or burrs as one gains confidence.

Incising the dura

The dura is diathermied with a bipolar in the midline and an incision using a retractable blade in a cruciate fashion is made (Fig. 22.28).

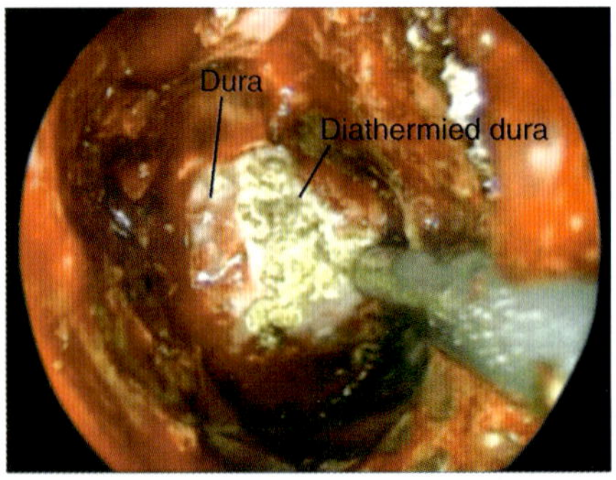

Fig. 22.28. Diathermy of dura.

Tumour removal

As soon as the dura is incised the tumour will protrude forward under pressure, a Nicola Forceps is used to collect specimen for frozen biopsy (Fig. 22.29).

The remaining tumour is removed using various size ring curettes in an organized fashion, starting infero-laterally and gradually superiorly (Fig. 22.30).

The object of the procedure is to visualize the complete descent of the diaphragma sella thus confirming complete tumour removal (Fig. 22.31).

22

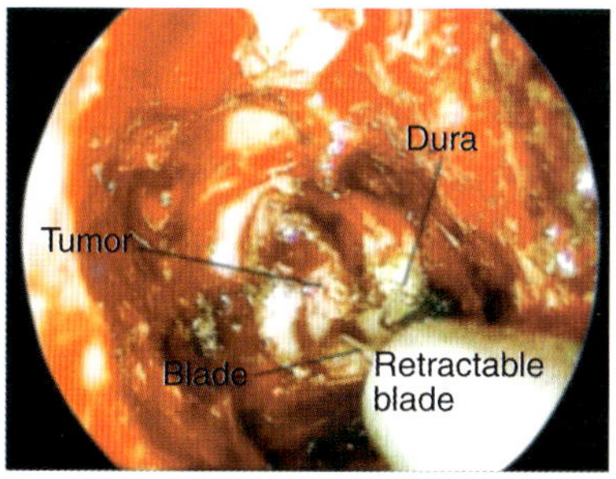

Fig. 22.29. Incision of the dura.

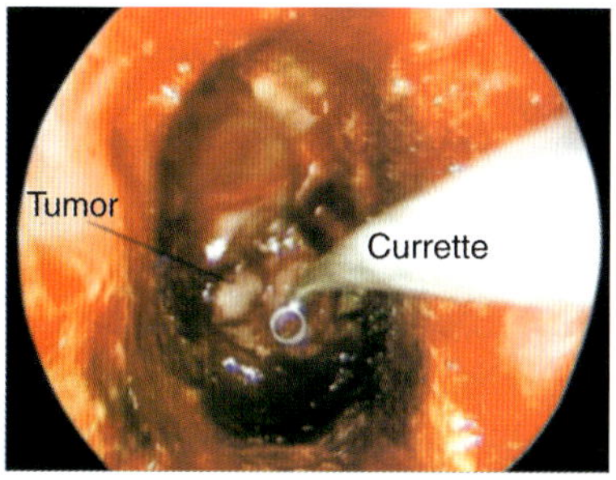

Fig. 22.30. Tumour removal with ring currette.

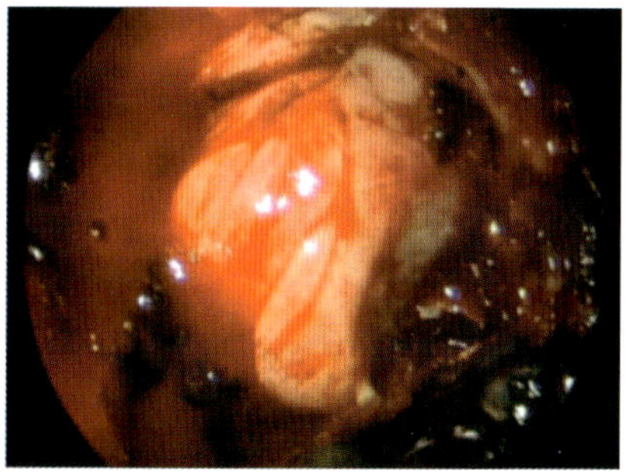

Fig. 22.31. Descent of diaphragma sella.

30 or 45 degree endoscopes can be used to confirm the same.

HINT: It is important to be extremely gentle while using the curette to avoid accidental CSF leaks or injury to the cavernous sinus and carotid artery. It is also advisable to restrict the use of forceps to hold and pull tumour in the sella. It is important to use the suction to remove blood and tumour superficially and not deep inside the sella.

Reconstruction/closure of sella

Post removal of tumour, the sella is plastered with 1 cm × 1 cm surgicel in a single layer followed by a layer of 1 cm × 1 cm gelfoam.

In cases of large empty sella, the diaphragma sella is supported with fat (Fig. 22.32).

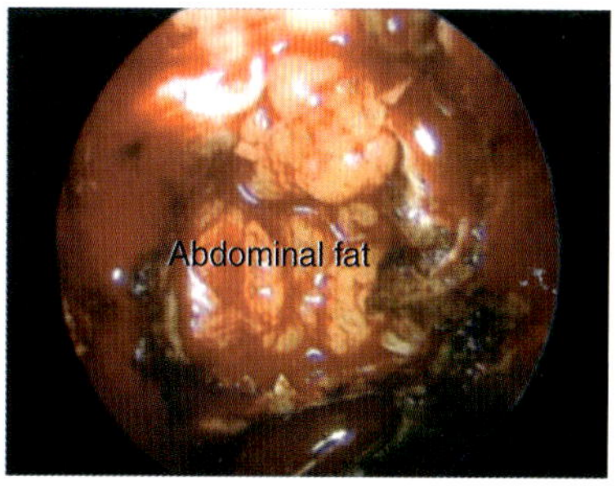

Fig. 22.32. Abdominal fat in sella.

In cases with intraoperative CSF leaks, the leak is repaired endoscopically and the sella is packed with fat and fibrin glue is poured over the edges of the sella wall (Fig. 22.33), followed by gelfoam or the Vascular Pedicle Nasoseptal Flap depending on the size of the defect.

The sphenoid is left unpacked.

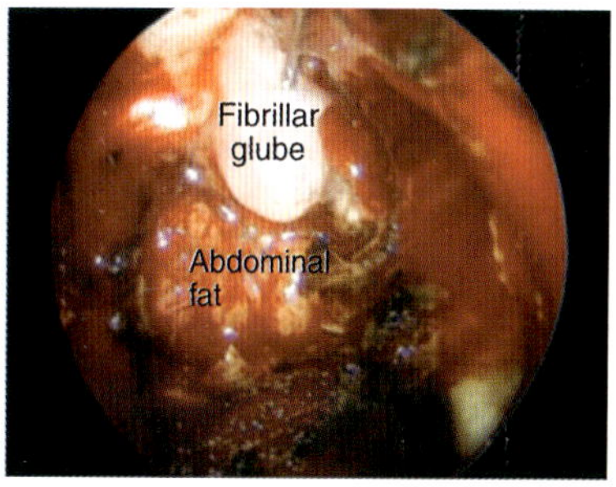

Fig. 22.33. "Glue" poured over the edges of sella and abdominal fat.

Completion of surgery

- Meticulous attention is paid to any bleeding sites and the same arrested.
- The middle turbinate is medialised and secured into position via placement of a gelfoam into the middle meatus.
- The nasal septum is relocated.
- If the Vascular Pedicle Nasoseptal Flap has not been used, it is repositioned against the opposing mucoperichondrium and the edges supported with surgicel.
- Nasal packing is generally not used unless oozing is anticipated.

ADVICE

This procedure has a steep learning curve and the quicker the learning surgeon masters the eye hand technique the easier the road to mastery and confidence.

Albeit, it is best that the apprentice surgeon finds a mentor who will guide him/her along this journey of learning.

MEDICOLEGAL PITFALLS

- Pituitary apoplexy is a potentially life-threatening condition and should be considered in patients presenting with sudden collapse, particularly patients known to have a pituitary tumour.
- Acute sterile meningitis has been reported as a primary manifestation of pituitary apoplexy and should be considered in patients with a pituitary adenoma who present with features of meningitis.

SUGGESTED READINGS

1. Jho HD, Carrau RL. Endoscopic endonasal transsphenoidal surgery: experience with 50 patients. *J Neurosurg*, 1997; 87: 4451–3.
2. http://neurosurgery.ucla.edu/body.cfm?id=699
3. http://www.ncbi.nlm.nih.gov/bookshelf/br.fcgi?book=endocrin"=A1257
4. emedicine.medscape.com/article/343207
5. Kachhara R, Menon G, Bhattacharya RN, et al. False aneurysm of cavernous carotid artery and carotid cavernous fistula: complications following transsphenoidal surgery. *Neurol India*, 2003; 51(1): 81–3.
6. Sethi DS, Pillay PK. Endoscopic surgery for pituitary tumours. *Operative Technique in Otolaryngol Head Neck Surg*, 1996; 7(3): 264–8.
7. Har-El G. Endoscopic transnasal transsphenoidal pituitary surgery – comparison with the traditional sublabial transseptal approach. *Otolaryngol Clin North Am*, 2005; 38(4): 723–35.
8. Shah N, Navnit M, Deopujarl CE, Mukerji SS. Pituitary surgery – A beginner's guide. *Indian J Otolaryngol Head Neck Surg*, 2004; 56: 71–8.
9. Indrajit IK, Chidambaranathan N, Sundar K, Ahmed I. Value of Dynamic MRI Imaging in Pituitary Adenomas. *Ind J Radiol Imag*, 2001; 11 (4): 185–90.
10. Kennedy DW, Cohn ES, Papel ID, et al. Transsphenoidal approach to sella: the Jones Hopkins experience. *Laryngoscope*, 1984; 94: 1066–74.
11. Kelley RT, Smith JL, Rodzewicz GM. Transnasal endoscopic surgery of pituitary: modifications and results over 10 years. *Laryngoscope*, 2006; 116(9): 1573–6.
12. Koren I, Hadar T, Rappaport ZH, Yaniv E. Endoscopic transnasal transsphenoidal microsurgery versus the sublabial approach for the treatment of pituitary tumours: endonasal complication. *Laryngoscope*, 1999; 109(11): 1838–40.
13. Jho HD. Endoscopic pituitary surgery. *Pituitary*, 1999; 2: 139–54.
14. Jho HD, Alfieri A. Endoscopic Endonasal Pituitary Surgery: Evolution of surgical technique and equipment in 150 operations. *Minim Invas Neurosurg*, 2001; 44: 1–12.
15. Sethi DS, Stanley RE, Pillay PK. Endoscopic anatomy of the sphenoid sinus and sella turcica. *J Laryngol Otol*, 1995; 109: 951–5.
16. Cappabianca P, Cavallo LM, de Divitis O, Solari D, Esposito F, Colao A. Endoscopic pituitary surgery. *Pituitary*, 2008; 11(8): 385–90.
17. De Divitiis E, Cappabianca P, Cavallo LM. Endoscopic transsphenoidal approach. Adaptability of the procedure to different sellar lesions. *Neurosurgery*, 2002; 51(3): 699–707.
18. Nasseri SS, Kasperbauer JL, Strome SE, McCaffery TV, Atkinson JL, Meyer FB. Endoscopic transnasal surgery: report on 180 cases. *Am J Rhinol*, 2001; 15(4): 281–7.
19. Uren B, Vrodos N, Wormald PJ. Fully endoscopic transsphenoidal resection of pituitary tumours: technique and results. *Am J Rhinol*, 2007; 21(4): 510–14.

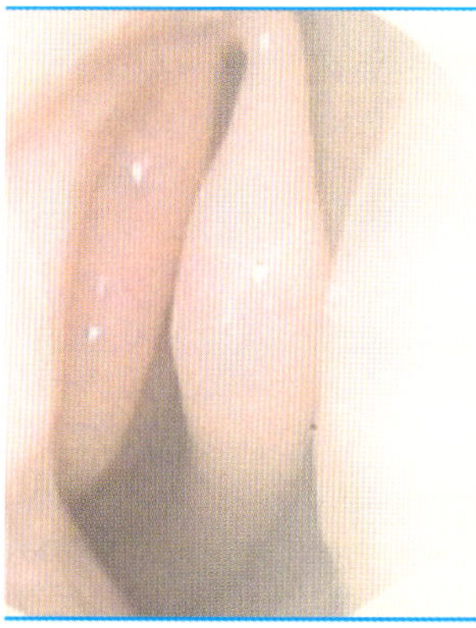

CHAPTER 23

Optic Nerve Decompression

Ashok K. Gupta, Shruti

ANATOMY

The optic nerve is the second of twelve paired cranial nerves but is considered to be part of the central nervous system as it is derived from an outpouching of the diencephalon during embryonic development. Consequently, the fibers are covered with myelin produced by oligodendrocytes rather than the Schwann cells of the peripheral nervous system. Similarly, the optic nerve is ensheathed in all three meningeal layers (dura, arachnoid, and pia mater) rather than the epineurium, perineurium, and endoneurium found in peripheral nerves. The outer sheath of dura mater and an inner sheath from the arachnoid are attached to the sclera around the area where the nerve fibres pierce the choroid and sclera of the bulb. The fibre tracks of the mammalian central nervous system (as opposed to the peripheral nervous system) are incapable of regeneration and hence optic nerve damage produces irreversible blindness.

The optic nerve carries about 1.2 million axons derived from retinal ganglion cells to the optic chiasma spanning a length of approximately 50 mm. It can be divided into 4 anatomical segments. The intraocular segment is about 1 mm long and is supplied by choroidal and ciliary vessels. The intraorbital segment is 23–30 mm long and the blood supply is via dural and central branches of ophthalmic artery. The intracanalicular segment is approximately 8 mm long and is fixed within the bony canal. The blood supply is from the pial branches of the internal carotid artery. The intracranial segment varies from 3–16 mm and extends from the proximal origin of optic canal to the optic chiasma (Table 23.1).

Table 23.1

Division of optic nerve	*Length*	*Blood supply*	*Mode of injury*
1. Intraocular	1 mm	Ciliary/ choroidal artery	Avulsion injury
2. Intraorbital	23–30 mm	Ophthalmic artery	Compression injury
3. Intra-canalicular	8 mm	Internal carotid artery	Compression injury
4. Intracranial	15 mm	Intracranial artery	Tears/ vascular disruption

The average length of optic canal is 9.1 mm (range 5.5–11.5 mm). The canal runs in an anterior, inferior declination to the Frankfort plane at an average angle of 15.5 degree. The canal also courses in an anterolateral angle to the midline at an average of 39.1 degrees (33–44.4 degree). Tao (1999) based on computer-aided three-dimensional reconstruction of optic canal divided it into anterior (orbital), middle and posterior (cranial part). The cranial opening of optic canal is elliptical in shape and the horizontal width is consistently greater than its height. The orbital opening is also elliptical, with its widest diameter oriented vertically. The subarachnoid space transverse area in the optic canal of the cranial opening, middle and orbital part is $4.45 + 0.46\ mm^2$, $2.68 + 0.54\ mm^2$ and $1.23 + 34\ mm^2$ respectively.

The optic canal consists of optic nerve and ophthalmic artery along with the meningeal extension. The dural sheath wraps the optic nerve, subarachnoid space and ophthalmic artery. The subarachnoid space considered to be compensatory space for distension incurred by the hemorrhage, optic nerve edema or hematoma is $21.16 + 4.13\ mm^2$ and this space gradually deceases from posterior to anterior.

In the optic canal, ophthalmic artery is located mainly on the inferomedial side and is rotated to the inferolateral side at the orbital end. However, 15.5% of patients may have the ophthalmic artery entering on the medial side of the orbital aperture of the optic canal and is susceptible to injury by medial approach.

Because of limited compensatory space and limited transverse area in the middle and anterior parts of optic canal, these parts are critical in optic nerve decompression.

The optic nerve is composed of retinal ganglion cell axons and support cells. It leaves the orbit (eye) via the optic canal, running posteromedially towards the optic chiasm where there is a partial decussation (crossing) of fibres from the temporal visual fields of both eyes. Most of the axons of the optic nerve terminate in the lateral geniculate nucleus from where information is relayed to the visual cortex in the occipital lobe of the brain.

The optic canal shares its medial wall with the ethmoid and sphenoid sinuses. The posterior most ethmoidal air cell may reach the optic canal and therefore share a portion of its posterolateral wall with the optic canal. In 12–25% of specimens ethmoid air cells pneumatize the sphenoid bone and are known as Onodi cells. These cells abut or may even surround the optic nerve, thereby placing this nerve at risk when surgical excisions of these cells is performed. The CT anatomic study by Delano et al. (1996) described four discrete classifications of the various relationships that exist between the optic nerve and the posterior paranasal sinuses. Type I optic nerves include those which course immediately adjacent to the sphenoid sinus, without indentation of the wall or contact with the posterior ethmoid air cell (76%). Type II nerves course adjacent to the sphenoid sinus causing indentation of the sinus wall, without contact with the posterior ethmoid air cells (15%). Type III nerve courses through the sphenoid sinus with at least 50% of the nerve surrounded by air (6%). Type IV nerve courses immediately adjacent to the sphenoid sinus and posterior ethmoid sinus (3%). The incidence of bony dehiscence over optic nerve has been found to be around 4% whereas the incidence of bony dehiscence around the presellar and juxtasellar portions of the internal carotid artery ranges from 12–22%.

Traumatic optic nerve injury is a relatively uncommon but disabling cause of permanent visual loss, commonly seen in closed head injuries. Injury to the optic nerve can occur either as a result of direct trauma, in the form of a penetrating injury to the nerve, or due to avulsion, laceration or fracture of the optic nerve canal leading to impingement of the bony fragments on the nerve.

Indirect injury is usually seen in cases of blunt head trauma which leads to hematoma formation within the optic nerve sheath or nerve edema, thus increasing the intracanalicular pressure and blocking the direct axoplasmic transport. Optimal management of cases is also far less defined ranging from corticosteroids, surgical decompression of the optic canal, to observation alone. It is of utmost importance to identify the predictors of a successful outcome correlating clinical presentation with neuroophthalmological examination and radiological evidence and to be able to differentiate which patients would benefit from conservative management and which would require an early surgical intervention.

Traumatic injury to the optic nerve can occur anywhere along the course of the nerve from intraorbital to intracranial region. It can manifest as decreased visual acuity, loss of colour vision, or visual field defects. The visual loss may be temporary or permanent and may range from no perception of light to finger counting at a few metres. Clinical and radiological pointers can help a surgeon to prognosticate visual outcome and decide the course of management in the form of medical or surgical intervention.

Approximately 2% of all closed head injuries affect the optic nerve with intracanalicular segment being most common, followed by intracranial segment. The average length of the optic canal is 9.22 mm (range: 5.5–11.5 mm) and is about 6.5 mm in diameter. The medial wall of the canal is the thinnest and averages about 0.21 mm behind the optic ring. The optic canal transmits the optic nerve (diameter: 3–4 mm), within its dural sheath along with the ophthalmic artery and fibres of sympathetic choroids plexus. The compensatory space, i.e., the volume of intracanalicular subarachnoid space available for distension incurred either by haemorrhage, optic nerve edema or hematoma is only 21.16 + 4.31 mm^3 and this space gradually decreases from posterior to anterior. Thus, even slight amount of edema or blood can cause optic nerve compression and disrupt the axoplasmic flow. The rationale of using high dose corticosteroids is based on studies which suggest that steroids have a neuroprotective effect by inhibition of oxygen-free radical-induced lipid peroxidation, support of aerobic energy metabolism, prevention of post-traumatic ischemia, reversal of intracellular calcium accumulation and inhibition of neurofilament degradation and membrane lipid hydrolysis.

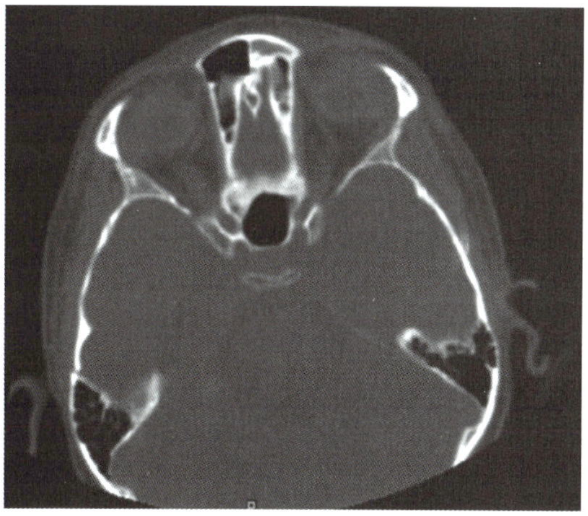

Fig. 23.1. NCCT of nose and PNS showing the compression of optic nerve.

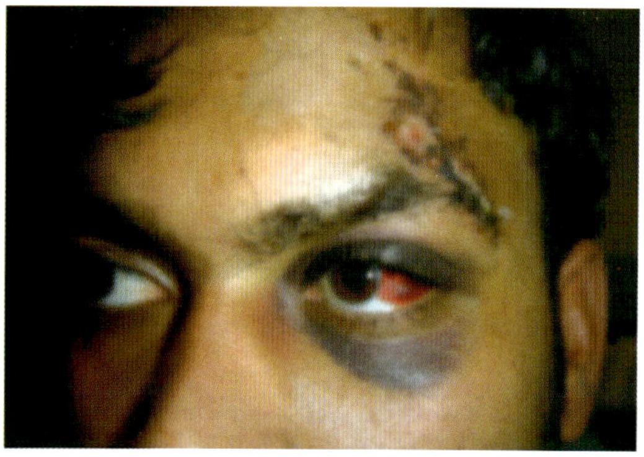

Fig. 23.2. Patient's photograph showing injury on forehead with sub-conjunctival haemorrhage and dilated pupils.

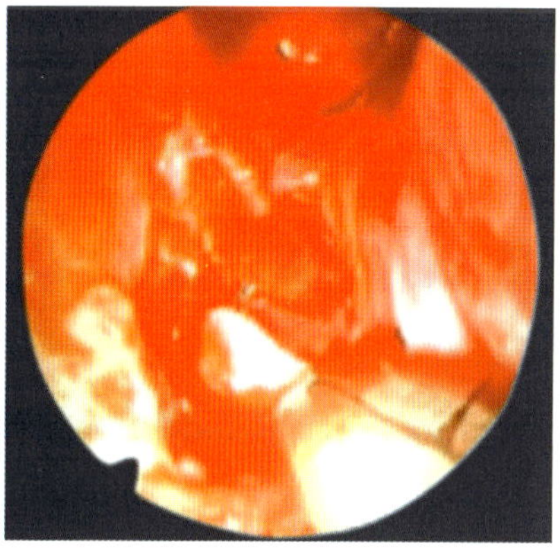

Fig. 23.3. Operative photograph showing fractured optic canal.

DIAGNOSIS

The characteristic clinical presentation of indirect optic nerve injury includes history of blunt trauma to forehead, diminished or absent vision, and proof of relative afferent papillary defect (RAPD) with the swinging – Flashlight test. Loss of colour perception or colour desaturation is another important clinical symptom indicating optic nerve compression.

Concussion and epistaxis occur in 75% patients and loss of consciousness in 60% patients. In cooperative patients Snellen's acuity chart or Rosenbaum near vision can document acuity, however, photophobia and lid closure indicates light perception in the uncooperative patients. Optic disc pallor or papilledema may be present, although the disc is usually normal in the early post-traumatic period.

Diagnosis and ancillary testing

The diagnosis of optic nerve injury is usually established on the basis of clinical assessment, but imaging studies are essential for complete understanding of the nature of the canalicular injury and the surrounding structures. High resolution computed tomography of the orbit is the diagnostic procedure of choice for patients who have suspected traumatic optic neuropathy. Preoperative planning for endoscopic optic nerve decompression (ENDOND) requires high resolution computed tomography (CT) of orbit to provide detailed maps on anatomical variants and also to know the extent of injury in traumatic optic neuropathy.

High resolution CT scan allows identification of canalicular pericanalicular fractures and extent of

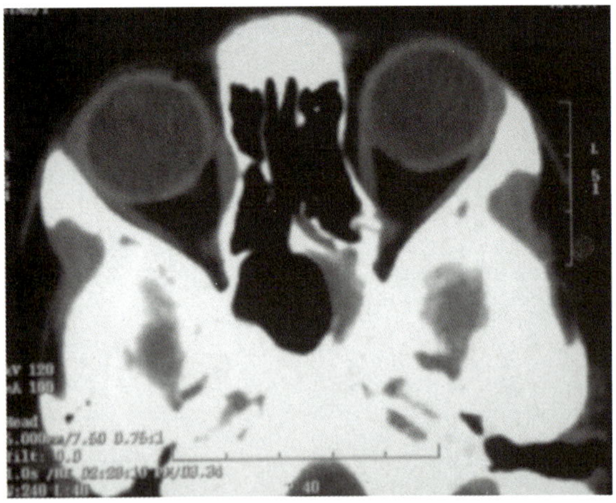

Fig. 23.4. CCT nose and PNS showing fractured optic canal.

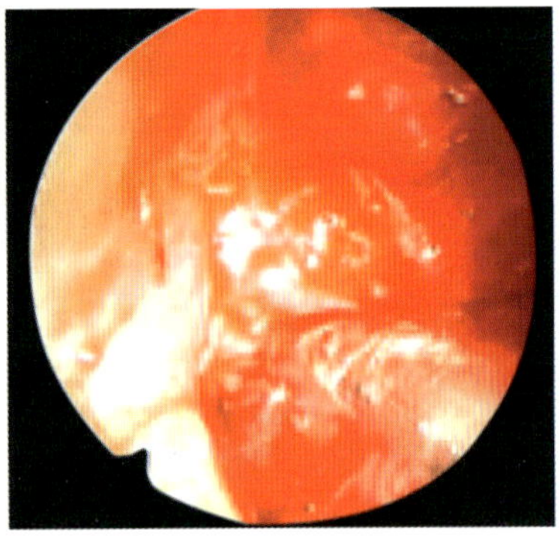

Fig. 23.5. Decompression posterior one-third of orbit and optic nerve.

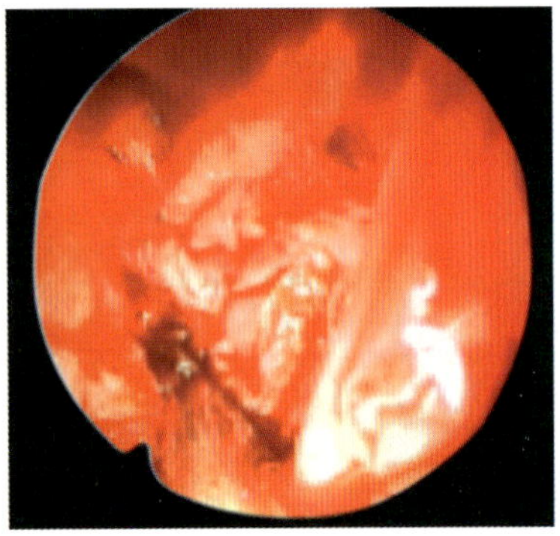

Fig. 23.6. Fractured bone chip in the optic canal.

injury. Skull fracture is documented in approximately 60% of patients, most of whom sustain only a closed injury. The incidence of optic canal fracture has varied significantly from series to series, yet the importance is unclear. The incidence of concomitant feature of the optic canal in traumatic blindness has been variably reported from 6%–92%. Hughes reported canal fracture in 5 (6%) of 90 patients studies, Edmund reported in 5 (23%) in 22 patients and Fukado in 460 (92%) of 500 patients. These data support that fracture is not necessary for nerve damage to occur but is merely an indication to the excessive energy delivered to the region of the optic canal and subsequently transmitted to the optic nerve.

Visual evoked potential (VEP) performed to assess the integrity of anterior visual pathways. It may be helpful in the assessment of optic nerve function in an unresponsive patient suspected of having a traumatic optic neuropathy. This is especially true in bilateral cases where an RAPD may not be present. Diagnostic criteria are based on latency and amplitude of VEP. Sometimes its shape is also taken into account. Patients with normal VEP show good recovery whereas patients with repeatedly absent VEP had shown poor recovery.

TREATMENT

The treatment of traumatic optic neuropathy is controversial. Available studies have documented spontaneous improvement of vision in 20–40% of untreated cases. Various treatment modalities, including steroids, surgery or both have been used with variable results. However, recent data have demonstrated that the recovery of vision is significantly better when treated with corticosteroids, optic nerve decompression, or both, compared with observation alone. Studies have shown that early use of steroids can reduce the edema and tissue damage resulting from ischemic and traumatic injuries. Steroid (methyl prednisolone) is given in a loading dose of 3 mg/kg body weight for 3 days followed by 1 mg/kg for one week. When treatment is initiated within 7 days of injury, the outcome is much better. A detailed ENT and ophthalmological examination should be done for all patients pre- and postoperatively. Subconjunctival haemorrage, black eye, restriction of extraocular movements, pupillary reflexes and relative afferent pupillary defect should be noted. Besides this, visual evoked potentials, field of vision and fundoscopic examination is very essential to compare postoperative benefit from surgery.

Of the various approaches available for optic nerve decompression, including transcranial, transantral, transethmoidal and intranasal microscopic, most ENT surgeons now prefer the transnasal endoscopic approach. The endoscopic approach offers various advantages including decreased morbidity, preservation of olfaction, no risk of scarring or injury to developing teeth in children and a shorter recovery time. More importantly, it provides a clear, detailed and an unobstructed view of the orbital apex and is the most familiar approach for the endoscopic surgeon. In case of a deviated nasal septum obstructing the view of the surgeon an endoscopic septoplasty can be performed in the same sitting. However, this approach also has some disadvantages and limitations. An iatrogenic injury to the nerve fascicle can occur during any surgical procedure that involves the orbital apex. Endoscopic optic nerve decompression carries additional risks and therefore requires the skills of an experienced endoscopic surgeon. Conchal pneumatization is a relative contraindications to this procedure.

Surgical Decompression (Endoscopic Optic Nerve Decompression)

Aurbach et al. (1991) described endonasal, endoscopic-microscopic decompression of the optic nerve in surgical anatomical specimens. Kountakis (1993) first used this approach to optic nerve decompression in a case of optic neuritis secondary to sphenoethmoiditis and total blindess. Since then various authors have used endoscopic approach for optic nerve decompression commonly for traumatic blindness (Table 23.2).

Table 23.2. Literature on endoscopic optic nerve decompression for TON

First Author (year)	*Endon (No.)*	*Improvement (%)*	*Major complication*
1. Lieb (1996)	13	53	Nil
2. Kountakis (1997)	8	75	Nil
3. Luxenberger (1998)	15	46	Nil
4. Shi (1998)	14	64	Nil
5. Kountakis (2000)	17	82	Nil
6. DeGanseman (2000)	8	50	Nil
7. Jiang (2001)	17	52	Worsening (11%)

There is a controversy regarding slitting of the optic nerve sheath during optic nerve decompression. Slitting the sheath increases the risk of cerebrospinal fluid leakage, injury to ophthalmic artery and secondary injury to the optic nerve. Moreover, literature mentions fenestration of the optic nerve sheath causes no significant improvement in vision. The optic nerve sheath should not be incised in any of the cases, except those which showed evidence of an intrasheath hematoma.

Endoscopic optic nerve decompression is safe and effective without any significant morbidity in expert hands. Early intervention gives a better prognosis in cases presenting with traumatic optic nerve injury. Patients who present with complete loss of vision at initial presentation have a poor prognosis for visual outcome when compared to those who have some residual vision at initial presentation. Patients in whom visual evoked potential shows an absent response tend to have a poorer prognosis than those with an "abnormal response". Intraoperative evidence of laceration or transection of the nerve heralds a poorer prognosis.

Optic nerve decompression relieves intracanalicular pressure and any angular strangulation. Steroid being used as initial treatment of choice with varying duration (12 to 48 hours) before surgery. We have given high dose methylprednisolone for 72 hours as there is evidence of improvement with steroid alone 20–100%.

Total blindness, time lapse of treatment and CT evidence of canalicular and pericanalicular fracture were found to be poor prognostic factor. We advise combine therapy with steroid and ENDOND in patients presented before 7 days of injury.

CONCLUSION

Opic nerve decompression is a rewarding procedure in expert hands more so if patient presents early and put on high doses of steroids preferably in first 72 hours. The results depend on time of presentation, residual eyesight at the time of presentation and associated injuries which may jeopardise early intervention.

SUGGESTED READING

1. Habal MB, Maniscalco JE, Lineaweaver WC et al. Microsurgical anatomy of the optic canal. Anatomical relations and exposure of the optic nerve. *Surgical Forum*, 1976; 27: 542–4.
2. Hai Tao, Zhizhong Ma, Pu Dai, Li Jiang. Computer Aided Three Dimensional Reconstruction and Measurement of Optic Canal and Intracanalicular Structure. *Laryngoscope*, 1999; 109: 1499–1501.
3. Luxenberger W, Stammberger H, Jebeles JA et al. Endoscopic optic nerve decompression: The Graz experience. *Laryngoscope*, 1998; 108: 873–82.

4. Delano MC, Fun FY, James Zinreich S. Relationship of the optic nerve tot he posterior paranasal sinuses. A CT anatomic study. *AJNR*, 1996; 17: 669–75
5. Sofferman RA, Burlington. Sphenoethmoid approach to the optic nerve. *Laryngoscope*, 1981; 91: 184–96.
6. Walsh and Hyodt. Clinical Neuro-ophthalmology. 5th edition.
7. Kountakis SE, Maillard AA, Richard Urso, Stiernerg CM. Endoscopic approach to traumatic visual loss. *Otolaryngol Head Neck Surg*, 1997; 116: 652–5.
8. Kountakis SE, Maillard AA, EI – Harazi SM et al. Endoscopic optic nerve decompression in traumatic blindness. *Otolaryngol Head Neck Surg*, 2000; 12: 34–7.
9. Scuderi AJ, H. Ric Harnsberger, Boyer RS. Pneumatization of paranasal sinuses: Normal features of importance tot he accurate interpretation of CT scan and MR images. *AJR*, 1993; 160: 1101–4.
10. Elwany S, Yacout YN, Tallat M, et al. Surgical anatomy of sphenoid sinus. *J Layrngol Otol*, 1983; 97: 227–41.
11. Seiff SR, Berger MS, Guyon J. Pitts LH. CT evaluation of optic canal in sudden traumatic blindness. *Am J Ophthalmol*, 1984; 98: 751–5.
12. Ramsay JH. Optic nerve injury in fracture of the canal. *Br J Ophthalmol*, 1979; 63: 607–10.
13. Cook MW, Levin LA, Joseph MP, Pinczower EF. Traumatic Optic Neuropathy. *Arch Otolaryngol Head Neck Surg*, 1996; 122: 389–92.
14. Unger JM, Orbital apex fractures. The contribution of Computed Tomography. *Radiology*, 1984; 150: 713–7.
15. Aurbach G. Reck R, Mihm B. Endonasal, Endoscopic microscopic control of the decompression of the optic nerve. An anatomic endoscopic presentation of the operation. *HNO*, 1991; 39: 302–6.
16. Lieb WE, Maurer J, Muller-Forell W, Mann W. Microsurgical endonasal decompression in traumatic and neoplastic optic nerve compression. *Ophthalmology*, 1996; 93: 194–8.
17. Shi J, Xu G, Li Y. Research of optic canal decompression by transnasal endoscopic approach. *Zhonghua Er Bi Yan Hou Ke Za Zhi*, 1998; 33: 225–7.
18. De Ganesman A, Lasudry J, Choufani G et al. Intranasal endoscopic surgery in traumatic optic neuropathy the Belgian experience. *Acta Otorhinolaryngol Belg*, 2000; 54: 175–7.
19. Jiang RS, Hsu CCY, Shen BH. Endoscopic optic nerve decompression for the treatment of traumatic optic neuropathy. *Rhinology*, 2001; 39: 71–4.
20. Warner JEA, Simmons Lessell. Traumatic optic neuropathy. *Int Ophthalmol Clin*, 1995; 35: 57–62.

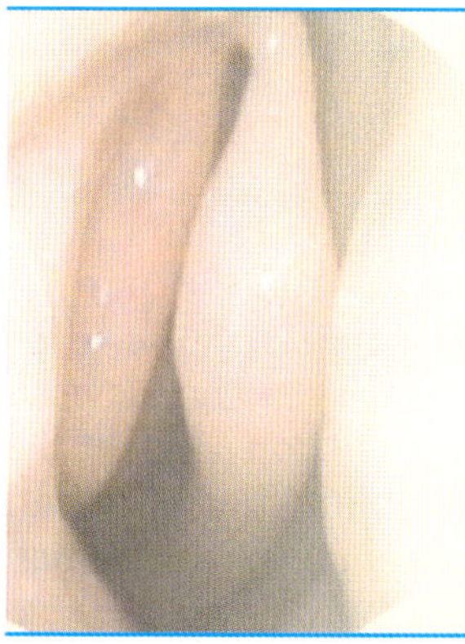

CHAPTER 24

Sinonasal Tumours

Surinder K. Singhal

Although exact incidence of sinonasal tumours is not known in Indian population but various authors quote the incidence as less than 1% of all the neoplasms. These tumours grow initially silently till they cause obstruction to the airflow and encroach upon the surrounding structures like orbit, cheek, palate and intracranial structures. Once the patient presents, the diagnosis is established by endoscopic examination, radiology and biopsy. The treatment is excision of the benign tumour. In malignant tumours, the excision may be combined with radiotherapy and/or chemotherapy. In the modern era with the available instrumentation particularly Hopkins telescope combined with three-dimensional navigation systems and modern imaging make the evaluation and management of these tumours through a transnasal approach feasible though technically challenging.

ANATOMIC CONSIDERATIONS

To understand the pattern of spread and behaviour of the sinonasal tumours, one must be thorough with the knowledge of anatomy of nose and paranasal sinuses. The exact and finer details of the anatomy of nose and paranasal sinuses are beyond the scope of this article. But anatomic relations which are important clinically as well as surgically are discussed.

Nasal cavity

The nasal cavity starts from the external nares anteriorly and continues posteriorly till the choanae, where it becomes continuous with the nasopharynx. The nasal septum is a midline structure which divides the nasal cavity into two halves. The roof is formed by the cribriform plate of the ethmoid bone from where the olfactory nerves enter the nose. The olfactory region corresponds to the upper third of the nasal cavity bounded by the superior turbinate, upper part of the septum and the cribriform plate. The floor of the nose is superior surface of hard palate and formed by palatine processes of maxillae and horizontal process of palatine bones. The lateral wall is formed by nasal bone, inferior turbinate bone, maxillary bone, lacrimal bone, ethmoid bone, palatine bones, and medial pterygoid plates of the sphenoid bone. The lateral wall has the three turbinates namely superior, middle and inferior. The inferior turbinate is the largest of three and extends full length of the nasal cavity. There are three meati corresponding to the turbinates. Sometimes a supreme turbinate may also be found. The inferior meatus has the opening of nasolacrimal duct in the anterior part. The middle meatus has the openings of frontal, anterior ethmoids and maxillary sinus. Posterior ethmoids open in superior meatus and sphenoid sinus opens into the sphenoethmoidal recess.

Maxillary sinuses

These are paired sinuses located anteriorly on either side of the nose just below the orbits. They are the largest of the sinuses and are contained within the body of maxilla. They have a pyramidal structure with the apex directed laterally extending into the zygomatic processes. The bases lie medially and form the lateral wall of the nose. The roof is formed by the orbital surface of maxilla and slopes downwards from medial to lateral. The medial wall is thin and made of medial wall of the maxilla, maxillary process of the inferior turbinate, perpendicular plate of the palatine bone, uncinate process of the ethmoid bone and descending process of lacrimal bone. The floor of the sinuses consists of alveolar and palatine processes of maxilla. The anterior and posterior walls of the sinuses are the corresponding surfaces of maxilla and are directly related to the facial surface of cheek and the infratemporal fossa respectively.

The size of the maxillary sinuses varies considerably and the average dimensions in an adult are 34 mm anteroposteriorly, 23 mm in width and 33 mm in height. The approximate volume is 14.75 ml but a large antrum may hold up to 30 ml.

Ethmoid sinuses

The ethmoid sinuses are a series of variably interconnected air cells within the ethmoid bone situated between the nasal cavity and orbit. On average, 10 such air cells compose each of the paired ethmoid sinuses. The ethmoid sinuses are the most variable of all the paranasal sinuses. Roof of the ethmoid sinus is formed by fovea ethmoidalis and frontal bone and is related superiorly to anterior cranial fossa. On its lateral aspect lies the lamina papyracea which is a thin papery bone separating the orbit from the ethmoids. It articulates with maxilla inferiorly, posteriorly with lesser wing of sphenoid bone and frontal bone superiorly. The latter suture line is an important landmark in external ethmoid surgery as it indicates the plane of roof of ethmoid air cells. Medially the sinus is bounded by the middle and superior turbinates. Middle turbinate is continuous superiorly with fovea ethmoidalis and lateral aspect of cribriform plate.

The ethmoid sinuses are divided by internal septae called basal lamellae. These septae traverse the sinuses from the medial aspect of the lamina papyracea to the middle and superior turbinate. They divide the ethmoid sinuses into anterior and posterior air cells and their ostea drains into middle meatus and superior meatus respectively. Bulla ethmoidalis is the group of cell which lies behind the hiatus semilunaris and forms a prominent bulge just lateral to the middle turbinate. They are sometimes called middle ethmoid cells and vary in number from one to four.

Frontal sinuses

The frontal sinuses are usually paired, but may show focal fusion. They are of unequal size and are divided by a thin inter sinus septum which is seldom in midline. Superiorly the sinus may extend between the inner and outer table of frontal bone. In fact, the frontal sinuses are remarkable for their size and shape variations. These are usually larger in man than in women. Occasionally they may be absent. The roof of the sinus has incomplete septae giving it a scalloped radiological appearance in the occipitofrontal projections. Anterior wall of the sinus is a diploic bone which is fairly thick but the posterior wall is thinner and formed by compact bone. The floor separates the sinus from the orbit and slopes downwards and medially to the nasofrontal duct which opens into the middle meatus.

Sphenoid sinuses

The sphenoid sinuses are unique among the paranasal sinuses because they do not arise as invaginations of the nasal cavity. Instead, they originate from embryonic rests in the nasal capsule. These are rudimentary at birth but begin to grow after the third year. They expand within the body of the sphenoid and occasionally into the greater and lesser wing of the sphenoid bone. Posterior extension may occur into the basilar part of the occipital bone. The two sinuses are separated by a bony septum which is rarely in midline. The overall size of the sinuses varies and its capacity may vary 0.5 to 30 ml with an average of 7.5 ml.

The sphenoid sinus lies immediately beneath and often anterior to the sella turcica, which encases the pituitary gland. Because of this the sinus forms the most accessible route to the pituitary gland. The gland lies in the sella turcica in the roof of the sinus posteriorly. On either side of this are the optic nerves and sometimes indent the roof anteriorly. Laterally, the sinus is directly related to the cavernous sinus, the internal carotid artery, and branches of trigeminal nerve. Inferiorly the floor of the sinus is related to the nasopharynx. Posterior wall is usually thick and separates the sinus from the pons and basilar artery. The sinus ostium is situated in the anterior wall and usually present above the floor. It opens into the sphenoethmoidal recess above the superior turbinate.

Lymphatic drainage

The lymphatic drainage of the sinuses and nasal cavity include levels I–III. In addition, the retropharyngeal lymph nodes can be site of drainage for the posterior ethmoids, posterior nasal cavity, and sphenoid sinuses.

EPIDEMIOLOGY

Because cancer of the paranasal sinuses is uncommon, it is more difficult than usual to identify promoting and initiating factors. Despite this, up to 44% are attributed to occupational exposures, including nickel, chromium, isopropyl oils, volatile hydrocarbons, and organic fibers that are found in the wood, shoe, and textile industries. In addition, human papillomavirus can be a cofactor, and in one series, human papillomavirus 6 or 12 was documented in 24% of inverting papillomas and 4% of squamous cell carcinomas. Specific associations found include squamous cell carcinoma in nickel workers and adenocarcinoma in workers exposed to hardwood dusts and leather tanning. Cigarette smoking and heavy alcohol consumption has long been known to increase the risk of head and neck malignancy. Their association with sinonasal neoplasms has been harder to establish. It has long been thought that there was no association with sinonasal cancer but Zhenget et al. have proposed an increased risk of nasal cancer, particularly in the maxillary sinus in smokers and alcoholics.

FREQUENCY

Sinonasal malignancies (SNM) are rare. They are more common in Asia and Africa than in the United States, where about 2000 Americans develop these malignancies each year. In parts of Asia, sinonasal malignancies (SNM) are the second most common head and neck cancer behind nasopharyngeal carcinoma. Men are affected 1.5 times more often than women, and 80% of these tumours occur in people aged 45–85 years.

Approximately 60–70% of sinonasal malignancies (SNM) occur in the maxillary sinus and 20–30% occurs in the nasal cavity itself. An estimated 10–15% occurs in the ethmoid air cells (sinuses), with the remaining minority of tumours found in the frontal and sphenoid sinuses.

ETIOLOGY

There have been extensive investigations to know the risk factors for sinonasal malignancies. The results of these investigations are complex and controversial. Exposure to nickel dust, mustard gas, thorotrast, isopropyl oil, chromium, or dichlorodiethyl sulfide is well established. The squamous cell carcinoma (SCCA) and adenocarcinoma in this area are associated with these products. These products are commonly found in the furniture-making industry, the leather industry, and the textile industry. Wood dust exposure, in particular, is found to increase the risk of SCCA 21 times and the risk of adenocarcinoma 874 times. Hence it is very important to elicit a careful social and employment history of these patients.

Human papillomavirus (HPV) and Epstein-Barr virus (EBV) infection may also be an early event in a multistep process of malignant transformation of inverting papilloma (IP). Viral infections and their relationship to malignancy is an interesting area that has not received sufficient investigation. Preliminary studies show that epidermal growth factor receptor (EGFR) and transforming growth factor-alpha (TGF-alpha) in elevated levels of expression may be associated with early events in inverting papilloma (IP) carcinogenesis.

PRESENTATION

The diagnosis of sinonasal malignancies is challenging. Not only are they rare, but they are difficult to distinguish from their benign counterparts. The similarities of benign and malignant disorders at initial presentation lead to a significant delay in the diagnosis of malignancy. It is estimated that a span of 6 to 8 months passes on average from the time of initial symptoms until diagnosis is established. Presentations such as cranial neuropathies and proptosis are uncommon at initial presentation and signify advanced disease. Patients presenting with sinonasal symptoms not responding to medical treatment should be viewed with high index of suspicion.

Signs and symptoms of maxillary sinus carcinoma fall into several major categories: oral, nasal, ocular, facial, and auditory. Oral presentations occur in 25–35% and include pain involving the maxillary dentition, trismus, palatal and alveolar ridge fullness, and frank erosion into the oral cavity. Nasal findings are seen in up to 50% of patients and include obstruction, discharge, stuffiness, congestion, epistaxis, and extension into the nasal cavity. Ocular findings occur in approximately 25% and arise from upward extension into the orbit, where unilateral tearing, diplopia, fullness of lids, pain, and exophthalmos are seen. Facial signs include infraorbital nerve hypoesthesia, cheek swelling, pain, and facial asymmetry. Auditory complaints include hearing loss secondary to serous otitis media due to nasopharyngeal extension.

DIAGNOSIS

The physical examination should be thorough. The sinonasal, ocular, and neurologic systems should be studied in detail. In particular, evidence of infraorbital nerve hypoesthesia, diplopia, proptosis, and loose dentition should be carefully evaluated. Nasal endoscopy should be performed after adequate topical anesthesia so that examination is not limited by patient's discomfort. Any suspicious lesions found on nasal endoscopy should be biopsied, however, Caldwell-Luc approach is not recommended because of the potential to seed the gingivobuccal sulcus and cheek skin with tumour. These days with the advent of endoscopy the biopsy can be done without breaching the anterolateral wall of maxilla.

Plain radiographs are rarely used currently and have been replaced by computed tomography (CT) scans. The CT scans should be done axial, coronal and sagittal plane. These scans give the 3-dimensional view of extent of the tumour and one can approach these tumours with the endoscope also.

The CT scan can detect the bony erosion due to the spread of tumour in areas like orbital walls, cribriform plate, fovea ethmoidalis, posterior wall of the maxillary sinus, pterygopalatine fossa, the sphenoid sinus, and the posterior table of the frontal sinus. The accuracy of CT in determining tumour spread to these areas is in the order of 85%. One should be careful in interpreting the bony destruction in areas having very thin bones like lamina papyracea. The partial volume averaging in these areas can sometimes be misleading. Despite the significant amount of information, CT has certain limitations also. It is difficult to differentiate secretions and soft tissue swellings because of their similar densities. Also it is difficult to find out on CT scan whether the tumour has invaded the periorbita or dura. Administration of contrast offers only marginal assistance in these situations.

MR imaging is useful and complementary to CT scan in places where CT alone is not sufficient. It can differentiate tumour and secretions within the sinuses. On T1 imaging edema of inflamed tissue and retained secretions would be of low intensity and high intensity on T2 secondary to increased water content. Whereas sinonasal tumours are highly cellular and has very less water and hence give low to intermediate signal intensity on both T1 and T2 imaging. Intravenous injection of gadolinium provides additional information. Majority of the sinonasal tumours enhance diffusely on injection of contrast in comparison to the inflamed mucosa which enhances intensely and in a peripheral fashion.

Squamous cell carcinoma accounts for more than 70 percent of malignant neoplasms in the nose and paranasal sinuses. The maxillary sinus is involved in 70 percent of cases, followed by the nasal cavity (20 percent) and other sinuses (10 percent). Unfortunately, the presentation of the disease is late and a localized growth in maxillary sinus is found only in less than 25 percent of cases. The tumour tends to spread faster through the natural foramina and eroding the bony walls some of which are papery thin.

Majority of the patient may have a long-standing history suggestive of sinusitis before the actual diagnosis is made. However, it is not clear whether the chronic inflammation is a contributing factor in the development of carcinoma or not. The basic rule to follow is if a patient presenting with complaints of sinus disease does not respond to a routine course of medical management, a further workup is necessary to rule out neoplastic disease. It is important to keep a high index of suspicion so that the diagnosis of malignancy in the nose or paranasal sinuses can be made early in the course of the disease. The average delay from onset of symptoms to diagnosis is 8 months. In order to confirm the diagnosis, biopsy material is needed. This is usually obtained through a transnasal approach, if there is visible tumour present, or with a nasal endoscope enlarging the natural ostium of maxillary sinus. Metastases to the neck nodes occur in 17 percent of patients.

Maxillary sinus carcinoma is twice as common in men than in women, and more than 95 percent of patients are older than 45 years of age. Patient may start with the history of sinus disease. In addition, oral symptoms ranging from pain in the maxillary teeth or loosening of the teeth, swelling of the hard palate or gingivobuccal sulcus and inability to wear previously well-fitting dentures may be present. Some patients may present with oroantral fistula following extraction of tooth. There can be difficulty in opening the mouth which is a symptom of advanced disease and means that the tumour has invaded pterygoid fossa.

A unilateral blood stained nasal discharge is present in 35 percent of patients, and nasal obstruction is present in half. When large tumours erode the medial wall of the antrum, the tumour may be visualized within the nasal cavity. Patient may present with ocular symptoms as a result of extension of the tumour through the floor of the orbit and may include diplopia, decreased visual acuity, periorbital edema, or proptosis.

Growth of the tumour through the anterior wall of the maxilla will result in symptoms referable to the soft tissue of the face. Erosion through the orbital floor will lead to proptosis and extension through the posterolateral wall will lead to cheek swelling and trismus (Fig. 24.1). Asymmetry of the face may occur and is often associated with facial numbness secondary to invasion of the infraorbital nerve. In advanced cases, the tumour may erode through the skin. During the course of the disease, cervical node metastases develop in approximately 35 percent of patients and distant metastatic disease in 10 percent. The survival rates becomes dismal with the appearance of neck nodes.

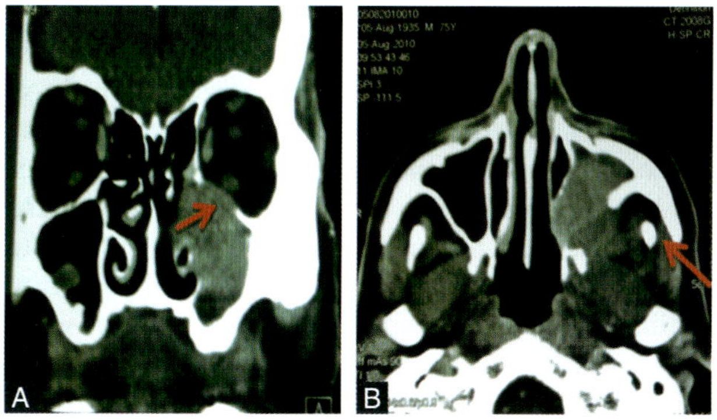

Fig. 24.1. CT scan showing squamous cell carcinoma of maxilla eroding orbital floor (**A**) and posterolateral wall (**B**).

Carcinoma of the nasal septum is much less common than its counterparts in paranasal sinuses. The mucocutaneous junction is the most common site. The patient tends to present early in such cases hence diagnosed early. Small lesions can be excised surgically with good results. Radiation therapy provides equally good results. For larger lesions, combination therapy is necessary to control the disease. Cervical spread can occur to either side and is found in approximately 10 percent of cases. As a result, 5-year survival statistics for nasal cavity carcinomas are approximately double those for tumours located in the paranasal sinuses.

Primary ethmoidal carcinomas are very rare and relatively ethmoidal sinus involvement is generally the result of spread from the maxillary antrum. Unlike maxillary sinus carcinoma, there is only a slight male preponderance. Nasal obstruction with epistaxis is more common than in antral carcinomas. Extension through the cribriform plate occurs early and is usually accompanied by anosmia. A craniofacial resection is required to allow removal of the tumour with good surgical margins. Survival statistics parallel those of large maxillary sinus carcinomas.

Frontal or sphenoid sinuses are the rare sites for primary carcinomas. They account for less than 1 percent of all paranasal sinus tumours. However, they are secondarily involved as direct extension from the other sinuses, primarily the ethmoidal sinuses.

STAGING

Maxillary sinus is divided into a "suprastructure" and an "infrastructure" by Ohngren. Using this he correctly reasoned that tumour above this line is harder to resect and therefore carries a worse prognosis. One caveat with this is that although inferior extension through the palate is more easily resected than other structures, some consider this to be more correctly considered an oral cavity tumour which carries a higher rate of cervical node involvement.

American Joint Committee on Cancer has proposed the staging of maxillary tumours. It consists of the following:

- T1 Tumour limited to the antral mucosa with no erosion or destruction of bone.
- T2 Tumour with erosion or destruction of the infrastructure, including the hard palate and/or the middle meatus.

T3 Tumour invades any of the following: skin of cheek, posterior wall of maxillary sinus, floor or medial wall of the orbit, anterior ethmoid sinus.

T4 Tumour invades orbital contents and/or any of the following: cribriform plate, posterior ethmoid or sphenoid sinuses, nasopharynx, soft palate, pterygomaxillary or temporal fossae, or base of skull.

Nodal (N) and metastatic (M) designations are similar to other head and neck malignancies.

TREATMENT

Most sinonasal tumours present at advanced stages due to the relative lack of specific symptoms. Seventy-five percent of tumours will be of T3 or T4 status at diagnosis leading to difficulty in resections. Resection of many of these lesions will lead to permanent disfigurement and still may not provide much hope of disease control. Use of preoperative or postoperative radiation is often used for positive margins and/or attempts to limit the size of resection. Chemotherapy is usually reserved for palliation of unresectable lesions, metastatic lesions, or with recurrences. Recently chemoradiotherapy has been shown to be successful but the results of these treatment protocols are still awaited.

Surgery

Surgery is the mainstay of treatment and usually consists of enbloc resection of the tumour. Depending upon the extent of the tumour as seen on CT scan and MRI examination, the surgical excision is decided which may be partial maxillectomy, total maxillectomy. If the lesion is localized to inferior wall one can do inferior partial maxillectomy. For a lesion on the medial wall, medial maxillectomy may be done. However, the surgeon should be confident about the extent of the tumour before embarking upon any type of partial maxillectomy. Total maxillectomy is a standard procedure and can be combined with orbital exenteration if orbital invasion is present. Patient undergoing total maxillectomy has a palatal defect which needs to be rehabilitated with an obturator so that patient can swallow food without nasal regurgitation and enable him to speak properly (Fig. 24.2). Those patients where orbital exenteration has been done are fitted with artificial eyeball to cover up the ugly-looking orbital socket. These procedures can be

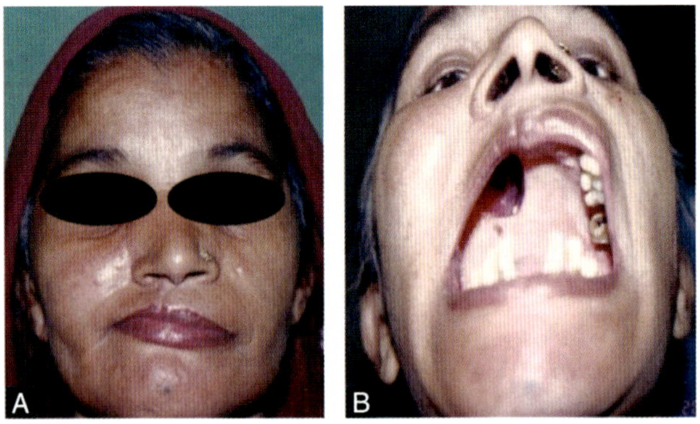

Fig. 24.2. Clinical photograph of patient after total maxillectomy showing healed Weber-Fergusson's incision (**A**) and palatal defect (**B**).

combined with neck dissection depending upon the nodal status of the patient. However, the prognosis falls drastically with the appearance of nodes.

Nasal septal lesions can be treated by wide-local excision of the lesion. Medial maxillectomy was described by Sessions and Larsen in 1977 and is most amenable to inverting papilloma or limited lesions involving the lateral nasal wall. Maxillectomy has been the standard approach towards sinus neoplasia with bone cuts through the palate, lateral maxilla, and ethmoids below the skull base. Tumours with extensive spread or tumours of the ethmoids and frontal sinuses with involvement of the skull base require craniofacial resections with neurosurgical assistance. There are numerous approaches and procedures described for these more complicated resections.

Radiation

Surgery as a single modality is only used at our center for lesion which falls into stage I, and stage II. However, number of such patients is extremely small as most of the patients present in advanced stage. So, most of our cases receive combined modality, i.e., surgery followed by radiotherapy. The use of RT alone as primary treatment modality is no longer considered a viable option except for palliation. Five-year survival for RT alone is said to be 23% and for surgery and RT 44%. The use of palliative high-dose irradiation alone for unresectable disease offers 5-year survival rates of 10 to 15%.

There is no convincing evidence as to the superiority of preoperative versus postoperative irradiation. Most select postoperative irradiation because tumour margins are easier to discern and wound complications are less. When radiographic evaluation indicates tumour in proximity to the periorbita or dura mater preoperative irradiation may be preferred.

In order to avoid damage with irradiation to the central nervous system and globe, ports must be carefully designed while treating the neoplasm. About 12 to 20% of patients lose their useful vision after treatment with irradiation alone for sinus neoplasms.

Chemotherapy

Previously, chemotherapy was usually reserved for palliative treatment of advanced or recurrent paranasal malignant neoplasms. But recently, it has been used concomitantly with radiotherapy with encouraging results. The usual protocols in sinonasal tumours are cisplatin-based regimens for squamous cell carcinoma, and with doxorubicin or fluorouracil for glandular malignant neoplasms. High risk patients for recurrence such as those presenting with positive margins, perineural spread, or extracapsular spread in regional metastasis, as well as patients who represent a poor surgical risk and those who refuse surgery, could be considered for enrolment in protocols that include combinations of radiation and chemotherapy. Combined treatment with both surgery and radiation therapy, is given either pre- or post-surgery.

Adenoid cystic carcinoma

Mucous glands are distributed all over the upper respiratory tract. Adenoid cystic carcinoma can arise within these mucous glands. The most common site of occurrence is the palate, followed by the major salivary glands and the paranasal sinuses. The paranasal sinuses comprise 14–17% of all cases. Perineural spread along cranial nerves is believed to be responsible for the high rates of local recurrence even with negative surgical margins. Despite aggressive surgical resection and radiotherapy, most adenoid cystic carcinomas tend to grow insidiously over several years, resulting in multiple local recurrences and distant metastases. So it is important that all patients, regardless of the status of their margins, receive regular long-term follow-up. Neck nodal metastases are extremely rare with this type of tumour. Distant metastases most commonly occur in the lungs. Unlike other tumours, the distant metastasis doesn't mean a dismal prognosis. If in the lung, the metastatic lesion which is usually circumscribed can be excised with good results.

Mucoepidermoid carcinoma

These are extremely rare in the sinuses and tend to present in later stages. The propensity for widespread local invasion makes resection with negative margins difficult so combination treatment with radiation is often recommended.

Adenocarcinoma

This is the second most common malignant tumour in the maxillary and ethmoid sinuses being seen in up to 5 to 20% of cases. Most of the patients have had occupational exposures as it is believed that dust particles will travel along the middle turbinate and the larger particles will be deposited there. As a result of this the tumour has a propensity for ethmoidal region.

Hemangiopericytoma

Sinonasal hemangiopericytomas are considered neither malignant nor benign, but "intermediate" in behaviour. Hemangiopericytoma is a well-recognized but uncommon vascular tumour that arises from the pericytes of Zimmerman. These cells are found spiraling around the outside of blood capillaries and postcapillary venules. About 1/3rd of the tumours arise in head and neck, with a small proportion involving the nose and paranasal sinuses. More than 80% of these are said to involve the ethmoids. Metastases are rare. Clinically, intranasal part presents as pale, gray-white, well-circumscribed mass with a soft, rubbery consistency, resembling nasal polyps. Nasal obstruction with epistaxis is common. The mean age of onset is 55, and the gender distribution is roughly equal. Treatment is complete surgical resection followed by radiation if the margin is positive.

Melanoma

The incidence of new cases of malignant melanoma is two per 100,000 populations annually. Of these, 15 to 20 percent occur in the head and neck region. Less than 2 percent of all melanomas originate in the nose or paranasal sinuses. Metastasis to the nose or paranasal sinuses is quite rare. These lesions are predominantly found in the nasal cavity. The anterior part of the nasal septum is the most common location followed by the middle and inferior turbinates. The maxillary antrum is the most frequently involved sinus. Even though the olfactory area has pigmented cells, there have been no cases reported of melanomas arising from this area. Mucosal melanomas are thought to arise from melanocytes in the mucosa of the nose and sinuses and not from a precursor nevus. Although melanocytes are present in the nasal cavities of both white and black persons, this is primarily a disease of white persons. Mucosal melanomas in general are rare before puberty. There is no sexual predilection.

Sinonasal melanoma presents with the same symptoms as other neoplasms; however, 80 percent of these patients complain of epistaxis. Typically it is seen as a polypoid fleshy mass and its pigmentation varies. There is no difference in the clinical course between melanotic and amelanotic tumours. Mucosal melanomas have a poorer prognosis than their cutaneous counterparts. The clinical course is one of aggressive local tumour with regional node metastasis and distant metastasis. The treatment is surgical and involves wide local excision of the involved structures (Fig. 24.3). If nodal involvement is evident at the time of surgery, a neck dissection is included in the procedure. Radiation therapy is not beneficial, and there is currently no efficacious chemotherapeutic regimen. Nasal melanomas appear to have a slightly better prognosis than do other mucosal melanomas.

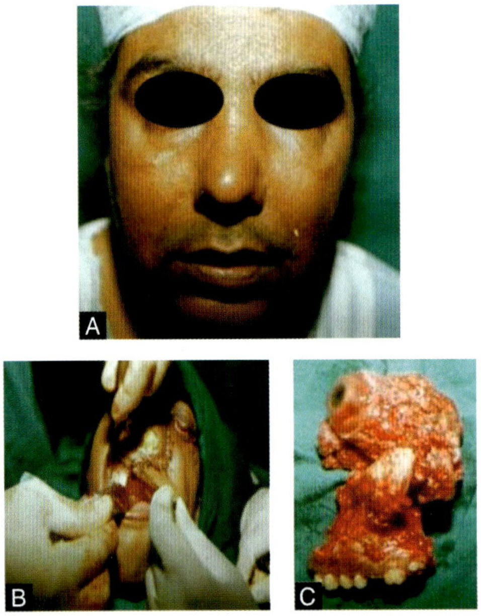

Fig. 24.3. (**A**) Clinical photograph, (**B**) intraoperative photograph, and (**C**) surgical specimen of melanoma patient.

Olfactory neuroblastoma

Berger and Luc first described "L'esthesioneuroepitheliomeolfacti" in 1924. To date, barely 300 cases have been recorded in the world literature. These are rare lesions arising in the upper part of the nasal cavity from stem cells of neural crest origin that differentiate into olfactory sensory cells. The tumour can occur at any age, but almost two thirds of these patients are between the ages of 10 and 34 years. There is a slight male predominance. As with all, intranasal tumours, symptoms are nonspecific and include epistaxis, anosmia and nasal obstruction. Because of this lack of symptoms, most patients are diagnosed late in the course of the disease. Esthesioneuroblastoma usually appears as a red or fleshy mass in the nasal vault. Symptoms of local invasion, such as proptosis or headaches, are usually evident at diagnosis. The diagnosis is made by biopsy. Adequate tissue is needed to prevent confusion with other undifferentiated round cell tumours of the nasal cavity. Although slow growing, all esthesioneuroblastomas are locally invasive and carry a 20 percent rate of metastasis. The cervical lymph nodes and lungs are most frequently involved.

Kadish proposed a clinical staging system with "Group A tumours being confined to the nasal cavity, Group B involving the paranasal sinuses, and Group C extending beyond these limits". Rosettes of the neuroblastoma cells are the hallmark of diagnosis but the histology varies widely and these tumours are sometimes classified mistakenly as undifferentiated carcinoma. It appears that combined surgery and radiation therapy provides the highest survival statistics. Baily and Barton (1975) demonstrated a 45 percent 5-year survival for patients treated with either surgery or radiation. Because of the location of esthesioneuroblastomas, preferred surgical excision is usually accomplished through a craniofacial approach (Fig. 24.4).

Recently an attempt has been made to treat these tumours endoscopically. Endoscopic resection has been advocated for tumours of Kadish stage A or B with no evidence of intracranial extension. Endoscopically, it is possible to resect the cribriform plate, the crista galli, the olfactory bulb and their surrounding dura along with the superior part of the septum and middle turbinate where they are attached to the skull base. Sporadic case reports mention the endoscopic resection of olfactory neuroblastoma with intracranial extension but long-term follow-ups are required to see their effectiveness. However,

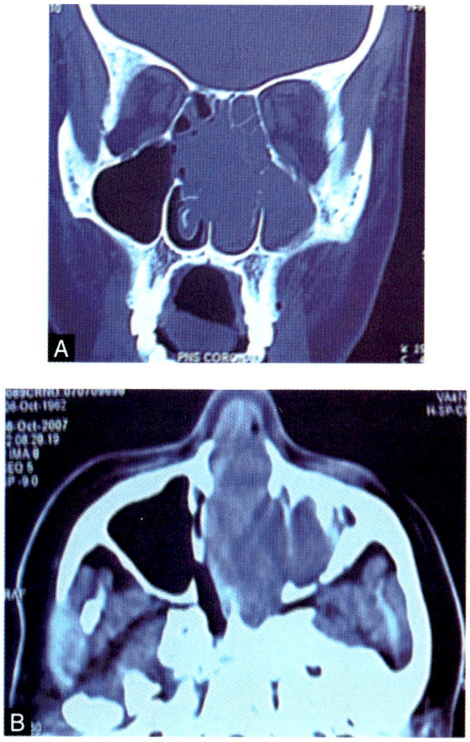

Fig. 24.4. CT scan showing olfactory neuroblastoma. Axial section (**A**), Coronal sections (**B**).

the primary determining factor affecting the prognosis is the degree of differentiation. So in cases of poorly differentiated tumours having the poor prognosis, surgical morbidity and mortality should be reduced by endoscopic resection. The complication rates are one in four in cases of craniofacial resections.

Osteogenic sarcoma

A rare tumour in the nose and paranasal sinuses, osteosarcoma is the most common primary malignant tumour of bone. Only about 5% occur in the head and neck where the mandible is more commonly affected than the maxilla. The patient presents with history of nasal obstruction and bleeding. Nasal endoscopy reveals a bony hard mass in the frontoethmoid region. X-ray paranasal sinuses may show a bony dense shadow in the nose. CT is more informative in terms of extent of the tumour. The treatment is wide excision followed by radiotherapy. There is a 30–40% chance of distant metastases and the five-year survival is 15–20%.

Chondrosarcoma

These are seen in the third to fifth decades with an equal male : female incidence. Histologic differentiation between benign and malignant types can be difficult but the malignant variety predominates. Distant metastases are rare. Death is by slow erosive destruction of the skull base. Treatment is often inadequate because of difficulty in establishing margins.

Rhabdomyosarcoma

This is the most common paranasal sinus malignancy seen in children but can affect older individuals as well. Occurrence in the head and neck accounts for more than 40 percent of cases. Rhabdomyosarcoma of the nasopharynx and paranasal sinuses accounts for 20 to 25 percent of all extra-orbital cases. Rhabdomyosarcoma is much more common in whites than in blacks. In the head and neck, the most prominent type of tumour is the embryonal form, followed distantly by the alveolar form. Because of the age group involved, early nasopharyngeal rhabdomyosarcoma is usually misdiagnosed as adenoidal hypertrophy. The correct diagnosis is usually considered only after regional spread has already occurred. The prognosis for patients with rhabdomyosarcoma of the head and neck is poorer than for those with peripheral tumours. The prognosis for patients with rhabdomyosarcomas in the parameningeal areas (nasopharynx, paranasal sinuses, and middle ear) is especially poor. The Intergroup Rhabdomyosarcoma Study advocates the use of combination therapy (radical surgery, radiation therapy, and chemotherapy) for the treatment of all rhabdomyosarcomas. They have demonstrated an increase in the 2-year survival rate from less than 30 percent to 70 percent for all head and neck tumours.

Lymphoma

Extranodal non-Hodgkin's lymphoma is said to affect 10 percent patients in head and neck. The majority of lymphomas in the nose and paranasal sinuses are of the histiocytic and diffuse lymphocytic types. The symptoms age and sex distribution are similar to those of squamous cell carcinoma, requiring a biopsy to differentiate between the two. Systemic symptoms are unusual. The antrum and ethmoidal sinuses are most frequently involved, but there is usually local extension to the soft tissue of the face at the time of diagnosis. Current treatment for early lesions with favorable histologic features consists of radiation therapy to the primary site and the neck. For lesion with a poorer prognosis, radiation is combined with chemotherapy. Five-year survival rates depend on the histologic grade of the lymphoma. Most authors quote a 5-year survival of 50 to 70 percent after radiation therapy.

Extamedullary plasmacytoma

The large majority of these occur in the head and neck with 60% developing in the nasal cavity, nasopharynx and paranasal sinuses. There is a male to female ratio of 4 : 1, and most patients present between the ages of 40 and 70 years. These tumours may be either polypoid or sessile, are red, and rarely ulcerate. The more aggressive lesions tend to be soft and friable. After the diagnosis of plasmacytoma has been returned, the patient must undergo a thorough evaluation to determine that this is not a local manifestation of multiple myeloma. The clinical course with this tumour is variable, and histologic appearance is not a useful criterion in determining aggressiveness. The disease may remain localized or evolve into systemic multiple myeloma after a latent period. Because of this, there is no one treatment of choice. Most surgeons would favour excising the tumour widely. Radiation can be given as part of a planned combination therapy or may be held in reserve for recurrences.

Benign lesions

Papillomas

Nose and paranasal sinuses are a common site of papillomas. Most papillomas are nonkeratinizing squamous cell lesions, and although they are histologically similar to the lesions found in recurrent respiratory papillomatosis, there is no pathogenic relationship. In the vestibule, a squamous papilloma similar to that found elsewhere on the skin. Simple excision with knife or Laser is effective.

Inverted papilloma

24

Inverted papilloma is a true epithelial neoplasm characterized by hyperplastic endothelium inverting into the underlying stroma. A single layer of respiratory columnar epithelium lining the surface is usually present. Most common site of origin is lateral nasal wall in the area of the middle meatus and rarely may arise from nasal septum or the paranasal sinuses. At diagnosis, it is often found completely filling the nasal cavity and may involve adjacent structures. The maxillary antrum and the ethmoidal sinuses are most frequently involved, but the orbit and sphenoidal and frontal sinuses may also contain tumour. Inverted papilloma has a peak incidence in the fifth and sixth decades of life. There is a male to female ratio of 3 : 1. Patient presents with unilateral nasal obstruction, often in association with rhinorrhea and bleeding from the nose. On rhinoscopy they look different from the usual polypi and an experienced rhinologist will be able to identify the tumour. Although there is no pathognomonic radiologic finding, a large nasal mass with destruction of the lateral nasal wall is suggestive of inverting papilloma. Bony sclerosis secondary to synchronous chronic sinusitis may be present. CT scan is must to know the exact extent of the tumour and planning the excision (Fig. 24.5). MRI is specifically used for inverted papilloma as it can differentiate simple nasal polypi and inverted papilloma (Fig. 24.5). However, the diagnosis is confirmed by biopsy. The tumour can be staged as per Krause staging which is as under:

- Stage 1 Papilloma confined to nasal cavity
- Stage 2 Papilloma involving ethmoid sinuses, medial and superior region of maxillary sinus
- Stage 3 Papilloma involving all para nasal sinuses, but confined to nose and paranasal sinuses.
- Stage 4 Papilloma not confined to nose and paranasal sinuses.

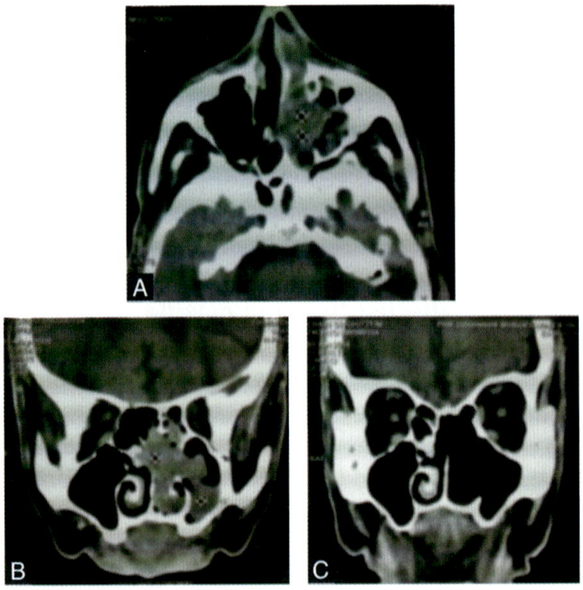

Fig. 24.5. CT scan showing inverted papilloma arising from the septum. **(A)** Axial section, **(B)** Coronal sections, **(C)** Two-year postoperative view after endoscopic medial maxillectomy.

The treatment of inverting papilloma is surgical. Complete excision is necessary to prevent recurrence. The type of resection performed is dependent upon on the size and extent of the tumour. Previously the excision used to be done by open surgery with lateral rhinotomy or Weber Fergusson's approach but nowadays endoscopic excision can be done safely for any extent of tumour. The high rates of recurrence quoted in the literature represent incomplete excision of the tumour. Extension of the tumour into the nasofrontal duct, supraorbital ethmoid cells, lacrimal fossa, or infraorbital recess of the maxillary antrum are associated with high recurrence rates. Most recurrences occur within 2 years.

It is necessary to understand the underlying pathophysiology of the disease to justify a conservative excision as suggested by Chee and Sethi. This has been well documented by Hyams, who reviewed 315 cases and found the origin of tumour from a single wide base. Multifocal disease was only present in 4.6% cases. He further concluded that all recurrences occurred at the same anatomic site. This suggests that recurrence is related to inadequate resection rather than other factors. The addition of powered instruments like the shaver can help in identifying the origin of the tumour and chances of recurrence are reduced. The endoscope is also useful for follow up to see any recurrence. In most instances a medial maxillectomy is required to remove the entire tumour. For very small lesions, a more conservative excision may be attempted if one can identify the site of origin of the tumour. Unless there is associated malignancy, mutilating surgery should be avoided. McCary et al. reported on a smaller number of primary and recurrent cases treated endoscopically with no recurrences with a maximum of 19 months follow-up. Waitz and Wigand reported on a series of 51 patients comparing endoscopic treatment with open treatment and found recurrence rates essentially identical and in conformation to with reports in general literature. Radiotherapy is ineffective in controlling these tumours and may promote malignant transformation. There is known association between inverting papilloma and malignancy. Unfortunately, the quoted incidence ranges from 2–50 percent. Hyams, in his large series from Armed Forces Institute of Pathology (1971), found a recurrence rate of 13 percent. It is still not clear whether this association represents malignant degeneration of an inverting papilloma or the simultaneous presentation of carcinoma and inverting papilloma.

Haemangioma

Haemangiomas can present as mucosal lesion in the nose and paranasal sinuses or intraosseously in the nasal bones. The former are more common. The male to female ratio is 1 : 4, and most patients are middle-aged. These patients present with history of bleeding and pain and often a history of local trauma is elicited. They can originate from the septum or turbinate and may alarm the general physician by bleeding who may think it to be a malignancy. They can emulate pyogenic granuloma. Endoscopic examination and palpation with blunt probe can clinch the diagnosis. These small lesions can be excised with the endoscope after infiltration and by taking a margin of the healthy tissue around the lesion. Haemangiomas of the mucosa may be difficult to differentiate from inflammatory polyps. The polypoid lesions may be treated with local excision, including septal perichondrium. Haemangiomas are often associated with Osler-Weber-Rendu disease or von Hippel-Lindau disease and are difficult to control. These patients often present with a history of frequent copious epistaxis. In these patients, a septodermoplasty, excision of the involved nasal mucosa, and reconstruction by placing a dermal graft over the bare septal cartilage, can be attempted.

Intraosseus nasal haemangiomas appears as translucent area with spicules of bone radiating out from a central core on X-ray film. Complete excision is curative.

Chordoma

Chordomas probably arise in detached remnants of the notochord, and these tumours tend to occur at the skull base. They account for 0.2 percent of nasopharyngeal tumours. Patient usually presents with diplopia, frontooccipital headache visual field defects and nasal obstruction. The peak incidence is in the third and fourth decades of life with a slight male predominance. A mass in the nasopharynx covered with normal mucosa may be visualized on endoscopy. Extensive bone destruction and the presence of a soft tissue mass in the nasopharynx may be evident on X-ray film and CT scan. The diagnosis is confirmed by biopsy. Because of its location, it is almost impossible to completely excise a skull base chordoma. A multicenter phase II clinical trial has confirmed the clinical efficacy of imatinib mesylate in the treatment of chordoma. Treatment with imatinib was successful in stabilizing tumour growth (84%) or shrinking tumour size (16%) in a cohort of patients with progressing, advanced chordoma. Imatinib is a tyrosine kinase inhibitor targeting several enzymes including platelet-derived growth factor receptor – (PDGFRB), which can be expressed in chordomas. However, research is ongoing, and surgery remains the standard treatment for chordomas. Adjuvant radiation therapy is used in cases in which incomplete resection is suspected. Traditional chemotherapy has not been shown to be effective.

Surgery is the preferred treatment for chordomas. Success often depends on the extent and location of the tumour. In general, a more complete removal with wide excision delays the time interval between surgery and eventual recurrence. The natural history and the effectiveness of different kinds of therapy are not well understood in chordomas because of their rare incidence and slow-growing nature.

Radical resections of tumours with clean margins are associated with a longer disease-free interval. If subtotal excision is the only option (generally due to location and proximity to delicate anatomy), the addition of radiation therapy can lengthen the interval to recurrence. In cases in which radiation therapy is utilized without surgical resection, an average of only 50% for 10-year local control is seen for skull-based and cervical spine tumours.

The preferred surgical treatment at many centers in U.S. for chordomas of the skull base is the Endoscopic Endonasal Approach (EEA) to remove the tumour. This innovative, minimally invasive technique uses the nose and nasal cavities as natural corridors to access hard-to-reach or previously inoperable tumours. EEA offers the benefits of no incisions to heal, no disfigurement to the patient, and a faster recovery time. If complementary treatments such as radiation therapy or chemotherapy are needed, those therapies can begin soon after surgery.

Juvenile nasopharyngeal angiofibroma

Juvenile nasopharyngeal angiofibroma (JNA) is benign, but locally destructive, tumour seen exclusively in males. It accounts for 0.05 percent of head and neck tumours. JNA can grow to a large size before overt symptoms are present, which include unilateral nasal obstruction, epistaxis, rhinorrhea, and facial swelling. The mean duration of symptoms is 6 months. Angiofibromas originate at the posterolateral wall of the roof of the nose at the point at which the sphenoidal process of the palatine bone joins the vomer and the pterygoid process of the sphenoid bone. Grossly tumour is usually seen to fill one or both sides of the nasopharynx and extends into the nasal cavity. Ulceration of the overlying mucosa is uncommon unless the tumour has been previously biopsied. The tumour is pink to red, lobulated, and rubbery. The main blood supply in JNA is the ipsilateral internal maxillary artery. However, in recurrent tumours and in tumours for which embolization has been attempted, bilateral arterial supplies are common. The tumour tends to spread through the paths of least resistance. From the site of origin it can spread anteriorly filling the nasal cavity, posteriorly into the nasopharynx, laterally to pterygopalatine fossa and infratemporal fossa. From pterygopalatine fossa it can go superiorly to orbit and intracranial cavity. From the nasal cavity superiorly it can go to ethmoids, sphenoid and medial to cavernous sinus intracranially. Extension into the infratemporal fossa causes cheek fullness and orbital symptoms. Intracranial extension through the lateral route is more common and is amenable to resection; involvement of the cavernous sinus is difficult to manage surgically (Fig. 24.6).

The diagnosis can usually be arrived at preoperatively based on the physical and roentgenographic findings. Opacification of one or more sinuses is generally seen on X-ray studies, most commonly of the maxillary sinus. The presence of anterior bowing of the posterior wall of the maxillary sinus is considered pathognomonic of JNA. Other signs include erosion of the greater wing of sphenoid bone with characteristic widening along the lower lateral margin of the superior orbital fissure, erosion of the medial wall of the antrum or hard palate and displacement of the nasal septum. Because the blood supply in unoperated tumours is constant, some groups no longer advocate the use of preoperative angiography.

The tumour is staged depending upon the CT scan extent and treatment plans have been devised as per the stage of the tumour. There are many

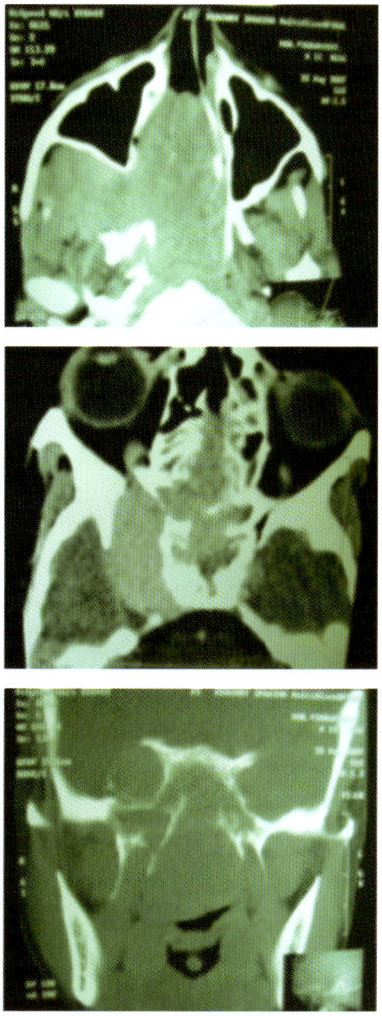

Fig. 24.6. CT scan sections of a patient showing huge angiofibroma with intracranial extension.

staging systems for angiofibroma like Session's, Chandler's, Radkowski, Andrews and Fish's classification, etc. The staging system proposed by Chandler is based on the AJCC classification for nasopharyngeal carcinoma and doesn't truly reflect the clinical behavior of the JNA. The treatment of angiofibromas has changed over the years and has become more refined by more accurate diagnostic radiological investigations such as CT and MRI. Familiarity with the skull base approaches combined with three dimensional navigation systems has facilitated the management of these tumours. Currently surgery is the preferred treatment. The surgical approach is decided primarily on the location extent, and expertise of the surgeon. The surgical approaches include transpalatal transoral route, transoral tranpharyngeal route, Lateral rhiniotomy approach, Weber Fergussion's approach and midfacialdegloving approach. Most of these approaches include elevation of soft tissues and periosteum from, dissection of mucoperiosteum of the palate, medial maxillectomy, ethmoidectomy and facial osteotomies. The procedures might affect the growth of craniofacial skelton of the young patients. Hence the endoscopic endonasal excision of JNA is becoming popular. However it needs expertise of the surgeon, preoperative embolization and good anesthetist's team.

Using endoscopic approach, successful treatment has been achieved by various surgeons (Fig. 24.7). Rogers reported 20 patients of JNA with successful outcome without preoperative embolization and suggested that highly vascular and extensive cases may leave residual tumours. Andrade et al. reported a series of 12 patients of JNA. The age ranged between 9–22 years. Eight patients were stage 1, and 4 patients were stage II according to Andrew's classification. Three patients were taken up by open approach and rest were operated endoscopically. There were no significant differences in mean operative time between endoscopic and open groups (312 versus 365 minutes). In the endoscopic group, the intraoperative blood loss was almost half that of the open group (506 cc versus 934 cc). And the average hospital stay was one day less in endoscopic group (3 versus 4 days). Blood loss and hospital stay were important difference giving

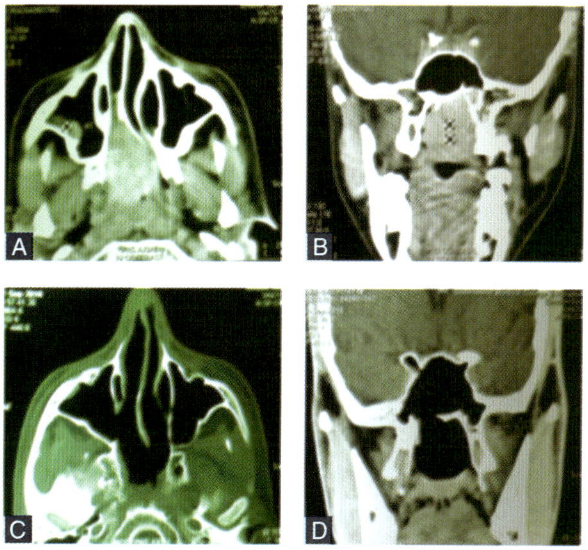

Fig. 24.7. Preoperative (A & B) and 4 years postoperative (C & D), CT scans after endoscopic excision of angiofibroma.

credibility to endoscopic removal of JNA in his series.

In the series of Bremer and associates (1986), there was an overall recurrence rate of 17 percent. Only 5 percent of patients with extracranial disease had recurrent disease, but 50 percent of patients with intracranial extension demonstrated recurrent disease. Residual intracranial disease can be treated with radiation.

Osseous tumours

Osteomas

Osteomas are slow-growing, benign tumours composed of mature bone and are found almost exclusively in the head and neck. The mandible is the most frequent location for osteomas. In order of frequency, the frontal, ethmoidal, and maxillary sinuses can be involved (Fig. 24.8). Sphenoidal sinus osteomas are very rare. Symptoms are related to the site of the tumour and are usually present for more than a year before the patient seeks help. These tumours are occasionally diagnosed incidentally during the workup for an unrelated complaint. The treatment for osteomas is surgical but is not warranted unless the patient is symptomatic. At surgery, the tumour is attached to underlying bone by a pedicle. Often a rim of normal bone must be removed to allow extraction of the tumour. Osteomas in the frontal sinus are best removed through an osteoplastic flap approach. External ethmoidectomy is performed to provide access to osteoma in the ethmoidal sinuses. For maxillary sinus tumours, Caldwell-Luc approach affords adequate exposure for removal of the osteoma. Complete excision is curative.

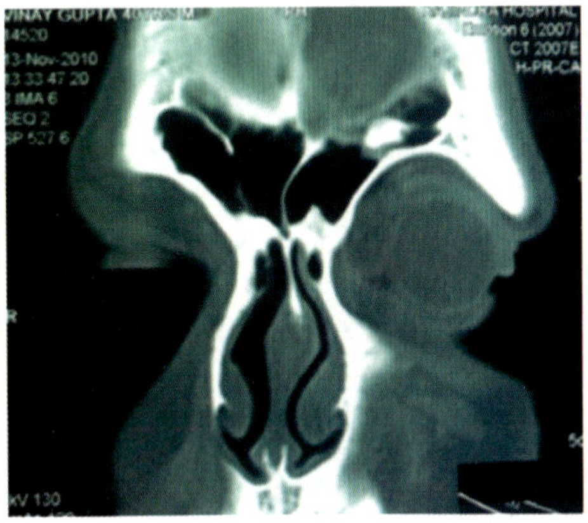

Fig. 24.8. CT scan showing asymptomatic osteoma in the frontal sinus.

With the advent of intranasal drill and endoscope the osteomas can be removed from all these sites without any significant morbidity. As these tumours are slow growing so partial excision can be done to give symptomatic relief. The author has the experience of one such case who presented with nasal obstruction and proptosis. A partial excision was done and patient is happy. The residual tumour has not grown either.

Meningioma

Extracranial meningiomas, excluding orbital meningioma are very rare. Although there are different histologic types, all meningiomas arise from meningothelial arachnoid cells. Extracranial meningiomas are histologically idenentical to their intracranial counterparts, and most are the result of extracranial arachnoid cell clusters. These clusters tend to occur along the tracts of the cranial nerves and in association with skull foramina. The treatment for these tumours is surgical, usually involving a medial maxillectomy. Complete removal is curative; there is no role for radiation therapy in the primary treatment of nasal meningiomas.

Neurogenic tumours

Neurogenic tumours are very rarely seen in nose and paranasal sinuses. Literature search shows only sporadic case reports. Neurofibromas arise from within nerve fibers, and may occur as solitary lesion or multiple tumours. They may occur as part of von Recklinghausen's disease also. They have been described within facial bones and undergo malignant change in 15% of cases. These tumours are treated by complete surgical excision unless vital surrounding structures are involved in which partial excision is acceptable. Schwannomas have been described within facial bones and along the branches of the trigeminal nerve and nerves of the autonomic nervous system. In the nose septum is the common site and simple excision of the tumour is effective.

CONCLUSION

Due to the common clinical presentation it is difficult to diagnose a sinonasal neoplasm early. The treating surgeon should have a high index of suspicion so that the diagnosis is not delayed. Once diagnosed, the treatment should be commenced early in order to have good results. The surgical morbidity has been reduced due to the advent of endonasal endoscopic-assisted surgeries being reported as successful in many cases. This can be combined with postoperative radiotherapy and or chemotherapy to further enhance the survival rates.

SUGGESTED READING

1. Rice DH. Endonasal approach for sinonasal naso-pharyngeal tumours. *Otolaryngol Clin North Am*, 2011; 34: 1087–93.
2. Evans PHR. Anatomy of the nose and paranasal sinuses. In Scott Brown's Otolarngology, 5th edition, Vol. I. Alan G Kerr (eds.), 138–61.
3. Zheng W et al. Risk factors for cancers of the nasal cavity and paranasal sinuses among White men in the United States. *Am J Epidemiol*, 138: 965–72.
4. Robin PE, Powell DJ, Stansbie JM. Carcinoma of the nasal cavity and paranasal sinuses: Incidence and presentation of different histological types. *Clin Otolaryngol Allied Sci*, 1979; 4: 431–56.
5. Bridger GP, Mendelsohn MS, Baldwin M, Smee R. Paranasal sinus cancer. *Aust NZ J Surg*, 1991; 61: 290–4.
6. Golabek W, Drop A, Golabek E, Morshed K. Site of origin of paranasal sinus malignancies [in Polish]. *Pol Merkuriusz Lek*, 2005; 19: 413–4.
7. Larsson LG, Martensson G. Carcinoma of the paranasal sinuses and the nasal cavities; a clinical study of 379 cases treated at Radiumhemmet and the Otolaryngologic Department of Karolinska Sjukhuse. *Acta Radiol*, 1954; 42: 149–72, 1940–50.
8. Bornholdt J, Hansen J, Steiniche T, et al. K-ras mutations in sinonasal cancers in relation to wood dust exposure. *BMC Cancer*, 2008; 20; 8:53.
9. Klintenberg C, Olofsson J, Hellquist H, Sokjer H. Adenocarcinoma of the ethmoid sinuses. A review of 28 cases with special reference to wood dust exposure. *Cancer*, 1984 ; 54: 482–8.
10. Luce D, Gerin M, Leclerc A, Morcet JF, Brugere J, Goldberg M. Sinonasal cancer and occupational exposure to formaldehyde and other substances. *Int J Cancer*, 1993; 53: 224–31.
11. Katori H, Nozawa A, Tsukuda M. Markers of malignant transformation of sinonasal inverted papilloma. *Eur J Surg Oncol*, 2005; 31: 905–11.
12. McKay SP, Gregoire L, Lonardo F, Reidy P, Mathog RH, Lancaster WD. Human papillomavirus (HPV) transcripts in malignant inverted papilloma are from integrated HPV DNA. *Laryngoscope*, 2005; 115: 1428–31.
13. Ott G, Kalla J, Ott MM, Muller-Hermelink HK. The Epstein-Barr virus in malignant non-Hodgkin's lymphoma of the upper aerodigestive tract. *Diagn Mol Pathol*, 1997; 6: 134–9.
14. Gallagher TM, Boles R. : Symposium: Treatment of malignancies of paranasal sinuses. *Laryngoscope*, 1970; 80: 924–32.
15. Batsakis JG. Tumours of the Head & Neck. Baltimore. The Williams & Wilkins Company, 1979.
16. Tabb HG, Barranco SJ. Cancer of the maxillary sinus. *Laryngoscope*, 1971; 81: 818–27.
17. Sessions RB, Larsen DL, Enbloc ethmoidectomy and medial Maxillectom. *Arch Otolaryngol*, 1977; 103: 195–202.
18. Batsakis JG, Sciubba JJ. Pathology. *In:* Blitzer A et al. (eds.): Surgery of the paranasal sinuses. Philadelphia, W.B. Saunder's Company, 1985.
19. Blatchford SJ, Koopman CF, Coulthard SW. Mucosal melanomas of the head & neck. *Laryngoscope*, 96: 929–34.
20. Berger L, Luc C, Richard CL. Esthesioneuroblastoma olfactif. *Bull Asso Fr Etude Cancer*, 1924; 13: 410–21.
21. Bailey BJ, Barton S. Olfactory neuroblastoma: Management & prognosis. *Arch Otolaryngol*, 1975; 101: 1–5.
22. Kadish S, Goodman M, Wang CC. Olfactory neuroblastoma: A clinical analysis of 17 cases. *Cancer*, 1976; 37: 1571–6.
23. Casiano RR, Numa WA, Falquez AM. Endoscopic resection of olfactory neuroblastoma. *Am J Rhinol*, 2000; 15: 271–9.
24. Gupta AK, Grover M, Virk RS et al. Giant esthesioneuroblastoma: Is there any scope of endoscopic approach. *Clinical Rhinol*, 2010; 3: 31–4.
25. Levine PA, Gallagher R, Cantrell RW Esthesioneuroblastoma: reflection on a 21-year experience. *Laryngoscope*, 109: 1539L–3.
26. Donaldson SS, Castro JR, Wilbur JR et al. Rhabdomyosarcoma of the head & neck in children: Combination therapy by surgery, irradiation and chemotherapy. *Cancer*, 1973; 32: 26–35.
27. Lawson W, Biller HF, Jacobson A, Som P. The role of conservative surgery in the management of inverted papilloma. *Laryngoscope*, 1983; 93: 148–55.
28. Vrabec DP. Schneiderian Inverted papillomas. A clinical and pathological study. *Larnygoscope*, 1975; 85: 186–220.
29. Chee LWJ, Sethi DS: The Endoscopic management of sinonasal papilloma. *Clin Otolaryngol*, 1999; 24: 61–6.
30. Hyams V: Papillomas of the nasal cavity and paranasal sinuses: A clinicopathological study of 315 cases. *Ann Otol Rhinol Laryngol*, 1971; 80: 192–206.
31. McCary WS, Dross CW, Raffel JF, et al. Preliminary report: Endoscopic versus external surgery in the management of inverted papilloma. *Laryngoscope*, 1998; 108: 1320–4.
32. Waitz G. Wigand ME. Results of endoscopic sinus surgery for the treatment of inverted papilloma. 2000; 110: 39–42.
33. Mills RP. Chordoms of skull base. *J Roy Soc Med*, 1984; 77: 10–16.
34. Casali PG, Stacchiotti S, Sangalli C, Olmi P, Gronchi A. Chordoma. *Curr Opin Oncol*, 2007; 19(4): 367–70.

35. Bremer NW, Neel HB, DeSanto LW, Jones GC. Angiofibroma: Treatment trends in 150 patients during 40 years. *Laryngoscope*, 1986; 96: 1321–9.
36. Neel HB. Juvenile angiofibroma. *In:* Blitzer A, Lawson W, Freidman WH (eds.): Surgery of the paranasal sinuses. Philadelphia, W.B. Saunder's Company, 1985.
37. Sessions RB. Radiographic staging of juvenile angiofibroma. *Head Neck Surg*, 1981; 3: 279–83.
38. Chandler's, Chandler JR. Nasopharyngeal angiofibroma: staging and management. *Ann Otorhinolaryngol*, 1984; 93: 322–9.
39. Radkowski D, McGill T, Healy GB et al. Angiofibroma: Changes in staging and treatment. *Arch Otolarygol Head Neck Surg*, 1996; 112: 122–9.
40. Andrews JC, Fish U, Valavanis A, Aeppli et al. The surgical management of extensive nasopharyngeal angiofibromas with the infratemporal fossa approach. *Laryngoscope*, 1989; 99: 429–37.
41. Rogers G, Huy PT, Froelich P et al. Exclusively endoscopic surgery for juvenile nasopharyngeal angiofibroma. Trends and limits. *Arch Otolaryngol Head Neck Surg*, 2002; 128: 908–35.
42. Andrade NA, Pinto JA, Gerraro T et al. Exclusively endoscopic surgery for juvenile nasopharyngeal angiofibroma. *Otolaryngol Head Neck Surg*, 2007; 137: 492–6.
43. Granich MS, Pilch BZ, Goodman ML. Meningiomas presenting in the paranasal sinuses and temporal bone. *Head Neck Surg*, 1983; 5: 319–28.

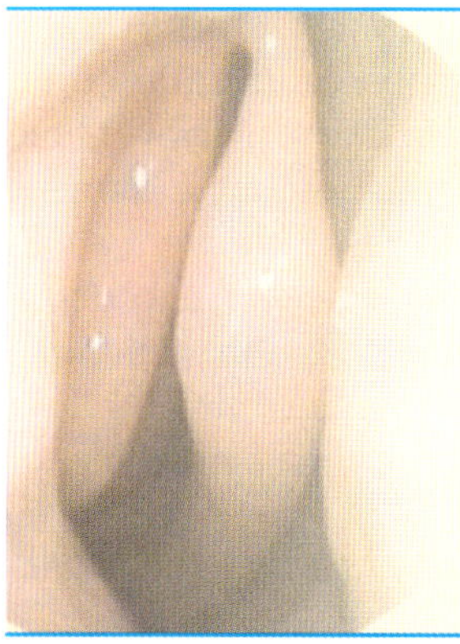

CHAPTER 25

Update on Snoring and Sleep Apnoea

Jagdeepak Singh

Snoring is the low frequency sound produced in the oropharyngeal area during sleep or sleep-like states like alcoholic slumber, deep sedation and post anaesthetic recovery period. It indicates obstruction to the free flow of air somewhere between the opening of the nose and into the trachea. Depending upon the degree of obstruction, the patient either exhibits partial collapse of the soft tissue and produces a noise – called snoring or with total obstruction of any portion of the collapsible airway, experiences a condition called sleep apnoea (total cessation of breathing for 10 seconds or longer) or hypopnoea (50% or greater decrease in air exchange for 10 seconds or longer).

INCIDENCE

Snoring affects 19 to 37% of the general population and more than 50% middle-aged men. Normal adults (45%) snore at least occasionally while 25% are habitual snorers. It is estimated that 20% of men and 5% of women between 30–35 years of age snore, this rate increases to 50% in men and 30% in women above 60 years of age.

As a direct consequence of obstruction, the CO_2 in blood increases and the O_2 level in the patient's blood decreases proportionate to the severity of the airway obstruction. This disruptive pattern of breathing generates disruptive sleep pattern, the consequences of which being increased fatiguability, lethargy, decreased ability to concentrate, increased irritability, morning headaches and decreased libido in these patients.

SNORING, SLEEP APNOEA AND ENT ABNORMALITIES

People with sleep apnoea syndrome can be grouped according to the mechanism of apneic episodes. In a patient who has central aponea, there is cessation of airflow through either the nasal or oral cavities in conjunction with absence of any thoracic or other respiratory movement. Patients with obstructive sleep apnoea will also have no nasal or oral air flow, but will exhibit this persistent and vigorous thoracic and other respiratory effort. Some people will have both types of apnoea termed as mixed sleep apnoea. The obstructive type of sleep apnoea is the most common form. It is unusual for a patient with obstructive sleep apnoea to have a single anatomic abnormality that could be surgically corrected to the extent that it totally cures the patient of the sleep disorder. However, it has been noted that one patient can have a variety of anatomic abnormalities that collectively result in reduction of the volume of the upper airway. Abnormalities such as abnormally large tongue, retrognathic mandible, long palate, shallow pharynx, hyperactive gag reflex, short neck, floppy epiglottis and large tonsils can contribute to "disproportionate anatomy" that results in a decreased oral and hypopharyngeal volume and predisposes to airway obstruction while the patient is in a supine position during sleep.

SNORING AND CARDIOVASCULAR STATUS

The immediate consequence of OSA are readily recognizable. However, not so easily recognizable are the long-term cardiovascular effects secondary to OSA that lead to an estimated 30,000 to 40,000 cardiovascular/cerebrovascular deaths per year. Untreated OSA ultimately leads to an increased incidence of pulmonary and systemic high blood pressure and ventricular hypertrophy. Multiple studies reveal a positive co-relation between loud snoring and risk of heart attack (about 34% chance) and stroke (about 67% chance). Significant decreases in O_2 saturation of blood during apneic episodes can lead to potentially lethal arrhythmia. New studies associate loud snoring with the development of carotid artery atherosclerosis, risk of brain damage and of stroke. Researchers hypothesise that loud snoring creates turbulence in carotid artery blood flow which is closest to the airway. Increased turbulence irritates blood cells which has been implicated as a cause of atherosclerosis.

SLEEP APNOEA AND STROKE

Stroke is the second most common cause of death worldwide and leading cause of disability among adults. Therefore, an understanding of the underlying pathophysiology, promotion of preventive behaviours and the development of novel therapeutic approaches for stroke is of crucial importance. Understanding the link between the obstructive sleep apnoea and stroke may be one such approach. Several case control and cross-sectional epidemiological studies show a strong association between snoring (a surrogate for sleep apnoea) and stroke. The presence of sleep apnoea in the setting of stroke is associated with unfavourable clinical course including early neurological worsening, delirium, depressed mood, impaired functional capacity, impaired cognition and a longer period of hospitalization and rehabilitation.

SNORING AND PSYCHOLOGICAL STATUS

It has also been suggested that snoring can cause significant psychological and social damage to sufferers. Though snoring is often considered as minor affliction, snorers sometimes suffer severe impairment in lifestyle. Snoring is an impediment to partner's sharing/sleeping in the same room and is seen as a fault of the snorer. This can lead to low self esteem and strained marital relationship.

SNORING AND GLAUCOMA

Sleep disordered breathing characterized by snoring, excessive day time sleepiness and insomnia is considered as one of the risk factors for the development of primary open angle glaucoma (POAG). It is the second leading cause of irreversible blindness in the US. Chronic hemodynamic changes and recurrent severe hypoxia resulting from sleep disordered breathing (SDB) may contribute to anoxic optic nerve damage implicated in glaucoma. Normal tension glaucoma patients contribute to a high risk population of sleep apnoea syndrome.

SNORING IN CHILDREN

Recent studies show that 3–12% of children between the ages of 1 to 9 snore. Loud and regular nightly snoring is usually abnormal in otherwise healthy children. Contributing factors to sleep apnoea include obesity, nasal allergies, asthma, GERD, abnormality in the physical structure of face or jaw, medical and neurological conditions in children and the most common physical problem causing sleep apnoea is large tonsils and adenoids.

Sleep is essential for children from the proper maturation and development of the brain. Anything that disrupts the integrity of a child's sleep can result in significant impairment of mental and physical development.

Warning signs in children include snoring or "squealing" during sleep, difficulty in breathing during sleep, sleeping in abnormal position with head in unusual position, experiencing night terrors, sleep walking, bed wetting, mouth breathing, daytime hyperactivity, being irritable/agitated/aggressive and problems in school.

Consequences of OSA in children

- Attention Deficit Hyperactivity Disorder (ADHD).
- Emotional problems.
- Behavioural and social problems.
- Delayed mental and physical development.
- Poor academic performance.
- Raised BP and cardiovascular problems.

SNORING AND WOMEN

Recent studies show that in metros it is the women doing the heavy snoring more often than not, while there are higher numbers of men finding themselves upon the suffering end. Stressful and overdemanding lifestyle of modern-day women is considered as one of the causes for high incidence of snoring in women recently. Other causes include obesity, hypertension, hypothyroidism and diabetes mellitus type II. Women are at a higher risk of heart disease, diabetes and many other health issues even without problem of snoring.

SNORING AND PREGNANCY

Snoring and OSA in pregnant women can be a real problem for the mother as well as the foetus. Cessation of breathing during sleep leads to deprivation of O_2 in maternal blood which in turn leads to heightened increase in the appropriate growth formation. The risks include the brain development for the child's future learning abilities and proper growth of all body organs.

Hence, snoring and OSA can lead to cluster of complications which can take a toll on one's health. Hence, the goal should be early detection and appropriate management of these conditions to enable the individual to lead a healthy, disease-free life.

A multidisciplinary approach is essential to manage the scores of sleep disorders and its many manifestations and, for this, a close collaboration is required amongst an otolaryngologist, general physician, neurologist, eye specialist, psychiatrist, dentist, anaesthetist and marriage counsellors.

Role of anaesthetists

Role of pre-anaesthetic checkup (PAC)

- Peri- and postoperative status of patients with snoring can be a source of worry for the anaesthetists.
- Special protocol for pre-operative pre-medication.
- All sedatives are avoided.
- Preoperative C-PAP not only acclimatizes the patient to the instrument but also reduces the oedema of the cheek mucosa in the upper airway.
- C-PAP is discontinued after the effect of the anesthesia is worn off.

Eye checkup

Regular visits to an eye specialist is extremely important in patients with snoring in order to detect any rise in intraocular pressure and diagnose chronic simple glaucoma at the earliest, thus preventing irreversible blindness due to optic nerve atrophy. Sleep apnoea is known to affect oxygenation, neurohumoral factors and circulatory haemodynamics which together have an effect on the integrity of optic nerve. A close co-relation between chronic simple glaucoma and sleep disordered breathing has been suggested by a study conducted. Out of 83 patients with confirmed sleep apnoea, 33% had glaucoma. Hence, sleep apnoea is considered as a risk factor for glaucoma.

Psychiatrists and marriage counsellors play a major role in boosting the self-confidence of the patient by modifying his lifestyle. This leads to improved marital relationship and better social life.

TREATMENT

Once the diagnosis of clinically significant OSA/hypopnea is made by a sleep lab polysomnogram (sleep study), treatment aiming at clearing the blockage in the breathing passage are initiated.

Snorers are advised to:

- Lose weight.
- Stop smoking.
- Sleep on side.
- Avoid alcohol before going to bed.
- Avoid sleeping pills.
- Yoga, medication, laughter exercises and even loud singing or playing a musical instrument (digderidoo) has been found to curb snoring and relieve stress to a great extent.

Various treatment options available include:

- Nasal sprays.
- Nasal strips.
- Nose clips.
- Anti-snore clothing and pillows.
- Lubricating sprays.

Treatment modalities include:

1. Drugs

Drugs like protryptilline (antidepressant), modalert (wakefulness promoting agent), combination of pseudoephedrine and domperidone have been used in treatment of severe snoring and satisfactory results have been obtained. Other drugs include intranasal steroid like fluticasone furuoate, mometasone furuoate which are used to relieve snoring in cases associated with allergic rhinitis. During snoring the uvula, soft palate, tonsillar pillars and the walls of the pharynx are exposed to the traumatizing suction force. Inflammatory mediators play an important role in leading to injury of sensory, motor nerves in the upper airway and are also known to impair muscle contractility, thus contributing to upper airway muscle dysfunction in OSA. Corticosteroid receptors are present in the uvular tissue and nasal mucosa. Thus nasal steroids have an effect on reducing the development of vibration related edema and snoring and also influence the swelling of the soft palate caused by vibrations of the tissues. In a study started in 2010, effect of mometasone furoate nasal spray is being evaluated in 75 patients of snoring selected at random from the OPD of Govt. Medical College. The patients are assessed for snoring by the 'snoring score', daytime somnolence by 'sleepiness score', daytime activities by 'Epworth sleepiness scale' and nose and throat discomfort by 'nose and throat trouble score', both before and after treatment with mometasone furoate nasal spray. The results are awaited.

2. Positive airway pressure

A continuous positive pressure airway (C-PAP) machine is often used to control sleep apnoea and snoring associated with it.

3. Dental appliances

Specially made dental appliances called mandibular advancement splints, which advance the lower jaw slightly and thereby pull the tongue forwards are a common mode of treatment for snoring. Typically, a dentist specializing in sleep apnoea dentistry is of immense value. These splints are often tolerated much better than C-PAP machines.

4. Surgery

It is also available as a method of correcting social snoring, procedure include turbinectomy, septoplasty, stiffening procedures of soft palate by excision, diathermy, laser, e.g., Laser-assisted Uvulopalatopharyngoplasty (LAUP) and somnoplasty. The most commonly performed surgical procedure for the treatment of pediatric OSA is adenotonsillectomy. It is important to emphasise that both tonsillectomy and adenoidectomy should be performed if the objective is to improve airway obstruction in OSA.

5. Regular medical checkup

It is of paramount importance in patients with snoring in order to deal with conditions like hypertension, obesity, insulin resistance and other cardiovascular complication at the earliest possible.

CONCLUSION

Snoring should no longer be considered as a harmless habit but a new health warning and a wake up call for action. Close association of OSA with a cluster of disorders like obesity, hypertension, high cholesterol, risk of developing POAG, psychological and emotional problems can take a huge toll on health. Hence, management of snoring and sleep apnoea require close collaboration amongst all these fields at the earliest possible.

ACKNOWLEDGEMENT

I am grateful to Dr. Inderjit Kaur, Associate Professor, Department of Opthalmology for her constant support in preparing the manuscript. I would also like to thank Dr. Jasveen Kaur, Junior Resident of E.N.T. for her contribution.

SUGGESTED READING

1. Kushida CA. Obstructive sleep apnea: Diagnosis and treatment. Informa Healthcare, New York, 2007.
2. Kereiakes TJ. Indication for UPPP in snoring and sleep apnea. *In:* Pensak ML, editor. Controversies in otolaryngology. Thieme, New York, 2001; 56–62.
3. Barthel SW, Stome M. Snoring, obstructive sleep apnea surgery. *Med Clin North Am*, 1999; 83: 85–96.
4. Fujita S, Conway W, Zorick F. Surgical correction of anatomic abnormalities in obstructive sleep apnea syndrome: Uvuloplatopharyngoplasty. *Otolaryngol Head Neck Surg*, 1981; 89: 923–34.
5. Shang CY, Gau SS, Soong WT. Association between childhood sleep problems and perinatal factors, parental mental distress and behavioral problems. *J Sleep Res*, 2006; 15: 63–73.
6. Peppard P, Young T, Palta M, Shatrud J. Prospective study of the association between sleep disordered breathing and hypertension. *New Engl J Med*, 2000; 342: 1378–84.
7. Hung J, Whitfard EG, Parsons RW, Hillman DR. Association of sleep apnea with myocardial infarction in men. *Lancet*, 1990; 336: 261–4.
8. Farney RJ, Lugo A, Jensen RL et al. Simultaneous use of antidepressant and antihypertensive medication increases likelihood of diagnosis of obstructive sleep apnea syndrome. *Chest*, 2004; 125: 1279–85.
9. Pien GW, Fife D, Pack AI et al. Changes in symptoms of sleep-disordered breathing during pregnancy. *Sleep*, 2005; 28: 1299–305.
10. Schmidt-Nowara W, Lowe A, Wiegand L et al. Oral application for the treatment of snoring and obstructive sleep apnea: A review. *Sleep*, 1995; 18: 501–10.

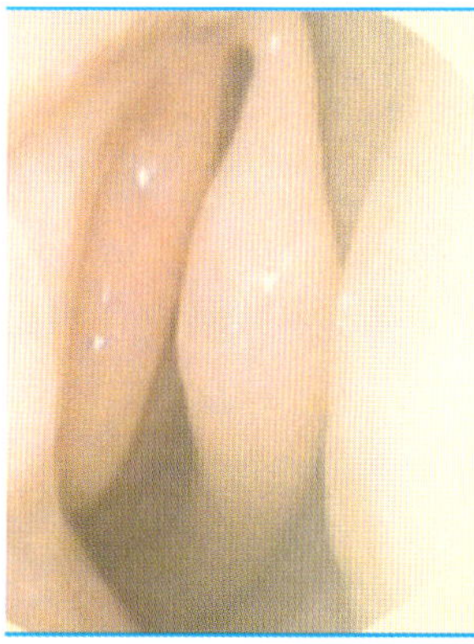

CHAPTER 26

Cosmetic Surgery in ENT Practice

Firdous Quader Minu, S.A. Siddiky

With greater exposure to the outer world our knowledge has expanded, and so has our ability to recognize what we like and don't like. People everywhere are getting more and more conscious about their looks. It plays a great role in how we feel about ourselves. Cosmetic surgery can now play a great role in improving the way someone looks; and is therefore becoming more and more popular with time. It used to be in the domain of plastic surgeons alone but now some head and neck surgeons are also dealing with patients desiring cosmetic surgery. As our population has a longer life expectancy, rejuvenation of the aging face is becoming a common concern for all.

Some of the common procedures done in cosmetic surgery of the head and neck have been outlined here. Of course, it should be remembered that before attempting any of the procedures, text-book should be consulted. Also adequate training is needed for the procedures to be successful.

Patient counselling is very important; as there are many patients who have unrealistic expectations. Patient has to be explained about the procedure and its outcome. It is of utmost importance that pre- and postoperative pictures are taken at all relevant angles.

SCAR REVISION

Scar formation comes hand in hand with any kind of surgery. The head-neck area is one of the most exposed parts of the body. So, the bad scar in this area is a matter of concern. Some factors are beyond the surgeons' control – these are mode of injury, position of the wound, patients' skin type and history to form hypertrophied scars. But, the factors that a surgeon can control are proper realignment of wound edges, conservative and meticulous handling of injured tissues during primary repair and use of proper suture material and dressing.

As cosmetic surgeons, we are often faced with the challenge of revising these scars. The surgeon should be familiar with the location of the relaxed skin tension line (RSTL) on face (Fig. 26.1). These are curvilinear lines that are naturally formed on the skin. Also knowledge of facial aesthetic units and blood supply as well as nerve supply of the face is important. An ideal scar is a fine line that is level with the skin and blends with the RSTL. Scars, which are raised, depressed, stretched, pigmented or misaligned with the RSTL, are unpleasant to look at.

Before doing a scar revision, the scar has to be examined properly. Scars can take a long time to heal; it may take 6 months to one year to mature. But in some cases where functional impairment is involved early scar revision can be done. The goal of scar revision is to position a scar into the RSTL and dispersing a long scar into smaller indiscreet scars. Patients should be informed that cosmetic surgery cannot make the scar disappear completely, but there can be significant improvement in its appearence.

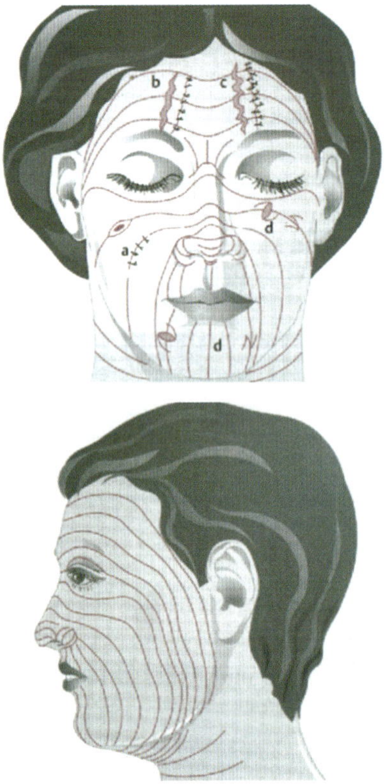

Fig. 26.1. Relaxed skin tension lines and scar revision.

Fusiform elliptical excision

The simplest method of scar revision is the re-excision of the scar in a linear or curvilinear fashion with 30 degree angle ends. The scar should be positioned within the RSTL (Fig. 26.2A). Undermining of 1–2 cm around the periphery will allow for re-approximation of skin edges without tension. Proper closure with deep and superficial sutures will ensure proper wound eversion. Vertical mattress sutures improve wound edge eversion when needed. Interrupted sutures by 6/0 or 7/0 monofilament are commonly used.

In larger scars/skin lesions, serial excision can be done in steps (Fig. 26.3). This is done on the principle of the ability of skin to stretch. Time is taken between excisions for the wound tension to subside and elasticity to return. The final result is often very gratifying; although it may take a long time for the excision to be complete.

Scars which are long, linear and not in alignment with RSTLs are most visible to the eye. These scars can be broken down to make them less visible. This can be done by Z-plasty or W-plasty (Fig. 26.4). In some cases geometric broken lines are also created for a good closure (Fig. 26.5).

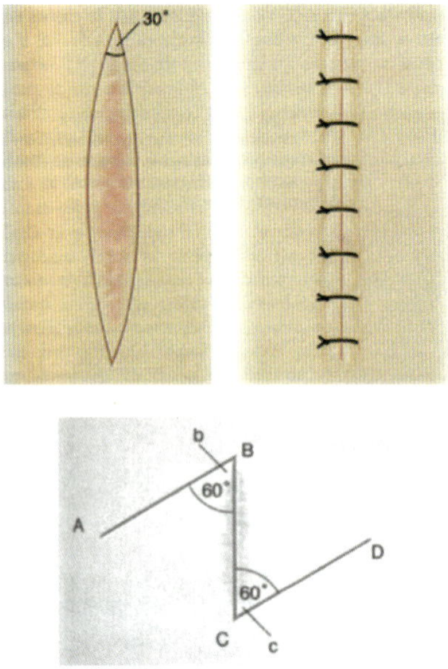

Fig. 26.2. A. Fusiform elliptical excision, **B.** Z-plasty.

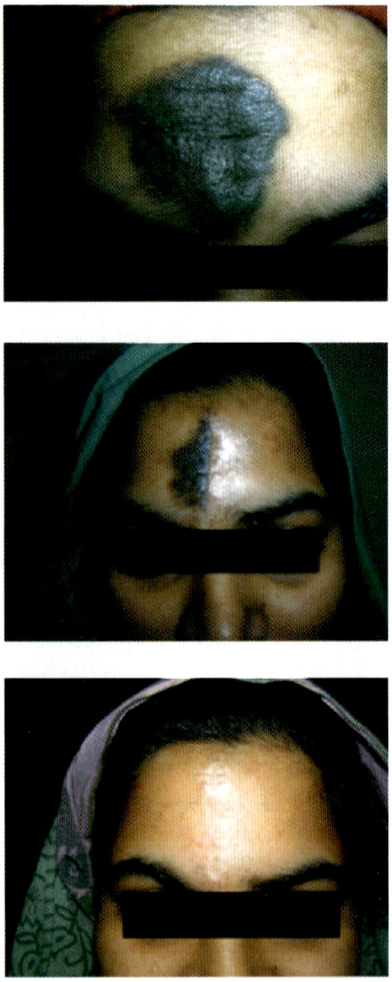

Fig. 26.3. Serial excision in two steps.

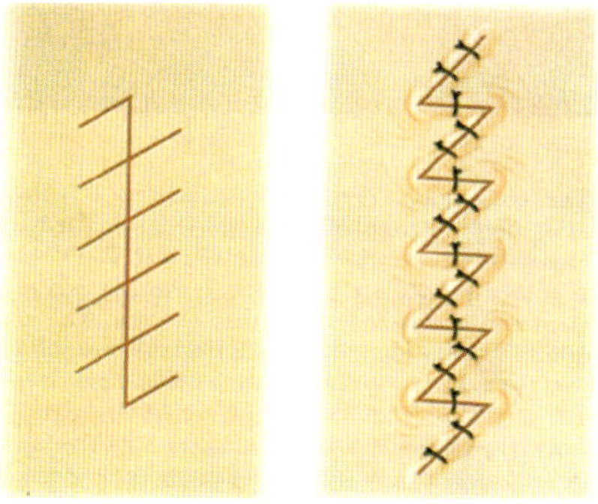

Fig. 26.4. W-plasty.

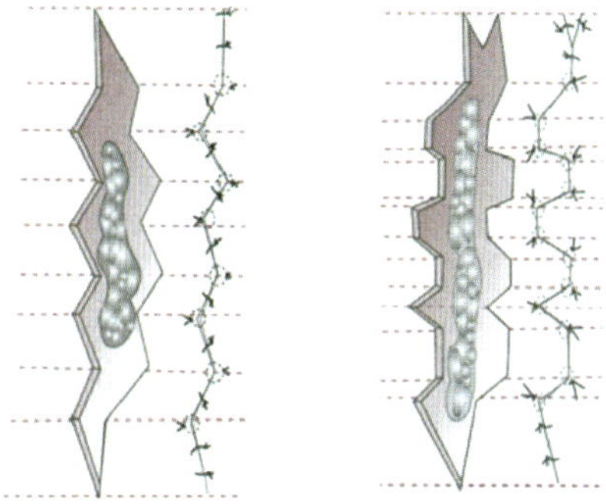

Fig. 26.5. Geometric broken line closure.

Z-plasty lengthens the scar and can be used to redirect scars into RSTL's. The scar is excised and two incisions are given in opposite direction on both ends at 60 degree angles (Fig. 26.2B). The skin is undermined and the tips of the triangular flap are transposed, thus changing the direction of the scar as well as lengthening it. Multiple Z-plasties can be done for long scars.

After excision and undermining, suturing is done in two layers. Steristrips are used, as it causes immobilization of the wound and helps in better healing. Tissue expanders are used now-a-days as a means for scar revision for large scars. Healthy tissues on the sides of the scar is expanded by inserting expanders under the skin and inflated using normal saline for a period of time. When the size of tissue expanded is enough to cover the defect, the expander is taken out and the flap replaces the scar.

Dermabrasion and ablative lasers can be used to smooth out irregular margins of scars and blend them into surrounding area. Care should be taken not to overtreat with these, as there may be excessive scarring.

Steroids are sometimes used intralcisionally to treat thick, bulky scars. Overdosing may cause hypopigmentation and atrophy.

DEALING WITH KELOIDS AND HYPERTROPHIED SCAR

Besides dealing with scars, the cosmetic surgeon also has to deal with keloids and hypertrophied scar. When there is excessive local tissue response to injury it causes an irregular deposition of extra-cellular matrix and collagen and causes a hypertrophied scar or keloid to develop.

Keloids can occur in all skin types but is seen most in dark-skinned people with a family history. It appears mostly on areas with high skin tension like anterior chest, upper back and deltoid areas. Postsurgical skin tension can be a cause in keloid formation. Endocrine factors may also contribute to keloid formation. Melanocyte-stimulating hormone has been said to contribute to keloid formation.

It is difficult to treat keloids and hypertrophied scars as there are no definitive treatment protocols which could ensure that it will disappear or not recur. Some treatment options available are:

Silicone gel or sheeting

When applied for 8–9 hours for 2 months reduction in size can occur up to 30%. It lightens hypertrophied scars and reduces erythema. The mechanism of action is not clear.

Compression therapy

Applying pressure causes reduction in soft tissue celllularity. It can be applied by tight dressing or garment or pressure ear rings in case of ear lobule. If worn for 24 hours for at least 6 months it gives a good result. Caution must be taken that it doesn't cause necrosis of tissues due to excess pressure.

Intralesional steroids

It is used frequently to treat keloids and hypertrophied scars. The response rate is quite good. Corticosteroids are injected into the lesion and this can be used as monotherapy or postsurgically after removal of keloid.

Surgery

Surgery alone has a recurrence rate of 50–90% and should be done very selectively. It usually depends on size, shape and location of the keloid. Large keloids on the jaw, neck and anterior chest can cause dysfunction as patient has difficulty turning head, or to extend or flex neck. These lesions are excised partially to improve mobility and high doses of corticosteroids injected to intentionally cause atrophy of scar tissue.

Keloids in the ear lobule are very common and we ENT surgeons get to deal with it a lot. It is seen in 4 different shapes – anterior and posterior buttons, wraparound, dumbbell, and lobular. Button keloids can be shaved off completely but leaves very little lobule tissue. Dumbbell keloids have a component within the lobe that must be removed. Wraparound and lobular keloids usually require wedge excision of the entire keloid and closed primarily (Fig. 26.6). In all cases, as much keloid material possible is removed and dermis should be kept intact. Closure should not be too tight using monofilament sutures. I/L steroids are given post-operatively at 3–4 weeks interval for at least 3 months.

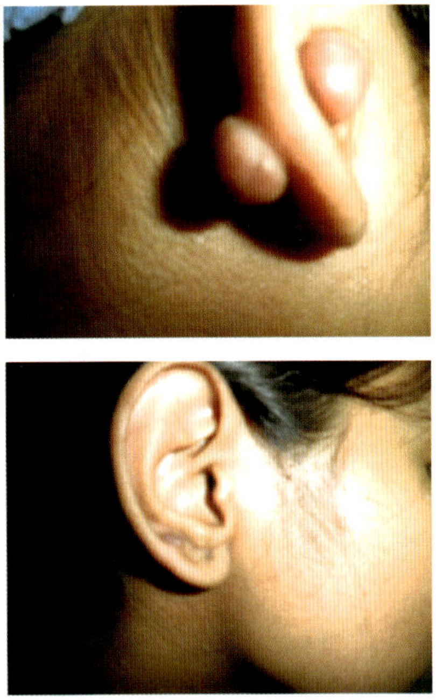

Fig. 26.6. Ear lobule keloid treated by surgery.

Radiation therapy

In radiation therapy, up to 400–2000 rads is used in some cases. The results are debatable.

Laser surgery

Using CO_2 laser, argon laser, or pulse dye laser for keloid excision is not very popular.

It is seen that although keloids are hard to treat, if surgery and I/L steroids along with compression is applied, the best result is seen.

THE AGING FACE

Rejuvenation of the aging face can be done in many ways. These include surgical as well as non-surgical procedures.

The surgical procedures include blepharoplasty, facelift, rhinoplasty, brow lift, liposuction just to name a few.

Non-surgical techniques include botox injection, fillers, lipoinjection, lasers, etc.

BLEPHAROPLASTY

Blepharoplasty is a popular surgical procedure when dealing with the aging face. Swollen puffy eyelids and bagginess under the eyes gives a person a tired and older look. Blepharoplasties can achieve aesthetic improvement of the periocular face.

Applied anatomy

A surgeon performing blepharoplasty should have thorough understanding of the surgical anatomy of the eyebrow and eyelids.

Fig. 26.7 demonstrates certain sectional anatomic structures of the upper and lower lids. The inferior oblique and inferior rectus should be identified as these can be injured during lower lid blepharoplasty. Beneath the skin lies the orbicularis muscle, deep to this above the crease line lies the orbital septum. Posterior to the septum lies the preaponeurotic orbital fat. There are two main fat pads in the upper eyelid (Fig. 26.8). It is important to distinguish the lacrimal gland from orbital fat.

The lower eyelid skin crease lies approximately 4–5 mm below eyelid margin. The lateral canthal angle is 1.5 mm higher than the medial canthal angle. In the lower lid the orbicularis muscle is immediately deep to the skin of lower lid. Deep to the orbicularis occuli muscle like in the upper lid lies the orbital septum which retains the orbital fat. There are three compartments of fat in the lower lid.

Pathophysiology

The changes seen in both upper and lower eyelids are similar to normal aging changes of the skin. There is thinning of the epidermal tissue with loss of elastin, resulting in laxity and hypertrophy of the skin. Repeated facial expressions combined with effect of gravity also contribute to the changes.

Indication

1. To remove an appropriate amount of excess skin and muscle in both upper and lower lids.

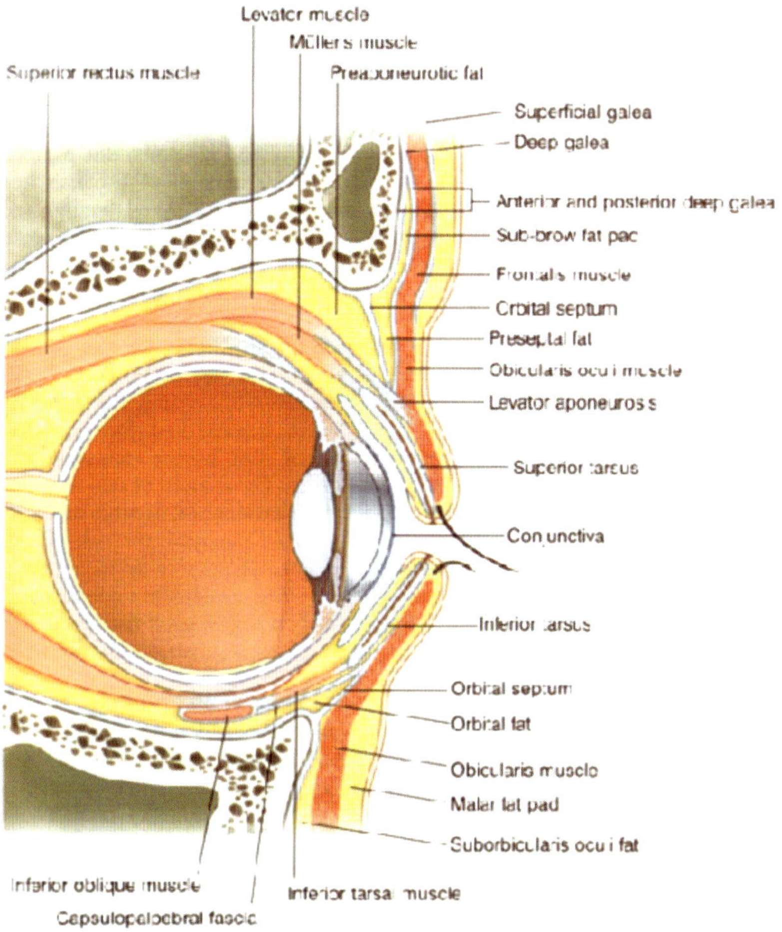

Fig. 26.7. Cross-sectional anatomy of upper and lower eyelid.

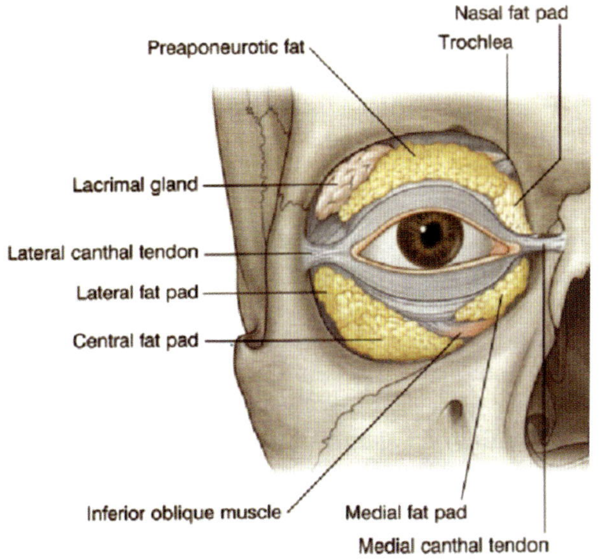

Fig. 26.8. Upper and lower eyelid fat pads and tendons.

2. To remove orbital fat where appropriate.
3. To create a symmetrical upper lid skin crease at an appropriate height.
4. In cases where there is excess upper eyelid skin causing a loss of superior visual fields.
5. In cases of dark circles under the eyes, skin wrinkles and malar bags.

Upper lid blepharoplasty

The degree of eyelid laxity is assessed and measured. The upper lid skin crease is marked. Both eyelids should be marked simultaneously so that there is symmetry. The skin centrally above the crease is gently pulled with fine toothed forceps. The superior aspect of pinched skin is marked in an ellipse. In women, the planned incision is approx. 8–10 mm above the lash line. It is divided into 3 parts to maintain good aesthetic appearance (8 mm medially, 10 mm centrally, and 9 mm laterally), and 10–15 mm below the eyebrows. In men, the excision

26

should be 6–8 mm above lash line and 15–20 mm below the eyebrow. Any temptation to remove more than 10 mm of skin should be resisted.

The procedure can be done under local or general anesthesia.

Surgical procedure

Using a surgical blade, electrosurgical needle or CO_2 laser, the skin and underlying orbicularis occuli are incised. A myocutaneous flap is dissected off the orbital septum. If no fat needs to be extracted then skin closure is performed by 7.0 vicryl by continuous or interrupted stitches. If the fat needs to be removed then the orbital septum needs to be opened along the entire length. Fat is excised making sure proper haemostasis is done. Skin closure is done by 7.0 vicryl.

Lower lid blepharoplasty

Lower lid blepharoplasty can be performed alone or in combination with upper lid surgery. It can be done by a transcutaneous approach as well as trans-conjunctival route. The surgical approach selected depends upon proper assessment of the patient. For patients who only have excess fat, the conjunctival approach is best as it does not leave any external scars. For the rest the transcutaneous route is preferred.

Lid laxity should be tested. Distraction test is performed by pulling the lower lid anteriorly from the globe, if there is more than 6–8 mm distraction then here is indication for surgery, also if the skin is pulled down and it does not go back to normal position within the next blink then laxity is present.

The procedure can be done by local or general anesthesia.

Transconjunctival approach

Corneal shields are used to protect the eyeball. Conjunctival incision is placed 2–3 mm below the inferior tarsal edge, and will run lateral to medial. The plane between the orbicularis and septum is entered. Dissection along this plane is done to the level of inferior orbital rim, and then the septum is opened. The septum is entered and fat pads identified and extracted ensuring haemostasis. The conjunctival edges can be left open or sutured with 7.0/8.0 vicryl.

Transcutaneous approach

A subcilliary incision is made 1–3 mm below the eyelid margin to avoid damage to the eyelid follicles. It extends from the medial punctum in a curved manner to beyond the lateral canthus. Skin and orbicularis muscle are incised and dissected up to orbital rim. Orbital septum is opened and fat pad identified. After removal of fat the skin and muscle flap are draped across lid margin in a manner to avoid tension. The excess skin and muscle are excised, closure is with 7.0 vicryl.

Postoperative care

Compressive bandage for 30 minutes post-operatively will prevent oozing. Ice-pack can be applied to reduce swelling and bruising.

Complications

The following complications may arise:

- Complications due to anesthesia
- Haemorrhage
- Lower eyelid retraction
- Lower eyelid ectropion
- Rounding of the lateral canthus,
- Hollowing of eyelids – asymmetry of lid creases
- Epiphora, diplopia
- Chemosis, corneal abrasion.

Blepharoplasty is a very successful surgery in the management of rejuvenation of the upper face, especially if done in conjunction with other procedures.

FACELIFT

Facial aging although a natural process is sometimes hard to accept, new procedures are developed everyday to counter this process. It has progressed with modern medicine to the stage it is today.

Applied anatomy

Understanding of the facial anatomy specially that related to the SMAS (superficial musculoapo-neurotic system) and its retaining ligaments, the platysma, superficial muscle of expression and motor nerve branches is essential. The SMAS is a complex mesenchymal tissue system that is most broadly defined as the superficial muscles of facial expression, fascial planes continuous with these muscles, and the myrad septal attachments between these fascial planes and the dermis. In most parts of the face the SMAS lies just deep to the subcutaneous fat. The SMAS includes the platysma in the neck and a robust fascia in the lateral cheek area. It is attached to the dermis above and bone below via two distinct ligaments – the zygomatic and mandibular ligaments. There are also several other ligaments attached between SMAS and dermis, like in the masseteric, preauricular, and infraauricular areas (Fig. 26.9). These are surrounded by perforating vessels and sensory nerve branches, and may bleed during dissection.

The most important structure at risk of damage during facelift surgery is the facial nerve (Fig. 26.10). Inferior to the zygomatic arch the facial nerve branches travel below the SMAS. In a typical facelift undermining is done superficial to the SMAS, so the branches are protected. Within the superior temporal fascia and above the zygomatic arch lies the temporal branch of facial nerve, which can be injured during dissection in this area.

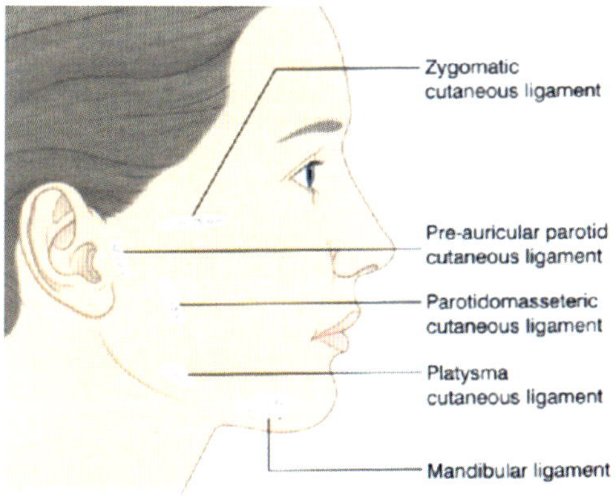

Fig. 26.9. Facial retaining ligaments.

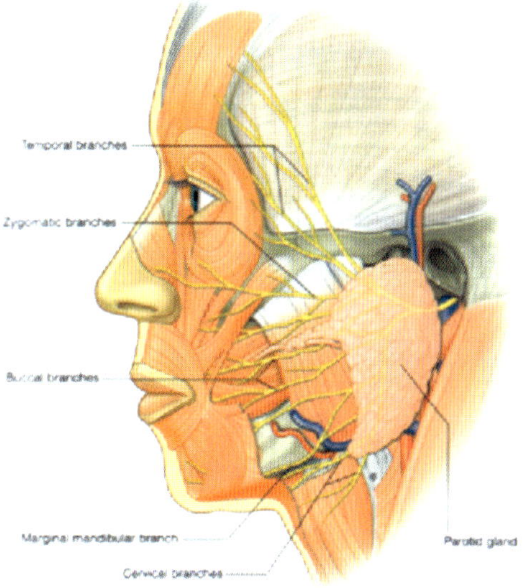

Fig. 26.10. Branches of facial nerves.

Pathophysiology

Facial aging involves both intrinsic and extrinsic mechanism. Intrinsic aging involves atrophy of the facial skin and subcutaneous fat, as well as changes in the facial skeleton. There are significant changes in the density of keratinocytes and melanocytes in the epidermis, which causes thinning and abnormal pigmentation of skin. Gravity plays a role in manifesting the sagging of soft tissues specially those of the musculoaponeurotic system.

Extrinsic factors include skin damage due to sun exposure also known as photoaging. This causes disorganization of dead elastic tissue fibres which contribute to further wrinkling.

Indication

This mainly depends on patients' complaints. Usually they will complain of early signs of aging, sagging of facial skin and prominence of nasolabial folds.

The procedure is usually done under general anesthesia. Preoperative preparation has to be taken accordingly.

Technique

Facelift operations involve undermining along one or more tissue planes of the face and neck and the resuspension of tissue planes to reverse gravitational sagging. The most superficial plane is subcutaneous (supra-SMAS), the next level is sub-SMAS, and deeper still is subperiosteal dissection. This includes release of deep retaining ligaments that bind the SMAS to the dermis, and gives the flap better mobility.

A S-shaped skin incision starting from the temporal hairline downwards along preauricular crease up to the root of lobule and upwards and backwards onto the postauricular area is given. Raising of the flap starts at the postauricular area in an avascular plane and continues up to neck in the supraplatysmal plane. The preauricular flap is raised up to nasolabial folds approximately 7–9 cm in radius from the tragus. It continues along the jaw line and neck. Dissection in the neck should be in subcutaneous plane. SMAS is identified and a horizontal incision is made along zygomatic arch and connects to a vertical limb coursing 2 cm anterior to the tragus. SMAS flap is elevated approximately 3–5 cm and pulled in a superior and slight posterior direction. A triangular segment of

SMAS is excised and then sutured to the dense fibrous tissue at inferior margin of zygomatic arch. After that, the skin flap is draped over face and preauricular area and pulled superiorly and slightly posteriorly. In all steps proper haemostasis needs to be ensured. After careful measurement excess skin is excised. Closure is with 5/0 prolene. Compression by head band is applied over the bandage and kept for at least 3 days.

Postoperative care

Analgesics and antibiotics are prescribed for 7 days. Sutures are removed after 7–10 days of surgery. Swelling and bruising will take several weeks to disappear.

Complications

- Haemorrhage or haematoma formation.
- Overexcision of skin flap resulting in tight skin closure – so-called mask-like face.
- 'Pixie ear' deformity.
- Asymmetry of both sides.
- Infection of the operative area.
- Flap necrosis.
- Facial nerve palsy.

Facelift operation can be a very rewarding surgery and makes a person look at least 5–8 years younger than before.

RHINOPLASTY

As ENT surgeons we are very familiar with this procedure, so we will not elaborate on it. Mostly we do reconstructive rhinoplasty in our regular practice. There is a huge demand for aesthetic rhinoplasty even here in the Indian subcontinent. The types of aesthetic rhinoplasty that can be done are augmentation, reduction, tip-plasty, and alar base reduction. Usually one or two procedures need to be combined to get good aesthetic result (Fig. 26.11).

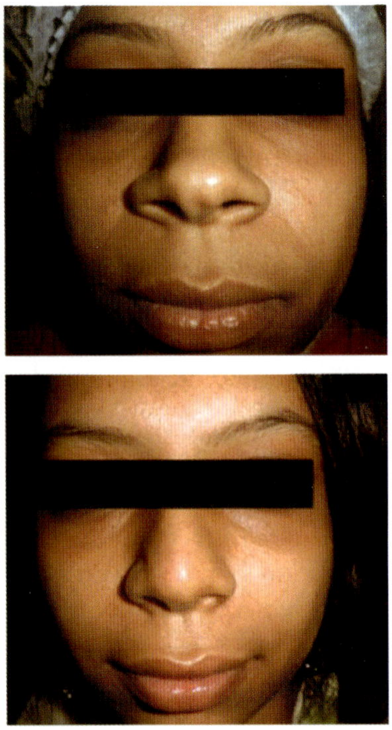

Fig. 26.11. Aesthetic rhinoplasty – tip plasty with ABR.

LIPOSUCTION/LIPOSCULPTING IN THE HEAD-NECK AREA

Sometimes we see that there is excess fat accumulation in the neck, submental and jowl area. This is due to many factors including ptosis of fatty tissue in the elderly and also accumulation of fat in the young overweight patient. Evaluation of the patient should be done carefully; the ideal candidate is one who has good skin elasticity, full jowl and palpable submental fat pad (Fig. 26.12).

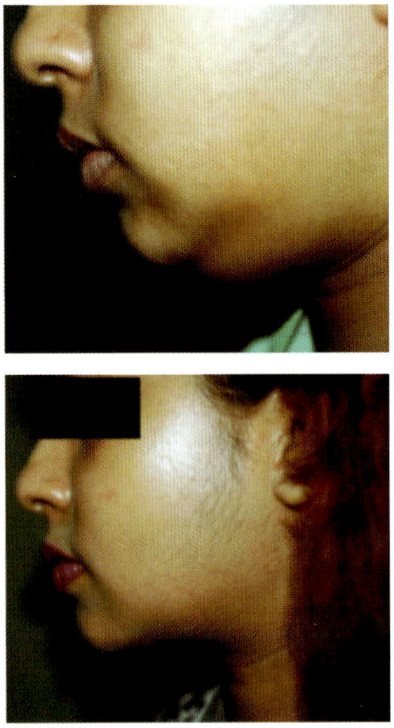

Fig. 26.12. Liposuction of double chin.

Positioning of the patient is done with head gently extended posteriorly, and the chin raised with a supportive small pillow for neck support. Tumescent fluid is infused into the area to be suctioned. It is ideal to wait for 20 minutes as this allows proper vasoconstriction, anesthesia, and diffusion of tumescent fluid. Entry site is placed in the submental crease, additional points may be needed if excessive fat pads are present in the neck area. Suctioning is done using small cannulae. Care should be taken to avoid injury to the marginal mandibular branch of facial nerve, which drops below the angle of the mandible. Oversuctioning should be avoided as it will cause dimpling and depressions. A compression bandage has to be applied for a few days.

Heavyness of the jowl area can make a person look older and heavy. Recontouring this area is done by removal of buccal fat. This can be done externally or intraorally. It is easier if done by intraoral route unless patient is also opting for mini-facelift. Intraorally an incision is made along the upper gum border against 2nd and 3rd molars and buccal space is opened. Fat is identified and extracted. Wound is closed by using 4/0 vicryl or catgut.

NON-SURGICAL PROCEDURES OF THE AGING FACE

Lipoinjection

The use of fat as a filler is becoming popular day-by-day. It is not only used as a corrective technique for soft tissue defects and rhytids but also to correct atrophy due to aging process. It is specially ideal for use on face and neck area as not large amounts are needed. Defects like tear-trough deformity, depressed perioral regions, prominent nasolabial folds can be corrected (Fig. 26.13), also augmentation of lips and other areas can be done. Proper patient counselling is to be done to explain that this is not a permanent method and touch ups may be needed after some time.

Fat can be harvested from thigh, buttocks, knee, and lower abdomen. Gentle suctioning has to be done, so as not to damage the fat cells and their viability. After injecting with tumescent fluid syringe aspiration using a small cannulae with low negative pressure is most often recommended. Not much fat is needed in the facial region so 10 ml syringe can be used. Harvested fat is centrifuged at 3500 r.p.m. for 5–7 minutes to separate the fluid portion and fat. The fluid portion is discarded and the concentrated fat is ready for use. Now a days PRP platelet-rich plasma is mixed with the fat and then injected into the recipient site. PRP is believed to increase the viability of the fat cells by releasing growth factors present in the plasma. Taking blood from the patient and adding coagulating factors and then leaving upright for about half an hour can prepare PRP. Then the plasma along with the buffy coat is taken and centrifuged for 5 minutes. The lower portion of fluid is taken and mixed with the harvested fat. After marking and preparing the area by undermining at subcutaneous level, syringe with blunt tipped cannulae of about 14–25 gauge is used to inject the fat under low pressure.

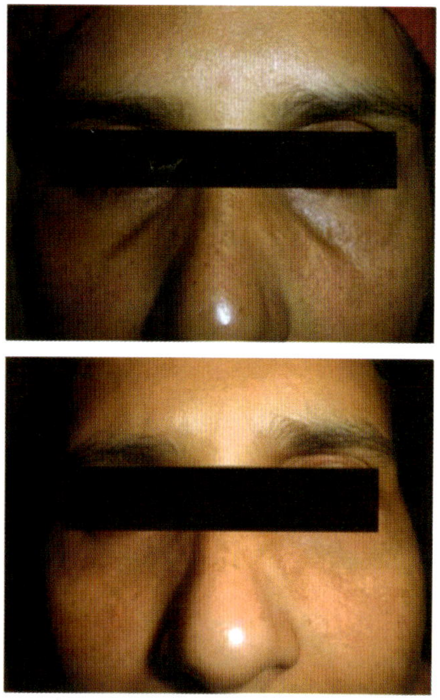

Fig. 26.13. Lipoinjection with PRP for tear-trough deformity.

Injectable fillers

Soft tissue augmentation has become a popular means of addressing volume loss and contour defects that result from ageing, photodamage, trauma and/or scarification and disease. Dozens of filling agents (Table 26.1) now exist in our armamentarium with varying degrees of durability and viscosity. The fillers are injected into areas where there is a filling defect. No anaesthesia is required and the injection can be given as an office procedure.

Botulinum toxin

Also known as Botox injection, it is a very popular procedure used for rejuvenation of the face and neck. It is routinely used as a remedy for wrinkle

Table 26.1

Product	*Trade/Brand Name*
Dermal fillers	
Superficial/mid-dermis	Cosmoderm I
	Zyderm I
Mid-dermis	Autologen (Cosmoderm II)
	Hylaform
	Restylane
	Zyderm II
Deep dermis	Artecoll
	Cosmoplast
	Dermalive
	Hylaform Plus
	Perlane
	Reviderm Intra
	Zyplast
Versatile dermal levels	Fascian
	Hylan Rofilan Gel
	Isolagen
	Juvederm 18, 24, 30
Subdermal fillers	Cymetra
	Radiesse (calcium hydroxyl-apatite)
	Dermadeep
	New-Fill/Sculptra
Subdermal implants	Advanta
	Alloderm
	Gore-Tex
	Softform/Ultrasoft
	Autologous grafts (fat, dermis, dermis-fat, tendon, scar, fascia)

lines on the upper, middle and lower face and neck. It is a neurotoxin produced by *Clostridium botulinum*. It acts by selectively blocking the release of acetyl-choline causing prolonged transitory muscle paralysis. When used at recommended doses it does not induce systemic clinical effects.

The product is freeze-dried and should be stored at 2–8 degree Celsius. The injection is prepared with sterile, non-preserved 0.9% saline solution.

26

The areas to be injected are cleaned and the points marked. It can be used for forehead wrinkles, crow's feet, glabellar folds, perioral rhydids, and chin area and necklace line. Units injected depend on the concentration of the solution. No injection should be given within 1 cm above the central bony orbital rim as it causes ectropion, diplopia, upper lid ptosis, or drooping lateral lower lid. In the lower face injection should be low dose and not too close to the mouth area as there may be drooling, incompetent mouth and asymmetry. Manipulation of the area should be minimal for at least a few hours.

Thread facelift

Correction of facial ptosis with threads is a minimally invasive procedure that can be done in the early stages of change. It can be done for soft tissue lifting including mandibular/submandibular ptosis, and eyebrow ptosis. These threads are composed of polypropylene and have multiple microhooks. The hooks are oriented in opposite direction on both halves. This helps the thread to anchor itself in tissues and then lifting it. Local anesthesia is used. The thread is placed by a 16–20 gauge flexible metal cannula in the subcutaneous plane according to marking. The cannula is with-drawn leaving thread in place. The remainder of thread is cut off. There is almost no swelling or bruising over the area. Fibrosis occurs in around 4–6 weeks. Complications are rare accept there may be asymmetry between both sides. Now-a-days absorbable threads (PDS) with atraumatic needles are available which makes them less traumatic to the tissue and easier to handle.

Chemical peels, microdermabrasion, CO_2 ablation, and NdYag laser according to need can also help in rejuvenation of the face. These can be done in combination with other procedures to give better results.

ACKNOWLEDGEMENT

Pictures are courtesy of Cosmetic Surgery Centre Ltd., Dhaka, Bangladesh.

CONCLUSION

Facial plastic surgery is concerned with improving the appearance and function of facial structures. Scar revision, laser surgery, blepharoplasty, face lift, rhinoplasty, liposuction in head and neck area, lipo injection, injecting fillers like botulinum toxin and thread face procedure are discussed. A variety of injections are used to reduce lines and wrinkles on the face to enhance the appearance. Chemical peels, microdermabrasion, CO_2 ablation, and NdYag laser according to the need can also help in rejuvenation of the face. These can be done in combination with other procedures to give better results.

SUGGESTED READING

1. Weerda, H. Reconstructive Facial Plastic Surgery, 1st Edition, Thieme, Stuttgart-New York, 2001.
2. Robinson JK, Hanke CW, Senglemann RD and Siegel DM (Editors): Surgery of the Skin – Procedural Dermatology, 1st Edition, Elsevier Mosby, 2005.

3. Gleeson M et al. (editors): Scott-Brown's Otorhinolaryngology, Head and Neck Surgery, 7th Edition, Vol 3, Hodder-Arnold, UK, 2008.
4. Furnas DW. "The Retaining Ligament of the Cheek", *Plast Reconstr Surg*, 1989; 83: 11–6.
5. Stucker F, Shaw G. An approach to management of keloids. *Arch Otolaryngol Head Neck Surg*, 1992; 118: 63–67
6. Levine MR. Manual of oculoplastic surgery. Philadelphia: Butterworth Heinemann; 2003
7. Siddiky SA, Minu FQ. Rejuvenation of the Aging face. Vol. 1, p. 50, Dec. 2009.
8. Roberta D Senglemann, Stacey T, Sheldon V Pollack. Soft tissue augmentation, Surgery of the Skin, *Procedural Dermatol*, 2005; 28: 440
9. Meunier FA, Schiavo G, Molgo J. Botulinum neurotoxins: From paralysis to recovery of functional neuromuscular transmission. *J Physiol Paris*, 2002; 96: 105–13.

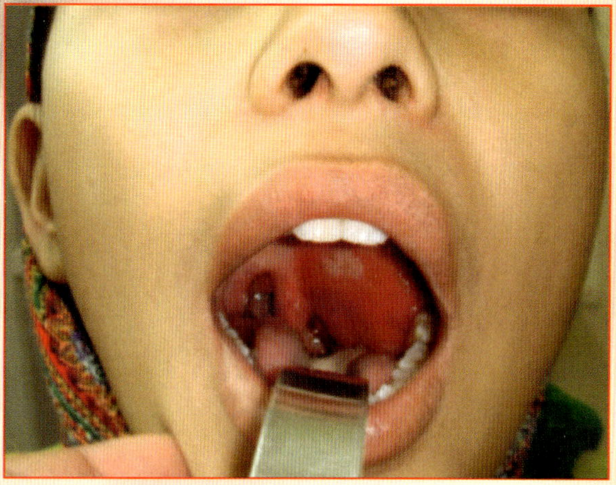

SECTION 4

Oropharynx and Esophagus

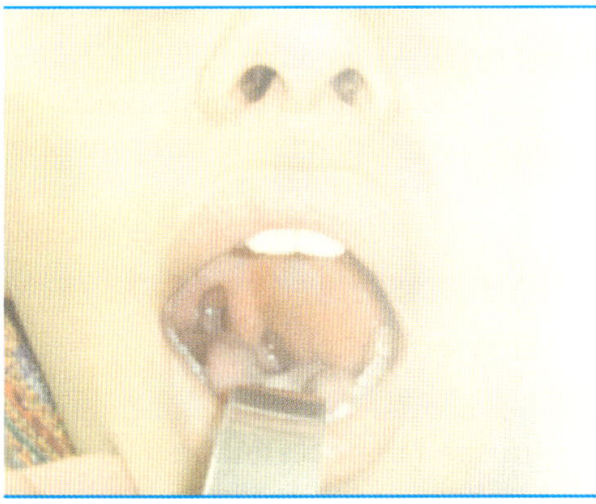

CHAPTER 27

Diseases of Tonsils

Anil K. Monga, Rajeev Gupta

The word tonsil actually derives from Latin word tonsilla meaning a mooring post. There are three such structures. They are: palatine or faucial tonsils between the palatopharyngeus and palatoglossus muscles; lingual tonsils one on each side between base of tongue and valleculla; and single naso-pharyngeal tonsil named adenoids in the roof of nasopharynx. In practice the word tonsil refers exclusively to the palatine tonsils. In the following description we shall follow the same nomenclature. This chapter is specifically included because of the fact that tonsillar diseases are so common that every otorhinolaryngologists encounter and treat them. Further tonsillectomy may not make your reputation but it can definitely mar your reputation as a surgeon in the city.

Embryology

The second branchial pouch is visible in the 4th post-conceptional week and demonstrates canalization and branching in the 8th week. The pharyngeal tonsils arise as aggregation of mesenchymal cells which later are invaded by lymphocytes which arise in situ or are derived from blood stream. The ventral pouch of second arch is almost completely obliterated by proliferation of endodermal lining later invaded by mesodermal tissue to form primordium of palatine tonsils. Unobliterated part persists as intratonsillar cleft. Lymphoid infiltration of the lamina propria occurs in the seventh month of intra-uterine life. Primary follicles form late in gestation, but germinal center stimulation does not occur until shortly after birth. During the first year of life, there is rapid proliferation of lymphoid elements and formation of active germinal centers. During the phase of maximum tonsillar hyperplasia, the lymphoid elements proliferate rapidly, increasing tonsillar bulk.

Gross anatomy

A ring of lymphoid tissue surrounds the naso-pharynx and oro-pharynx. These lymphoid tissues are collectively known as the Waldayer's ring which has two components, namely the inner and outer rings. The cervical lymph nodes constitute the outer ring, while the inner ring is constituted by:

(a) adenoids at the roof of nasopharynx;

(b) tubal tonsils or tonsil of Gerlac (part of adenoids) which surround the pharyngeal ends of eustachean tube.

These lymphoid tissues surround the nasopharynx.

The lymphoid tissues surrounding the oropharynx also constituting the components of the inner Waldayer's ring are:

1. Lingual tonsil in the posterior 1/3 of the tongue,
2. Palatine tonsils on either side of oro pharynx, and
3. Subepithelial lymphoid tissue found in the posterior pharyngeal wall. All these structures of the inner Waldayer's ring are interlinked.

The faucial tonsils are the largest and most important moieties of the inner ring of lymphoid tissue. The medial surface of the tonsil is free and faces the oropharynx. It is covered by non-keratinizing stratified squamous epithelium which is continuous with that of the lining of the oropharynx The mucosa covering the palatine tonsils is thrown into numerous crypts about 18–20 in each tonsil. These crypts serve to increase the surface area of mucosa covering the tonsil. These crypts can harbor pus and microorganisms. Clothing the lateral two-thirds of each tonsil is the capsule, a well-defined structure composed of fibrous and elastic tissue, and muscle fibers. The medial third of the tonsil lies between the pillars of the fauces and, being bereft of covering, is accessible to clinical examination.

Tonsil lies in a triangular space, bounded by the anterior and posterior pillars of the fauces and the tongue.

The tonsillar bed is formed by four thin sheets of which two are areolar & two fleshy. From within outwards they are:

1. Pharyngobasillar fascia
2. Palatopharyngeus
3. Superior constrictor. Both of which are deficient below
4. Buccopharyngeal fascia

The glossopharyngeal nerve and the stylohyoid ligament pass downwards and forwards beneath the lower edge of the superior constrictor in the lower part of the tonsillar fossa

Attachments of the tonsil

The tonsils are continually exposed to forces tending to dislodge them, and to resist these forces appropriate attachments are developed. Every time swallowing occurs, a powerful downward and backward pull is exerted on the tonsil as they lie within the grasp of the pharyngeal constrictors. To counteract this force there are two attachments, one fibrous and one muscular. The first is a band of fibrous tissue connecting the capsule of the anterior angle of the tonsil to the base of the tongue, where it blends with the muscle sheaths. This fibrous 'suspensory ligament' is always present, and as might be expected is most marked in large and prominent tonsils

The second anchorage is the insertion of the decussating fibers of the palatoglossus and palatopharyngeus muscles into the lower third of the tonsillar capsule. This is not a mere adherence, but a definite insertion with the object of lifting the tonsil up past the descending bolus as the soft palate rises in the act of swallowing. This action may have some importance in the production of mouth breathing in children, in many of whom the tonsils are so large that an airway in the pharynx can only be obtained when the tonsils are lifted by contracting the soft palate, at the price of shutting off the nasal airway.

Blood supply of the tonsil

The tonsil has an exceptionally good blood supply. It is well to bear in mind that a tortuous facial artery may be closely related to the lower pole. A vein unaccompanied by an artery – the paratonsillar vein – is often a source of serious venous bleeding following tonsillectomy. When divided, the bleeding end retracts into the upper part of the tonsillar fossa, and must be found and ligated before the patient leaves the theatre.

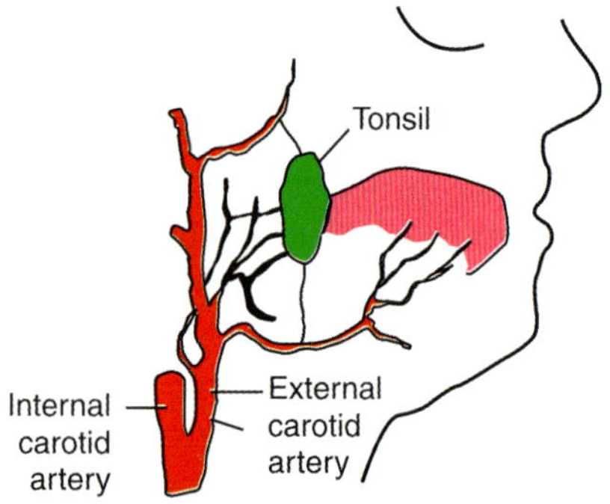

Fig. 27.1. Blood supply of tonsil.

The traditional description of the blood supply is that it comes from half a dozen arteries, and that on the deep surface there is a peritonsillar venous plexus. It is believed that the tonsil is supplied like an ordinary lymphatic gland, from a single artery entering a definite hilum, from which the veins emerge. In this case the hilum is always in the lower part of the buried surface close to the tongue, The main artery of the tonsil is the tonsillar branch of the facial artery which enters the tonsil near its lower pole by piercing the superior constrictor just above the styloglossus muscle. Other arteries supplying the tonsil are lingual artery through its dorsal lingual branches, ascending palatine branch of facial artery, and ascending pharyngeal vessels.

The other tonsillar arteries described ramify in the muscles and mucous membrane round about,

27

but do not pierce the capsule. There are usually two veins, which run out from the hilum through the superior constrictor close to where the artery passes through it, to end in the common facial trunk. In consequence of this arrangement of the blood vessels the tonsil may be separated over two-thirds of its buried surface during tonsillectomy for the loss of only a few drops of blood. When the hilum is divided the artery may spurt freely, but then like all arteries of that size, it quickly retracts and stops bleeding. The veins are very small and never allow any considerable backflow of blood.

(Where then does the bleeding, that is often so free and occasionally so dangerous, come from? The dangerous vessel is a vein, inconstant in its course and form as the lesser veins tend to be, which runs down from the soft palate in the areolar tissue between the capsule of the tonsil and the muscles of its bed. Below, it pierces the superior constrictor near the hilum, and enters the common facial vein. This vein is very variable: it may take the form of several small trunks, it may run in the muscles of the tonsillar bed, or it may be absent altogether. But in its most dangerous form it is a large, single trunk running close to the capsule and often adherent to it. When the tonsil is dragged out it appears to a casual glance to be running into it, and has been so described.)

Nerves of the tonsil

The glossopharyngeal nerve is only separated from the lower pole of the tonsil by a thin layer of superior constrictor fibers, and the plexus which it forms with the palatine branches of the sphenopalatine ganglion gives off some surprisingly large filaments which enter the hilum. The glossopharyngeal nerve passes downward medially and forward in the tonsillar bed. It is probably through Jacobson's nerve that the referred pain in the ear after tonsillectomy arises.

Mucous glands near the tonsil

There is a very constant small group of mucous glands on the anterior surface of the upper angle pole of the tonsil. They are adherent to the capsule on their deep surfaces, and have their ducts discharging through the mucous membrane of the anterior pillar, so that they always cause a slight difficulty in separating the tonsil at this point. It has been suggested that their removal may cause the feeling of dryness in the throat that occasionally follows tonsillectomy, but this is difficult to believe when one considers the numbers of similar glands close by.

Surgical application of these points

This is obvious. The "suspensory ligament" may be divided early in the operation, thus doing away with the main anchorage of the tonsil without increasing the bleeding. It is of importance also in that when a piece of tonsil is left behind by the guillotine, its center is almost invariably the part of the capsule fixed by this inextensible band. The "paratonsillar vein", if it should be cut, retracts into the upper angle of the tonsillar bed, where it may be caught and ligatured.

Functions of palatine tonsils

Local immunity

Tonsillar B cells can mature to produce all the five major Ig classes. They produce specific antibodies against diphtheria toxoid, poliovirus, Streptococcus pneumoniae, Haemophilus influenzae, Staphylococcus aureus, and the lipopolysaccharide of *E. coli.*

In addition to humoral immunity elicited by tonsillar and adenoidal B cells following antigenic stimulation, there is considerable T-cell response in palatine tonsils. Thus, natural infection or intranasal immunization with live, attenuated rubella virus vaccine has been reported to prime tonsillar lymphocytes much better than subcutaneous vaccination. Also, natural infection with varicella zoster virus has been found to stimulate tonsillar lymphocytes better than lymphocytes from peripheral blood.

Combined tonsillectomy and adenoidectomy had a profound detrimental effect on the local IgA response in the nasopharyngeal fluid against poliovirus. These immunological observations paralleled the increased incidence of paralytic poliomyelitis after this operation. Thus, it is obvious that the tonsil have an important role to play in the defense of the host against bacterial and viral infections,

Altogether, therefore, several pieces of direct and indirect evidence indicate that the palatine tonsils are continuously engaged in local immune responses to microorganisms. If the tonsillar lymphocytes became overwhelmed with this persistent stimulation they may be unable to respond to other antigens; the immunological response, particularly in recurrent tonsillitis, may then be impaired. Once this immunological impairment occurs, the tonsil is no longer able to function adequately in local protection nor can it appropriately reinforce the secretory immune system of the upper respiratory tract.

DISEASES OF TONSILS

The pathogenesis of infectious/inflammatory disease in the tonsils most likely has its basis in their anatomic location and their inherent function as organ of immunity, processing infectious material, and other antigens and then becoming, paradoxically, a focus of infection/inflammation. No single theory of pathogenesis has yet been accepted, however. Viral infection with secondary bacterial invasion may be one mechanism of the initiation of chronic disease, but the effects of the environment, host factors, the widespread use of antibiotics, ecological considerations, and diet all may play a role.

Acute tonsillitis

Tonsillitis is the inflammation of tonsils. Acute tonsillitis is the most common manifestation of tonsillar disease. It may be bacterial or viral in nature.

The most common causes of tonsillitis are the common cold viruses (adenovirus, rhinovirus, influenza, coronavirus, respiratory syncytial virus). It can also be caused by Epstein-Barr virus, herpes simplex virus, cytomegalovirus, or HIV. The second most common causes are bacterial. The most common bacterial cause is Group A β-hemolytic Streptococcus (GABHS), which causes strep throat. Less common bacterial causes include: Staphylococcus aureus, Streptococcus pneumoniae, Mycoplasma pneumoniae, Chlamydia pneumoniae, pertussis, Fusobacterium, diphtheria, syphilis, and gonorrhea.

Under normal circumstances, as viruses and bacteria enter the body through the nose and mouth, they are filtered in the tonsils. Within the tonsils, white blood cells of the immune system mount an attack that helps destroy the viruses or bacteria, and also causes inflammation and fever. The infection may also be present in the throat and surrounding areas, causing inflammation of the pharynx. Sometimes, tonsillitis is caused by an infection of spirochaeta and treponema, in this case called Vincent's angina or Plaut-Vincent angina.

Acute tonsillitis may present as follicular tonsillitis, coalescent tonsillitis.

Follicullar tonsillitis

The disease usually begins with high temperature and possibly chills, especially in children. The patient complains of a persistent pain in the throat, and pain radiating to the ear on swallowing. Opening the mouth is often difficult and painful, the tongue is coated, and there is a mouth odour. The patient may also complain of headache, thick speech, marked feeling of malaise, as well as swelling and tenderness of the neck glands (lymph nodes). Both tonsils and the surrounding area including the posterior pharyngeal wall are deep red and swollen. Later, whitish spots (follicles) form on the tonsils, hence the name follicular tonsillitis (Fig. 27.2). There is also swelling of the neighboring organs such as the faucial pillars, the uvula, and the base of the tongue. Multiple follicles of whitish exudate cover the tonsils. Ultimately, the follicles coalesce to form a white patch over the tonsils. This is called coalescent acute tonsillitis.

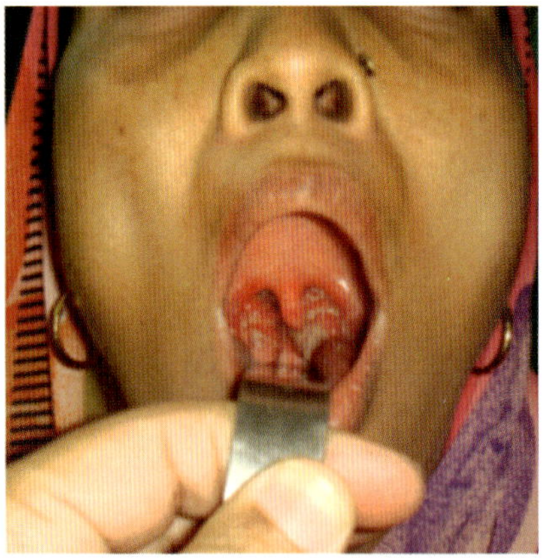

Fig. 27.2. Whitish spots (follicles) on the tonsils.

Bacterial tonsillitis shows higher fever, higher WBC, Granulocytic shift and is more exudative

Viral tonsillitis shows lower grade fever, lower WBC, lymphocytic shift, less tonsillar exudate.

Differential diagnosis

Infectious mononucleosis, EBV, scarlet fever, *Corynebacterium diptheriae*, malignancy.

Recurrent tonsillitis

Recurrent infection has been variably defined as from four to seven episodes of acute tonsillitis in one year, five episodes for two consecutive years or three episodes per year for 3 consecutive years.

Treatment

Treatments to reduce the discomfort from tonsillitis symptoms include:

- Pain relief, anti-inflammatory, fever reducing medications (acetaminophen, ibuprofen but not Aspirin)
- Sore throat relief (salt water gargle, lozenges, warm liquids)

If the tonsillitis is caused by group A Streptococcus, then antibiotics are useful with penicillin or amoxicillin being first line. A macrolide such as erythromycin is used for patients allergic to penicillin. Patients who fail penicillin therapy may respond to treatment effective against beta-lactamase producing bacteria such as clindamycin or amoxicillin-clavulanate. Aerobic and anaerobic beta lactamase producing bacteria that reside in the tonsillar tissues can "shield" group A streptococcus from penicillins. When tonsillitis is caused by a virus, the length of illness depends on which virus is involved. Usually, a complete recovery is made within one week; however may last for up to two weeks. Chronic cases may be treated with tonsillectomy (surgical removal of tonsils) as a choice for treatment.

Complications of acute tonsillitis may be:

Local

Chronic tonsillitis: Incomplete or inadequate antibiotic therapy in case of follicular tonsillitis may result in recurrence. If there are multiple such episodes then the patient may end up with chronic tonsillitis.

Peritonsillar abscess: An abscess may develop lateral to the tonsil during an infection, typically several days after the onset of tonsillitis. This is termed a peritonsillar abscess or quinsy (Fig. 27.3). Rarely, the infection may spread beyond the tonsil resulting in inflammation and infection of the internal jugular vein giving rise to a spreading septicaemia infection (Lemierre's syndrome).

Parapharyngeal abscess: Infection may spread through superior constrictor and pus may form between the muscle and the deep cervical fascia.

Features: Pain in the throat and neck with marked dysphagia. There is toxemia leading to high fever (103–105°C) with or without rigors. There is diffuse tender swelling of neck below angle of mandible.

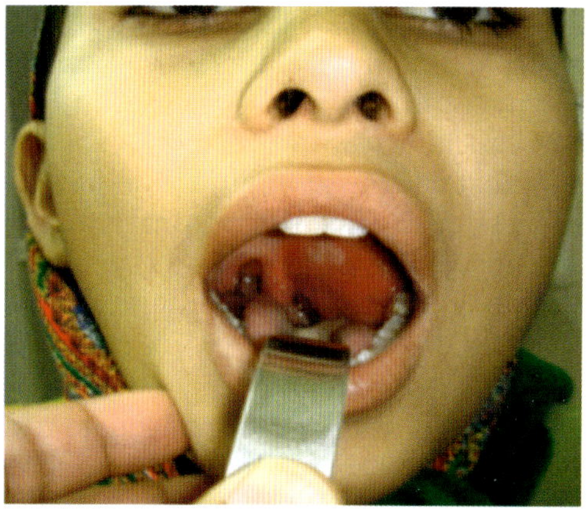

Fig. 27.3. Left side peritonsillar abscess.

There may be apparently visible quinsy or infected tonsil pushed medially.

Treatment. It is a dangerous condition as there is risk of thrombosis in nearby internal jugular vein or necrosis of wall of vein or carotid artery leading to massive fatal haemorrhage. Therefore early external drainage through incision in the neck under adequate injectable antibiotic cover is a must

Systemic

In very rare cases of strep throat, diseases like rheumatic fever or glomerulonephritis can occur. These complications are extremely rare in developed nations but remain a significant problem in poorer nations. Tonsillitis associated with strep throat, if untreated, can also lead to pediatric autoimmune neuropsychiatric disorders associated with streptococcal infections (PANDAS). Tonsilloliths occur in up to 10% of the population frequently due to episodes of tonsillitis. Complications may rarely include dehydration and kidney failure due to difficulty swallowing, blocked airways due to inflammation, and pharyngitis due to the spread of infection.

Chronic tonsillitis

Incomplete or inadequate antibiotic therapy in case of follicular tonsillitis may result in recurrence. If there are multiple such episodes then the patient may end up with chronic tonsillitis. This happens because inflammatory debris gets trapped in the crypts due to fibrous occlusion of openings. Germinal centers become hyperplastic with marked thickening of septa thus there is chronic infection due to lowered resistance.

Clinical features: Bad taste in mouth, halitosis, discomfort in throat. Very large tonsils lead to thick voice, at times difficulty in swallowing and snoring. The most clinching features irrespective of their size are sore throat with history of multiple such attacks. There may be enlargement of regional lymph nodes. In children there may be enlarged mesenteric lymph nodes leading to pain abdomen and episodes of vomiting.

Treatment: As can be understood, chronicity is result of trapped disease and inadequate response to antibiotics. Tonsillectomy remains the only certain cure.

Tonsillar hypertrophy

Tonsillar hypertrophy is the enlargement of the tonsils, but without the history of inflammation (Fig. 27.4). Obstructive tonsillar hypertrophy is currently the most common reason for tonsillectomy. These patients present with varying degrees of disturbed sleep which may include symptoms of loud snoring, irregular breathing, nocturnal choking and coughing, frequent awakenings, sleep apnea, dysphagia and/or daytime hypersomnolence. These may lead to behavioral/mood changes in patients and facilitate the need for a polysomnography in order to determine the degree to which these symptoms are disrupting their sleep. Treatment is partial or complete tonsillectomy.

Peritonsillar abscess (Quinsy)

The clinical picture is that of a rapidly increasing difficulty in swallowing that occurs after a streptococcal tonsillitis (strep throat). The tonsillitis may seem to be improving for a day or two, but then, one side of the throat becomes increasingly painful. The pain is severe and radiates to the ear. Opening the mouth is difficult and so painful that the patient refuses to eat or swallow. There is drooling of saliva and bad breath. The voice is indistinct and muffled It is referred to as "hot potato or plummy voice".

On examination, there is a tense swelling of the soft palate and anterior pillar above the tonsil. The uvula may be displaced to the opposite side. It is often difficult to know at first whether the swelling is an abscess or a peritonsillar cellulitis. In the early

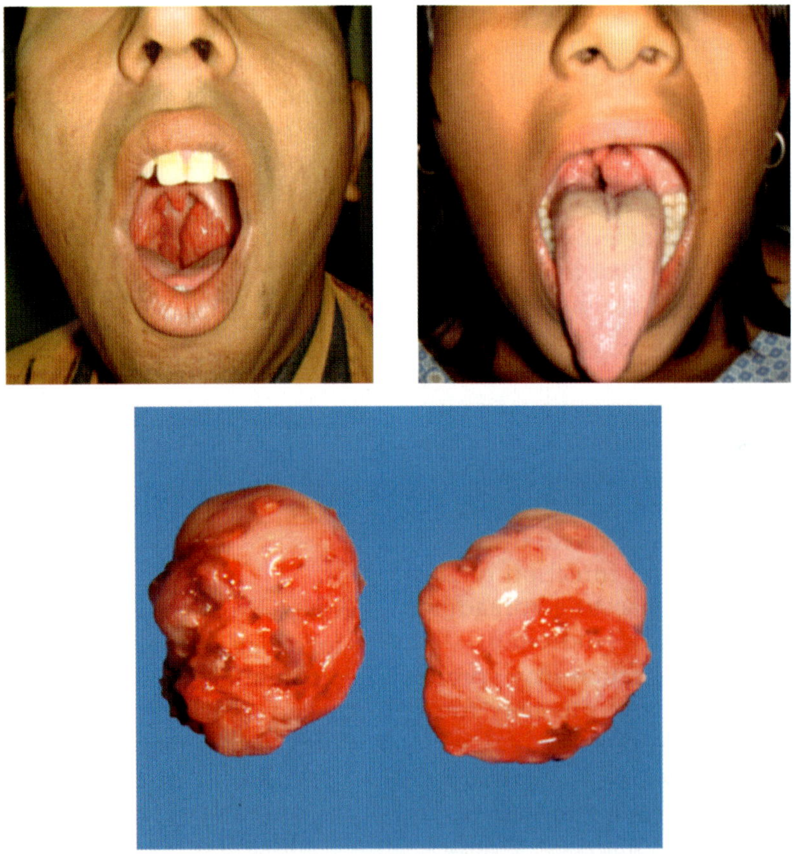

Fig. 27.4A, B & C. Unilateral and bilateral tonsillar hypertrophy and specimen of tonsillectomy.

27

phase the treatment is similar to that of acute tonsillitis. Finally, when the abscess points in the region adjacent to the tonsil, it is incised and drained. Occasionally, the abscess ruptures spontaneously and foul-smelling thick pus drains through a crater in the anterior pillar.

Infectious mononucleosis/glandular fever/ kissing disease

The Epstein-Barr virus, best known for causing infectious mononucleosis, or "kissing disease, " has also been implicated in a number of cancers, particularly among people who have undergone organ transplants. In addition, the virus has been linked to several specific cancers, including nasopharynx cancers, stomach cancers and lymphomas: cancers in the lymphatic system including the spleen, tonsils and thymus.

Epstein-Barr virus is one of the most common human viruses. The virus occurs worldwide, and most people become infected with EBV sometime during their lives. Many children become infected with EBV, and these infections usually cause no symptoms or are indistinguishable from the other mild, brief illnesses of childhood. When infection with EBV occurs during adolescence or young adulthood, it causes infectious mononucleosis 35% to 50% of the time

Clinical features

Symptoms of infectious mononucleosis are fever, sore throat, and swollen lymph glands (Fig. 27.5). Sometimes, a swollen spleen or liver involvement may develop. There may also be tonsillitis, headache, rash, malaise, loss of appetite, jaundice, heart problems or involvement of the central nervous system occurs only rarely, and infectious mononucleosis is almost never fatal. Symptoms usually develop between four to six weeks after exposure to the EBV. In younger children, the symptoms may be more subtle and may additionally include irritability and poor feeding.

Although the symptoms of infectious mononucleosis usually resolve in 1 or 2 months, EBV remains dormant or latent in a few cells in the throat and blood for the rest of the person's life. Periodically, the virus can reactivate and is commonly found in the saliva of infected persons. This reactivation usually occurs without symptoms of illness.

Infectious mononucleosis generally resolves without medical help, though it may last from weeks to months. Treatment is aimed at easing the symptoms of the illness, and it can usually be done at home with plenty of rest, fluids, and over-the-counter medications. Serious complications only rarely occur.

Vincent's angina

It is an acute necrotizing infection of the pharynx caused by a combination of fusiform bacilli (*Bacillus fusiformis* – a Gram -ve bacillus) and spirochetes (*Borrelia vincentii*). These are the same organisms that cause a gingivostomatitis known as "trench mouth".

The patient complains of unilateral sore throat that increases in intensity over several days with an associated referred earache on the same side. In addition, the patient complains of a bad taste in the mouth and a fetid bad breath.

On examination, there is a deep well circumscribed unilateral ulcer of one tonsil (Fig. 27.6). The base of the ulcer is gray and bleeds easily when scraped with a swab. There may also be an associated submandibular lymphadenopathy.

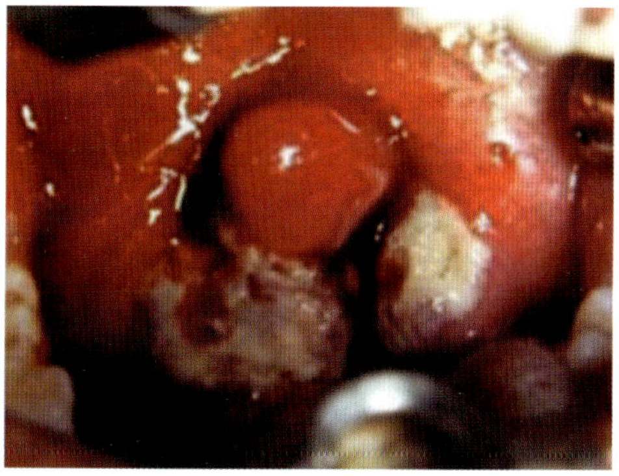

Fig. 27.5. Infectious mononucleosis lesion on tonsillar area.

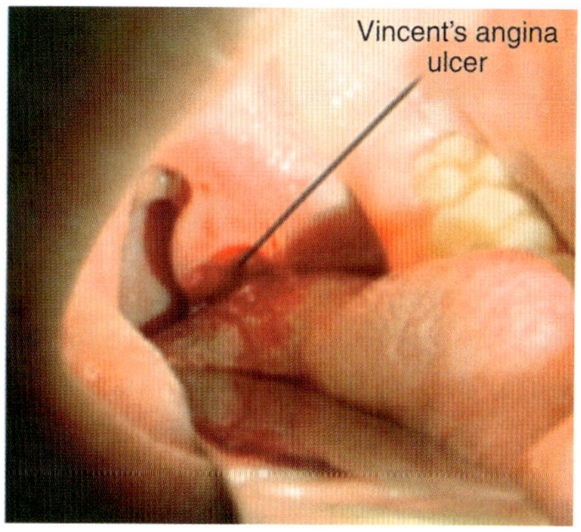

Fig. 27.6. Circumscribed unilateral ulcer on left tonsil.

Vincent angina is diagnosed using a gentian violet-stained smear of the pharyngeal exudate, which demonstrates the presence of Fusobacterium and spirochetes.

Penicillin or clindamycin and surgical debridement are the recommended treatment.

Scarlet fever

Scarlet fever is a disease caused by infection with the group A Streptococcus bacteria (the same bacteria that cause strep throat) which produce a toxin that leads to the hallmark red rash of the illness.

Symptoms: The time between becoming infected and having symptoms is short, generally 1–2 days. The illness typically begins with a fever and sore throat. The rash usually first appears on the neck and chest, and then spreads over the body. It is described as "sandpapery" in feel. The texture of the rash is more important than the appearance in confirming the diagnosis. The rash can last for more than a week. As the rash fades, peeling (desquamation) may occur around the fingertips, toes, and groin area.

Other symptoms include abdominal pain, bright red color in the creases of the underarm and groin (Pastia's lines), chills, fever, feneral discomfort (malaise), headache, muscle aches, swollen, red tongue (strawberry tongue) and vomiting.

Investigation: Throat culture positive for group A streptococcus. Rapid antigen detection (throat swab).

Treatment: The treatment is on lines similar to acute tonsillitis. This is crucial to prevent rheumatic fever, a serious complication of strep throat and scarlet fever. With proper antibiotic treatment, the symptoms of scarlet fever should get better quickly. However, the rash can last for up to 2–3 weeks before it fully goes away.

Tonsillolith

Concretions of varying size and consistency can form within the substance of the tonsils. Repeated episodes of inflammation may produce fibrosis at the openings of the tonsillar crypts. Food, epithelial and bacterial debris then accumulates within these crypts and produces a chronic inflammation. Calcification occurs subsequent to the deposition of inorganic salts, and contributes to the gradual growth of the concretion. This process may be facilitated by the oral flora and may include fungi and actinomyces-like organisms. The resultant calculus may reach a significant size and even ulcerate through the surface of the tonsil.

Tonsilloliths occur more frequently in adults and may cause symptoms of recurrent sore throats, chronic cough or otalgia. There is also a sensation of constant irritation, foreign body sensation in the back of the throat, and above all, halitosis (bad breath). Initially, these concretions are soft and cheesy, but with time, they calcify and become hard calculi. It is not uncommon for patients to pick them with various sharp objects, such as crochet needles, knitting needles, pencils, etc. Patients invariably complain about the foul smell that emanates from these cheesy concretions.

Examination of the throat demonstrates a whitish tonsillolith within the tonsil. There may be local inflammation and enlargement of the affected tonsil.

Treatment includes the removal of these concretions from the tonsillar crypts when possible, by the use of curettes and probes. Larger calculi may require incision and extraction. Tonsillectomy is reserved to patients who suffer from chronic recurrent infection, bad breath and persistent pain.

Epithelial cysts of the tonsils are quite common. They are glistening, smooth white or yellowish sessile masses (Fig. 27.7). Small cysts do not produce any symptoms. Larger cysts that cause a sensation of a "lump in the throat" may require removal.

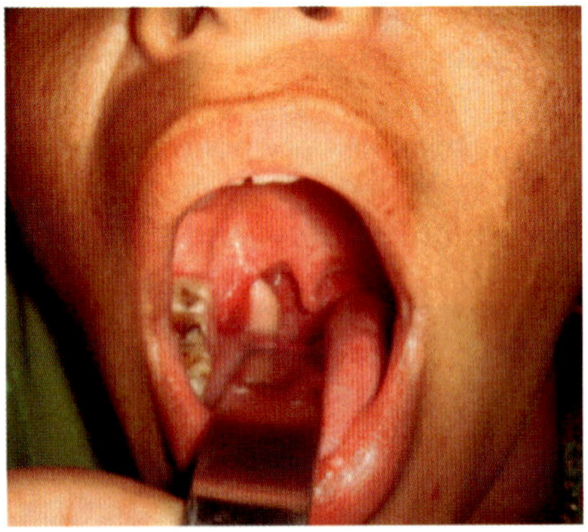

Fig. 27.7. Right tonsillar epithelial cyst.

Tonsillectomy

History

The tonsillectomy has been practiced for 3, 000 years. The procedure was first mentioned in "Hindu medicine" about 1000 BC. Galen (121–200 AD) was the first to advocate the use of the surgical instrument known as the snare. In the 7th century Paulus Aegineta (625–690) described a detailed procedure for tonsillectomy, including dealing with the inevitable post-operative bleeding. The Middle Ages saw tonsillectomy fall into disfavor. In 1828, Philip Syng Physick modified an existing instrument originally designed by Benjamin Bell for removing the uvula; the instrument, known as the tonsil guillotine (and later as a tonsillotome), became the standard instrument for tonsil removal for over 80 years. By 1897, it became more common to perform complete rather than partial removal of the tonsil. Removal of the tonsil with a scalpel and forceps were much better than partial removal; tonsillectomy using the guillotine fell out of favor.

Tonsillectomy is being performed less frequently than in the 1950s, This has been due in part to more stringent guidelines for tonsillectomy and adenoidectomy, however, it remains one of the most common surgical procedures in children.

Indications for tonsillectomy

1. Recurrent attacks of acute tonsillitis Paradise in 1983 defined recurrent tonsillitis warranting surgery by the attack frequency standard as "Seven or more in a year, five or more per year for two years, or three or more per year for three years". However according to the current guidelines (2000) of the American Academy of Otolaryngology & Head and Neck Surgery (AAO-HNS), tonsillectomy is indicated if a patient contracts "Three or more attacks of sore throat per year despite adequate medical therapy".
2. Chronic tonsillitis, consisting of persistent, moderate-to-severe throat pain.
3. Multiple bouts of peritonsillar abscess.
4. Sleep apnea (stopping or obstructing breathing at night due to enlarged tonsils or adenoids).
5. Difficulty in eating or swallowing due to enlarged tonsils.
6. Recurrent tonsillolith.
7. Abnormally large tonsils with crypts.
8. Chronic infection with beta-haemolytic streptococcus.
9. As a surgical approach to other structures like styloid process, glossopharyngeal nerve.

Preop considerations

With the aim of making the procedure safe and reducing the probability of complications certain precautions are to be taken.

- Proper selection of cases – preferably operates during cold stage, i.e., when infection and inflammation have subsided. This reduces per operative bleeding.
- Adequate course of preop antibiotics
- Haematological investigations:
- Hb, TLC, DLC
- BT/CT, platelet count, APTT, INR
- In cases of Down's syndrome cardiac disorder is a probability

Surgical procedure

The generally accepted procedure for tonsillectomy involves separating and removing the tonsils from the subcapsular plane – a fascia of tissue that surrounds the tonsils. Removal is typically achieved using a scalpel and blunt dissection or with electrocautery. Bleeding is stopped with electrocautery, ligation with sutures, and the topical use of thrombin, a protein that induces blood clotting. Dissection and snare method is also known as cold blunt steel dissection method (CBSD).

The procedure is carried out with the patient lying flat on the back, with the shoulders elevated on a small pillow so that the neck is hyperextended – the so-called 'Rose' position. A mouth gag is used to prop the mouth open; pharyngeal packing should be done preferably by the surgeon even with a cuffed ET tube. This further reduces chances of aspiration. If an adenoidectomy is also being performed, the adenoids are first removed with a curette; the nasopharynx is then packed with sterile gauze. A tonsil is removed by holding it by the upper part, pulling it slightly medially, and making a cut over the mucosa just medial to the anterior faucial pillar with a scissor or Waugh tenaculum forceps or a no. 12 blade. This incision is carried along the upper pole and to the posterior pillar. Plane for dissection is found between the capsule and the bed using a tonsillar scissors. This may be obliterated in case of an adult or fibrosed tonsils. It is important to maintain adequate traction medially. It is advisable to separate the upper pole first so that the tonsil can be pulled down and medially thus putting fibers at a stretch. This makes dissection easier. Once the dissection reaches the inferior pole (the pedicle) a snare can be used to cut it to remove the tonsil. The bed is packed with gauze and the procedure repeated on the other side. After removal of both tonsils, packs are removed and meticulous haemostasis is carried out using bipolar cautery/ligating of bleeders. Pharyngeal pack(s) should be removed after complete haemostasis.

Other methods

Electrocautery: Electrocautery uses electrical energy to separate the tonsillar tissue and assists in reducing blood loss through cauterization. Research has shown that the heat of electrocautery (400°C) may result in thermal injury to surrounding tissue. This may result in more discomfort during the postoperative period.

Harmonic scalpel: This medical device uses ultrasonic energy to vibrate its blade at 55 kHz. Invisible to the naked eye, the vibration transfers energy to the tissue, providing simultaneous cutting and coagulation. The temperature of the surrounding tissue reaches 80°C. Proponents of this procedure assert that the end result is precise cutting with minimal thermal damage.

Radiofrequency ablation: Monopolar radiofrequency thermal ablation transfers radiofrequency energy to the tonsil tissue through probes inserted in the tonsil. The procedure can be performed in an office (outpatient) setting under light sedation or local anesthesia. After the treatment is performed, scarring occurs within the tonsil causing it to decrease in size over a period of several weeks. The treatment can be performed several times. The advantages of this technique are minimal discomfort, ease of operations, and immediate return to work or school. Tonsillar tissue remains after the procedure but is less prominent. This procedure is recommended for treating enlarged tonsils and not chronic or recurrent tonsillitis.

Thermal welding: A new technology which uses pure thermal energy to seal and divide the tissue. The absence of thermal spread means that the temperature of surrounding tissue is only 2–3°C higher than normal body temperature. Clinical papers show patients with minimal post-operative pain (no requirement for narcotic pain-killers), zero edema (swelling) plus almost no incidence of bleeding. Hospitals in the US are advertising this procedure as "Painless Tonsillectomy" also known as Tissue Welding.

Carbon dioxide laser: Laser tonsil ablation (LTA) finds the otolaryngologist employing a hand-held CO_2 or KTP laser to vaporize and remove tonsil tissue. This technique reduces tonsil volume and eliminates recesses in the tonsils that collect chronic and recurrent infections. This procedure is recommended for chronic recurrent tonsillitis, chronic sore throats, severe halitosis, or airway obstruction caused by enlarged tonsils. The LTA is performed in 15 to 20 minutes in an office setting under local anesthesia. The patient leaves the office with minimal discomfort and returns to school or work the next day. Post-tonsillectomy bleeding may occur in 2–5% of patients. Previous research studies state that laser technology provides significantly less pain during the post-operative recovery of children, resulting in less sleep disturbance, decreased morbidity, and less need for medications. On the other hand, some believe that children are adverse to outpatient procedures without sedation.

Microdebrider: The microdebrider is a powered rotary shaving device with continuous suction often used during sinus surgery. It is made up of a cannula or tube, connected to a hand piece, which in turn is connected to a motor with foot control and a suction device. The endoscopic microdebrider is used in performing a partial tonsillectomy, by partially shaving the tonsils. This procedure entails eliminating the obstructive portion of the tonsil while preserving the tonsillar capsule. A natural biologic dressing is left in place over the pharyngeal muscles, preventing injury, inflammation, and infection. The procedure results in less post-operative pain, a more rapid recovery, and perhaps fewer delayed complications. However, the partial tonsillectomy is suggested for enlarged tonsils – not those that incur repeated infections.

Bipolar radiofrequency ablation (coblation tonsillectomy): This procedure produces an ionized saline layer that disrupts molecular bonds without using heat. As the energy is transferred to the tissue, ionic dissociation occurs. This mechanism can be used to remove all or only part of the tonsil. It is done under general anesthesia in the operating room and can be used for enlarged tonsils and chronic or recurrent infections. This causes removal of tissue with a thermal effect of 45–85°C. It has been claimed that this technique results in less pain, faster healing, and less post-operative care. However, studies give conflicting results about levels of pain, and its comparative safety has yet to be confirmed. This technique has been criticized for a higher than expected rate of bleeding presumably due to the low temperature which may be insufficient to seal the divided blood vessels.

Postoperative care

- It is important to make sure that complete haemostasis is achieved. Few extra minutes spent for this can save a lot of risk, embarrassment and time which would occur in case of immediate postop haemorrhage. It is equally important to make sure that the count of packs used is complete to ensure that no packs have been left behind.
- Extubation is done only when cough reflex has returned.
- Patient should be turned on the side.
- Regular watch for pulse and oxygen saturation should be kept
- Very frequent swallowing and/or rattle in the breath sound and increasing pulse rate may be a warning sign of bleeding.
- Plenty of cold liquids should be given to reduce swelling and to prevent bleeding. This also prevents dehydration which would otherwise increase pain, make swallowing difficult and initiate a vicious cycle.
- Patient can be given soft /semi solid non spicy food from 3rd post-op day.
- The pain is bothersome for 7–10 days, but not aspirin analgesics are given and a course of antibiotics is prescribed

Complications of tonsillectomy

These can be classified in to immediate, intermediate and delayed.

Immediate complications

Mostly encountered on the table during surgery. The most common of them being the complications of general anaesthesia.

Troublesome intraoperative bleeding. This is common in poorly prepared tonsillectomies (i.e., patients who have been taken up for surgery without a pre-op course of antibiotics), hot tonsillectomy (i.e., quinsy tonsillectomy). Bleeding can be controlled by proper dissection, staying in the correct plane (i.e., subcapsular plane) during dissection, ligation of bleeders, using bipolar cautery to coagulate the bleeding vessels.

Trauma to the anterior and posterior pillars. Trauma to posterior pillar causes nasal regurgitation whenever the patient attempts to drink fluids after surgery. It may also cause undesirable changes in the voice, i.e., rhinolalia aperta.

Intermediate complications

Haemorrhage during immediate post op period is also known as reactionary haemorrhage. This is caused due to

1. Wearing off of the hypotensive effect of the anaesthesia during the immediate post op period.
2. Slipping of ligature

These patients must be taken to the operation theatre, reanaesthetised and the bleeders must be ligated or cauterised.

If bleeding is diffuse and uncontrollable pillar suturing can be resorted to. This is done by suturing both the anterior and posterior pillars after placing a gauze or gelfoam in the tonsillar fossa. If gauze is used to pack the tonsillar fossa, silk is used to suture the pillars and these sutures must be removed after 48 hours and the gauze is removed.

Delayed complications

They occur mostly due to infections and when the slough is seperating. These commonly occur a week after the surgery. Bleeding during this period is known as secondary haemorrhage. Minor bleeding can be contolled by asking the patient to suck ice cubes. Antibiotics are used to control infections. If the bleeding is severe then cautery under anaesthesia may be required.

CONCLUSION

Tonsillar disease is a common problem in all age groups with symptom of pain, inflammation and redness in throat. Most of the time diagnosis is clinical, howeve, X-ray soft tissue nasopharynx lateral view is diagnostic for adenoidal hypertrophy. There are certain indications for tonsillectomy such as persistent infection, obstructive and suspected unilateral neoplastic tonsillar hypertrophy. There are many methods for tonsillectomy like cold blunt steel dissection method, electrocautery, harmonic scalpel, radio-frequency ablation, thermal welding, carbon dioxide laser, microdebrider and bipolar radio-frequency ablation. Common complication of tonsillectomy is haemorrhage. Tonsillectomy may not make, however, it can definitely mar your reputation in the city.

SUGGESTED READING

1. Benign Tonsillar Masses: Tonsillopharyngitis. The Merck Manuals: The Merck Manual for Healthcare Professionals. http://www.merck.com/mmpe/sec08/ch090/ch090i.html.
2. Wetmore RF. Tonsils and adenoids. *In:* Bonita F Stanton, Kliegman Robert, Nelson Waldo E, Behrman Richard E, Jenson Hal B. Nelson Textbook of Pediatrics. Robert M Kliegman, Richard E Behrman, Hal B Jenson, Bonita F Stanton. Philadelphia: Saunders, 2007.
3. Thuma P (2001). Pharyngitis and tonsillitis. *In:* Hoekelman Robert A. Primary pediatric care. St. Louis: Mosby, 2001.
4. Simon HB (2006). Bacterial infections of the upper respiratory tract. *In:* Dale, David. ACP Medicine, 2006 Edition (Two Volume Set) (Webmd Acp Medicine). WebMD Professional Publishing, 2006.
5. Tonsillitis and Adenoid Infection MedicineNet.
6. van Kempen MJ, Rijkers GT, Van Cauwenberge PB (May 2000). The immune response in adenoids and tonsils. *Int Arch Allergy Immunol,* 122 (1): 8–19. doi:10.1159/000024354. PMID 10859465.
7. Perry M, Whyte A (September 1998). Immunology of the tonsils. *Immunology Today,* 19 (9): 414–21. doi:10.1016/S0167-5699(98)01307-3. PMID 9745205.
8. Tonsillitis Overview Medline Plus. Putto A (1987). Febrile exudative tonsillitis: viral or streptococcal? *Pediatrics,* 80 (1): 6–12. PMID 3601520.
9. Renn CN, Straff W, Dorfmüller A, Al-Masaoudi T, Merk HF, Sachs B (2002). Van Cauwenberge P (1976). Significance of the fusospirillum complex (Plaut-Vincent angina) (in Dutch; Flemish). Acta Otorhinolaryngol Belg 30 (3): 334–45. PMID 1015288. - fusospirillum complex (Plaut-Vincent angina) Van Cauwenberge studied the tonsils of 126 patients using direct microscope observation. The results showed that 40% of acute tonsillitis was caused by Vincent's angina and 27% of chronic tonsillitis was caused by Spirochaeta
10. Medline Plus, http://www.nlm.nih.gov/medlineplus/ency/article/001043.htm
11. Boureau, F. et al. Evaluation of Ibuprofen vs Paracetamol Analgesic Activity Using a Sore Throat Pain Model. Clinical Drug Investigation, 1999; 17: 1–8. doi:10.2165/00044011-199917010-00001.
12. Praskash, T. et al. Koflet lozenges in the Treatment of Sore Throat. *The Antiseptic,* 2001; 98: 124–7.
13. Touw-Otten FW, Johansen KS. Diagnosis, antibiotic treatment and outcome of acute tonsillitis: Report of a WHO Regional Office for Europe study in 17 European countries. *Fam Pract,* 1992; 9: 255–62. doi:10.1093/fampra/9.3.255.PMID 1459378.
14. http://www.ncbi.nlm.nih.gov/pmc/articles/PMC2804585/pdf/1471-2334-9-202.pdf Brook I. The role of beta-lactamase-producing-bacteria in mixed infections. *Bio Medical Central Infect Diseases,* 2009; 9: 202.
15. Brook I. Microbiology and principles of antimicrobial therapy for head and neck infections. *Infect Dis Clin North Am,* 2007; 21: 355–91.
16. Scottish Intercollegiate Guidelines Network. Referral Criteria for Tonsillectomy. Management of Sore Throat and Indications for Tonsillectomy. Scottish Intercollegiate Guidelines Network. ISBN 1-899893-66-0, 1999.
17. Paradise JL, Bluestone CD, Bachman RZ, et al. Efficacy of tonsillectomy for recurrent throat infection in severely affected children. Results of parallel randomized and nonrandomized clinical trials. *N Engl J Med,* 1984; 310 (11): 674–83. doi:10.1056/NEJM198403153101102. PMID 6700642.
18. Wolfensberger M, Mund MT (2004). Evidence based indications for tonsillectomy (in German). *Ther Umsch,* 61 (5): 325–8. PMID 15195718. - review of literature of the past 25 years concludes "No consensus has yet been reached, however, about the number of annual episodes that justify tonsillectomy".
19. Del Mar CB, Glasziou PP, Spinks AB (2004). Antibiotics for sore throat. *Cochrane Database Syst Rev,* (2): CD000023.doi:10.1002/14651858.CD000023.pub2. PMID 15106140. - Meta-analysis of published research.
20. Zoch-Zwierz W, Wasilewska A, Biernacka A, et al. (2001). The course of post-streptococcal glomerulonephritis depending on methods of treatment for the preceding respiratory tract infection (in Polish). *Wiad Lek,* 54 (1-2): 56–63. PMID 11344703.
21. American Academy of Pediatrics (2006). Group A streptococcal infections. *In:* Pickering, Larry K. (2006). Red Book: 2006 Report of the Committee on Infectious Diseases (Red Book Report of the Committee on Infectious Diseases). Amer Academy of Pediatrics, ISBN 1-58110-194-5.
22. Bisno AL, Stevens DL. Streptococcus pyogenes. In: Mandell GL, Bennett JE, Dolin R, eds. Principles and Practice of Infectious Diseases. 7th ed. Philadelphia, Pa: Elsevier Churchill Livingstone; 2009: Chap 198.
23. Singh I, Gathwala G, Pathania R, Singh J, Yadav SPS. Hypertrophic tonsils causing articulation defect. *Indian J Pediatr,* 1994; 61: 106–7.
24. Yadav RS, Yadav SPS, Lal H. Immunoglobulin E levels in children with chronic tonsillitis. *Int J Pediatr Otoshinolaryngol,* 1992; 24: 131–4.

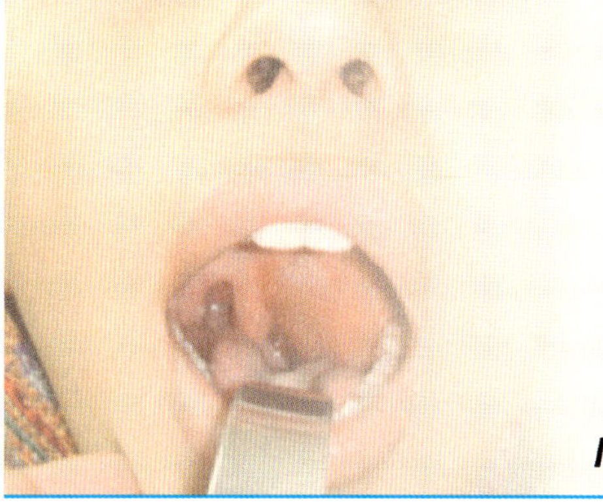

CHAPTER 28

Styloid Process

Inder Pal Nangia, Ashutosh Nangia, Dipti Jain Nangia

The name 'Styloid' is derived from the Greek word "stylos" meaning "pillar". The styloid process is a slender, pointed, bony projection on the inferior aspect of the temporal bone. Its length varies from a few millimeters to an average of 2.5 cm. It is considered elongated if the length is more than 4 cm. An elongated styloid can give rise to troublesome symptoms, first described by Eagle (1937), and known as "Eagle's syndrome". This chapter discusses the clinical aspects and surgical management of the elongated styloid process, with special emphasis on ring curette method styloidectomy, a minimally invasive procedure, devised by the author.

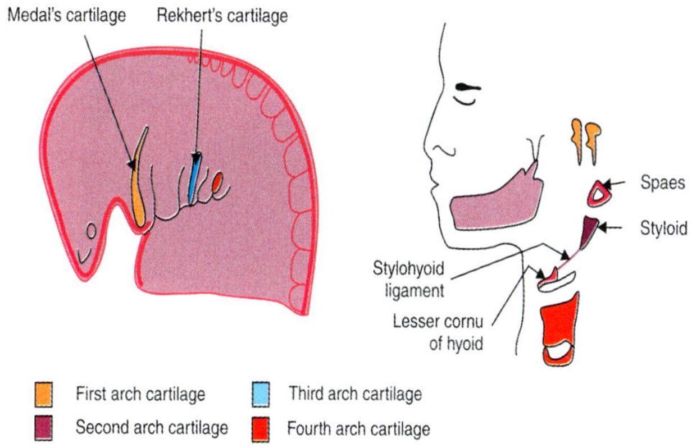

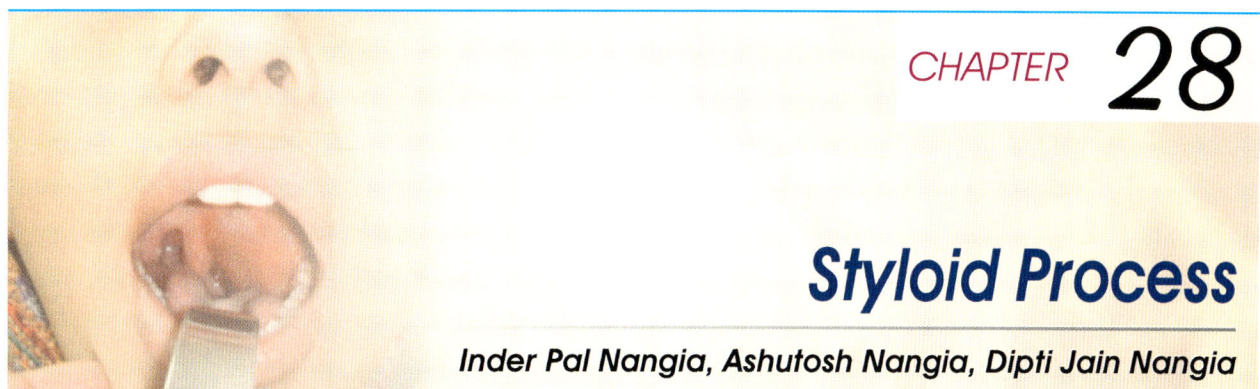

Fig. 28.1. Pharyngeal arches and their derivatives.

DEVELOPMENT

An independent cartilage anlage near the dorsal end of the second pharyngeal arch cartilage (Reichert cartilage) ossifies to form the styloid process of the temporal bone, and the stapes. The part of cartilage between the styloid process and hyoid bone regresses and its perichondrium persists as the stylohyoid ligament. The ventral end of Reichert's cartilage ossifies to form the lesser cornu and the superior part of the body of the hyoid bone (Fig. 28.1).

The styloid process develops from two centres. The centre for the proximal tympanohyal part (part ensheathed by the tympanic plate) appears before birth, and for the distal stylohyal part, appears after birth. The tympanohyal part fuses with the petromastoid portion during the first year of life. The stylohyal part may unite with the rest of the process only after puberty or may remain separate. Ossification may sometimes extend to include the stylohyoid ligament (Fig. 28.2).

ANATOMY

The temporal bone consists of four parts: the squamous, petromastoid, tympanic and the styloid. Projecting downwards, the styloid process is often almost straight but may be curved, commonly anteromedially (Fig. 28.3). Its proximal part (tympanohyal) is ensheathed by the tympanic plate in the anterolateral aspect, while muscles and ligaments are attached to its distal part (stylohyal).

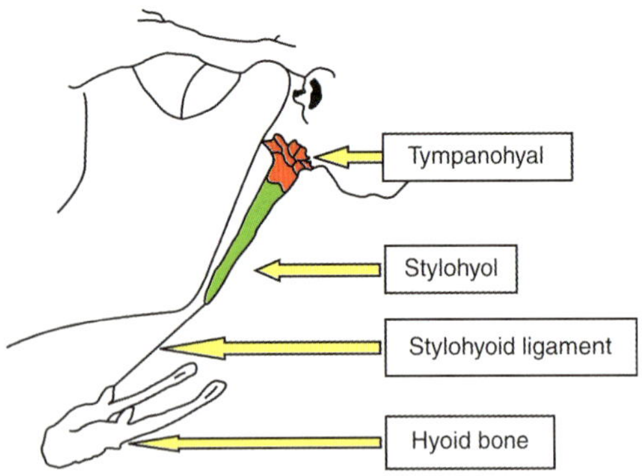

Fig. 28.2. Ossification centres for styloid process.

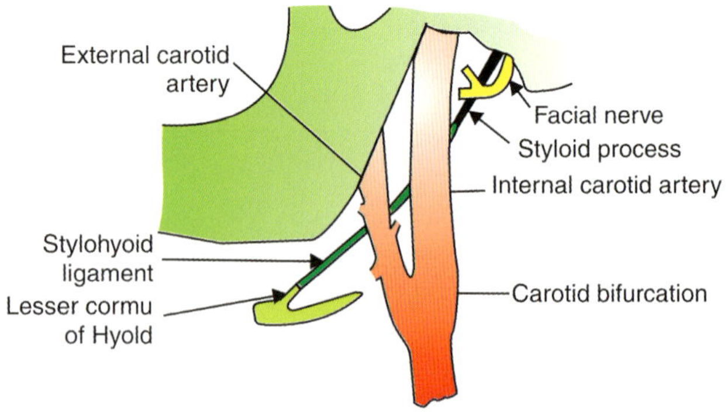

Fig. 28.4. Relation of the styloid process and the stylohyoid ligament with the carotid arteries and facial nerve.

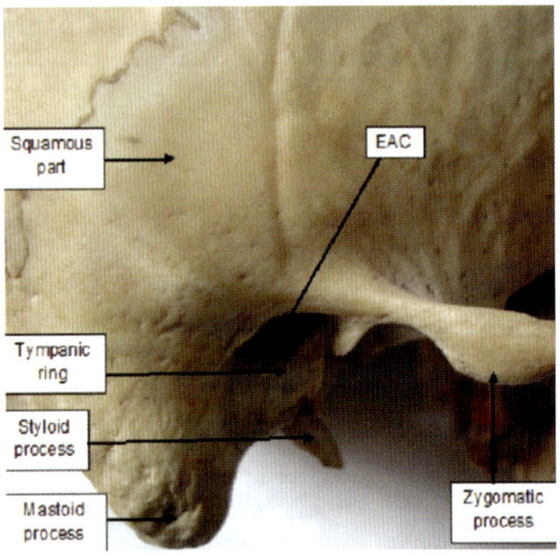

Fig. 28.3. Temporal bone.

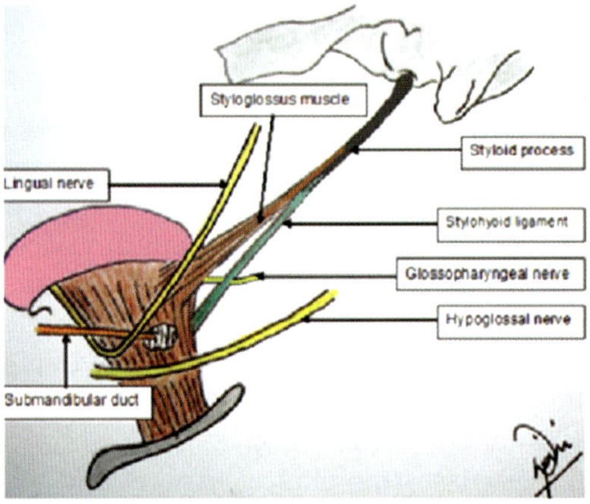

Fig. 28.5. Relation of the styloid process and the stylohyoid ligament with surrounding nerves.

RELATIONS

The styloid process lies anteromedial to the mastoid process. The two are separated from each other by the stylomastoid foramen, through which the facial nerve exits the temporal bone and then curves anteriorly to cross the styloid process, lateral to it, near its base. Laterally the styloid is covered by the parotid gland and posterior border of mandibular ramus. The tip and the attached stylohyoid ligament pass between the external and internal carotid arteries (Fig. 28.4). Medial to the process is the internal jugular vein.

The styloid projects down from the base of the skull into the parapharyngeal space, and divides it into a pre-styloid and a post-styloid compartment.

The glossopharyngeal nerve lies in relation to the styloid process. After leaving the jugular foramen, it passes forwards between the internal jugular vein and internal carotid artery and then descends anterior to the ICA, deep to the styloid process, to reach the stylopharyngeus (Fig. 28.5).

ATTACHMENTS

The styloid process gives attachment to two ligaments and three muscles, which together with the styloid form the styloid apparatus (Fig. 28.6). The ligaments are stylohyoid and stylomandibular and the muscles are styloglossus (XII CN), stylohyoid (VII CN) and stylopharyngeus (IX CN).

ELONGATED STYLOID PROCESS

Elongated styloid process and calcification of the stylohyoid ligament have long been recognized in literature. Eagle in 1937 described a pain syndrome and attributed it to an elongated styloid and differentiated it from primary glossopharyngeal neuralgia. This was termed "Eagle's syndrome". It is also known by several other names such as Stylalgia, Elongated Styloid Process Syndrome, Styloid Process-Carotid Artery Syndrome, Stylohyoid Syndrome, and Styloid Process Neuralgia.

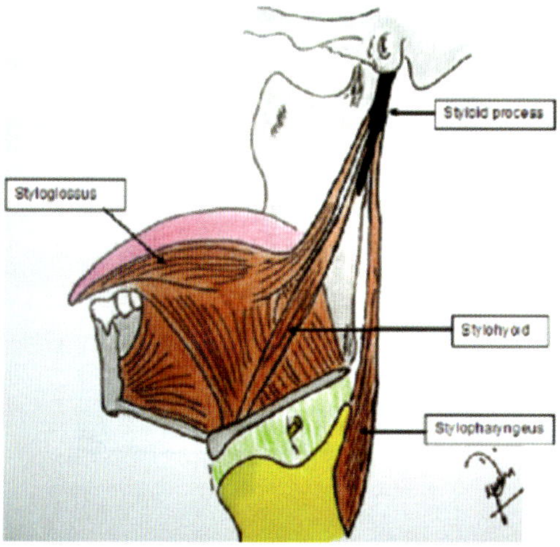

Fig. 28.6. Muscular attachments of styloid process.

ETIOPATHOGENESIS

The pathophysiology of elongation of styloid process is not clearly defined. Ossification of the stylohyoid ligament, as mentioned earlier, as an extension of the normal fusion of styloid process is the commonly accepted theory. The stylohyoid ligament may retain some embryonic cartilage rests and hence the potential to get ossified. The abnormal length and angulation of styloid process lead to pain by compression of the adjacent structures, particularly the IX cranial nerve. Impingement of the pharyngeal mucosa or carotid vessels and sympathetic chain can also cause pain. Irritation of mechanoreceptors by the enlarged styloid in the distribution of cranial nerves V, VII, IX and X has been described as the underlying pathologic process. Similar mechanical irritation may also be caused by trauma or inflammatory edema by increasing intracompartmental pressure which may affect the neurovascular contents of the para-pharyngeal space.

EPIDEMIOLOGY

The incidence of elongated styloid process in the general population has been reported to be around 4 percent. Out of these, only a few, 4–10 percent, are symptomatic. So, in the general population, a very small percentage, 0.16%, are symptomatic, making this a relatively rare condition. The male to female ratio has been reported to be around 1 : 3. In a study conducted by the author over a period of 15 years, in 151 cases that underwent styloidectomy the male to female ratio was found to be 1 : 1.96.

CLASSIFICATION

Elongated styloid process is classified into three types (Fig. 28.7):

Type I	Elongated
Type II	Pseudoarticulated
Type III	Segmented

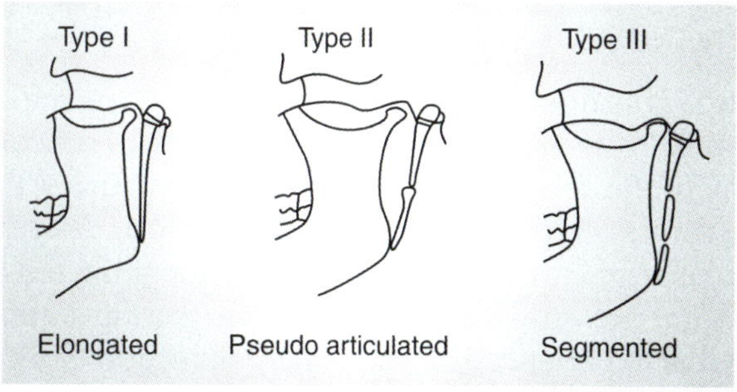

Fig. 28.7. Classification of enlarged styloid process.

CLINICAL FEATURES

Styloid elongation presents usually after the second decade. By this time the fusion of the styloid process has occurred and calcification of the stylohyoid ligament comes into the picture. The most common symptom is recurrent pain throat, seen in around 85 to 90 percent of the cases in the author's series. Other common symptoms are difficult or painful swallowing, foreign body sensation throat and pain in the tongue, ear, temporal region, neck and infra-orbital region. Another common symptom is painful neck movements.

Eagle described two variants, the Classical Eagle syndrome, which was seen in post-tonsillectomy/trauma patients. The symptoms were dysphagia, FB sensation, pain throat and otalgia. These were attributed to surgery or trauma induced scarring which causes neural stretching or compression as well as induced mineralization of the stylohyoid ligament.

The second variant, stylocarotid syndrome, comprised of a group of patients presenting with supra- or infraorbital pain, parietal headache and cervicofacial pain. These occur due to the stretching of perivascular sympathetic fibres around the carotid.

DIFFERENTIAL DIAGNOSIS

Many conditions giving rise to cervicofacial pains can be considered in the differential diagnosis of Eagle's syndrome. These include cranial nerve neuralgias (trigeminal neuralgia, primary glossopharyngeal neuralgia), temporomandibular joint disorders, chronic tonsillopharyngitis, unerupted or impacted molar teeth, improperly fitting dental prostheses, pharyngeal and tongue base tumours, otitis media, salivary gland disease, and laryngopharyngeal reflux.

DIAGNOSIS

The diagnosis of elongated styloid process, clinically, is made by a thorough history to rule out any of the above mentioned conditions causing the patients symptoms. On examination, a bony projection can be palpated in the tonsillar fossa. Digital pressure over this area leads to pain similar to that experienced by the patient. Injection of local anesthetic solution into the tonsillar fossa relieves the symptoms. These findings are confirmed radiographically by an X-ray or CT scan which show enlargement of the styloid process, as well as tell us its exact length.

Common methods of imaging styloid process are plain X-rays of the skull, Towne's view (anteroposterior view with cephalocaudal angulation of 30 degrees) and lateral view. An orthopantomogram (OPG) gives a panoramic view of the mandible and shows both styloid processes well. Lateral oblique view of mandible can also be used to visualize the styloids. Computed tomography scans show the styloid well in the coronal sections. 3-dimensional reconstruction of the CT shows the size as well as spatial orientation of styloid (Fig. 28.8).

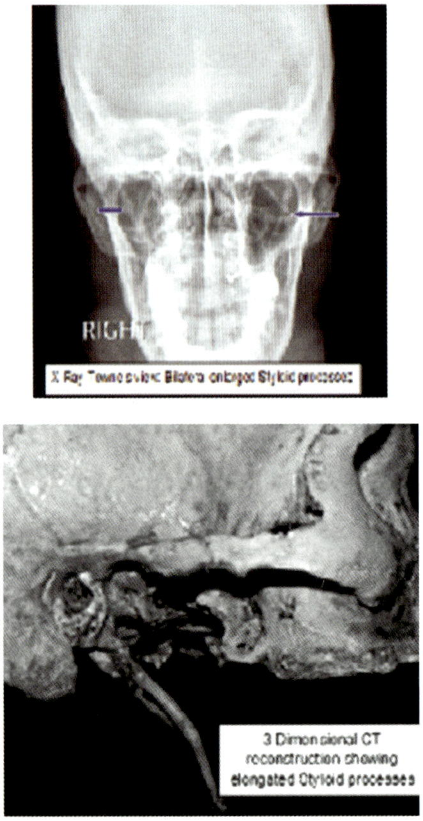

Fig. 28.8. Styloid process imaging.

TREATMENT

Treatment of the enlarged styloid process is staged. An initial trial of conservative management is widely advocated. Similar to the diagnostic procedure, local infiltration of the tonsillar fossae with long-acting local anaesthetics or steroids provides relief to the patient. This approach is effective but requires repeated injections. Drug therapy with antidepressants and anticonvulsants like carbamazepine, which have a neural membrane stabilizing effect, is also proposed but the efficacy is doubtful. Analgesics like NSAIDs are quite effective for temporary pain relief, but are not recommended for prolonged use. Another conservative measure especially advocated by the lead author, particularly in patients with painful neck movements and concurrent spondylosis of cervical spine, is neck exercises, which have been found effective in a large majority of patients.

Surgical treatment is considered in cases not responding to conservative methods. Styloid may be approached via an external or an intraoral approach.

External approach via a cervical incision has the advantages of a wide exposure and a sterile operative field. Incision extends from upper two-thirds of the anterior border of sternocleidomastoid to the hyoid bone. The posterior belly of the digastric muscle is retracted to reach the parapharyngeal space where the styloid can be accessed after separating the muscular and ligamentous attachments. The disadvantages of this external approach are increased operative time and hospital stay, external scar and risk to the facial nerve and major neck vessels.

The intraoral approach is via the bed of the tonsil. The styloid process is palpated and incision given over it. The pharyngeal musculature is split, the styloid process identified, its mucoperiosteum incised, elevated, the styloid process fractured and excised. This approach necessitates performing a

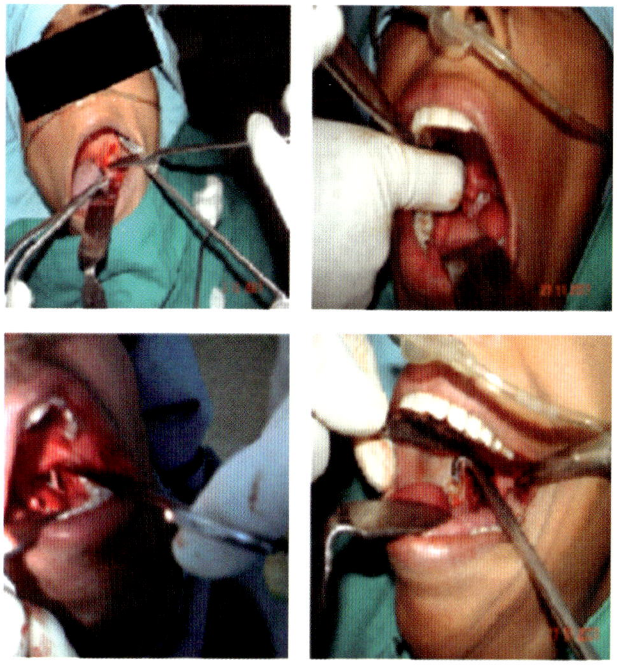

Fig. 28.9. Surgical photographs of ring curette method styloidectomy. (**A**) Dissection of tonsil under LA. (**B**) Palpation of tonsillar fossa. (**C**) Styloid process arrested in ring curette. (**D**) Removed with curved artery forceps.

tonsillectomy before the styloid is removed. It can also be approached via the anterior pillar, without removing the tonsil. This method is safe, simple, less time-consuming, and an external scar is avoided. The disadvantages are risk of deep neck space infection, vascular injury, poor visualization and postoperative pain.

Ring curette method styloidectomy is a minimally invasive intraoral approach that has been devised by the author (Fig. 28.9). In this method, a preliminary tonsillectomy is done. The styloid is then digitally palpated in the tonsillar fossa to confirm the position of the tip. A ring curette (Fig. 28.10) is then employed to arrest the styloid process and using a sliding motion, the periostium is stripped off the styloid along with the muscle and ligament attachments. The styloid is then fractured using a curved Negus artery forceps and removed. After removal of the styloid, the retracted pharyngeal tissues automatically fall back into their normal anatomical position. If the tip of the styloid is projecting anteriorly into the anterior tonsillar pillar, the same technique can be utilized without removing the tonsil. The advantages of this procedure are:

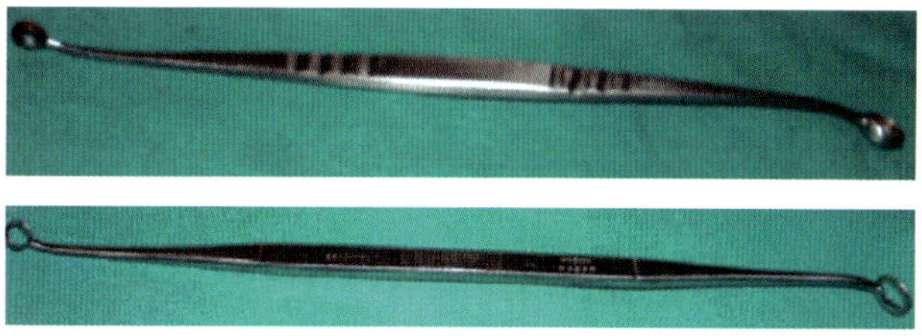

Fig. 28.10. Ring curette employed to arrest the styloid process. The instrument was originally designed to be used as a 'D&C' curette by the gynaecologists.

- The procedure is performed under local anesthesia.
- Daycare procedure.
- Ease of operative technique.
- Minimum operative time of around 1–2 minutes per side.
- Minimal risk of injury to facial nerve and major vessels.
- No splitting of pharyngeal musculature. Hence, reduced risk of infection, no suturing required, much lesser post operative pain.

The disadvantage of this technique is that in case of incomplete mineralization of stylohyoid ligament, leading to an elongated but 'soft' styloid process, it becomes difficult to arrest the styloid in the ring curette. Also, if the elongation is going beyond the inferior limit of the tonsillar fossa, the tip of the styloid may not be palpable. In cases of post-tonsillectomy stylalgia, this technique is difficult to employ because of fibrosis of the tissues.

POSTOPERATIVE CARE

After surgery, antibiotic cover is given as per the operating surgeon's protocol. In cases of intraoral approach, meticulous vitals monitoring as for any tonsillectomy case is required as is ensuring good oral hygiene. If ring curette method is used, the patient can be discharged the same day as per the author's protocol.

CONCLUSION

Styloid process elongation is a clinicoradiologically proven entity. Despite this only a small proportion of these patients are symptomatic, casting a shadow of doubt over the existence of stylalgia or Eagle's syndrome. In the author's experience, the symptom severity is unrelated to the length of styloid process. Majority of the patients respond to conservative treatment. In those requiring surgery, the ring curette method is the most suitable.

SUGGESTED READING

1. Baddour HM, Anear JT, Tilson AB. Eagles Syndrome, Case report. *J Oral Surg,* 1978; 36: 486.
2. Balbuena L Jr, Hayes D, Ramirez SG, Johnson R. Eagle's syndrome (elongated styloid process). *South Med J,* 1997; 90: 331–4.
3. Flood LM. Otalgia. In Gleeson M, Browning GG editors. Scott-Brown's Otorhinolaryngology, 7th ed. Vol 3. London: Hodder Arnold 2008. p. 3526–36.
4. Gervicka A, Kubilius R, Sabalys G. Clinic, Diagnostics and treatment pecularities of Eagle's syndrome. *Stomatologija, Baltic Dental Maxillofacial J,* 2004; 6: 11–3.
5. Hilding DA. Fractures of elongated styloid process masquerading as foreign body. *Ann Otol Rhinol Laryngol,* 1961; 70: 689–92.
6. Maru YK, Patidar K. Stylalgia and its surgical management by intraoral route – clinical experience of 332 cases. *Indian J Otolaryngol Head Neck Surg,* 2003; 55: 87–90.
7. McGinnis JM Jr. Fracture of an ossified stylohyoid bone. *Arch Otolaryngol,* 1981; 107: 460.
8. Moore KL, Persaud TVN. editors. The Pharyngeal apparatus. *In:* The Developing Human. 8th ed. Philadelphia. Elsevier; 2008. pp. 159–60.
9. Naik SM, Naik SS. Tonsillo-Styloidectomy for Eagle's Syndrome: A Review of 15 Cases in KVG Medical College Sullia. *Oman Med J,* 2011; 26: 122–6.
10. Nangia IP. Stitchless tonsillostyloidectomy. *Indian J Otolaryngol Head Neck Surg,* 2002; 54: 59–61.
11. Rinaldi V, Meyers AD. Eagle Syndrome. [Online]. 2010 Mar 26; Available from: URL: http://emedicine.medscape.com/article/1447247-overview
12. Standring S. editor. External and middle ear. *In:* Gray's Anatomy. The anatomical basis of clinical practice. 40th ed. Spain. Churchill Livingston; 2008.
13. Yadav SPS, Chanda R, Gera A, Yadav RK. Styalgia: An Indian prospective. *J Otolaryngol,* 2001; 30: 304–6.

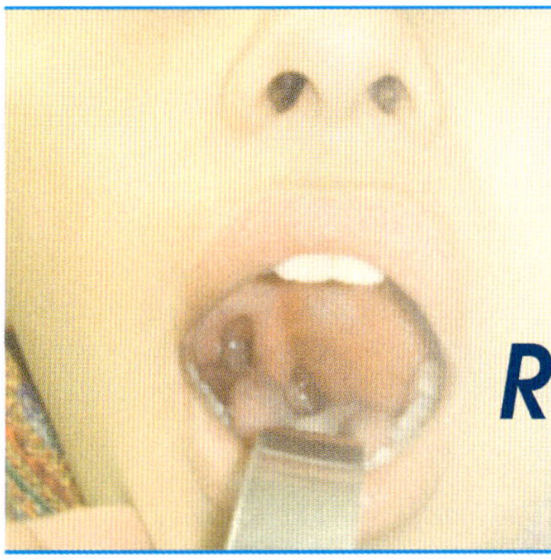

CHAPTER 29

Recurrent Aphthous Stomatitis

Ravi Mehar

Recurrent aphthous stomatitis (RAS) also called as mouth ulcers or canker sores and stress ulcers are a very common oral mucosal lesion. It is characterized by one or more painful oral ulcers at intervals ranging from days to months.

It usually begins in childhood or adolescence and may decrease in both frequency and severity with age.

RAS are confined to the non keratinized mucosa of the mouth, or keratinized mucosa that is not immediately adherent to bone. These can arise anywhere in the oral cavity except hard palate and gingiva.

RAS is subdivided into three categories based on the size of the ulcers and the disease severity.

1. Minor aphthous ulcers (80%).
2. Major aphthous ulcers.
3. Herpetiform ulcers.

Features of minor aphthous ulcer (i.e., Mikulicz ulcers) (Fig. 29.1)

- These are small round or ovoid ulcers 2–4 mm in diameter surrounded by an erythematous halo with single or in group of 1 to 6.
- Ulcer floor may be initially yellowish because of the slough but can have grayish hue as healing and epithelialization proceeds.
- Site – nonkeratinized mobile mucosa of the lips, cheeks, floor of the mouth, buccal and labial sulcus and ventral surface of the tongue.
- Heal spontaneously without any scarring in 7–10 days.
- Can recur at intervals of 1–4 months.

Features of major aphthous ulcer (i.e., Sutton ulcers, periadenitis mucosa necrotica recurrens (PMNR)) (Fig. 29.2)

- Larger and present for longer duration and often more painful than minor aphthous ulcers.
- Large around 1 cm or more in diameter round or ovoid ulcers with surrounding edema.
- Found on any area of the oral mucosa, including the keratinized dorsum of the tongue or palate.
- May be seen in groups of only a few ulcers (i.e., 1–6) at a time.
- Heal slowly over 10–40 days.
- Recur extremely frequently.
- May heal with scarring.
- Occasionally associated with a raised erythrocyte sedimentation rate.

Characteristics of herpetiform ulceration

- Age – slightly older age group than the other RAS.
- Consist of crops of up to 150 very small (1–3 mm) ulcers that heal completely in 7 to 10 days. Mainly found in females.

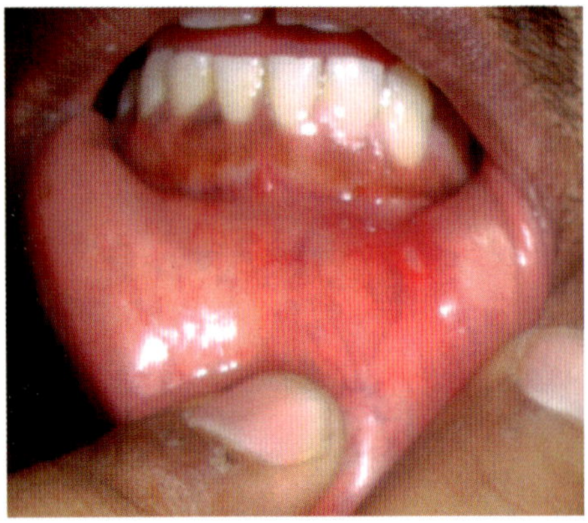

Fig. 29.1. Minor aphthous ulcer.

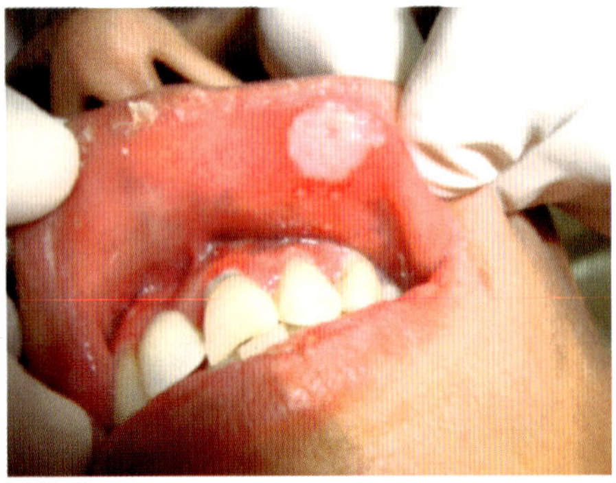

Fig. 29.2. Major aphthous ulcer.

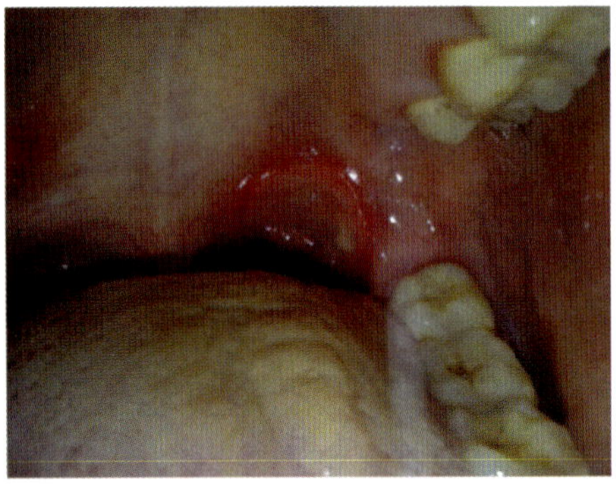

Fig. 29.3. Malignant ulcer.

29

- Begins with vesiculation that passes rapidly into multiple, minute, pinhead-sized, discrete ulcers.
- Can involve any oral site, including the keratinized mucosa, increase in size, and coalesce to leave large round ragged ulcers.
- Often extremely painful.
- Importantly these ulcers are completely unrelated to the herpes virus.
- The irregular and chronic nature of these lesions often necessitates a biopsy to rule out squamous cell carcinoma (Fig. 29.3).

Difference between minor and major aphthous ulcers

	Minor aphthous	*Major aphthous*
Size	2–4 mm in diameter surrounded by an erythematous halo	Large, around 1 cm or more in diameter with surrounding edema
Number	In a group of 1 to 6	1 to 3
Site	Nonkeratinized mobile mucosa of the lips, cheeks, floor of the mouth, buccal and labial sulcus and ventral surface of the tongue	Found on any area of the oral mucosa, including the keratinized dorsum of the tongue or palate
Healing	Heals in 7–10 days spontaneously	Heal slowly over 10–40 days
Scarring	Heals without any scarring	May heal with scarring
Recurrence	Can recur at intervals of 1–4 months	Recur extremely frequently
ESR	Normal	May be raised

Etiology

Exact etiology is not known and is said to be idiopathic, though various factors which are associated with the aphthous ulceration are:

1. An association with viruses such as adenovirus, herpes, and varicella-zoster has been suggested, but is not supported by the evidence. There is no report of successful treatment of RAS with antiviral therapy.
2. A bacterial association has also been suggested due to the fact that *Streptococcus* species have been cultured from patients with RAS. This has not been confirmed and it is clear that antibacterial drugs do not cure RAS.
3. RAS is clearly related to the progesterone level fall in the luteal phase of the menstrual cycle, and ulcers may then temporarily regress in pregnancy.
4. Found more in patients with high levels of anxiety, stress, and the "type A" personality.
5. Vitamins B_{12}, zinc, and iron deficiency has been implicated as the occurrence of RAS improved somewhat with replacements.
6. Sensitivities to foods such as nuts, chocolate, cereals, tomatoes, dairy products and citrus fruits have been implicated also, and the avoidance of such foods may decrease recurrences.

7. Trauma due to sharp tooth, dental appliances or hard food substances.
8. Nicotine in smoke seems to have a protective effect. Studies have shown that resumption of smoking after cessation caused pre-existing ulcers to heal within a few days. One hypothesis for the protective effect is the keratinizing action of nicotine on the oral mucosa.
9. Malabsorption in gastrointestinal disorders like celiac disease (gluten-sensitivity) and Crohn's disease.
10. Behçet syndrome, which may include genital, cutaneous, ocular, or other lesions.
11. Immunodeficiencies such as human immunodeficiency virus (HIV) infection, and neutropenia (Ulcers appearing on a regular 3-week cycle may indicate cyclic neutropenia).
12. Auto-inflammatory syndromes, such as periodic fever, aphthous stomatitis, pharyngitis, and cervical adenitis syndrome in children.
13. Drug use (e.g., nicorandil, aldreonate, NSAIDs, etc.).
14. Sweet syndrome, a rare immunologically mediated condition that belongs to the group of neutrophilic dermatoses and must be differentiated, particularly from Behçet disease. Sweet syndrome is characterized by red-brown plaques and nodules that are frequently painful and occur primarily on the head, neck, and upper extremities. Patients often also have neutrophilia and fever and may have oral ulceration.
15. A positive family history is there in about one third of patients with RAS with an increased frequency of HLA types A2, A11, B12, and DR2.
16. Food allergies like allergy to cow's milk.
17. Sodium lauryl sulphate (SLS): A detergent in some oral healthcare products that may aggravate or produce oral ulceration.
18. More common in medical student.
19. A number of diseases are reported to be associated in family like hypertension, diabetes, myocardial infraction, rheumatoid arthritis and peptic ulcer.

Sex

A slight female preponderance exists.

Age

RAS typically starts in childhood or adolescence.

Investigations

- There is no specific investigations for RAS.
- Also long-standing non-healing ulcer in oral cavity must be biopsied.
- Systemic disorders should be ruled out by following tests
  - Hemoglobin level
  - TLC and DLC
  - Red blood cell indices
  - Serum ferritin levels
  - Red blood cell folate assay
  - Serum vitamin B_{12} measurements
  - Serum antiendomysium antibody and transglutaminase assay (positive in celiac disease)

Histopathological examination

The histology is nonspecific. The surface of the ulcer is covered by a fibrinous exudate infiltrated by polymorphs. Beneath is a layer of granulation tissue with dilated capillaries and edema. Deeper still is a repair reaction, with fibroblasts in the surrounding connective tissue laying down fibrous tissue.

Medical Care

- Identify and correct predisposing factors like iron or vitamin deficiency.
- Ensure that patients brush atraumatically (super soft toothbrush).
- Avoid eating particularly hard or sharp foods (e.g., toast, potato crisps) and avoid other trauma to the oral mucosa.
- Patch testing may be indicated to reveal any allergies.
- Female patients in which ulcers are due to her menstrual cycle or to use of an oral contraceptive may benefit from suppression of ovulation with progesterone or a change in the oral contraceptive.
- In most cases, the natural history of RAS is one of eventual remission. Relief of pain and reduction of ulcer duration are the main goals of therapy.
- Topical corticosteroids (TCs) remain the mainstays of treatment. TCs reduce painful symptoms but not the rate of ulcer recurrence.

The commonly used preparations are as follows:
- Hydrocortisone hemisuccinate pellets.
- Triamcinolone acetonide in carboxymethyl cellulose paste.
- Betamethasone sodium phosphate.

- Hydrocortisone and triamcinolone preparations are popular because neither causes significant adrenal suppression; however, ulcers still recur.
- Betamethasone, fluocinonide, fluocinolone, fluticasone, and clobetasol are more potent and effective than hydrocortisone and triamcinolone, but they carry the possibility of some adrenocortical suppression and a predisposition to candidiasis.
- Topical tetracyclines may reduce the severity of ulceration, but they do not alter the recurrence rate. A doxycycline capsule of 100 mg in 10 ml of water administered as a mouth rinse for 3 minutes. Tetracyclines in children younger than 12 years is to be avoided.
- Chlorhexidine gluconate mouth rinses reduce the severity and pain of ulceration but not the frequency.
- Anti-inflammatory agents can help; a spectrum of topical agents such as benzydamine, benzocaine, lidocaine, diclonine, or benzydamine and amlexanox may help.
- Other therapies that have been reported include hydrogen peroxide, phenol, silver nitrate, topical antimicrobials, antivirals, and antiseptic mouthwashes. These treatments are generally not very effective
- If RAS fails to respond to local measures, systemic immunomodulators may be required. A wide spectrum of agents has been suggested as beneficial, but few studies have been performed to assess their efficacy (or their adverse effects are significant). Such agents include systemic corticosteroids, colchicine, clofazimine, and thalidomide. Teratogenicity, neuropathy, and other adverse effects dissuade most physicians from their use.
- If patients have a large number of lesions or long duration of attacks, a "burst regimen" of systemic steroid treatment may be used in addition to topical therapy.
- Aphthous major that is difficult to control, intralesional triamcinolone injection will often promote ulcer healing.

All patients with recurrent oral ulceration must be fully investigated to establish a definitive diagnosis and eliminate the possibility of an underlying systemic disorder or oral malignancy.

CONCLUSION

Recurrent aphthous ulcer usually presents as painful ulcer in the oral cavity and esopharynx. The etiology is unknown, however, bacterial, viral, stress, food allergy, immune reaction, vitamin deficiency, trauma, nicotine, gastrointestinal disorders, certain drugs used and familial history association are reported. For the management medical treatment as well as chemical cautery are effective.

SUGGESTED READING

1. Wilhelmsen NS, Weber R, Monteiro F, Kalil J, Miziara ID. Correlation between histocompatibility antigens and recurrent aphthous stomatitis in the Brazilian population. *Braz J Otorhinolaryngol*, 2009; 75(3): 426–31.
2. Gallo Cde B, Mimura MA, Sugaya NN. Psychological stress and recurrent aphthous stomatitis. *Clinics (Sao Paulo)*, 2009; 64(7): 645–8.
3. Shakeri R, Zamani F, Sotoudehmanesh R, Amiri A, Mohamadnejad M, Davatchi F, Karakani AM, et al. Gluten sensitivity enteropathy in patients with recurrent aphthous stomatitis. *BMC Gastroenterol*, 2009; 17: 9–44.
4. Meng W, Dong Y, Liu J, Wang Z, Zhong X, Chen R, Zhou H, et al. A clinical evaluation of amlexanox oral adhesive pellicles in the treatment of recurrent aphthous stomatitis and comparison with amlexanox oral tablets: a randomized, placebo controlled, blinded, multicenter clinical trial. *Trials*, 2009; 6: 10–30.
5. Lynde CB, Bruce AJ, Rogers RS 3rd. Successful treatment of complex aphthosis with colchicine and dapsone. *Arch Dermatol*, 2009; 145(3): 273–6.
6. Volkov I, Rudoy I, Freud T, Sardal G, Naimer S, Peleg R, Press Y. Effectiveness of vitamin B12 in treating recurrent aphthous stomatitis: a randomized, double-blind, placebo-controlled trial. *J Am Board Fam Med*, 2009; 22(1): 9–16.
7. Teixeira F, Taylor AM, Montaño S, Domínguez SL. Treatment of recurrent oral ulcers with mometasone furoate lotion. *Postgrad Med J*, 1999; 75: 574.
8. Ferguson MM, Wray D, Carmichael HA, Russell RI, Lee FD. Coeliac disease associated with recurrent aphthae. *Gut*, 1980; 21(3): 223–6.
9. Wray D, Ferguson MM, Mason DK, Hutcheon AW, Dagg JH. Recurrent aphthae: treatment with vitamin B_{12}, folic acid, and iron. *Br Med J*, 1975; 2(5969): 490–3.

10. Singh N, Scully C, Joyston-Bechal S. Oral complications of cancer therapies: prevention and management. *Clin Oncol*, 1996; 8: 15–24.
11. Shotts RH, Scully C, Avery CM, Porter SR. Nicorandil-induced severe oral ulceration: a newly recognised drug reaction. *Oral Surg Oral Med Oral Pathol Oral Radiol Endod*, 1999; 87: 706–7.
12. Albanidou-Farmaki E, Deligiannidis A, Markopoulos AK, Katsares V, Farmakis K, Parapanissiou E. HLA haplotypes in recurrent aphthous stomatitis: a mode of inheritance?. *Int J Immunogenet*, 2008; 35(6): 427–32.
13. Piskin S, Sayan C, Durukan N, Senol M. Serum iron, ferritin, folic acid, and vitamin B12 levels in recurrent aphthous stomatitis. *J Eur Acad Dermatol Venereol*, 2002; 16(1): 66–7.
14. Marakoglu K, Sezer RE, Toker HC, Marakoglu I. The recurrent aphthous stomatitis frequency in the smoking cessation people. *Clin Oral Investig*, 2007; 11(2): 149–53.
15. Akintoye SO, Greenberg MS. Recurrent aphthous stomatitis. *Dent Clin North Am*, 2005; 49(1): 31–47.
16. Yadav J. Apthous ulcer in medical students. *Indian J Clin Pract*, 2009; 19(8): 31–3.
17. Yadav J, Sood S, Shubhrica. Diseases associated with apthous ulcer. *Indian J Clin Pract*, 2010; 21: 194–6.

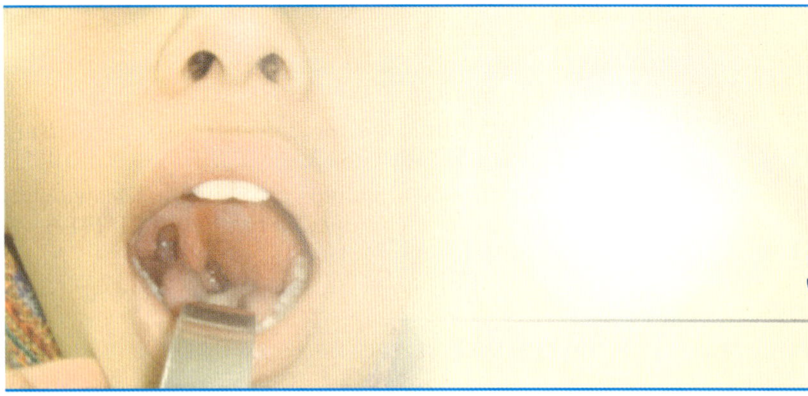

CHAPTER 30

Sialendoscopy

P.P. Singh, Vipin Arora

Sialendoscopy is the minimally access technique for direct visualization of the salivary ductal system. The advent of miniaturization of instrumentation and minimal access surgery has led to a paradigm shift in the management of salivary gland diseases from gland centric approach to the duct centric approach as latter is found to be the cause in most of the cases. Sialendoscopy has gradually established itself as an effective procedure for the diagnosis and treatment of both parotid and submandibular salivary gland diseases. It is also increasingly being used as a minimally invasive intervention for management of salivary duct obstructions. The basic principle of currently employed rigid sialendoscopy system is to visualize the salivary ductal system from its distal end, which is intraoral opening of the ducts, to proximal ductal system in the gland parenchyma by rigid endoscope, while keeping the ductal system patent by continuous saline irrigation. The pathologies of the ductal system calculi and strictures can be directly visualized and dealt accordingly.

Review of literature

Non-neoplastic salivary gland diseases are common in the otorhinolaryngological practice, with submandibular and parotid duct calculi contributing to a major chunk of these diseases. The conventional treatment of the non-neoplastic diseases of the salivary glands has been gland excision irrespective of the site of the pathology, in the gland parenchyma or the ductal system. Sialolithiasis is one of the major causes of sialadenitis. Salivary stones result in a mechanical obstruction of the salivary duct, leading to stasis of saliva, repetitive swelling during meals, which can be complicated by bacterial infections. The histopathology of these removed glands revealed them to be normal in several studies. This further strengthened the philosophy of saving these innocent glands which actually have ductal problems and outflow tract obstruction.

Increasing patient awareness and complications like facial scar, neural injury, particularly the facial nerve injury and postoperative infections in conventional surgery, led to the development of the minimal access approaches to selectively address the site specific pathology under direct visualization. In the early 1990s, Katz wrote about flexible endoscopy of the salivary ducts. A 0.8 mm passively flexible mini-endoscope was used to visualize intraductal anatomy and stone pathology. There were limitations of the flexible endoscopes to negotiate the tortuous ductal pathways and image quality was poor.

Nahlieli and his group started reporting their experiences with rigid salivary endoscopy in 1994. They reported using two endoscopes: a 1.1 mm diagnostic type and a 2.3 mm treatment type. Their overall success rate in removal of calculi was 82%. The group also proposed algorithms for treatment of salivary calculi.

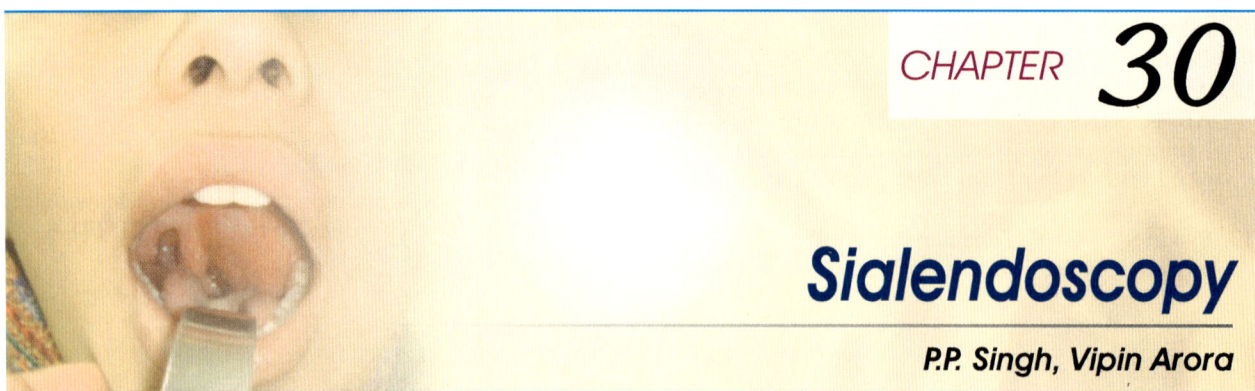

Marchal and colleagues in their study of removed glands found that most glands were near normal except for the ductal calculus, so it was important to preserve the gland if possible. As sialendoscopy gradually got established, Nahlieli and his group reviewed the management of chronic recurrent parotitis in 2004. They reported some treatable findings in these patients such as sausage-like ducts amenable to balloon dilatation, strictures helped by expansion with miniforceps and removal of mucous plugs with flushing. Several authors have reported their extensive experiences with sialendoscopy and the advanced techniques of sialendoscopy now being used. Overall, sialendoscopy has emerged as a safe and effective diagnostic and treatment modality. However, it has also been observed that despite its apparent simplicity, it is technically challenging and requires sequential learning.

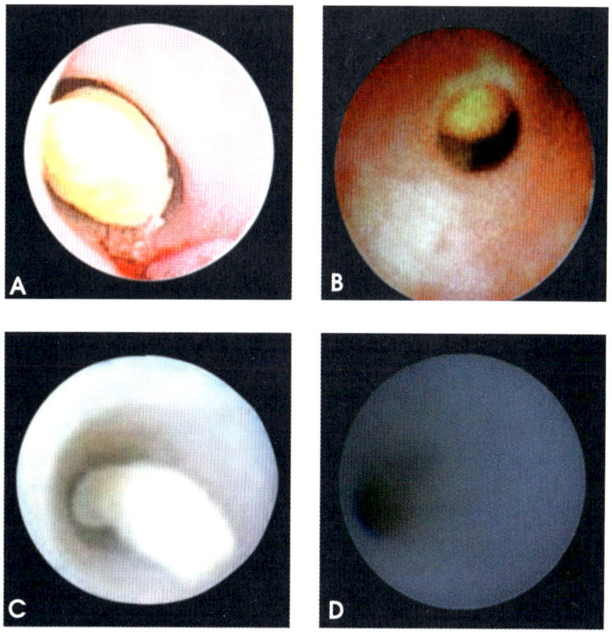

Fig. 30.1. A. Stone in the duct. **B.** Stone beyond a stricture. **C.** Mucous debris in duct. **D.** Stricture observed in whitish-appearing duct as seen in chronic inflammatory diseases of the salivary gland.

Indications

Diagnostic

1. Obstructive salivary disease.
2. Salivary gland swellings of unclear origin.

Various pathologies which can be diagnosed using sialendoscopy are shown in Fig. 30.1 A–D.

Therapeutic

1. Removal of salivary calculi.
2. Dilatation of strictures and localization of strictures for external approaches.
3. Management of chronic recurrent parotitis and juvenile recurrent parotitis.

SIALENDOSCOPY IN OPEN SURGERY

Sialendoscopy is often required to be combined with open salivary surgery both for submandibular and parotid sialolithiasis. The indications in open surgery are:

1. Localization of site for intraoral duct incision.
2. Multiple stones.
3. Too large a stone for endoscopic removal.
4. Stone at the hilum of the duct.
5. Stone associated with stenosis of the duct.

Sialendoscopy is a very useful tool in combined approach for removal of large stones in the parotid duct.

Contraindications

Acute sialadenitis is a relative contraindication because the swollen duct wall is more vulnerable to perforation.

Radiological investigations

Plain lateral view radiographs are not recommended for diagnosis of salivary calculus disease. Occlusal view is the minimum investigation for submandibular calculi, while axial CT scan localizes the stone inside the duct, hilum, gland parenchyma, number and size of the stones. CT scan is of value in treatment planning as well as in prognostication as hilar and intra-parenchymal stones and stones larger than 4 mm in size are difficult to remove by sialendoscopy. MRI particularly the MR sialography is gold standard for diagnosis of the salivary ductal and parenchymal diseases. MR sialography has replaced the conventional sialography as it is non- invasive and free from the radiation exposure. Virtual endoscopy is helpful in treatment planning, but is not routinely warranted in all the cases planned for sialendoscopy.

Instrumentation for sialendoscopy

A typical set up for sialendoscopy requires the connection of the endoscope to a camera system with a monitor, a light source and an irrigation

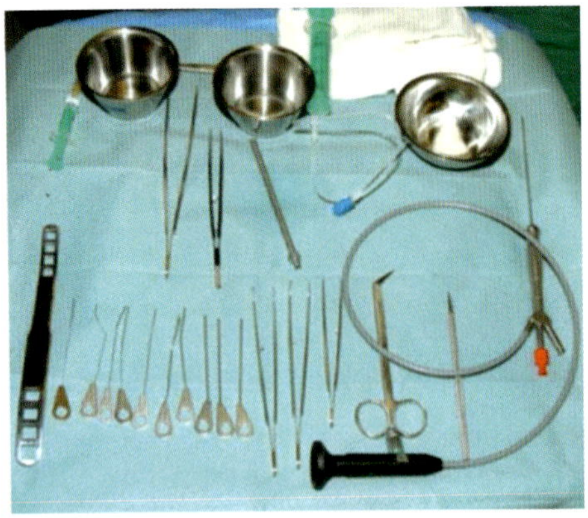

Fig. 30.2. Instruments used in sialendoscopy.

system. Fig. 30.2 shows the essential instruments required for diagnostic sialendoscopy.

The endoscopes currently available are the first generation endoscopes with sheaths, for diagnostic and interventional sialendoscopy. The second generation endoscopes are the all-in-one endoscopes with an integrated irrigation channel which can be used for introduction of operating instruments as

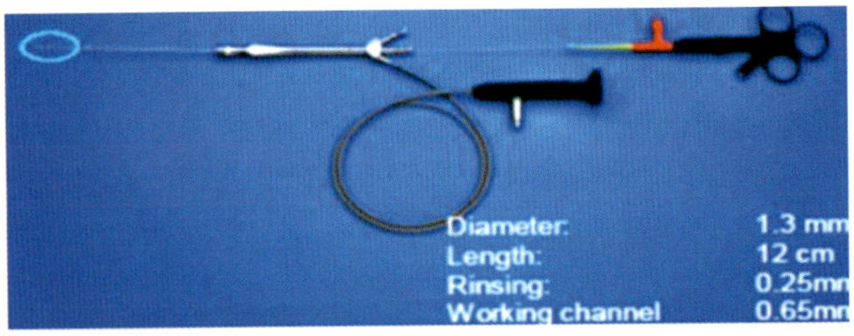

Fig. 30.3. Second generation sialoendoscope.

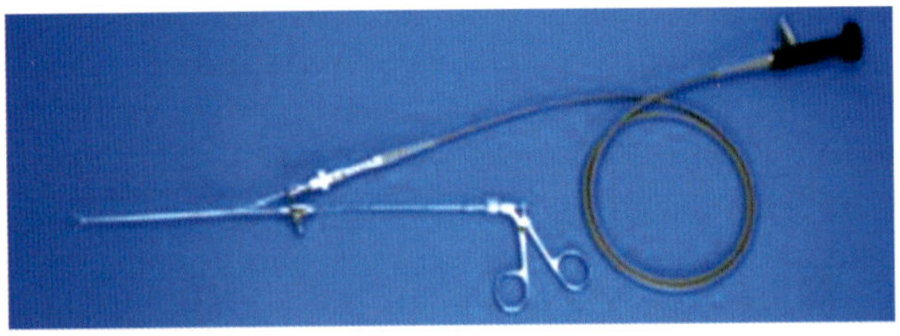

Fig. 30.4. Modular sialoendoscope.

seen in Fig. 30.3. A modular sialoendoscope is shown in Fig. 30.4.

The other equipments required are salivary probes, conic dilator, forceps, wire baskets, balloon dilators and boogies. The conic dilator (Fig. 30.5) is used for initial gentle dilatation of the papilla without trauma. Salivary probes have an atraumatic tip design, with a constant diameter along the entire length (Fig. 30.6). They are available in increasing

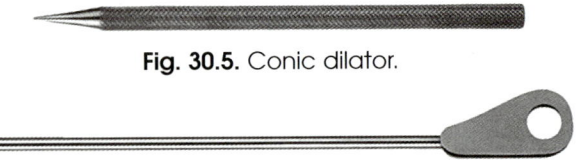

Fig. 30.5. Conic dilator.

Fig. 30.6. Salivary probe.

sizes from size 0 to size 6 for gradual dilation of the papilla and distal part of the duct.

Custom made forceps are available in different

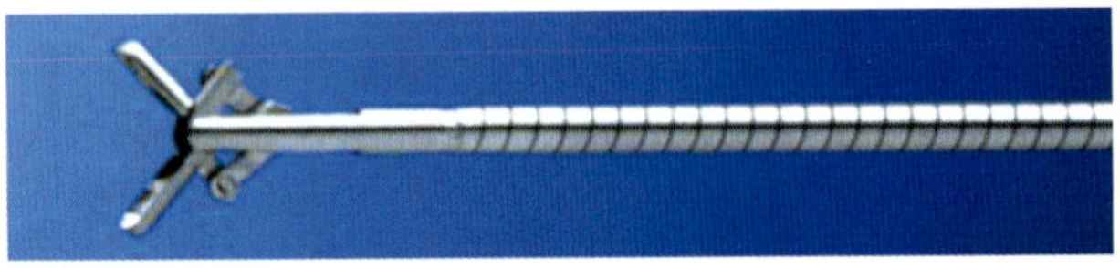

Fig. 30.7. Custom mode sialoendoscopic forceps.

sizes (Fig. 30.7). These may be used for removing small sialoliths from the ducts.

Wire baskets (Fig. 30.8) are available in various sizes with either three, four or six wires each. These are very delicate instruments and are extremely

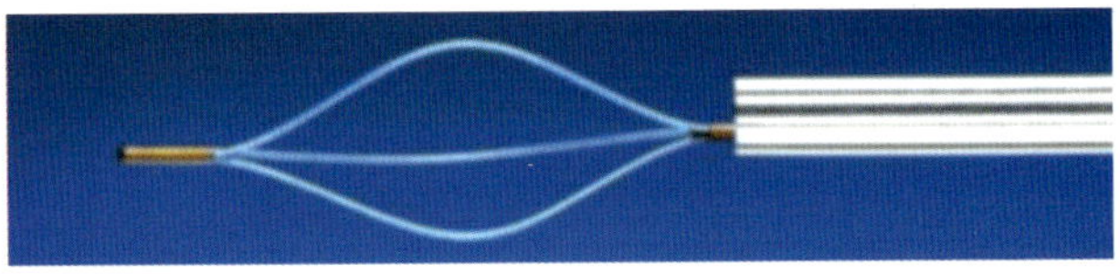

Fig. 30.8. Wire basket.

fragile so they need to be handled with utmost care and delicacy. The baskets are used for stone retrieval.

Balloon dilators (Fig. 30.9) are used when controlled dilatation of localized stenosis of the duct

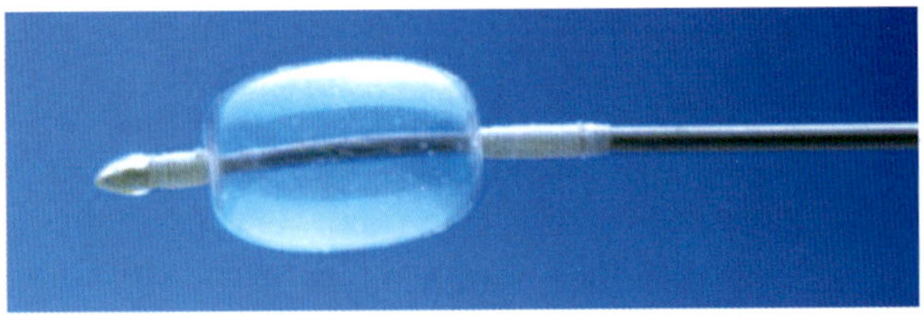

Fig. 30.9. Balloon dilator.

is required. This is mostly required in cases of chronic recurrent parotitis.

Boogies are also used in similar situations or when a stricture is encountered in the ductal system.

Technique of sialendoscopy

The normal parotid and submandibular ducts have diameters of about 1.5 mm with narrowing at the region of the papillae where the diameter is about 0.5 mm.

Diagnostic sialendoscopy can be easily performed under local anesthesia. Interventional sialendoscopy, apprehensive patients and children may require general anesthesia. The first step for a successful sialendoscopy is the choice of the appropriate endoscope. It is better to start with a scope of a smaller diameter and a scope appropriate to the age of the patient which will cause least trauma to the duct walls and provide adequate visualization of ductal system and subsequently an interventional sialendoscopy can be performed.

Diagnostic sialendoscopy

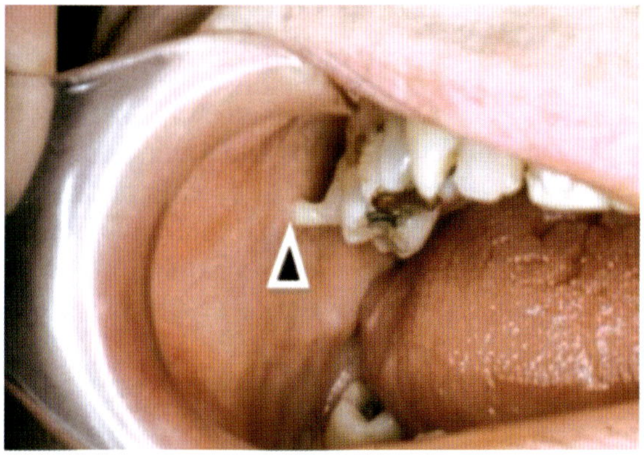

Fig. 30.10. Stensen's duct opening.

The Stensen's duct papilla opens in the buccal mucosa against the upper second molar (Fig. 30.10).

The Wharton's duct papilla opens in the floor of mouth at the anterior tip of the sublingual fold close to the midline. It may be difficult to visualize the papilla occasionally and magnification by operating microscope is helpful. To enhance the visibility of the papilla, the gland can be massaged to express saliva or secretions, conic dilator is used to gently dilate the papilla, a blunt probe can be used to identify the direction and dilatation of the duct. At times a small papillotomy may be required in case the submandibular duct opening is very small or scarred, whereby the mucosa is opened slightly dorsal to the expected position of the papilla under local infiltrative anesthesia.

The endoscope is gradually advanced into the duct along with continuous irrigation by saline mixed with xylocaine 2%. Apart from providing local anesthesia, the irrigation keeps the duct lumen patent so that the endoscope can be advanced under vision into the lumen of the duct and flushes out fibrin debris or sialomicroliths from the duct.

The ductal system is inspected systematically from distal to proximal for any pathology and the treatment can then be individualized based on the pathology.

Interventional sialendoscopy

Obstructive sialadenitis is the major cause of salivary gland disorders. The obstruction may be caused by presence of sialoliths, stenosis, strictures, intraductal fibromucinous plugs, polyps and foreign bodies, or rare cases such as extraductal stones or obstruction caused by salivary tissue and tumours that mimic stones.

After a diagnostic sialendoscopy, when a stone or stricture is localized, the intervention sialendoscope with two channels is used; one of the channels is for visualization by fiber-optic system and the other for introduction of grasping basket (Fig. 30.11) or LASER fiber or for a dilatation balloon. When the stone has a diameter smaller than 4 mm, the grasping basket is opened behind the stone. Once the stone is trapped, the whole device is removed. When the stone is larger than 5 mm, fragmentation before extraction is required which can be performed by external lithotripsy or by laser fragmentation. After the last stone is removed, the endoscope is introduced again to rinse the duct and confirm that the duct is intact.

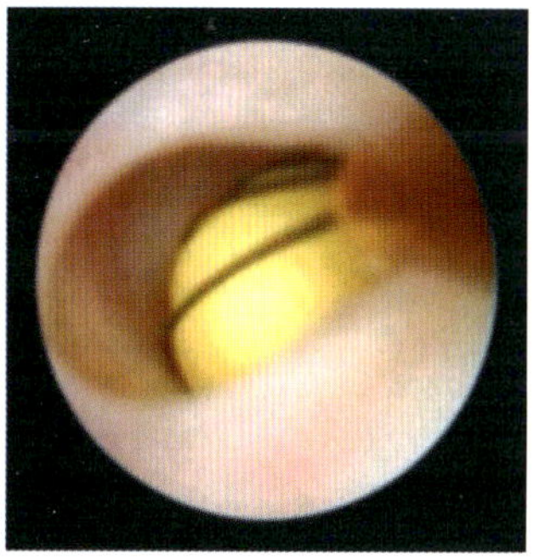

Fig. 30.11. Stone being removed using a wire basket.

The patient is given antibiotics in the postoperative period. Corticosteroids may be given for 48 hours. Self-massaging of the gland is advised.

The results of interventional sialendoscopy are directly related to the size of the stones in the parotid and submandibular glands, especially so in the parotid gland. Marchal reported that 97% of parotid stones smaller than 3 mm could be retrieved with the wire basket, without fragmentation, while for larger stones the success of this technique was 35%. For these larger sialoliths, fragmentation before extraction is necessary. It was observed that the smaller diameter of the parotid duct makes the procedure of interventional sialendoscopy more challenging.

Stones of soft consistency with a size of 5–7 mm may be fragmented within the ducts during interventional sialendoscopy by forceps and the fragments can then be removed. Stones that are not accessible using the sialendoscope, impacted stones, and intraparenchymal stones are disintegrated and fragmented using extracorporeal shock-wave lithotripsy (ESWL).

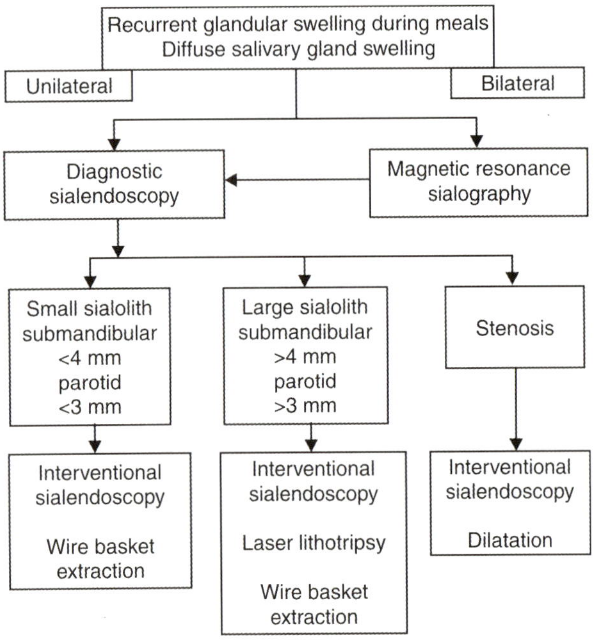

(Reproduced from Marchal F, Dulguerov P. Sialolithiasis management: The state of the art. *Arch Otolaryngol Head Neck Surg*. 2003; 129: 951–956.)

Marchal and colleagues suggested a decision tree for the evaluation and management of sialolithiasis.

Generally when the stone was considered too large to be fragmented or when the ductal stenosis was too tight to be dilated, the only solution was to remove the gland with its associated morbidity. Marchal reported two new techniques combining sialendoscopy and external surgery. He reported a symptomatic improvement of 92% in patients of parotid disease and a success rate of 69% in cases of submandibular stones.

Transoral duct slitting for submandibular duct stones is indicated if stone is larger than 5 mm or is impacted.

An advanced application of sialendoscopy for salivary calculi in the parotid duct includes the localization of the stone by skin transillumination as an aid to external approach for removal of stone (combined endoscopic transcutaneous approach).

Dilatation of stenoses and strictures

Endoscopically controlled procedures are especially helpful for short membrane like stenoses or where stenoses begin at duct branching. Dilatation is done using balloon dilatation.

Sialendoscopic management of chronic sialadenitis and recurrent juvenile parotitis

Sialendoscopy has been used successfully for treatment of chronic parotitis and juvenile recurrent parotitis. The mechanism proposed is perhaps the clearance of mucous plugs and dilatation of the duct by irrigation. Instillation of steroid solution in the duct has been found to give good results in recurrent parotitis. Insertion of a stent for three weeks can be done to ensure patency of the duct in postoperative period (Fig. 30.12).

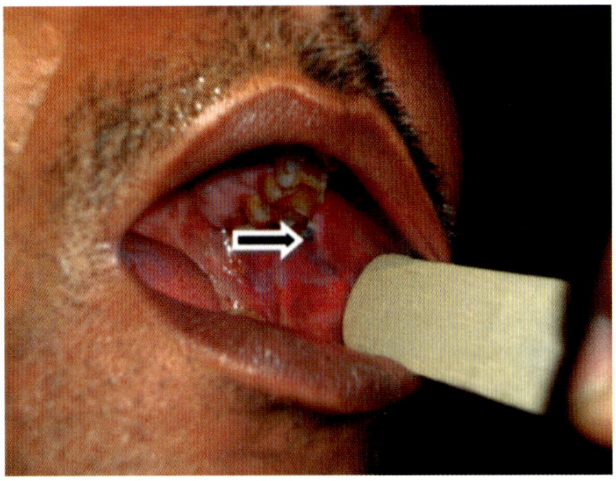

Fig. 30.12. Stent in-situ.

An endoscopic treatment protocol for recurrent parotitis was proposed by Nahlieli et al. The hydrostatic pressure of saline irrigation acts as a dilator for the strictures and a sialoballoon can be used. After the procedure, 100 mg of hydrocortisone solution is injected intraductally. A sialostent (Sialotechnology, Ashkelon, Israel) is inserted and kept in place for 4 weeks for prevention of recurrence of strictures.

Quenin et al reported preliminary therapeutic results of success in 89% cases (9 of 10) of juvenile recurrent parotitis with sialendoscopic dilatation of the duct. They performed sialendoscopy when patients reported a minimum of two episodes of swelling within 6 months. Sialendoscopy proved to be of a better diagnostic value than ultrasonography. They also confirmed the previously reported findings of a whitish ductal inner appearance without the natural proliferation of blood vessels in these cases of juvenile recurrent parotitis.

Complications

Complications are rare and are seen early in the learning curve, the technique is suitable and well tolerated by most of the patients. Marchal reported a much lower complication rate (12%) in his large series.

1. Temporary swelling of gland caused by saline irrigation.
2. Duct wall perforations.
3. Lingual nerve paresthesia.
4. Ranula formation.
5. Postoperative infection.
6. Ductal strictures.

Limitations of sialendoscopy

1. Extremely tortuous duct that hampers progression of endoscopes.
2. Difficulty in directing endoscope at the distal end of the canal system.

The indications of sialendoscopy are thus gradually expanding with new indication of salivary gland inflammatory disorders getting included in its scope. Though the technique is minimally invasive, safe and associated with minimal morbidity; it is technically challenging and requires skilled and gentle hands. As this technique gains popularity amongst the surgeons, in future the indications for gland removal will get restricted to salivary tumours and failed cases of sialendoscopy.

CONCLUSION

The technology of the endoscopes has been developed over the last 10 years evolved over four generations: free optical fiber, flexible endoscopes and two generations of semi-rigid endoscopic devices of various diameters. Recently 'all-in-one' sialendoscopes have been developed. Sialendoscopy can be either a diagnostic or an interventional procedure. Diagnostic sialendoscopy is an evaluation procedure that aims to replace most of the radiological investigations of salivary ductal system. Interventional sialendoscopy alone or combined with external surgery is an operation for obstructive salivary ductal pathology. It involves the use of miniature endoscopes (1–3 mm wide) to enter the small ducts of the salivary system in search of disease. The most common disease processes obstructing the salivary gland duct are stones (or calculi) and/or stenosis of the duct from chronic inflammation. Once diagnosis is finalized, it can be treated by a variety of methods, all of which spare total gland removal. This would include stone removal to relieve blockage or duct dilation to prevent recurrent obstruction. Avoid sialendoscopy during an acute inflammatory process because of the increased fragility of the ductal system. The overall success rate of the procedure is over 90%. Patients who suffer from sialadenitis or recurrent salivary gland stones will need to modify their lifestyles after sialendoscopy to help prevent recurrence. Advantages of this procedure include no surgical scar, no risk of nerve damage, no risk of bleeding, fast recovery time, preservation of normal salivary gland and duct, same day procedure in a safe outpatient setting and early return to normal diet

SUGGESTED READING

1. Fritsch MH. Sialendoscopy and lithotripsy: Literature review. *Otolaryngol Clin N Am*, 2009; 42: 915–26.
2. Nahlieli O, Baruchin AM. Long-term experience with endoscopic diagnosis and treatment of salivary gland inflammatory diseases. *Laryngoscope*, 2000; 110: 988–93.
3. Zenk J, Zikarsky B, Hosemann WG et al. The diameter of the Stensen's and Wharton ducts. Significance for diagnosis and therapy. *HNO*, 1998; 46: 980–5.
4. Geisthoff UW. Basic sialendoscopy techniques. *Otolaryngol Clin N Am*, 2009; 42: 1029–52.
5. Marchal F, Kurt AM, Dulguerov P, Becker M, Oedman M, Lehmann W. Histopathology of submandibular glands removed for sialolithiasis. *Ann Otol Rhinol Laryngol*, 2001; 110: 464–69.
6. Nahlieli O, Bar T, Shacham R, Eliav E, Hecht-Nakar L. Management of chronic recurrent parotitis: Current therapy. *J Oral Maxillofac Surg*, 2004; 62: 1150–5.

7. Walvekar RR, Razfar A, Carrau RL, Schaitkin B. Sialendoscopy and associated complications: A preliminary experience. *Laryngoscope*, 2008; 118: 776–9.
8. Iro H, Zenk J, Escudier MP, et al. Outcome of minimally invasive management of salivary calculi in 4691 patients. *Laryngoscope*, 2009; 119: 263–8.
9. Koch M, Zenk J, Iro H. Algorithms for treatment of salivary gland obstructions. *Otolaryngol Clin N Am*, 2009; 42: 1173–92.
10. Geisthoff UW. Basic sialendoscopy techniques. *Otolaryngol Clin N Am*, 2009; 42: 1029–52.
11. Marchal F, Dulguerov P, Beker M, Barki G, Disant F, Lehmann W. Specificity of parotid sialendoscopy. *Laryngoscope*, 2001; 111: 264–71.
12. Marchal F, Dulguerov P. Sialolithiasis management: The state of the art. *Arch Otolaryngol Head Neck Surg*, 2003; 129: 951–6.
13. Capaccio P, Torretta S, Pignataro L. The role of adenectomy for salivary gland obstructions in the era of sialendoscopy and lithotripsy. *Otolaryngol Clin N Am*, 2009; 42: 1161–71.
14. Nahlieli O. Advanced sialendoscopy techniques, rare findings, and complications. *Otolaryngol Clin N Am*, 2009; 42: 1053–72.
15. Marchal F, Becker M, Dulguerov P, Lehmann W. Interventional sialendoscopy. *Laryngoscope*, 2000; 110: 318–20.
16. Marchal F. A Combined endoscopic and external approach for extraction of large stones with preservation of parotid and submandibular glands. *Laryngoscope*, 2007; 117: 373–7.
17. Quenin S, Plouin-Gaudon I, Marchal F, Froehlich P, Disant F, Faure F. Juvenile recurrent parotitis: Sialendoscopic approach. *Arch Otolaryngol Head Neck Surg*, 2008; 134: 715–19.

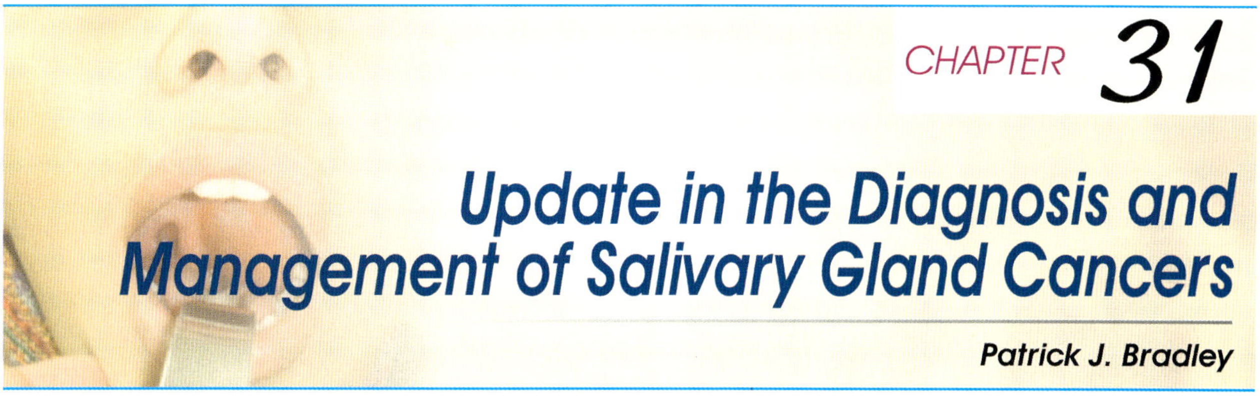

CHAPTER 31

Update in the Diagnosis and Management of Salivary Gland Cancers

Patrick J. Bradley

Primary salivary gland malignancy is uncommon, has a diverse histopathology spectrum and groupings, and as a result a varied biologic behaviour and a protracted risk of local and distant recurrence. The cause and epidemiology of salivary gland cancer has been associated with exposure to irradiation diagnostic, therapeutic or environmental. Occupational exposure (radiation/radioactive materials, nickel compounds/alloys, employment in the rubber industry has an increased risk. In men, smoking and heavy alcohol consumption is also associated with a higher risk, but these factors are not strongly related to salivary gland cancers in women. Of interest is intake of vitamin C > 200 mg/day and cholesterol intake are respectively, inversely and directly related with risk of developing salivary gland carcinoma. There exists an unproven association between the use of mobile or cordless phones and the development of salivary gland cancer. The controversies that arise concerning the diagnosis and management of salivary gland neoplasms reflect the necessity to achieve an accurate pathologic diagnosis in order to initiate the proper therapy.

Incidence

There are a number of reported large series from a number of departments who provide a salivary gland service for a general population, rather than taking series from large specialist centers with a tertiary practice, with a skewed clinical practice more towards the more rare cancers. The prevalence of salivary neoplasms is shown to be distributed between the parotid, submandibular, sublingual and minor salivary glands, 100 : 10 : 1 : 10, with the distribution between benign and malignant inversing from predominantly benign in the parotid gland to more likely malignant when the tumours present in a minor salivary gland.

Pathology

The majority of malignant salivary gland tumours arise from either the excretory duct or the intercalated duct reserve cell. Either of these two cells have the potential for differentiation into a variety of epithelial tumours.

Malignant salivary gland tumours are classified as low-grade and high-grade neoplasms, and are effective for clinical use and decision-making (Table 31.1).

Major salivary gland tumours

The parotid and submandibular glands are staged by the UICC/AJC separate from other head and neck malignant diseases. Malignant tumours of the sublingual gland and the other minor salivary glands are staged according to the staging system used for squamous cell carcinoma described for the site the tumour is located.

Table 31.1. Classification of salivary gland malignancy

High-grade	*Low-grade*
• High-grade mucoepidermoid • Adenoid cystic carcinoma • Salivary duct carcinoma • Adenocarcinoma NOS • Carcinoma ex-pleomorphic adenoma • Small cell carcinoma • Squamous cell carcinoma • Undifferentiated carcinoma	• Acinic cell carcinoma • Polymorphous low-grade adenocarcinoma • Epithelial-myoepithelial carcinoma • Basal cell carcinoma

Management

Surgery is the treatment of choice in the majority of cases with indications for adjuvant treatments such as radiotherapy in selected histopathologies and when certain pathological findings have been documented.

In most circumstances, the surgeon will not have all the definitive diagnostic information until the surgical specimen has undergone permanent section analysis by the histopathologist. Because of the above, the preoperative evaluation is aimed at minimizing the likelihood of encountering surgical surprises, the preservation of cranial nerve functions – facial, hypoglossal and lingual nerves, minimizing or preventing tumour recurrences, and to deal with a broad range of tumour aggressiveness.

Controversies

The controversies thus requiring discussion include:

1. The role of fine-needle aspiration cytology (FNAC).
2. Imaging salivary gland neoplasms.
3. Selection of the proper surgical procedure for the primary tumour.
4. Management of the neck.
5. Role of radiotherapy.
6. Role of chemotherapy.
7. Management of recurrent local disease.
8. Incidence of distant metastases.
9. Known prognostic factors.
10. Paediatric salivary gland malignancy.

Fine needle aspiration cytology and/or biopsy (FNAC or FNAB)

When the clinical suspicion is that the parotid gland is the location of a malignant tumour, one need to consider could this tumour be a secondary form either a local tumour in the head and neck region, or from a distant infraclavicular source – breast, lung and genitourinary tract, most commonly.

The use of FNAB is currently performed in the majority of head and neck clinical environments, either using a needle technique, sometimes a "core biopsy" with or without guidance being aided by the addition of ultrasound.

The diagnostic accuracy, sensitivity and specificity are in the region of high 80% in benign lesions, and 90% accuracy for diagnosing pleomorphic adenoma. There is a lower sensitivity, 85%, when the lesions are considered malignant and when considering a salivary malignancy there is also a higher risk of false positive and false negative diagnosis, thus adding to an increased risk of delaying treatment, errors in clinical advice or errors in subsequent applied surgical procedures. A recent paper reports the difficulties associated with the use of FNAB in primary parotid carcinoma, they had 72% recognition of malignancy, but could not be relied upon to provide an accurate tumour grading or type.

Thus FNAB can provide useful information that has value in planning therapy, but it should not be the sole basis for management decisions. One of the important benefits of FNAB is the opportunity to avoid unnecessary surgery and its risks for patients who have benign neoplasms but because of existing co-morbidities are poor candidates for an anaesthetic.

The clinical value of FNAB is a function of the experience of the cytopathologist; it must be combined with the impression gained from the history and physical examination.

Some clinicians consider that FNAB should be used in all salivary gland masses, emphasizing the diagnostic accuracy, rapidity, patient convenience, and cost-effectiveness of this study and feel that it is the single most important piece of information to be obtained. While others suggest that FNAC alone is not prone to determine the surgical management of parotid malignancies. Other clinicians advocate the use of FNAB only for three specific indications:

1. For patients who are poor surgical risks.
2. For patients with a history of previous malignancy/metastasis.
3. For patients in whom it is difficult to determine whether the lesion is neoplastic or inflammatory.

In lesions, located in the minor salivary glands, an incision biopsy or a punch biopsy is to be preferred.

Imaging studies

Options available for the imaging of salivary neoplasms include plain films, sialography, ultrasound (U/S), computed tomography (CT), magnet resonance imaging (MRI), and positron emission tomography scanning (PET). In Europe there is widespread usage of ultrasound in the clinic and employed by the diagnosing clinician and allows for FNAB at the time of presentation, thus minimizing delay in diagnosis and reducing the numbers of clinicians involved in the diagnostic process. However, in areas where U/S is not available CT and MRI is the most frequently used imaging for suspected salivary gland malignancies. There are advocates for both modalities, and frequently radiologists will request both imaging when investigating suspected malignancy. Both modalities outline the parapharyngeal space, the carotid artery and the possibility of the cervical nodal involvement. The advocates report that MRI is more sensitive for soft tissue and neurological involvement, and CT is better for identifying bony involvement. However, most surgeons, in patients suspected with a malignant salivary gland tumour, would insist on some imaging modality being performed, prior to proceeding to surgery.

Operative procedure of choice

The aim of surgery for the management of salivary gland malignancy is complete excision of the primary site and to consider preservation of cranial nerve and other functions should they not be involved in the tumours process.

In the parotid gland this should imply that if the facial nerve is working preoperatively it should be expected to work at some time postoperatively. The only indication to resection of the facial nerve is when the nerve is paralysed preoperatively or when, at the time of surgery, if leaving the facial nerve would result in incomplete excision of the tumour. Thus tumours usually small, < 3 cm it is possible, as most tumours are located in the lateral lobe, that a lateral lobe parotidectomy (superficial lobe!) can be performed, when the tumours are of a larger size, then a total parotidectomy should be performed, implying that the facial nerve and its functions are preserved. A radical parotidectomy is indicated when the facial nerve is paralysed preoperatively or when there is a need to sacrifice the facial nerve at the time of surgery. A sacrificed facial nerve should be reconstructed at the time of surgery, by a greater auricular nerve or sural nerve graft. While the results of facial nerve function are not normal, usually Grade II/III House-Brackman, they do return some tone to the facial muscles, the eye closure frequently requires the insertion of an upper lid "weight" or a tarsorrhaphy.

In the submandibular gland tumours, surgery is "more easy" – it is recommended that the best approach to malignancy is to perform a selective neck dissection including levels Ib, IIa and III for all neoplasms – benign and malignant.

In minor salivary glands – including the sublingual glands – incision biopsy initially is considered appropriate to confirm the true nature of the local pathology, determine its type and grade prior to recommending surgery. Surgery, in general, in minor salivary gland locations should be aggressive towards the tumour but functionally sparing, i.e., the removal of a painless functioning eye, or preservation of laryngeal function by performing a partial laryngectomy.

Management of the neck

It is reported that approximately 20% of parotid malignancy presents with a clinically apparent lymph node metastases. These patients require appropriate neck dissection and postoperative radiotherapy.

It must be emphasized that in parotid gland malignancy when the regional lymph nodes are not involved the 5-year survival is approximately 75%, while the presence of a positive lymph node decreases the survival to almost 10%. However, in the light of the above statement, these should be considered when dealing with parotid and other salivary gland malignancies that carry a high risk of nodal metastases, and also in some patients whose surgical approach to the primary disease may be facilitated by lymphadenectomy. Several factors are related to this high-risk group – histology, grade of tumour, primary stage of disease, size of tumour, presence or absence of facial nerve paralysis, age of the patient, extra-parotid extension and perilymphatic invasion. The reported incidence of metastases depends on the evaluation methods used and on their histological variants.

Three recent papers on the use of elective neck dissections on all patients who presented with a malignancy of the parotid gland in the main, but some submandibular gland tumours, were also included. They reported that there was significant difference between those patients considered to be clinically C1N+ (13.1%) and those with pathologically positive nodes C3N+ (52.5%). It was their recommendation that serious consideration be given to all patients who present with a malignant major salivary gland malignancy should undergo an elective neck dissection as a matter of routine. Zbaren et al. reported that in the observation group of patients recurrences developed in 16.8% of patients resulting in disease-free survival of 69% as compared to 86% in the elective neck dissection group. Klussmann et al. in a review of 142 parotid primary cancers and after reviewing the pattern of nodal spread concluded that total parotidectomy and radical-modified neck dissection is the treatment of choice to minimize loco-regional recurrence. Bradley has reviewed the evidence and indications for surgery to the neck in the management of malignancy of the salivary glands.

Role of radiotherapy

The primary treatment for malignant tumours of the salivary gland is surgery with radiotherapy being used in an adjuvant setting. Radiotherapy may be used as a definitive treatment when the patient either presents with an inoperable tumour or when the morbidity associated with a complete surgical extirpation is unacceptable. In general, should the tumour be proven a low-grade, if completely excised and thus unlikely to have evidence of regional metastases then surgery alone is the only treatment recommended. However, when the tumour is high-grade, close or incomplete excision, evidence of perilymphatic, perineural invasion, or evidence of lymph node metastases then postoperative radiotherapy is considered with the aim of controlling loco-regional disease. On some occasions all malignant tumours located deep to the facial nerve or parapharyngeal space are considered for postoperative radiotherapy, as the risk of complete excision is less than had the tumour being lateral to the nerve. The use of photons in the management of salivary gland malignancy remains controversial in spite of the good results reported by centers that have the facilities.

Role of chemotherapy

Spiro (1998) stated "at this time of writing, the only clear indication for chemotherapy is for palliation in symptomatic patients with recurrent and/or unresectable carcinoma". He also states, "the use of chemotherapy as a preoperative adjunct or concurrently with radiotherapy cannot be justified unless the drugs are administered as part of a well designed clinical trial".

A more recent review states "there are few data on the role of systemic therapies in the management of these cancers. The chemotherapy is generally reserved for the palliative management of advanced disease that is not amenable to local therapies such as surgery and/or radiation. The majority of patients for whom systemic therapy is considered will have adenoid cystic, mucoepidermoid, high-grade adenocarcinoma or salivary ductal carcinoma."

The identification of potential molecular markers c-Kit, a transmembrane cell surface receptor encoded by the c-Kit proto-oncogene, as well as EGFR and Her-2, has activated interest in the use of chemotherapeutic agents against certain salivary gland cancers – notably adenoid cystic carcinoma.

Management of local-regional recurrent disease

Many patients never experience relapse when the tumour is located in the major salivary glands. Whereas the same is not true when tumours are located in the minor salivary glands, including areas such as the paranasal sinuses and skull base.

The most common site for recurrences locally is in the surrounding soft tissues, including bone and cartilage, followed by cervical nodal failure, and some patients will have multifocal recurrences. The use of postoperative radiotherapy when there is evidence of high-risk factors, described above, has increased the clinician's ability to control loco-regional disease and prevent recurrences. The role of adjuvant chemotherapy alone or concurrent with radiotherapy in such a clinical scenario requires evidence from a randomized controlled trial (RCT).

Incidence of distant metastases

Distant metastases have become an increasingly common cause of death in cancer patients because of increasing therapeutic control of loco-regional disease. The incidence of failure at a distant site is

20–40% according to different histological types. It should be commented that survival of salivary gland cancers in the usual fashion of 5-year survival should not be reported, as frequently the tumour can recur by locally regionally and distally at times more than 10–20 years after treatment.

The conclusion of a large series reports that tumour stage at presentation, and local tumour aggressiveness were found to be the major prognostic factors in predicting the risk of distant failure. The lungs are the most frequent site for distant metastases followed by liver, bones and brain.

One peculiar tumour, adenoid cystic carcinoma (ACC) accounts for 25% of all malignant salivary gland tumours in most series and constitutes about 10–15% of all parotid malignancies. This cancer is more common in minor than major salivary glands. Patients with a pathologic solid type of ACC are more likely to develop distant metastases and die of their disease should they live a long period after treatment. In a review of ACC and distant metastases it was stated that the average time between the occurrence of lung metastases and death was 32.3 months and between the occurrence of metastases elsewhere and death 20.6 months.

Prognostic factors

A review of prognostic factors in salivary gland carcinoma determines patient's outcome has identified that for local control can be predicted by clinical T stage, bone invasion, site, resection margin, and treatment used. Regional control is dependant on N stage, facial nerve paralysis, and treatment used. The relative risk with surgery alone, compared with surgery plus postoperative radiotherapy, was 9.7 for local recurrence and 2.3 for regional recurrence. Distant metastases were independently correlated with T and N stage, sex, perineural invasion, histologic type, and clinical skin involvement. Overall survival depended on age, sex, T and pN stage, site, skin and bone invasion.

Another method has been to use prognostic indices for parotid carcinoma, which have been validated using the Dutch Head and Neck Oncology Cooperative Group Database and by a Belgian-German database. The findings confirmed that the prognosis of a parotid carcinoma patient can be quantified by using a weighted combination of the parameters of age, pain, clinical T (cT) classification, clinical N (cN) classification, skin invasion, facial nerve dysfunction, perineural growth, and involved surgical margins.

Pediatric salivary gland malignancy

Salivary gland neoplasms are rare in children and form less than 5% of all salivary gland tumours, with less than 8–10% of all pediatric head and neck tumours. Among salivary gland neoplasms, approximately 50% are malignant if vascular tumours are excluded. The majority of epithelial salivary tumours occur late in childhood, after 10 years of age. Most of these tumours, if malignant, are low-grade. However, if the tumour is malignant in a child less than 10 years, it is likely to be high-grade and with a poorer prognosis. The parotid gland is involved in more than 90% of all pediatric salivary gland tumours. Cumulative data from the literature suggests that benign : malignant is equal with a female : male 2 : 1. Surgery plays the mainstay for the treatment of salivary gland neoplasms in children as is performed in adults. Adjuvant therapy in the form of radiotherapy is generally reserved for high-grade tumours with residual disease, local or regional spread and recurrent disease.

CONCLUSION

Malignant salivary gland tumours are rare. The most common tumour site is the parotid gland. Aetiologic factors are not clear. Painless swellings of the salivary gland should always be considered as suspicious, especially if there are no signs of inflammation present. Signs and symptoms related to major glands differ from those of minor salivary glands, as their symptoms will depend on their different site location, but usually present with obstructive or blockage effects, or interference with local functions such as hoarseness. Surgical excision is the standard treatment for resectable tumours of both major and minor salivary glands. Neutron radiation may be a treatment option for inoperable locoregional disease. Surgery, radiation or re-irradiation are treatment options for local relapse, and neck dissection for regional relapse. Metastatic disease may be treated by either radiotherapy or palliative chemotherapy, depending on the site of metastases.

SUGGESTED READING

1. Horn-Ross PL, Ljung BM, Morrow M. Environmental factors and the risk of salivary gland cancer. *Epidemiology*, 1997; 8: 414–9.
2. Lonn S, Ahlbom A, Christensen HC et al. Mobile phone use and risk of parotid gland tumour. *Am J Epidemiol*, 2006; 164: 637–43.
3. Bradley PJ. General Epidemiology in a Defined UK Population. Chapter 1 (pp 3–13). *In:* Controversies in the Management of Salivary Gland Disease. Editors: McGurk M & Renehan A, Oxford University Press, 2001.
4. Brandwein MS, Ferlito A, Bradley PJ et al. Diagnosis and Classification of Salivary Neoplasms; Pathologic Challenges and Relevance to Clinical Outcome. *Acta Otolaryngologica*, 2002; 122: 758–64.
5. Hughes JH, Volk EE, Wilbur DC. Pitfalls in Salivary Gland Fine-Needle Aspiration Cytology: Lessons from the College of American Pathologists Inter-laboratory Comparison Program in Non-gynecologic Cytology. *Arch Path Lab Med*, 2005; 129: 26–31.
6. Zbren P, Nuyens M, Loosli H, Stauffer E. Diagnostic Accuracy of Fine-Needle Aspiration Cytology and Frozen Section in Primary Parotid Carcinoma. *Cancer*, 2004; 100: 1876–83.
7. Cristallini EG, Ascani S, Farabi R et al. Fine-Needle Aspiration Biopsy of Salivary Glands. *Acta Cytol*, 1997; 41: 1421–5.
8. Farrag TY, Lin FR, Koch WM, Califano JA, Cummings CW, Farinola MA, Tufano RP. The role of pre-operative CT-Guided FNAB for Parapharyngeal Space Tumours. *Otolaryngol Head Neck Surg*, 2007; 136: 411–4.
9. Zbaren P, Guelat D, Losli H, Stauffer E. Parotid tumours: fine-needle aspiration and/or frozen section. *Otolaryngol Head Neck Surg*, 2008; 139 (6): 811–5
10. Atula T, Grenman ST, Laippala P, Klemi PJ. Fine-Needle Aspirational Biopsy in the diagnosis of Parotid Gland Lesions. *Diagn Cytopathol*, 1996; 15: 185–90.
11. Howlett DC, Kesse KW, Hughes DV, Sallomi DF. The role of Imaging in the Evaluation of Parotid Disease. *Clin Radiol*, 2002; 57: 692–701.
12. Spiro JD, Spiro RH. Cancer of the parotid gland: Role of VII Nerve Preservation. *World J Surg*, 2003; 27: 863–7.
13. Bradley, PJ. Management of Submandibular and Minor Salivary Gland Neoplasms. *Current Opin ORL-HNS*, 1999; 7 (2): 72–8.
14. Munier N, Bradley PJ. The Management of Neoplasms of the Submandibular Gland Triangle. *Oral Oncology*, 2008: 44; 251–60.
15. Rinaldo A, Ferlito A, Bradley PJ et al. Management of Malignant Submandibular Gland Tumours – A Review. *Acta Otolaryngology*, 2003: 123 (8); 898–904
16. Rinaldo A, Shaha AR, Bradley PJ. Management of Malignant Sublingual Salivary Gland Tumors – A Review. *Oral Oncology*, 2004: 40: 2–5.
17. Spiro RH. Diagnosis and pitfalls in the treatment of parotid tumours. *Semin Surg Oncol*, 1991; 7: 20–4.
18. Ferlito A, Shaha AR, Rinaldo A, Mondin V. Management of Clinically negative Cervical Lymph Nodes in Patients with Malignant Neoplasms of the Parotid Gland. *ORL*, 2001; 63: 123–6.
19. Stennert E, Kisner D, Jungehuelsing M, Guntinas-Lichius O, Schroder U, Eckel HE, Klussmann P. High Incidence of Lymph Node Metastasis in Major Salivary Gland Cancer. *Arch Otolaryngol Head Neck Surg*, 2003; 129: 720–3.
20. Zbaren P, Schupbach J, Nuyens M, Stauffer E. Elective Neck Dissection versus Observation in Primary Parotid Gland Carcinoma. *Otolaryngol Head Neck Surg*, 2005; 132: 387–91.
21. Klussmann JP, Ponert T, Mueller RP, Dienes HP, Guntinas-Lichius O. Patterns of lymph node spread and its influence on outcome in resectable parotid cancer. *Eur J Surg Oncol*, 2008; 34 (8): 932–7.
22. Bradley PJ. Neck Dissection for Salivary Cancer. In: Neck Dissection – Management of Regional Disease in Head and Neck Cancer. Edited by Ferlito A, Robbins KT, Sliver CE. Plural Publishing Inc, USA. (Due publication September 2009).
23. Mendenhall WM, Morris CG, Amdur RJ, Werning JW, Villaret DB. Radiotherapy alone or combined with surgery for salivary gland carcinoma. *Cancer*, 2005; 103: 2544–50.
24. Terhaard CHJ, Lubsen H, Rasch CRN et al. The role of radiotherapy in the treatment of malignant salivary gland tumours. *Int J Radiat Oncol Bio Phys*, 2005; 61: 103–11.
25. Douglas JD, Lee S, Maramore GE. Neutron radio-therapy for the treatment of locally advanced major salivary gland tumours. *Head Neck*, 1999; 21: 255–63.
26. Spiro RH. Management of Malignant Tumours of the Salivary Glands. *Oncology*, 1998; 12: 671–80.
27. Laurie SA, Licitra L. Systemic Therapy in the Palliative Management of Advanced Salivary Gland Cancers. *J Clin Oncol*, 2006; 24: 2573–678.
28. Dodd RL, Slevin NJ. Salivary gland adenoid cystic carcinoma: A review of chemotherapy and molecular therapies. *Oral Oncol*, 2006: 42; 759–69.
29. Milano A, Longo F, Basile M, Iaffaioli RV, Caponigro F. Recent advances in the treatment of salivary gland cancers: emphasis on molecular targeted therapy. *Oran Oncol*, 2007; 43(8): 729–34.
30. Kirkbride P, Liu F-F, O'Sullivan B, Payne D, Warde P, Gullane P, Pintile M, Keane TJ, Cummings B. Outcome of Curative Management of Malignant Tumours of the Parotid Gland. *J Otolaryngol*, 2001; 30: 271–9.

31. Patel SG, Singh B, Polluri A et al. Craniofacial Surgery for Malignant Skull Base Tumours. *Cancer,* 2003; 98: 1179–87.
32. Vattemi E, Graiff C, Sava T, Pedersini R, Caldara A, Mandara M. Systemic therapies for recurrent and/ or metastatic salivary gland cancers. *Expert Rev Anticancer Ther,* 2008; 8(3): 393–402.
33. Bradley PJ. Distant Metastases from Salivary Glands. *Cancer, ORL,* 2001; 63: 233–42.
34. Gallo O, Franchi A, Bottai GV, Fini-Storcji G, Tesi G, Boddi V. Risk Factors for Distant Metastases from Carcinoma of the Parotid Gland. *Cancer,* 1997: 80; 844–51.
35. Bradley PJ. Adenoid Cystic Carcinoma of the Head and Neck – A Review. *Current Opinions ORL-HNS,* 2004: 12; 127–32.
36. van der Wal JE, Becking AG, Snow GB, van der Waal I. Distant Metastases of Adenoid Cystic Carcinoma of the Salivary Glands and the Value of Diagnostic Examinations during Follow-Up. *Head Neck,* 2002; 24: 779–83.
37. Terhaard CHT, Lubsen H, Van der Tweel I, Hilgers FJM, Eijkenboom WMH, Marres HAM, Tjho-Heslinga RE et al. Salivary Gland Carcinoma: Independent Prognostic Factors for Loco-regional Control, Distant Metastases, and Overall Survival: Results of the Dutch Head and Neck Oncology Cooperative Group. *Head Neck,* 2004; 26: 681–93.
38. Vander Poorten VL, Hart AAM, van der Laan BFA, de Jong RJB, Manni JJ et al. Prognostic Index for Patients with Parotid Carcinoma. *Cancer,* 2003; 97: 1453–63.
39. Poorten VV, Hart A, Vauterin T, Jeunen G, Schoenaers J, Hamoir M, Balm A, Stennert E, Guntinas-Lichius O, Delaere P. Prognostic index for patients with parotid carcinoma: international external validation in a Belgium-German database. *Cancer,* 2009; 115 (3): 540–50.
40. Bradley PJ, McClelland L, Metha D. Pediatric Salivary Gland Epithelial Neoplasms. *ORL,* 2007; 69: 137–45.

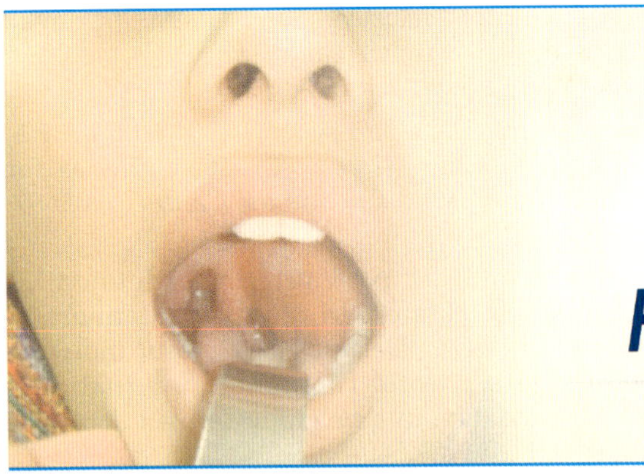

CHAPTER 32

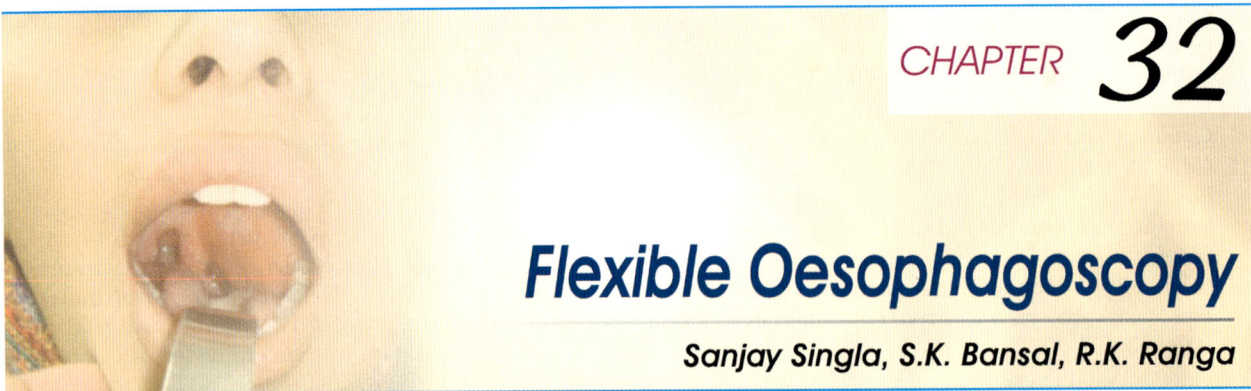

Flexible Oesophagoscopy

Sanjay Singla, S.K. Bansal, R.K. Ranga

Upper areodigestive tract is to deliver air to lungs and food to stomach. Food is to pass through oral cavity, oropharynx, hypopharynx and then oesophagus to reach the stomach. Process of digestion though starts in oral cavity by salivary enzymes, main digestion starts in stomach. Oesophagus mainly acts as a conduit. A complex nervous system has evolved to control its function of pushing food bolus by contraction and receptive relaxation. Upper aerodigestive tract is exposed to the largest number of foreign antigens as compared to other parts of the body. Therefore, malfunction of this organ by infection, neuromuscular incoordination, tumours, ulcers and vascular anomalies, etc., results in wide spectrum of pathology and symptoms noticed by the patient. Problem lies due to its inaccessibility to traditional examination of inspection by naked eye. Therefore, necessity of examining the interior of body organs led to the invention of endoscopy.

Development of endoscopy has to pass two initial barriers – one, no natural light shines beyond the most distal ends of the alimentary tube and second the tract is not straight. Though problem of illumination was solved in 1879 by Thomas Edison, it took pretty 25 years before a light source was incorporated into a rigid scope and oesophagus was looked in by making the upper tract straight by manoeuvering the cervical spine. It had its own limitations and complications. Further research by Hoffman in 1911 checked this problem of tortuosity and led to the development of a semiflexible gastroscope with articulated lenses and prisms by Wolf and Schindler in 1930s. Real breakthrough came when Hopkins made a model of flexible fibre imaging device which could transmit light and images beyond bends using flexible quarts fibres in 1954. Flexible endoscopy provided a quantum leap in the management of pathologies of internal tortuous tracts.

Before taking a patient for examination

A clinician must know the indications of endoscopy (oesophagoscopy), anatomy of the area and be well versed with the instrument, its handling, capabilities, limitations and proper care. One should know his or her strong and weak points too along with the capacity of his team and set-up.

Indications of oesophagoscopy

Diagnostic

- Symptoms evaluation
  - Dysphagia
  - Odynophagia retrosternal burning
  - Chest pain after evaluation of any cardiac cause
  - Regurgitation of food
  - Dyspepsia especially associated with weight loss and persistent despite medical management
  - Nausea and vomiting
- Malignancy check
  - Oesophageal ulcers and growths
  - Barrett's epithelium

- Evaluation of other conditions
  - Portal hypertension patients for oesophageal varices
  - Occult upper GI bleed patients
  - Evaluation for halitosis and cause for aspiration
  - To confirm the findings of Barium swallow
  - Endoscopic ultrasound to evaluate oesophageal tumours and periesophageal lesions in mediastinum

Therapeutic

- Acute upper GI bleed
- Foreign body removal
- Dilatation of stenosis, web and achalasia cardia
- Palliation for obstructing neoplasms
- Feeding tube placement
- Eradication of oesophageal varices
- Endoluminal therapy of gastroesophageal reflux disease (GERD) in cases which are on long-term medical management and do not require surgery right away.

Relevant anatomy of the area (Figs. 32.1 to 32.3)

All the distances are measured from incisor teeth and scopes are calibrated for that.

After the **incisors** teeth are crossed one enters the **oral cavity** passing over the tongue till one sees the **soft palate**. Next thing visible is lingual surface (upper end) of the **epiglottis**, a leaf-like structure which covers the larynx. Area between the soft palate and upper end of the epiglottis is known as the **oropharynx**. An area clinically called as **hypopharynx** (laryngopharynx) extends between the superior border of epiglottis to the inferior border of the cricoid cartilage, where it becomes continuous with upper end of the oesophagus (cricopharyngeaus sphincter). **The laryngeal inlet** lies anteriorly bounded above by the epiglottis, below by the arytenoid cartilages and laterally by the aryepiglottic folds.

A small **piriform fossa** lies on each side of the laryngeal inlet, bounded medially by the aryepiglottic folds and laterally by the thyroid cartilage and thyrohyoid membrane. Its mucous membrane covers the branches of internal laryngeal nerve.

Muscles of the pharynx

Pharynx extends from base of the skull up to upper end of the oesophagus. It is subdivided into naso-, oro- and hypopharynx. Posterior wall of pharynx is enveloped by superior, middle and inferior pharyngeal constrictor muscles in overlapping fashion. Inferior constrictor muscle is made of two parts, upper thyropharyngeus and the lower cricopharyngeus. Both the muscles join posteriorly with their contralateral parts.

The thyropharyngeus joins the median raphe and overlaps the middle constrictor while the cricopharyngeus blends with the esophagus.

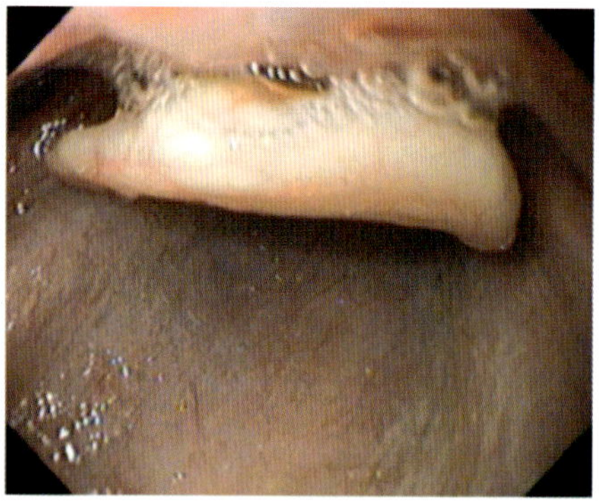

Fig. 32.1. Upper end of epiglottis.

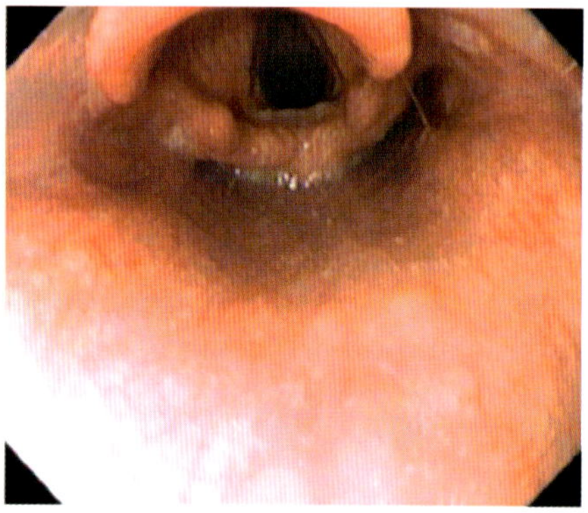

Fig. 32.2. Hypopharynx.

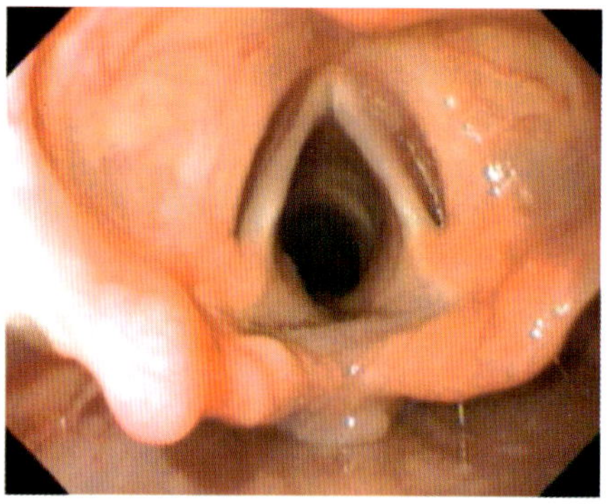

Fig. 32.3. Laryngeal inlet view.

Hypopharygeal diverticulum (Fig. 32.4)

The pharyngeal mucosa that lies between crico- and thyropharyngeus muscles is relatively unsupported

32

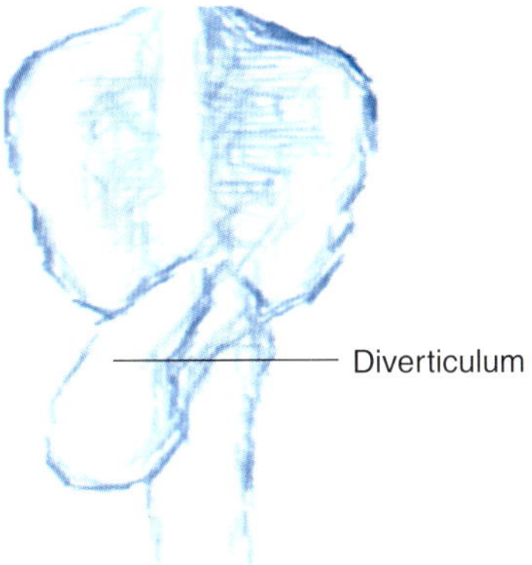

Fig. 32.4. Zenker's diverticulum through dehiscence of Killian.

and is called as **dehiscence of Killian**. Discoordination in relaxation of the cricopharyngeus muscle leads to prolapse of a pouch of mucosa through this weak area and is called as Zenker's diverticulum. This may trap portion of the food and may be a seat for abscess formation. It may be the cause for regurgitation of old food, halitosis, weight loss and aspiration pneumonia.

While doing endoscopy **avoid hyperextension of neck** as at the upper end near upper oesophageal sphincter mucosa is not well supported by the muscle and may be injured between scope and rigid spine.

As one negotiates upper sphincter, which is the narrowest part of upper GI tract, scope enters the oesophageal lumen which deviates slightly to the left in upper mediastinum where it is crossed by arch of aorta and left main bronchus about 27 cm from incisors. Here lumen deviates to right and then again to left where food passage leaves thorax to enter the abdominal cavity. Proximity of the oesophagus to the contents of mediastinum helps in using endo-ultrasound to detect abnormalities in mediastinum and take precise biopsy too.

Traction diverticulum can form in mid-oesophagus possibly due to some inflammatory node (tubercular mediastinitis) pulling on oesophageal wall. This is the only true diverticulum of oesophagus as it contains all layers of the oesophageal wall.

32

As one goes down the oesophagus whitish pinkish mucosa of oesophagus ends at so-called **Z line** and is replaced by more pinkish reddish gastric mucosa (Fig. 32.5).

Just below this Z line is lower physiological high pressure zone called **lower oesophageal sphincter**.

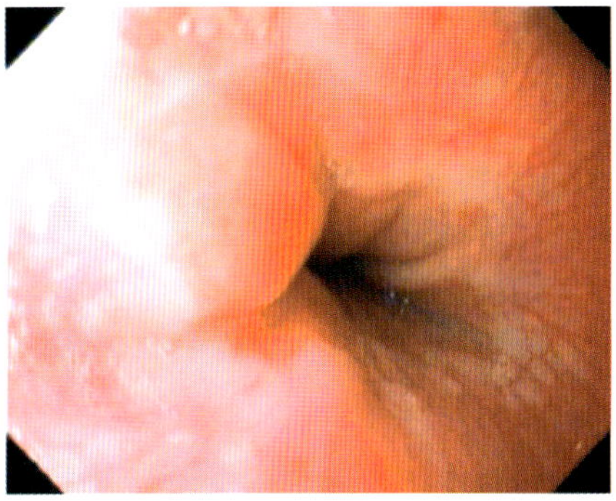

Fig. 32.5. Normal squamocolumnar junction Z line.

Diverticulae at lower end and sliding hernia (Fig. 32.6)

Pulsion diverticulum can form at the lower end of the oesophagus also. These epiphrenic (near the diaphragm) diverticulae usually form along with achalasia cardia due to incoordination in proximal propulsive and distal receptive relaxation of lower end of the oesophagus.

Abdominal part of the oesophagus can retract into chest leading to hiatal hernia (sliding type). Here one finds gastric rugae above the pinching action of diaphragm (Fig. 32.7).

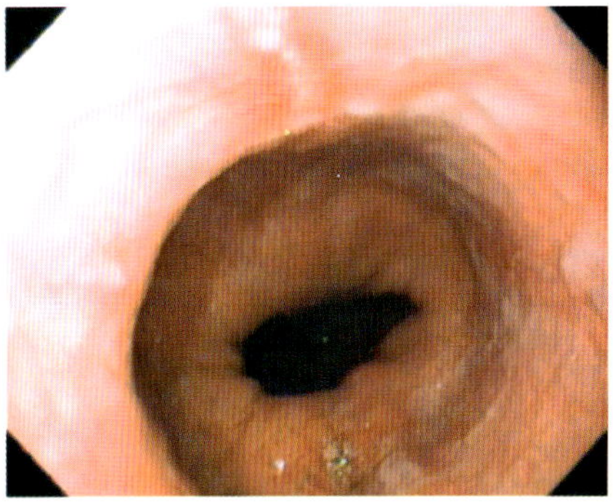

Fig. 32.6. Erosions lower end oesophagus with sliding hernia.

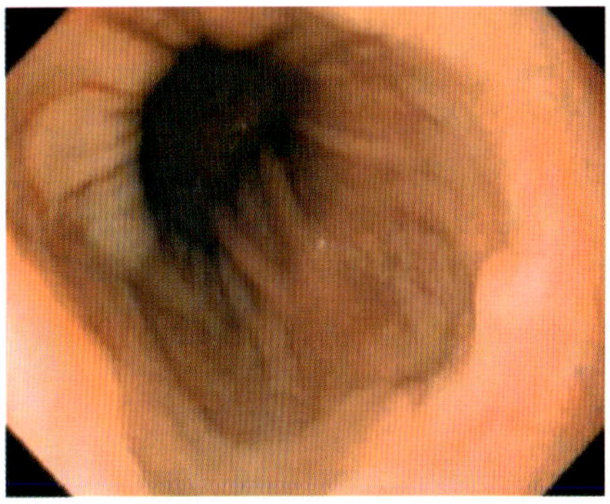

Fig. 32.7. Gastric rugae above the pinching action of LES in hiatus hernia.

Instrumentation

Two types of flexible scopes are available: Fiberoptic endoscopes and videoendoscopes.

Fiberoptic endoscopes

In fiberoptic endoscopes one bundle of around 20,000 plastic-coated glass fibres transmit light to illuminate internal organ by total internal reflection produced by that high optically dense coat.

Another bundle transmits image. As long as the spatial arrangement of fibres at both ends remains the same an image can be transmitted regardless of twists and turns.

These scopes have an eyepiece to directly view the image or a detachable camera can be attached over it. Picture quality is poor and scopes are fragile.

Videoendoscopes

Other type is videoendoscopes with CCD camera for transmission of images (Fig. 32.8).

In videoendoscopes light is transmitted through light bundles but image is captured by charged coupled device (CCD) located at the tip of the scope and a digital signal is transmitted to processor and video screen. The latter allows for a larger and better image which can be easily recorded digitally and reproduced.

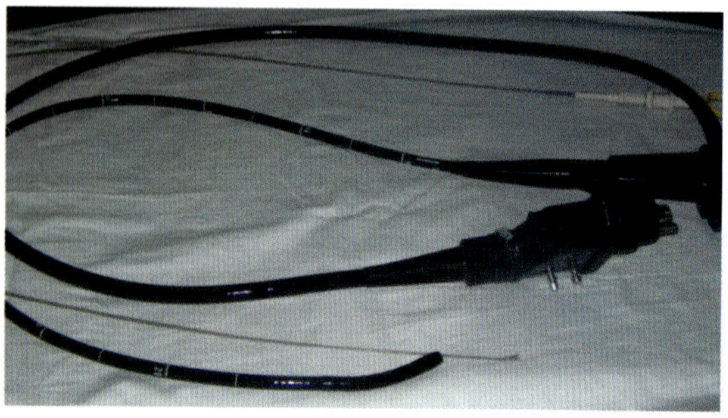

Fig. 32.8. Videoendoscope with biopsy forceps.

A large variety of scopes are available for diagnostic and therapeutic purposes.

- Small calibre scopes for children and 3.1 to 5.1 mm diameter scopes for transnasal oesophagoscopy.
- Double channel scopes for specific procedures.
- Side viewing scopes for ERCP are available.

Though initially endoscopic inspection of oesophagus were done as an isolated procedure, nowa-days usually gastro- and duodenoscopy are done along with. Thereby mother daughter scope combinations for complex procedures and thin slender scopes for small gut are also available.

Channels and accessories

- Air and water insufflation channels allow distension of bowel and cleansing of the lens. Other one or two channels permit accessories instruments for biopsy and other therapeutic procedures like sclerotherapy needle to pass through them.
- One can use biopsy forceps.
- Foreign body retrieval rat tooth forceps or a loop.
- Brush for cytology.
- Endo-ultrasound probe for diagnosis and mediastinal biopsy.
- Band applicators and sclerotherapy needles for control of varices.
- For chromo-endoscopy different dyes can be put on mucosa and lights of different wave bands can be utilised for better diagnosis. Many more accessories are available for complex upper GI procedures but we will restrict to esophagoscopy. Instrument tip control is achieved by two wheel knobs on the headpiece. Larger wheel allows for anterior and posterior deflection and smaller wheel helps in right to left movement of the tip (Fig. 32.9). The shaft of the instrument can also be rotated to change the deflection and an experienced endoscopist utilises all the three ways to its maximal potential and his or her fingers are always moving like a musician on a guitar.

Take proper care during handling, never force any instrument in its channel when tip is angulated acutely, little straighten the tip and then pass forceps and re-angulated the tip to desired angle.

Sterilisation and storage

High level of disinfection is sufficient for most of the procedures; it can be achieved by putting scope

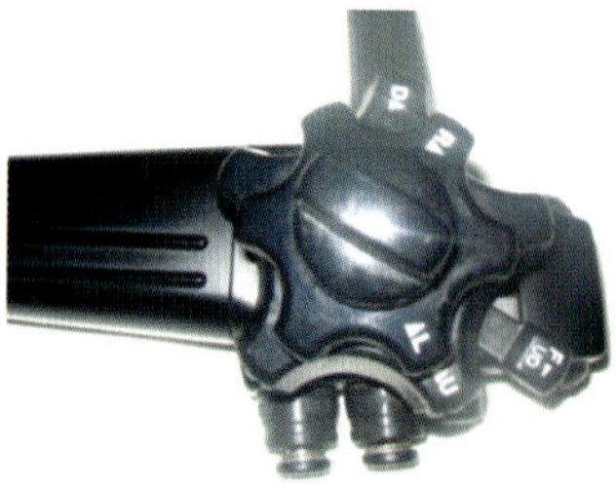

Fig. 32.9. Wheel knobs on head piece.

in glutaraldehyde solution for 15 to 30 minutes. Prior mechanical washing with soap and water is very important to get full effect of glutaraldehyde. One can use savlon or mild soap or detergent solution for the purpose. Always properly wash and dry the scope after use. One can use a padded hood to keep scope in vertical straight position in between the procedures. Brush the channels, flush with clean water and then dry the scope and hang over the pad. According to work load **leakage should be tested regularly and if there is any leakage do not immerse the scope in any liquid**, ask for repair. Tip and distal area of the scope which bends may need frequent change of a rubber coating over it.

Recording and documentation

Recording of findings is to be done for reporting and documentation. Various softwares are available to record on hard disk or portable digital media.

Technique of oesophagoscopy

Patient should be fasting for 6 hours or in emergency cases gastric lavage can be done. According to the procedure diagnostic or therapeutic, sedation or anaesthesia arrangements should be done. Patient should always be accompanied by one person and informed consent should be recorded.

The patient is positioned in left lateral position. Midazolam is administered intravenously for sedation, it leads to better toleration of the procedure as compared to throat local anaesthesia only (81% as compared to 44%). Propofol can cause deep sedation, so not used routinely. Even when using midazolam one should have access to assisted respiration technique and flumazenil as antidote to benzodiazepines. Flumazenil rapidly reverses the central effect of midazolam but may not completely reverse the respiratory depression. Resedation can occur after 1 to 2 hours.

Always balance camera for white colour.

Lubricate the tip of scope with xylocaine jelly. Ask the patient to hold the mouth gag in his jaws. Hold the scope from shaft about 20 cm from the tip so that one is not to change the grip before one negotiates the upper oesophageal sphincter. Advance the scope through the mouthpiece under vision. It may prevent inadvertent entry into Zenker's diverticulum. Pass the scope in oral cavity over the tongue when first thing to come under view is palate, leading to soft palate. After soft palate oropharynx starts with its distal limit at the upper end of epiglottis.

32

Observe epiglottis and then boundaries and contents of hypopharynx, i.e., aryepiglottic folds, piriform fosse etc. for any inflammation or growth. One can see laryngeal inlet and position of vocal cords. Foreign body may get lodged right there in hypopharynx (Fig. 32.10). Paralysis of vocal cord may give clue to underlying recurrent laryngeal nerve palsy.

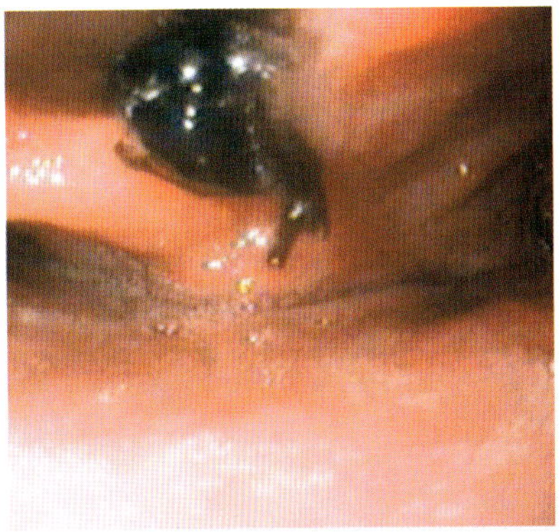

Fig. 32.10. A large ant trying to enter laryngeal inlet.

Neoplastic growth of uppermost part of oesophagus (upper oesophageal sphincter area) can be detected and biopsy can be taken to establish histopathological diagnosis (Fig. 32.11).

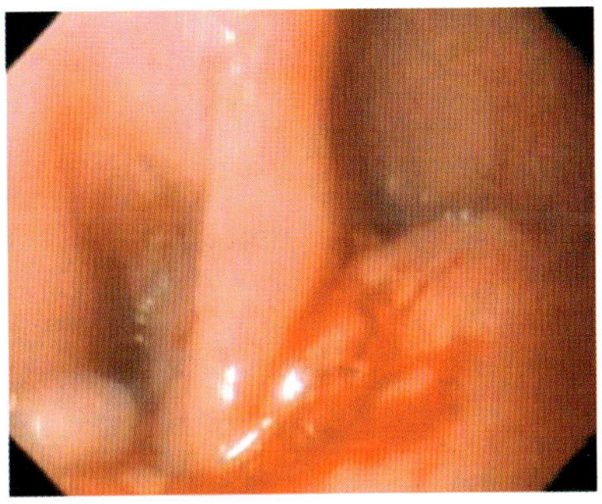

Fig. 32.11. Neoplastic growth UES area.

After this oesophageal lumen is entered. Asking a patient to swallow may help in entering oesophageal lumen; similarly entry from side, i.e., from piriform fossa instead of centre may facilitate entry in the lumen. Be gentle; never push hard as this is the narrowest and relatively blind area. One may find it difficult to enter the lumen because of postcricoid stricture as in Plummer-Vinson syndrome which is characterised by iron deficiency anaemia, dysphagia and postcricoid web (Fig. 32.12). Presence of angular cheilitis with dysphagia is a warning sign for postcricoid stricture.

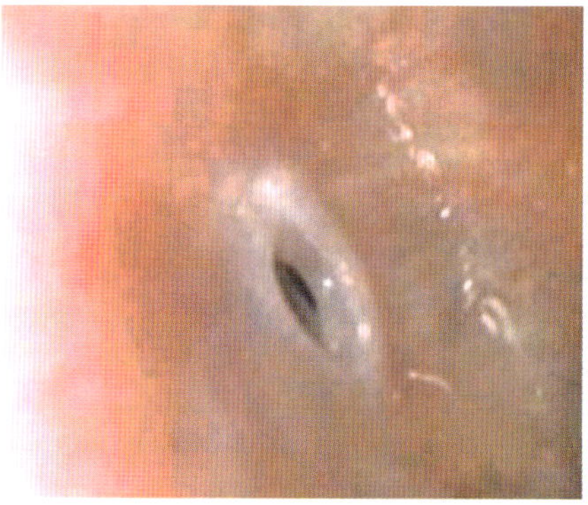

Fig. 32.12. Postcricoid web in a patient of PV syndrome.

Treatment of postcricoid web is dilatation by bougienage.

Once oesophageal lumen is entered insufflate air and slowly advance the scope. Observe for peristalsis, any inflammation, growth, foreign body or Barrett epithelium.

One may find white cotton wool of candidiasis which is common in immunocompromised patients (Fig. 32.13).

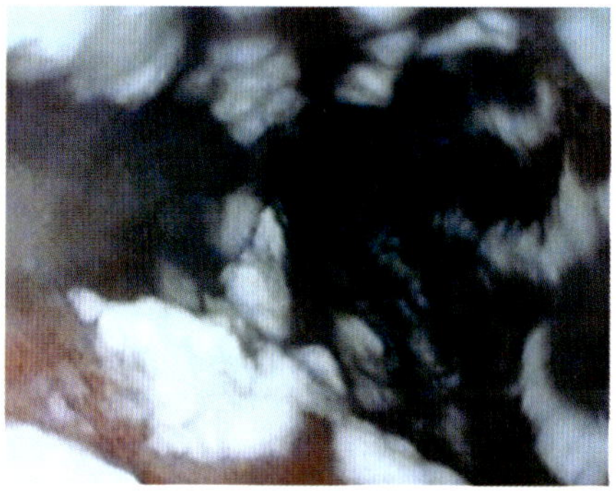

Fig. 32.13. Oesophageal candidiasis in a HIV positive patient.

Oesophageal candidiasis is taken as evidence of HIV infection. Such cases re-emphasise the need to take universal precautions while doing endoscopy. Other infections which can lead to oesophagitis are cytomegalovirus, herpes simplex virus, varicella zoster virus, EB virus, human papilloma virus, diphtheria, syphilis and human immunodeficiency virus.

A small **foreign body** may obstruct the passage in an already narrow segment of esophagus. In such cases, after removal of the FB always ascertain the cause of prior narrowing.

Foreign body in an old man in which the lower segment of oesophagus was stenosed due to inflammatory stricture (Fig. 32.14).

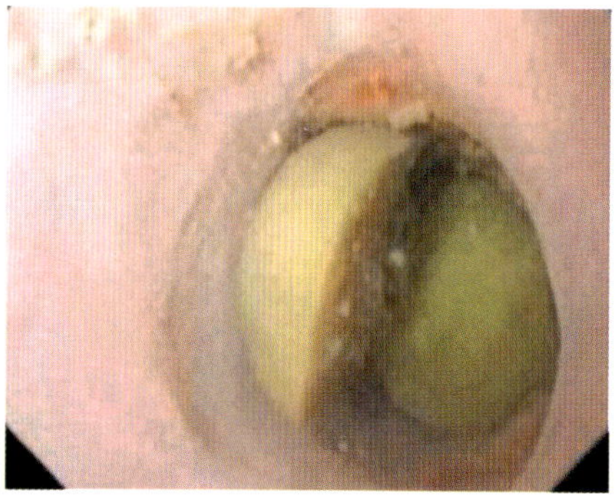

Fig. 32.14. Peanut over a stricture.

Breach in the normal mucosa by inflammation or suspected neoplasm should be investigated by brush cytology or biopsy (Fig. 32.15).

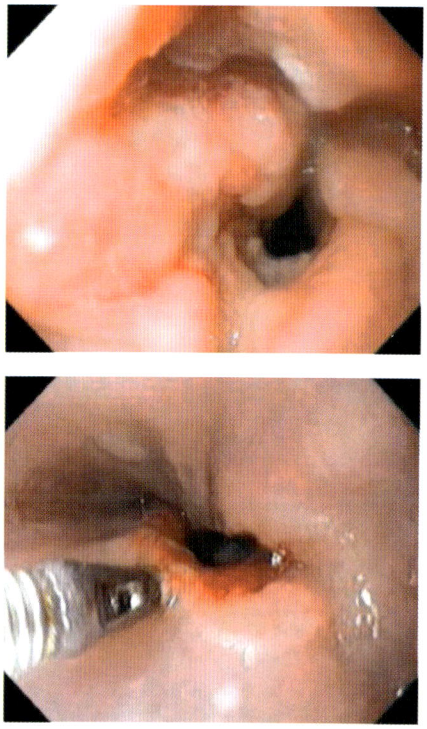

Fig. 32.15. Biopsy from a suspected neoplasm of mid oesophagus.

In cases of unresectable malignant lesions of oesophagus palliation can be done either by lasers or stents by endoscopic means to allow feeding by oral route (Fig. 32.16).

In case of dysphagia one may encounter severe lower end oesophagitis causing sloughing of superficial mucosal layers (Fig. 32.17).

Deep oesophageal ulcer may be caused by a pill sticking somewhere on the way, leading to dysphagia and odynophagia (Fig. 32.18).

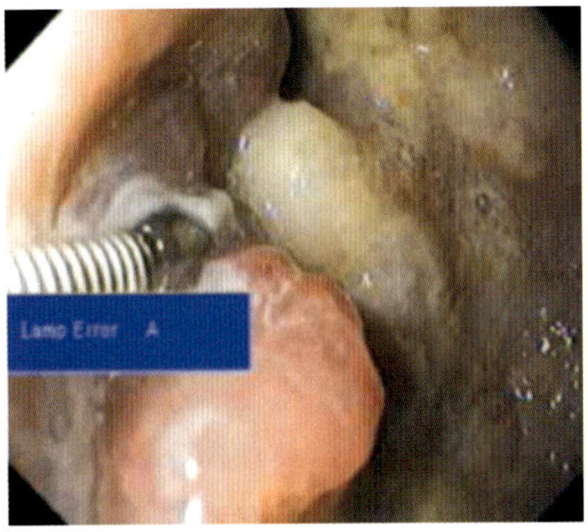

Fig. 32.16. Unresectable growth oesophagus.

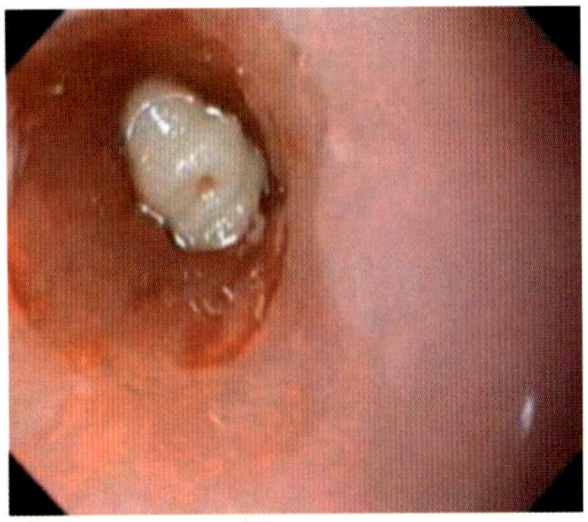

Fig. 32.17. Underlying Inflamed tissue in reflux oesophagitis after slough is separated.

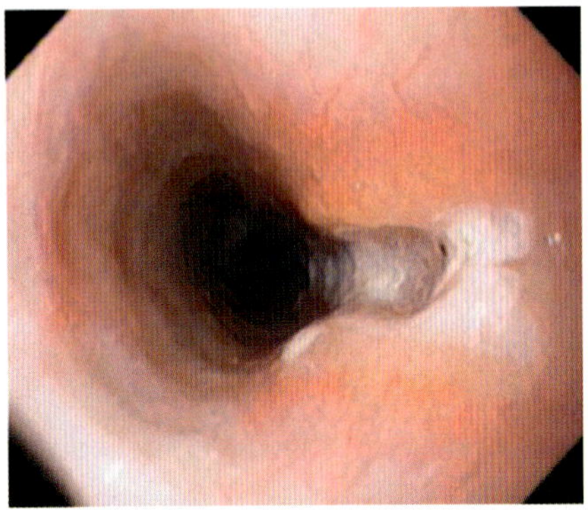

Fig. 32.18. Deep ulcer esophagus by a pill due to prolonged contact.

Pills damage the oesophagus by acidity, size, and contact time. The typical sites of pill-induced injury are at the level of aortic arch and lower end of esophagus, where there is anatomic narrowing. Drugs commonly involved in pill-induced injury are pottasium chloride, doxycycline, NSAIDs, iron tablets, quinidine and alendronate. To avoid pill-induced injury all medications should be taken with sufficient fluids.

Caustic ingestion can result in very severe injury to oesophagus and stomach. Strong alkalies cause more severe injuries as compared to acids as they cause liquefactive necrosis and cause rapid and deep injuries. Acids produce a coagulation necrosis in oesophagus that may limit penetration and injury.

Clinical features vary widely, oropharyngeal injuries may cause airway compromise and may need intubation. In all patients of caustic ingestion, upper GI endoscopy should be performed within first 24 to 48 hours to evaluate the extent of damage to oesophagus and stomach, which will guide therapy and prognosis. A grading system for oesophageal injury to predict subsequent clinical outcome has been developed.

Grading for caustic oesophageal injuries

Grade	*Features*
0	Normal
1	Mucosal oedema and erythema
2A	Superficial ulcers, bleeding and exudates
2B	Deep focal or circumferential ulcers
3A	Focal necrosis: deep ulcers with brown, black or grey discoloration
3B	Extensive necrosis
4	Perforation

Patients with grades 1 and 2A injury have excellent prognosis without immediate morbidity or late stricture formation. Strictures develop in 70% to 100% of patients with grades 2B and 3A injuries (Fig. 32.19). Grade 3B carries a 65% early mortality and a need for oesophageal resection. Strictures when develop are usually at the site of natural oesophageal narrowing, i.e., UES, at the level of aortic arch and LES (Fig. 32.20).

Lower end severe oesophagitis may be the cause of hametemesis as is evident from the following pictures (Figs. 32.20 & 32.21).

While investigating for hametemesis one may encounter growth, inflammation, tear in mucosa or esophageal varices (Fig. 32.22) as the cause for bleeding and this may modify and influence the mode of management. Variceal bleeding can be controlled by sclerotherapy or varices can be obliterated by bands. For prophylactic variceal obliterations bands are preferred over sclerotherapy. In fact sclerotherapy should not be done for varices which have never bled.

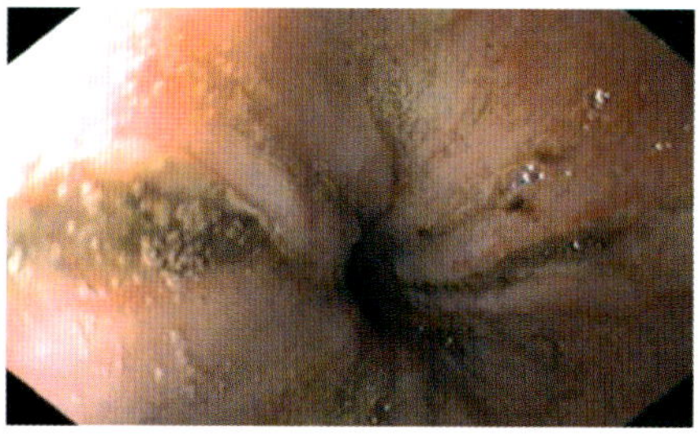

Fig. 32.19. Endoscopic view of 3A injury at LES.

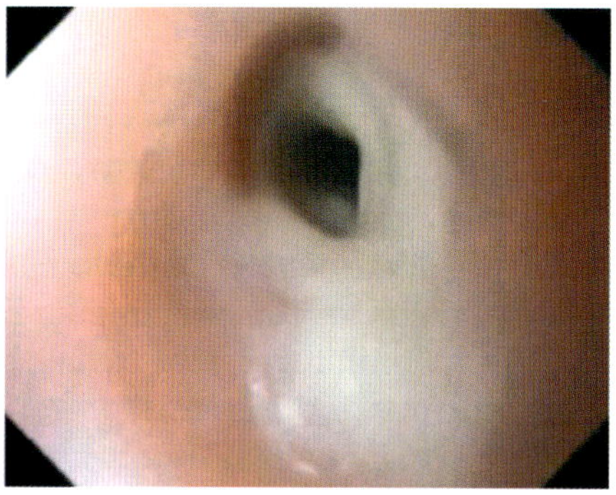

Fig. 32.20. Late stricture in a circumferential injury.

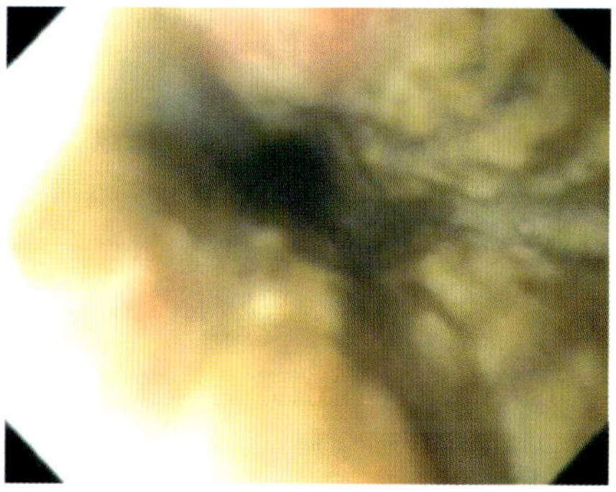

Fig. 32.21. Lower end esophagus on 1st day of bleeding.

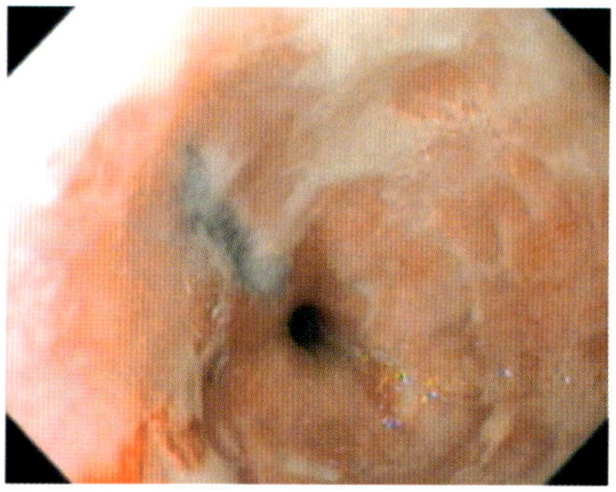

Fig. 32.22. View on fourth day after treatment.

In cases of reflux of gastric contents in esophagus (GERD, i.e., gastroesophageal reflux disease) lower end of esophagus may show isolated islands of pink red mucosa in between whitish squamous epithelium, there may be confluence of such abnormal mucosal patches or a strip of lower mucosa may change to abnormal epithelium (Fig. 32.23).

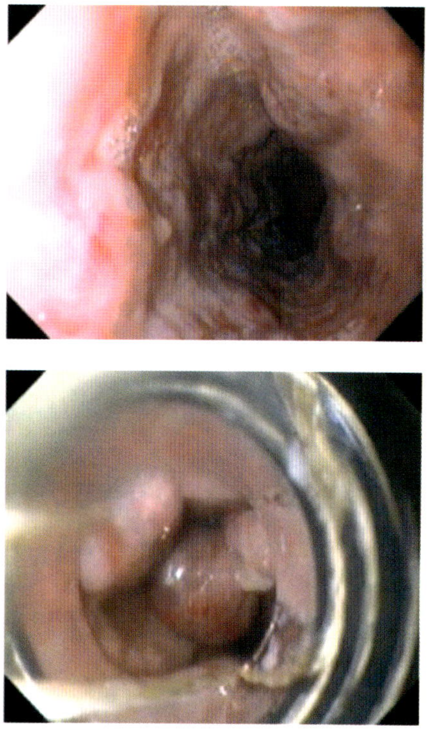

Fig. 32.23. Symptomatic esophageal varices in a patient of carcinoma colon with sec. liver. Ligated with bands.

Chromo-endoscopy can be utilized to detect neoplastic or pre-neoplastic abnormalities (Figs. 32.24 to 32.26). 20 ml of **Lugol's iodine** 1% to 2% solution can be applied over suspected area. Normal squamous epithelium of esophagus contains glycogen which takes up the iodine stain. Areas of inflammation and neoplasia remain unstained. These areas become apparent for biopsy sampling. **Methelyne blue (0.5% to 1% solution)** is another dye which is taken by intestinal metaplastic cells and then those areas can be biopsied selectively. Magnification endoscopy can magnify by X150, thereby showing cytological details on endoscopy itself. Another very promising technique is **narrow band imaging (NBI)**, it improves the quality of endoscopic images and enhances microvasculature visualization – a novel endoscopic technique that is based on the optical phenomenon that the depth of light penetration into tissues is dependent on the wavelength; the shorter the wavelength, the more superficial the penetration. Therefore, use of blue light or green light with the help of a special filter

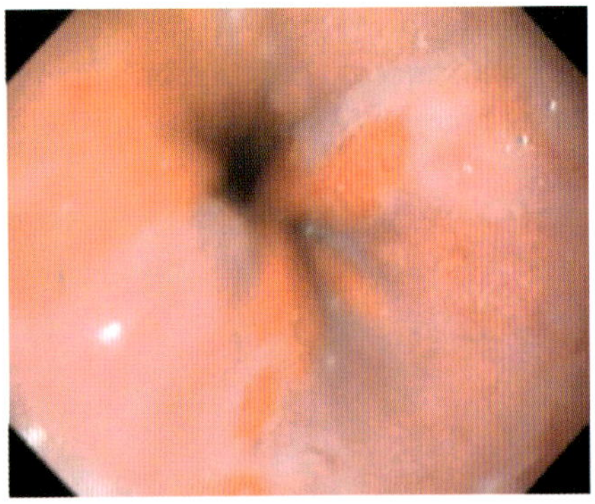

Fig. 32.24. Isolated patches of GERD.

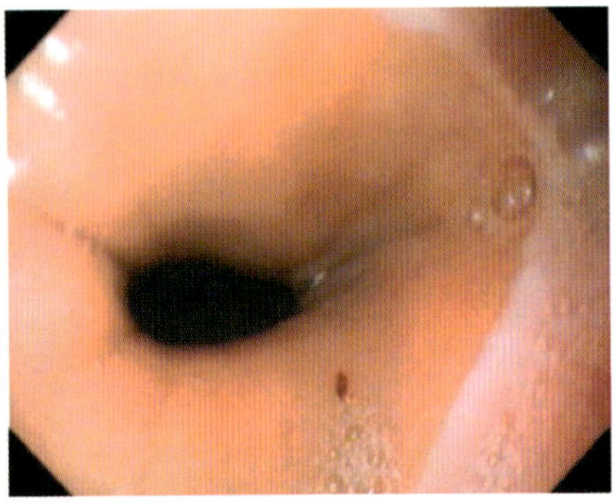

Fig. 32.25. Barrett epithelium (short segment < 3 cm).

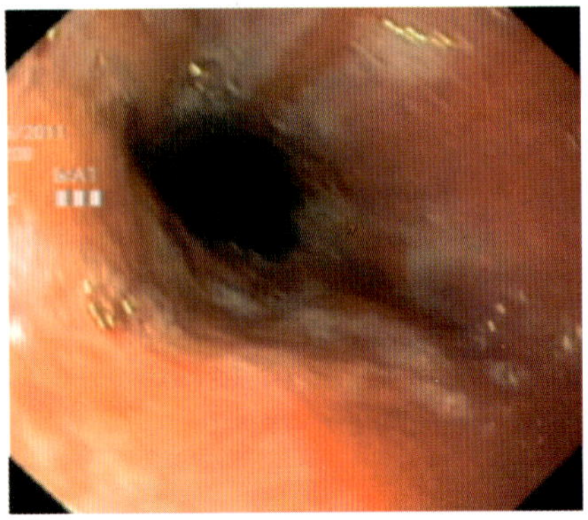

Fig. 32.26. GERD picture on standard endoscopy. (*Courtesy:* Dr. Sud Randhir)

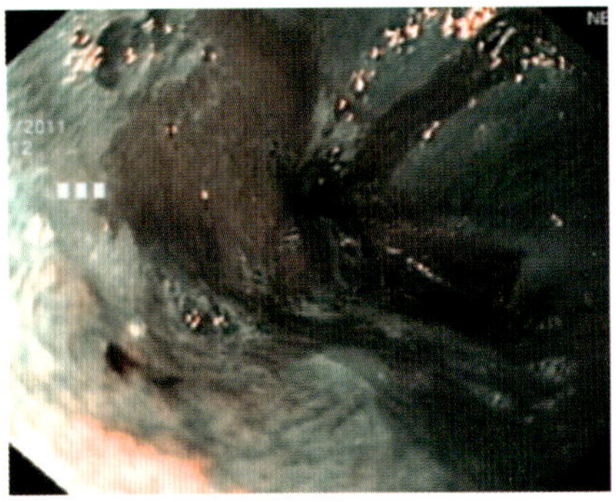

Fig. 32.27. Same picture when viewed by NBI.

can enable imaging of the superficial tissue surface structures without the need for chromo-endoscopy.

Preliminary studies suggest that NBI may represent a significant improvement over standard endoscopy for detection of metaplastic and neoplastic areas within the Barrett's epithelial segment. The mucosal (ridge/villous, circular, irregular/distorted) and vascular (normal, abnormal) patterns when correlated with histology showed excellent sensitivity and specificity for intestinal metaplasia and high grade dysplasia respectively.

Presence of **goblet cells** in suspected Barrett's epithelium confirms it. **Barrett's** is a pre-malignant condition and mucosa can be destroyed by laser before it changes to adenocarcinoma.

Patients with **documented pathological reflux disease**, especially those requiring ongoing therapy with proton pump inhibitors can be treated by **endoluminal techniques**. In general patients with complicated reflux disease such as Barrett's epithelium, erosive oesophagitis, reflux-associated strictures or dysphagia and patients with large hiatal hernias are reserved for surgical management. Of the currently available **endoluminal techniques**, which include **radiofrequency induction of localized thermal injury, endoscopic suturing and endoscopic submucosal injection or implantation of inert substances for LES augmentation**, radiofrequency technique (Stretta) has been most widely studied and applied.

While looking for **difficulty of taking liquids as compared to solids** one should suspect achalasia cardia. **Achalasia is inability of LES to relax**. The best way to diagnose achalasia is by manometry. Endoscopy may be reported normal if one is not suspecting achalasia in an early case before the procedure. In more obvious case one may find esophageal dilatation, presence of food, secretions and lack of esophageal contractions. Varying amount of mucosal inflammatory signs can be seen. A tight but elastic feel, as endoscope pops through the LOS area, is the hallmark of achalasia. **Achalasia can be treated by dilatation or injections of boutlinum** by endoscopy. Cardiomyotomy either open or by minimal access can be offered as definitive procedure. Exclusion of cancer at GE junction is very important as it can give similar picture.

Endoscopic ultrasound is a promising newer procedure where ultrasound transducer is attached at the tip of the scope and ultrasound images can be taken from very close proximity and FNAC can be done. **Current applications** include the **diagnosis and staging of the upper aerodigestive tract neoplasia, diagnosis of submucosal pathology, pulmonary and mediastinal lesions** (Fig. 32.27).

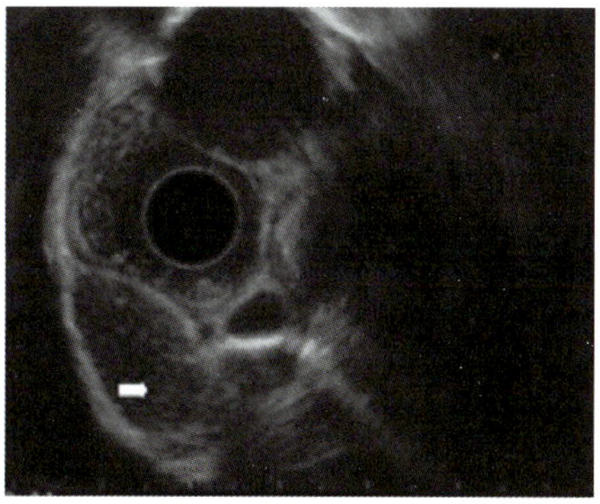

Fig. 32.28. Endo US showing layers of esophagus and mediastinal node (arrow mark). (*Courtesy:* Dr. Puri Rajesh)

Complications of flexible upper endoscopy

General complications

Cardiopulmonary complications

- **Hypoxia: Up to 15% patients experience** a decrease in SPO_2 below 85% during upper endoscopy. It is usually due to sedation and to encroachment upon the airway. Always use pulse oxymeter during endoscopy. Monitor the patient and give supplemental oxygen as required. A jaw thrust manoeuvre will increase airflow and oxygen saturation.
- **Bradycardia** can occur due to overdistention of stomach because of air used for insufflation. Decompress the stomach and if still bradycardia persists give atropine to combat vagal stimulation.
- **Hypotension** can occur due to bradycardia or hypovolemia. Maintain intravenous access and treat accordingly.
- **Bleeding diathesis due to medications.**
  Below is the list of medicines which can interfere in clotting mechanism of the body.
  - Aspirin, NSAIDs, warfarin, clopidogrel and ticlopidine.

  Careful history of drug intake especially in old age people and stopping drugs appropriately before the invasive procedure will help reduce the haemorrhage.

Infectious complications

- **Endocarditis and infection of prosthesis** can occur especially after dilatation of strictures and variceal sclerosis in susceptible individuals. Always note down previous history of endocarditis, valvular heart disease and valve replacement or vascular graft surgery and give prophylactic antibiotics to these patients. 2 gm of parenteral ampicillin and 80 mg of gentamycin followed by 1.5 gm of amoxicillin per oral, 6 hours after the procedure is fairly acceptable regimen.

Systemic Infections

- **Transmission of infection:** *Pseudomonas aeruginosa* infections spread by contaminated scopes has a high mortality rate. Contamination by *Salmonella, Helicobacter* and *Mycobacterium* have all been documented. There has been no convincing report of HIV colonizing endoscopes till date.
- **Aspiration:** Topical anesthesia, gastric distension and sedation all increase the risk of aspiration. Always keep the suction ready and left lateral position helps reduce the problem.
- **Complication of sedation:** Narcotics and benzodiazepines when given together have more sedation and cardiorespiratory complications as compared to either drug given alone. Flumazenil (antidote to midazolam) and narcan (antidote to narcotics) along with facility to access and maintain the airway with oxygen supplementation should be available.

Specific complications of diagnostic upper endoscopy

- **Esophageal perforation:** The cervical esophagus is the area at maximum risk and specific risk factors include anterior cervical osteophytes, Zenker's diverticulum, cervical rib and esophageal stricture or a web. Most esophageal perforations occur during rigid endoscopy or blind passage of a flexible endoscope.
- Retching with an overinflated stomach (Boerhaave syndrome) can lead to **Mallory-Weiss tears** or transmural perforation at lower end of the esophagus.
- **Cervical pain, crepitus and cellulitis are signs of high esophageal perforation. Distal breach** in esophageal continuity causes **chest pain**. A cervical soft tissue X-ray and a chest radiogram

may be helpful in detecting cervical air, air in mediastinum and pneumothorax and pleural effusions. CT scan and water-soluble contrast study of esophagus will confirm the diagnosis. Conservative management in the form of nil per oral, high dose appropriate antibiotics is reserved for minimal mucosal injury. Any sign of through and through breach in esophagus makes a patient candidate for surgical management in the form of early drainage of mediastinum, pleural space, closure of perforation with onlay patch of viable surrounding tissue, or diversion of proximal passage.

- **Dislodgement of teeth and dentures** can occur, beware of these precious possessions.

Specific complications of therapeutic upper endoscopy

- **Bleeding** may be variceal or non-variceal. It has to be controlled according to the principles laid down for their management.
- **Perforation** of a diseased esophagus may need immediate resection and replacement of the tube by appropriate tissue or for a very small perforation at least stenting beyond the obstruction is very essential.
- **Thermal injury** by heater probe or diathermy is best avoided.
- **Bacteremia** can occur during dilatation of strictures and variceal sclerosis and should be managed with antibiotics and support.
- **Recurrent obstruction and aspirations** due to stents in esophagus may need ablation of the tumour by lasers or replacement of the stent. ***Remember:*** These patients have short life expectancy; so do no more than the minimum required for the palliation.

CONCLUSION

Upper aerodigestive tract is gateway to respiratory and digestive system. **Out of all investigations to find out pathology of this area flexible endoscopy is the best and most productive tool. It not only helps in establishing the diagnosis, but has great therapeutic potential too.** In diseases like unrespectable malignant growths of esophagus endoluminal stenting can provide a useful palliation to the patient. This can be achieved at a very low complication rate though strict adherence to the basic principles of patient safety cannot be over-emphasized. Before performing complex and relatively new endoluminal procedures like suturing, radiofrequency treatment for GERD proper training and regular follow up of protocols are very essential. Results of therapeutic endoscopy are very gratifying if the surgeon and the patient have reasonable expectations and are ready for possible complications.

SUGGESTED READING

1. Andrus CH, Dean PA, Ponsky JL. Evaluation of safe, effective intravenous sedation for utilization in endoscopic procedures. Surg Endosc, 1990; 4; 179–83.
2. Assalia A, Ilivitzki A. Surgical complications of endoscopy. *In:* Schein's Common Sense Emergency Abdominal Surgery. Springer. Moshe Schein, Paul N. Rongers ed. 2006 2nd ed. 265–7.
3. Bordelon BM, Hunter JG. Endoscopic technology. *In:* Greene FL, Ponsky JL, eds. Endoscopic Surgery. Philadelphia: WB Saunders, 1994: 6–18.
4. Canto MIF, Setrakian S, Willis J, Chak A, Petras R, Powe NR, Sivak MV. Methylene blue-directed biopsies improve detection of intestinal metaplasia and dysplasia in Barrett's oesophagus. *Gastrointest Endosc*, 2000; 51: 560–8.
5. Cooper GS. Indications and contraindications for upper gastrointestinal endoscopy. *Gastrointest Endosc Clin North Am*, 1994; 4: 439–54.
6. DunkinBJ. Complication of upper gastrointestinal Endoscopy. *In:* The SAGES Manual Fundamentals of Laparoscopy, Thoracoscopy, and GI endoscopy. Springer. Carol E. H. Scott-Conner eds. 2007 2nd ed. 617–24.
7. Lindsay J. Gastrointestinal endoscopy in Bailey and Love's Short practice of surgery. Edward Arnold Ltd. Norman S. Williams, Christopher J. K. Bulstrode, P. Ronan O'Connell eds. 2008 25th ed. 151–61.
8. Sharma P, Bansal A, Mathur S, Wani S, Cherian R, McGregor D, Higbee A, Hall S, Weston A. The utility of a narrow band imaging endoscopy system in patients with Barrett's oesophagus. *Gastrointest Endosc*, 2006; 64(2): 167–75.
9. Trevisani et al. Evaluation of patient satisfaction in gastrointestinal endoscopy. *World J Gastroenterol*, 2004; 10(22): 3313–7.
10. Vaezi MF. The Esophagus: Anatomy, Physiology, and Diseases. *In:* Cumming's Otolaryngology: Head and Neck Surgery. Mosby. Paul W. Flint, Bruce H. Haughey, Valerie J. Lund et al. 2010; 5th. ed. 953–80.

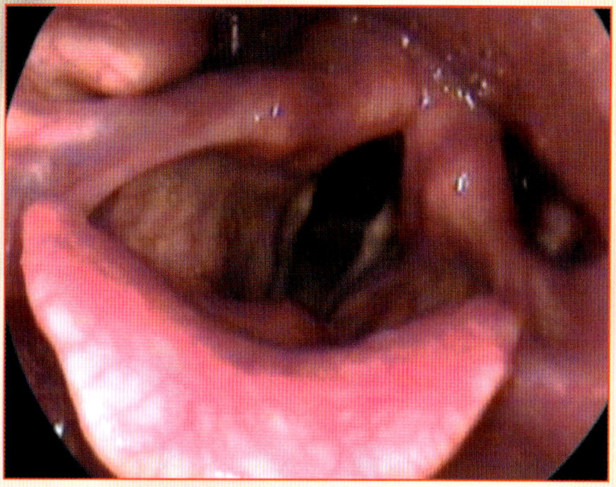

SECTION 5

Laryngology

CHAPTER 33

Recurrent Respiratory Papillomatosis

S.P.S. Yadav, Arpit Agrawal

Recurrent respiratory papillomatosis (RRP), also known as juvenile laryngeal papillomatosis, requires an adequate attention, as in addition to the high economic cost, there is high emotional burden on the patients as well as their families due to need for repeated surgery leading on to prolonged treatment.

RRP is the most common benign neoplasm of the larynx in children, but despite its benign histology, it has potentially fatal consequences as a result of its malignant conversion and involvement of airways. It is often difficult to treat 'as it has the tendency to recur and spread throughout the respiratory tract'.

NATURAL HISTORY

RRP is characterized by its waxing waning clinical course of remissions and exacerbations. After presentation the disease may remain stable or may undergo remission for which periodic surgical treatment is required. On the other hand it may become aggressive requiring frequent surgical treatment along with medical adjuvant therapy. Indicating that the nature of RRP is highly variable.

EPIDEMIOLOGY

RRP is a disease of viral etiology. Human papilloma virus (HPV), mostly types 6 and 11, which is characterized by proliferation of benign squamous papillomas within the aerodigestive tract. Although it most often involves the larynx, yet it may involve the entire aerodigestive tract. In the larynx glottis is most frequently involved followed by supraglottis and then subglottis. RRP may occur in two distinct forms depending on the onset of disease and aggression, juvenile onset recurrent respiratory papillomatosis (JORRP) – an aggressive form and adult onset recurrent respiratory papillomatosis (AORRP) – less aggressive form.

It may affect people of any age and has been reported in a 1-day-old infant. Three years age is watershed in RRP, those diagnosed at less than 3 years have been found to have four times more likely to have more than four surgical procedures per year and almost two times more likely to have two or more anatomic sites affected, as compared to children above three years age. Girls and boys are equally affected. The true incidence and prevalence of RRP are unpredictable.

HUMAN PAPILLOMA VIRUS (HPV)

It belongs to papovaviridae family and is a double-stranded DNA virus of 7900 b.p. long which is non-enveloped, icosahedral (20-sided), capsid virus. HPV is epitheliotropic (infects epithelial cells) and exhibit specificity for epithelium of different sites (i.e., oral mucosa, genital or skin).

Most common types of HPV causing RRP are HPV 6 and 11. Same types are responsible for more than 90% of genital condylomata. HPV-II seems to be associated with aggressive disease and greater likelihood of undergoing tracheotomy to maintain patent airway. HPV 16 and 18 tend to have malignancies in genital and respiratory tract, while HPV 31 and 32 exhibit transition to malignant potential.

PATHOPHYSIOLOGY

HPV enters the basal layer of mucosa to establish itself, and induce the proliferation of cells. HPV has been shown to activate the epidermal growth factor (EGF) receptor pathways for cellular proliferation. However, there may be other mechanisms too for induction of cellular proliferation by HPV.

Histologically, this cellular proliferation appears as 'Finger-like projections' or 'fronds' which is covered by stratified squamous epithelium and have a central fibrovascular core. When papillomas are microscopic they give a 'velvety' appearance, while when they are more macroscopic or exophytic growth pattern they give a 'cauliflower' appearance. Papilloma lesions are firm on palpation, may be sessile or pedunclated, pinkish to white in color and often occurs in irregular exophytic clusters. Due to repeated trauma ciliated epithelium undergoes squamous metaplasia, thus creating an "iatrogenic squamocellularity junction". GE reflux further flourishes RRP. Most RRPs do not exhibit dysplasia, abnormal mitoses or hyperkeratosis. Without any exception, RRP exhibit delayed maturation of the epithelium, resulting in significantly thickened basal cell layer and nucleated cells in the superficial layers. An intranuclear virus is evident in lesions by electron microscopy and HPV DNA may be found in laryngeal papillomas using Southern blot hybridization. Viral probes have identified HPV in virtually every papilloma lesion. During viral latency HPV DNA can be detected in normal-appearing mucosa in RRP patients who have been in remission for years.

TRANSMISSION

33

There has been well-established relationship between the cervical HPV infection in mother and RRP in their children. HPV is found in the genital tract of 25% of women with child-bearing age group. Of these, highest prevalence is in 20–24 years age.

Vertical transmission through an infected birth canal during delivery is the major mode of transmission of infection in children, while other modes appear to play minor role only, i.e., in utero, transplacental transfer, sexual abuse, etc. Support for this incidence lies in the fact that clinical condylomata is seen in more than 50% of the mothers of children with RRP.

Hence, some authors have suggested the role of cesarean section as the preventive measure to RRP, to some extent. Childhood onset RRP patients are mostly first-born child who is vaginally delivered as compared to controls of similar age, may be due to prolonged second stage of labour in primigravida. There is tendency of RRP to occur more in recently acquired genital HPV lesion as compared to long-standing cases, hence explaining the increased incidence in low socioeconomic status. Nearly 30-40% of the children exposed to HPV in the genital tract develop RRP. This tells us that other factors too are important determinants for the occurrence of RRP, i.e., patient immunity, timing, length and amount of virus exposure and local trauma.

Siblings of children with RRP do not seem to have an increased risk for RRP, hence excluding out genetic predisposition. Some cases of neonatal papillomatosis have been reported, which are thought to have occurred via transmission in utero.

CLINICAL FEATURES

Due to the involvement of glottis initially, hoarseness is the first and principal presenting symptom of a child with RRP. Second presenting symptom usually is stridor which begins with inspiratory noise which becomes biphasic as disease progresses. Other late symptoms may be cough, recurrent pneumonia, dyspnoea, dysphagia, failure to thrive, etc. Commonly before the definitive diagnosis of RRP is made it is usually mistaken as asthma, croup, vocal nodules or bronchitis. The clinical course of RRP is highly variable with remissions and exacerbation.

Due to rarity and slow progression of RRP, diagnosis is delayed and children finally come with respiratory distress or failure. These cases may need tracheotomy, but it is highly debatable, since it may activate or contribute to spread of disease to lower respiratory tract. Hence, most surgeons believe that in RRP tracheotomy to be avoided unless absolutely indicated and afterwards also decannulation should be considered as soon as disease is controlled effectively by endoscopic techniques.

Approximately 30% of children and 16% of adults with RRP present with extralaryngeal symptoms due to its spread. Most common extralaryngeal sites of involvement are oral cavity, trachea and bronchi in decreasing order of frequency. Pulmonary papilloma lesion involves parenchyma and leads to restrictive lung disease. It is seen as non-calcified peripheral nodule initially, which enlarges and undergoes cavitation with central liquefactive necrosis and seen as air fluid levels on CT scan. Clinically, these patients present as either bronchiectasis, pneumonia or respiratory failure. Malignant transformation of RRP into squamous cell carcinoma also has been reported.

CLINICAL VARIATIONS

Though hoarseness is first and chief complaint of RRP child, yet if the lesion's origin is in some other site then it may present as a late sign too. Variations are also individual dependent, as same papilloma that produces hoarseness in one patient may present as stridor or obstruction in the other. Quality of voice gives clue to the sites of involvement by papilloma lesions. A low pitched, coarse, fluttering voice suggests subglottic lesion; on the other hand high pitched cracky voice, aphonia or breathy voice suggests a glottis lesion. RRP child does not show much change in stridor with position change unlike laryngomalacia, vascular ring or a mediastinal mass.

DIAGNOSTIC ENDOSCOPY (Fig. 33.1)

Child should undergo flexible fibreoptic endoscopy and sequential inspection of pharynx, hypopharynx, larynx and subglottis to make the diagnosis of RRP, estimation of lumen size, vocal cord mobility and urgency of operative intervention. While performing the endoscopy topical decongestant of choice is 'oxymetazoline' because of less cardiac effects and topical pontocaine is used to enhance patient's cooperation.

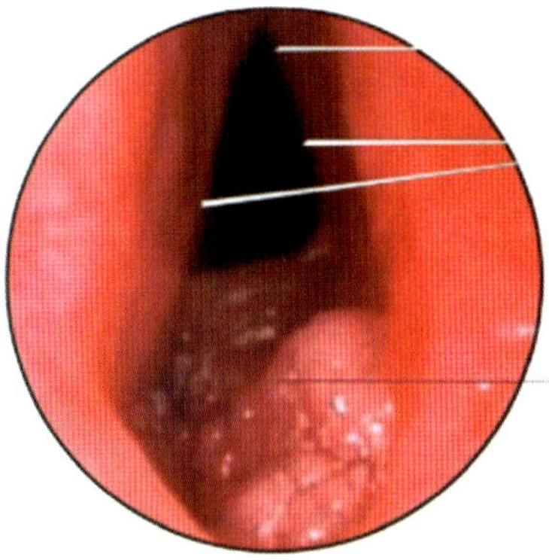

Fig. 33.1. Endoscopic view of laryngeal papilloma.

SURGICAL MANAGEMENT

There is no cure for RRP. No single or adjuvant therapy has been successful in eradicating RRP. The current standard of care for RRP is surgical therapy with the goal of complete removal of papillomas and preservation of normal structures. In aggressive diseases when anterior and posterior commisure get involved the goal sets down to subtotal removal of papillomas and preventing the complications of subglottic and glottic stenosis or web formation due to excessive scarring.

Surgical treatment in the past included the use of thermal cautery, cryosurgery and removal of papillomas with cup forceps. Now-a-days, CO_2 laser has been favoured. CO_2 laser vaporizes the cells by inspissating thermal energy intracellularly. CO_2 laser causes minimal bleeding. It also reduces the risk of vocal cords damage and limits scarring. CO_2 laser has its disadvantage of 'smoke plume' formation which can injure eyes or skin and it is also a potential source of infection to surgeon. Another significant disadvantage of the CO_2 laser is that the beam cannot be delivered through a flexible fibre endoscope. The KTP laser can be used in this way, hence KTP laser is more suitable for distal tracheobronchial disease. Frequent interval laser laryngoscopic excision is done to avoid tracheotomy and permit the child to develop good phonation by preserving normal vocal cords.

EVOLVING SURGICAL MODALITIES

To reduce the risk of scar formation in vocal cords 'cold steel excision' is being used successfully. Papillomata of the tracheobronchial tree often requires the use of 532 nm pulsed KTP (potassium titanium phosphate) laser coupled with bronchoscope for removal. Another recent advancement is removal of papillomas with endoscoic microdebrider, favouring the use of 'shaver' technology. The microdebrider can be manoeuvred to reach subglottis and tracheal lesions, area that are specially challenging for laser surgery.

ADJUVANT THERAPY

Role of adjuvant therapy starts when there are requirements of more than four surgical procedures per year, rapid papilloma regrowth with airway compromise or multisite spread of disease.

Interferon

These are class of proteins manufactured by cells in response to viral infection. Interferon binds to specific membrane receptors and alters cell metabolism. It affects the production of enzymes like protein kinases, endonuclease and has antiviral, antiproliferative, anti-tumour and immunomodulatory effects. It may be administered subcutaneously or intravenously. It is the most widely used adjuvant therapy and its most common side effect is 'Flu' like symptoms. Interferon produced by recombinant DNA technique has fewer side effects and better efficacy than blood bank harvested interferon.

Ribavarin

It is broad-spectrum antiviral agent, which has shown some results in aggressive laryngeal papillomatosis by increasing surgical interval. It is administered in nebulised form in dosages of 6 gm/50 ml over nine hours for three consecutive nights every two weeks over seven weeks and also administered orally 15 mg/kg/day.

Acyclovir

It is antiviral agent which inhibits thymidine kinase, an enzyme non-encoded by HPV, but shows good results when there are viral coinfections, i.e., herpes simplex virus, cytomegalovirus, Epstein-Barr virus. The dosage is 5 mg/kg/8 hourly for three months. Acyclovir delays the recurrence of RRP and results no recurrence.

Cidofovir

This antiviral agent is known as acyclic phosphonate nucleotide analog and it inhibits viral DNA polymerase. Cidofovir is directly injected into subepithelial vocal folds biweekly for six months with 2.5–37.5 mg (injection volume 0.5 ml). This regimes causes endomysial edema with muscle fibre separation, atrophy and scarring of vocal folds at the end of six month. Its possible adverse effects are nephrotoxicity, carcinogenesis, hypospermia.

Indole 3-carbinol

It is given as dietary supplement and found in cabbage, cauliflower and broccoli. It affects the ratio of estradiol hydroxylation. Since growth of RRP is oestrogen-dependent hence it is effective. It is safe and effective in dosages 200 mg twice a day over a period of five years to control the recurrence.

Celecoxib

It is selective inhibitor of cox-2 which is effective in controlling papilloma growth. Papilloma overexpress epidermal growth, increase expression of cyclooxygenase-2 and prostaglandin E2. Dosages 100 mg (paediatric weight between 12–25 kg) or 200 mg (weight > 25 kg) daily for long duration.

Retinoids

Its trials are being done on the basis that vitamin A in aerodigestive tract is the modulator of cellular proliferation and differentiation.

Mumps vaccines

In some trials, intralesional injections of mumps vaccine have shown some positive results.

Antireflux therapy

Several case reports have shown decrease in RRP following antireflux therapy specially 'cimetidine'.

Photodynamic therapy (PDT)

It is based on the transfer of energy to a photosensitive drug. PDT with dihematoporphyrin ether (DHE) uses the propensity of this substance to concentrate in papillomas as compared to surrounding normal tissue. Cell destruction occurs via production of toxic oxygen radicals. Patients are typically treated intravenously with 4.25 mg/kg of DHE prior to surface treatment of papillomas by photoactivation with an argon pump dye laser. This therapy should be specially considered for more aggressive cases who do not respond to other techniques.

Heat shock proteins (HSPS)

HspE7 is a recombinant fusion protein of Hsp56 from *Mycobacterium bovis* BCG and E7 protein from HPV16. It is administered subcutaneously. The effect is more marked in girls.

Radiation therapy has no role in RRP. In fact it increases the risk of malignant transformation.

PREVENTION

A new quadrivalent HPV vaccine is licensed and indicated for prevention of cervical cancer, vulval and vaginal intraepithelial neoplasias grades 2–3 and genital warts associated with HPV 6, 11, 16 and 18. With this vaccination there will be concomitant decrease in RRP and HPV associated head and neck cancers. The CDC Advisory Committee on Immunization Practices (ACIP) has recommended vaccination for all girls aged 11–12, girls and women 13–26 who have not yet been vaccinated and girls as young as age 9, in whom the physician believes it would be appropriate.

There is also a bivalent HPV vaccine which is under phase 3 trial. It provides protection against HPV 16 and 18 but not 6 and 11. Hence we can assume that it may reduce the risk of head and neck cancers associated with HPV and not RRP risk.

CONCLUSION

RRP is a frustrating disease with its potential morbid consequences of involvement of airway and risk of malignant degeneration. The goal of surgical therapy is to maintain safe and patent airway with serviceable voice. None of the therapy modalities to date has 'cured' RRP. There is a need for national or international registration of all RRP patients with exchange of data between centers. Such is the rarity of this condition that international collaboration among specialist centers may be required to establish the optimum management of these patient. The recent introduction of quadrivalent HPV vaccine offers hope for prevention of this devastating rare disease. Parental support and education are invaluable adjuncts to the safe care of children with RRP.

SUGGESTED READING

1. Mounts P, Shah KV, Kashima H. Viral etiology of juvenile and adult onset squamous papilloma of larynx. *Proc Natl Acad Sci USA*, 1982; 79: 5425–9.
2. Shykhon M, Kuo M, Pearman K. Recurrent respiratory papillomatosis. *Clin Otol*, 2002; 27: 237–43.
3. Derkay CS, Darrow DH. Recurrent respiratory papillomatosis. *Ann Otol Rhinol Laryngol*, 2006; 115: 1–11.
4. Shapiro AM, Rimell FL, Shoemaker D, et al. Tracheotomy in children with juvenile onset recurrent respiratory papillomatosis: the children's hospital of Pittsburgh experience. *Ann Oto Rhino Laryngol*, 1996; 105: 1–5.
5. Dedo HH, Yu KC. CO_2 laser treatment in 244 patients with respiratory papillomatosis. *Laryngoscope*, 2001; 111: 1639–44.
6. Zeitels SM, Akst LM, Burns JA, et al. Office based 532 nm pulsed KTP laser treatment of glottal papillomatosis and dysplasia. *Ann Otol Rhinol Laryngol*, 2006; 115: 679–85.
7. Pasquale K, Wiatrak KB, Wooley A, et al. Microdebridor versus CO2 laser for RRP: a comparative study. *Laryngoscope*, 2003; 113: 139–43.
8. Healy GB, Gelber RD, Trowbridge AL, et al. Treatment of RRP with human leucocyte interferon. *N Engl J Med*, 1988; 319: 401–7.
9. Yadav SPS, Gera A, Singh J, Ranga RK. Multiple papillomas larynx. *Indian J Pediatr*, 2000; 67: 567–69.
10. Pransky SM, Magit AE, Kearns DB, et al. Intralesional cidofovir for recurrent respiratory papillomatosis in children. *Arch Otolaryngol Head Neck Surg*, 1999; 125: 1143–8.
11. Derkay CS, Malis DJ, Zalzal G, et al. A staging system for assessing severity of disease and response to therapy in recurrent respiratory papillomatosis. *Laryngoscope*, 1998; 108: 935–7.
12. Freed G, Derkay CS. HPV vaccines and RRP. *Paediatr Otorhinolaryngol*, 2006; 70: 1–5.

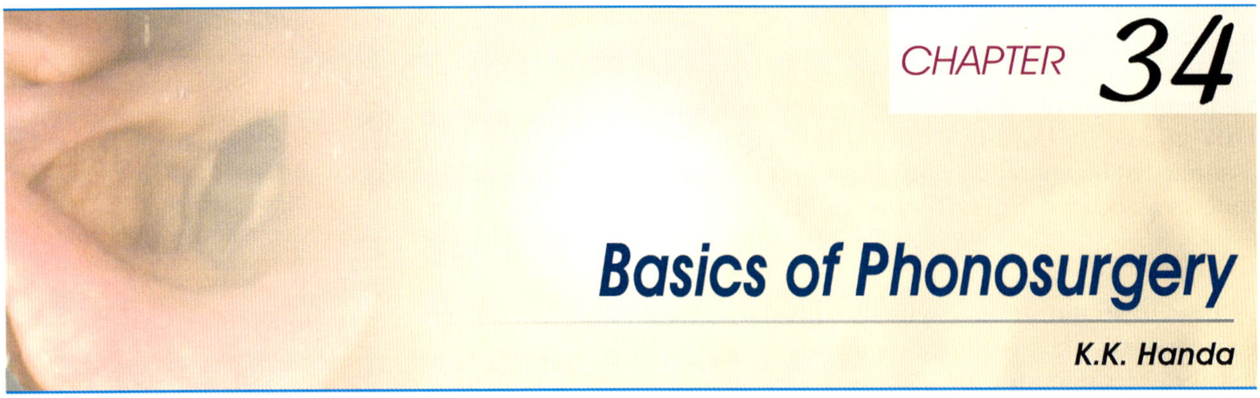

CHAPTER 34

Basics of Phonosurgery

K.K. Handa

It is the surgery to alter, modify or restore voice. This term has been used in a variety of ways. Some refer to external laryngeal surgery as phonosurgery. However, it is better to use the term in wider context and include phonomicrosurgery and allied procedures.

1. External laryngeal Framework surgery
2. Phonomicrosurgery

EXTERNAL LARYNGEAL FRAMEWORK SURGERY

It was the pioneering work of Isshiki[1] on dogs which laid the foundation of present day laryngeal framework surgery. Although the use of thyroid cartilage had been advocated before for the medialisation of a paralysed vocal cord (ref. Payr), it was only after the pioneering experimental work of Isshiki on dogs that external laryngeal framework surgery became popular. He applied the principles of external laryngeal framework surgery to alter not only the position but also the length and tension of the vocal cords.

He gave the following nomenclature.

Type 1	Thyroplasty	Medialisation
Type 2	Thyroplasty	Lateralization
Type 3	Thyroplasty	Cord shortening to reduce the pitch
Type 4	Thyroplasty	Cord lengthening to increase the pitch

In subsequent years there was a modification in the nomenclature by the American and European Laryngological Society

Type 1 Thyroplasty

Type 1 thyroplasty with or without arytenoid adduction is the international standard today for the treatment of unilateral vocal cord paralysis.

The procedure has undergone a lot of modifications after the initial description by Isshiki and different surgical techniques are used by different surgeons. The main steps are:

Anesthesia

Surgery is mostly preferred under local anesthesia as the improvement in voice can be assessed on the table. However, general anesthesia is given where patient has difficulty in tolerating local anesthesia and in certain cases where arytenoid adduction is being combined and the procedure time is likely to be prolonged.

The head is kept in neutral position without too much flexion or extension so that there is no modulation in voice.

Following landmarks are marked on the neck: superior thyroid notch, inferior thyroid notch and cricoid cartilage.

Incision

- A horizontal incision is given midway between superior and inferior thyroid notch extending till the anterior border of sternocleidomastoid muscle and crossing the midline for about 2 cm on the opposite side.

- Subplatysmal flaps are elevated.
- Anterior jugular vein often comes in the way and needs to be tied.
- Strap muscles are split in the midline and retracted. Normally the straps need not be cut. They only need to be cut occasionally when arytenoid's adduction is being combined with type 1 thyroplasty and better exposure is required.
- A posterior superior flap of external perichondrium is created and the thyroid cartilage is exposed. The exposure will have to be till the posterior border of thyroid cartilage if arytenoid's adduction is being combined with type 1 thyroplasty.

Making the window

There are several methods of making the window. The one we follow is Peak Woo's half and half rule. First the midpoint between the superior and inferior thyroid notch is marked. This is where the true vocal fold lies and any medialisation above this would medialise the ventricle. The superomedial angle of the window is marked about 5 mm from this. The window size is marked 15 × 6 mm in males and 13 × 6 mm in females. The other helpful indicator is that lower border of the window should be 2–3 mm above the lower border of the thyroid cartilage. One must be careful not to fracture the lower border of the cartilage.

Inner perichondrium

One has to be very careful in handling the inner perichondrium. A small plane of about 2 mm needs to be created between the cartilage and the inner perichondrium. If more than required inner perichondrium is elevated it can make the implant loose and the implant may migrate from the designated position. The cartilage must be very carefully separated from inner perichondrium using a fine periosteal elevator. Direct injury by knife should be avoided as it can lead to a haematoma formation. There are some surgeons who make a careful clean cut around the periphery of the perichondrium so that medialisation by the implant is more effective.

Implant

A variety of implants are being used. The author prefers to use either of the following three:

1. Silastic pre-carved implant (designed by Dr. Netterville).
2. A titanium implant (Kurz). Titanium is a good biocompatible material and with the Kurz implant the placement is easy and secure.
3. An implant carved out from silastic block. This is the cheapest option.

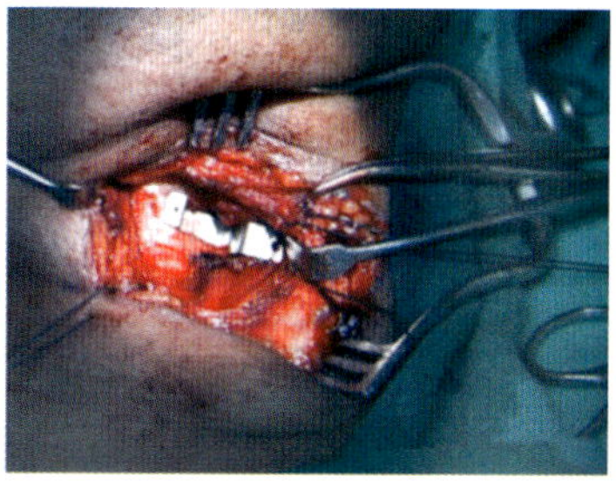

Fig. 34.1. Type 1 thyroplasty with titanium implant.

Arytenoid adduction

This procedure is often combined with type 1 thyroplasty especially when the posterior glottic gap is large. It consists of exposing the posterior border of the thyroid lamina and then making a window called Maragoss window and trying to feel the muscular process of arytenoid and passing a figure of 8 suture through it. This helps in closing the posterior glottic gap. However, today the arytenoid adduction is supposed to also help in mechanisms related to the vocal cord tension.

Complications

Thyroplasty is relatively a safe procedure.

(a) The commonest mistake is medialisation too far superiorly leading to a bulge of the false cord instead of the true cord. The voice will not improve.
(b) Haematoma: If inner perichondrium is breached and muscle is injured. It can also occur if there is extensive dissection during arytenoid adduction procedure.
(c) Abcess: Haematoma may get infected leading to abcess formation.
(d) Intrusion of the implant into the laryngeal lumen is rare.
(e) Extrusion of the implant: This may happen if the wound gets infected.

Type 2 Thyroplasty

This procedure was originally described by Isshiki for cord lateralization but now there are better procedures for abductor cord paralysis. Today it is being used in some cases of adductor spasmodic dysphonia who do not want repeated botulinum toxin injections. The effect of botulinum toxin injections only lasts for 5–6 months per injection.

In this procedure the thyroid cartilage is split anteriorly in the midline. Care is taken not to open into the laryngeal lumen. The thyroid ala is kept apart with silastic shims or titanium miniplates.

Type 3 Thyroplasty

In this procedure, on both sides of the thyroid ala a 2 mm vertical strip of the cartilage is removed. This has the effect of reducing the length of the vocal cord and hence there is reduction in tension in the vocal cord and lowering of the sound frequency.

The indications for this surgery are:

1. Cases of puberphonia who do not respond to speech therapy.
2. In sex change operations where one needs to change female voice to male voice.

Type 4 Thyroplasty

This procedure consists of carrying out cricothyroid approximation by passing sutures between thyroid cartilage lower end and the cricoid cartilage over either silastic shims or mini titanium plates.

This is used in cases where voice needs to be changed from a masculine to feminine voice.

PHONOMICROSURGERY

The first step in phonomicrosurgery is trying to understand the layered microstructure of the vocal cords and the 'body cover theory' as described by Hirano. The body-cover theory helps explain the mucosal wave. It states that there are two layers of the vocal folds with different structural properties. The cover is composed of stratified squamous epithelium and the superficial layer of the lamina propria (Reinke's space). The body of the fold is composed of the intermediate and deep layers of the lamina propria (vocal ligament), which is more fibrous than the superficial layer. The muscular layer is the thyroarytenoid (vocalis) muscle. The cover is pliable, elastic, and nonmuscular, whereas the body is stiffer and has active contractile properties that allow adjustment of stiffness and concentration of the mass. The mucosal wave occurs primarily in this loose cover of the fold. Changes in stiffness or tension in the fold alters the mucosal wave. As the stiffness in the fold increases with contraction of the cricothyroid muscle, the velocity of the wave increases and the pitch rises. Mucosal wave velocity also increases with greater airflow and greater subglottal pressure.

Phonomicrosurgery consists of preserving the layered microstructure of the vocal cords.

Steps of phonomicrosurgery

The technique consists of injecting 1 : 10000 adrenaline saline solution submucosally. This helps by:

- Causing vasoconstriction.
- Increasing the working space in the lamina propria.

Next, superior cordotomy is done by making a mucosal deep incision with a sickle knife. The cordotomy may be medial or lateral depending on the type of the lesion. Dissection is done in the Reinke's space with maximal preservation of the mucosa. Damage to the vocal ligament is avoided. The lesions which are very aptly addressed by this technique are intracordal cysts, sulcus vocalis, vocal polyps with broad peduncle and Reinke's oedema.

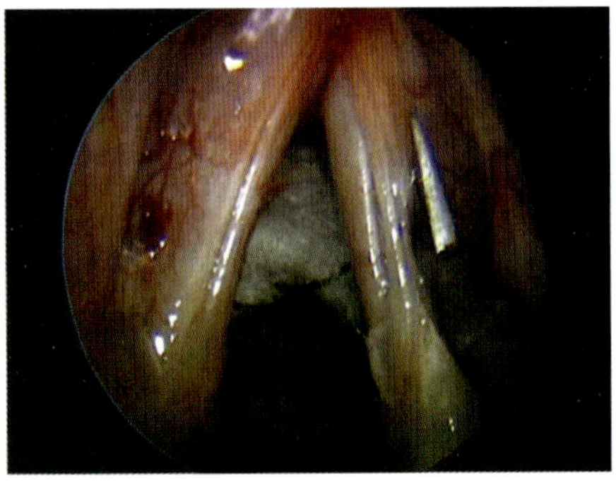

Fig. 34.2. Phonomicrosurgery for sulcus vocalis.

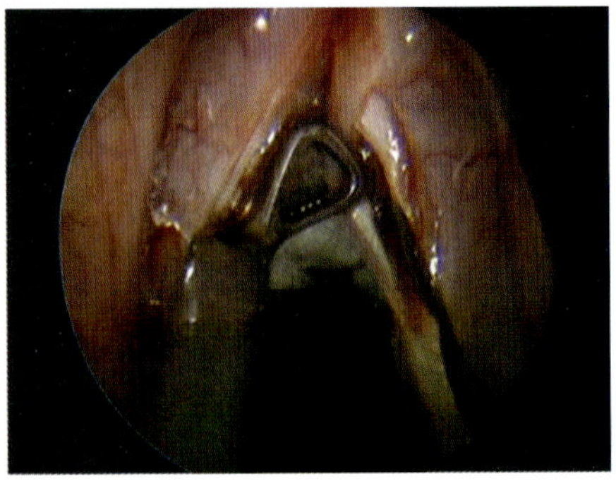

Fig. 34.3. Phonomicrosurgery: superior cordotomy.

Use of Laser

Carbon dioxide laser coupled to a microscope with a micromanipulator is the latest tool for laryngeal lesions. The type of lesions where laser has superiority over conventional instruments include juvenile papilloma, leukoplakia, early laryngeal cancer and haemorrhagic vocal polyp. The advantages are precision and better tissue healing with no fibrosis or scarring.

CONCLUSION

Phonosurgery is basically the surgery of vocal cords to maintain or improve the function or structure of the vocal cords by resecting its layer structure. This is achieved by minimal tissue excision, minimal disruption of superficial layer of lamina propria and preservation of epithelium especially at the vibrant edge. Laryngeal framework surgery is unique phonosurgical concept that enables us to influence the laryngeal biomechanics by changing the shape/position of the laryngeal cartilage, which is very soft, highly effective and long lasting method for voice improvement and adjustment.

SUGGESTED READING

1. Isshiki N. Folia Phoniatr (Basel). *Recent advances in phonosurgery*, 1980; 32(2): 119–54.
2. Crumley RL: Teflon thyroplasty versus nerve transfer: A comparison. *Ann Otol Rhinol Laryngol*, 1990; 99(Pt 1):759–63.
3. Gardner GM, Parnes SM: Status of the mucosal wave post-vocal cord injection versus thyroplasty. *J Voice*, 1991; 5:64–73.
4. Isshiki N, Taira T, Kojima H, Shoji K: Recent modifications in thyroplasty type I. *Ann Otol Rhinol Laryngol*, 1989; 98: 777–79.
5. Hirano M, Yoshida T, Tanaka S, Hibi S. Sulcus vocalis: functional aspects. *Ann Otol Rhinol Laryngol*, 1990; 99(9): 679–83.
6. Wanamaker JR, Netterville JL, Osoff RH. Phonosurgery: Silastic medialisation for unilateral vocal cord paralysis. *Oper Tech Otolaryngol Head Neck Surg*, 1993; 4: 207–17.
7. Koufmann JA. Laryngoplasty for vocal cord medialisation: An alternative to Teflon. *Laryngoscope*, 1986; 96: 726–31.

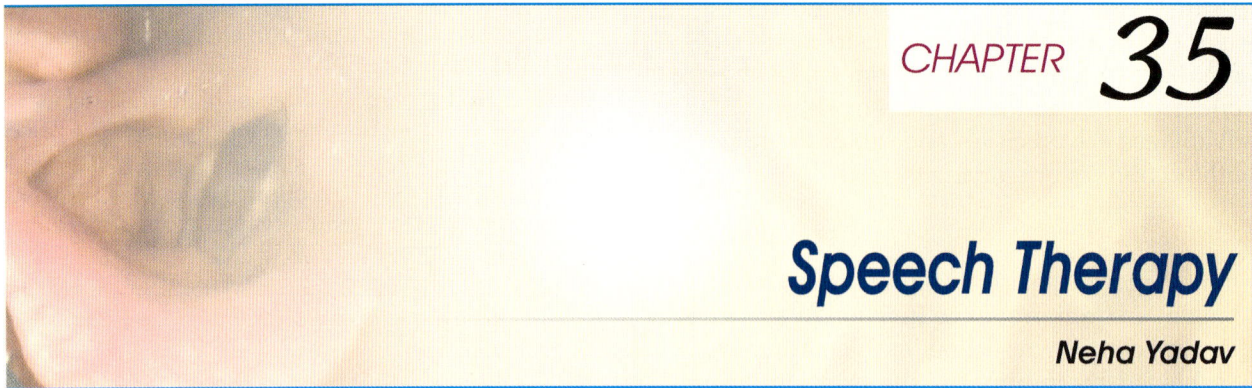

CHAPTER 35

Speech Therapy

Neha Yadav

Communication is the best gift given by God to mankind. We can share our views, ideas, jokes, laughter, education and knowledge via communication. Undoubtedly speech is an essential mode of human communication across the world. It can be defined as the dynamic production of voice sounds for communication through the process of respiration, phonation, resonation and articulation (Kent, 2000). Speech is the verbal/oral manifestation of language. The other two mediums or forms of language are writing and gestures. Verbal expression of thought and hearing are the building blocks on which our intricate human communication system is constructed. Thus, any impairment in the normal mechanism of speech production can cause a significant disability to an individual, performing routine and important activities with a resultant handicap. Thus, such individuals with faulty speech are bound to have difficulty in sustaining effective communication in day-to-day life. This makes it imperative for otorhinolaryngologists dealing with speech and hearing disorders to understand this handicap of the patient presenting with a speech and language disorder.

Any form of disruption in verbal thought formulation causes a speech and language disorder. Speech and language impairment are disorders that affect communication and/or oral functioning that affects speech. There are a number of these disorders and they range from sound substitution or inability to produce certain sounds to the inability to understand language or produce speech that can be understood.

What are the types of speech problems?

There are two types of communication disorders:

- Speech
- Language

With *speech disorders*, a person has trouble in producing speech. Speech disorders are again classified into *articulation, fluency and voice disorders.*

An **articulation disorder** is when a child has a problem making the sounds necessary for speech. Misarticulation/SODA Errors (**S**ubstitution, **O**mission, **D**istortion, **A**ddition errors) or a lisp would be an example of this type of disorder. In misarticulation people tend to substitute, omit, add or distort a speech sound. Whereas in lisp people have problems pronouncing certain sounds like /l/ or /r/. Articulation disorder is usually seen in patients with cleft lip and palate, tongue-tie, missing teeth, rugae, misocclusion, short velum or any other case with oral structure deformity.

Articulatory errors are also seen in adult patients with dysarthria, apraxia of speech and motor aphasia.

A phonological disorder is another form of articulation disorder which is a bit more complicated in nature. In this case, the person is capable of making all the sounds, but their speech is still not easily understood as they tend to have faulty representation of class of speech sounds. People with this type of disorder may have a voice that sounds very different; speak very softly or at a high pitch.

A **fluency disorder** is seen when smooth and easy flow of speech is disrupted by pauses, interruptions and repetition of linguistic elements such as sounds, syllables, words and phrases. Fluency may be hampered by speaker's hesitation, varying intonation rate of utterance. Stuttering and cluttering are the core disorders of fluency. Stuttering is interruption of the forward flow of speech by motoric disruptions or by the speaker reactions to the interruption itself (Wingate, 1962), whereas cluttering is the verbal manifestation of basic underlying central language imbalance, involving cerebral integration at the highest level of function (Weiss, 1964). It is characterized as speaking with excessive rate, where the person exceeds his/her ability to handle motor sequencing necessary for speech, which leads to distorted and jumbled speech. Fluency disorder is readily recognizable in severe cases of dysarthria and dyspraxia.

Voice disorder is seen where the quality, pitch, loudness, or flexibility are interpreted as being unpleasant or inappropriate to the age or sex of the speaker. Disorders of the voice may be classified as organic or non-organic. Organic disorders may be caused by disease, congenital disorders, injury, hyperfunction, or vocal abuse. Non-organic disorders include psychogenic and stress-related vocal dysfunction.

Pitch disorders are seen in young males, females and transsexuals who tend to have poor pubertal changes as they step into adulthood. These disorders are called as *puberphonia* (seen in males) and *androphonia* (seen in females). Puberphonia is characterized as high-pitch female-like voice whereas androphonia is characterized as low-pitch male-like voice.

Quality disorders such as harsh, hoarse and breathy voice are seen in professional voice users and in cases with hyper-functional voice usage such as in vocal nodules, vocal polyps, cysts, traumatic laryngitis and vocal cord palsy.

Resonance disorders such as hypernasality and hyponasality is seen in patients with cleft lip and palate, short velum, rhinolalia and individuals with congested airways.

Also voice disorders are seen in patients with neurological insult such as spasmodic dysphonia, vocal fold paralysis, essential tremor, paradoxical vocal fold movement (PVFM) disorder, ventricular dysphonia, hysterical aphonia and laryngectomy.

A *language disorder* is when a person cannot understand and/or communicate with other people. Language disorder can be developmental or acquired. Developmental language disorder is seen in children with autism, cerebral palsy, Down's syndrome, motor delay, cognitive impairment, and hearing loss whereas acquired language disorder is seen in adults with neurological insult such as stroke or traumatic brain injury. People with language disorders may have trouble matching a word with its meaning, be unable to create sentences, be unable to comprehend what another person is saying or be unable to express themselves through language. They may have a limited vocabulary as well. It is not unusual for people with a language disorder to have more than one of these symptoms.

What can be done?

For patients with various speech and language disorders, a speech-language pathologist can provide rehabilitative treatment with *speech therapy*.

Speech therapy is a rehabilitative treatment programme which is expected to restore speech to a person who has lost existing speech function (the ability to express thoughts, speak words, and form sentences) as a result of disease or injury.

In speech-language therapy, speech language pathologist will work with an individual one-to-one, in a small group, or directly in a classroom with children to overcome difficulties involved with a specific disorder.

Therapists use a variety of strategies including:

- Assessment and diagnosis of communication as well as swallowing disorders and identification of retained abilities.
- Advice and support of patient and caregiver to prevent, maintain, or improve communication and swallowing.
- Therapy to restore and improve impaired speech, language, voice, fluency and swallowing.
- Teaching compensatory strategies to improve intelligibility and general communicative effectiveness.

- Therapy to improve functional communication by using adaptive techniques, such as augmentative and alternative communication systems.
- Therapy to restore, improve and maintain social consequences of the speech disability.
- Manipulation of the environment, e.g., making physical surroundings more conducive to communication by amending carer's communication.
- **Language intervention:** The speech language pathologist will interact with a child by playing and talking, using pictures, books, objects, or ongoing events to stimulate language development. The therapist may also model correct pronunciation and use repetition exercises to build speech and language skills.
- **Articulation therapy:** Articulation, or sound production exercises, involve having the therapist model correct sounds and syllables for a child, often during play activities. The level of play is age-appropriate and related to the child's specific needs. The speech language pathologist will physically show the child how to make certain sounds, such as the "r" sound, and may demonstrate how to move the tongue to produce specific sounds using open-mouth approach.
- **Oral-motor/feeding and swallowing therapy:** The speech language pathologist will use a variety of oral exercises – including facial massage and various tongue, lip, and jaw exercises – to strengthen the muscles of the mouth. The speech language pathologist also may work with different food textures and temperatures to increase a child's oral awareness during eating and swallowing.
- **Voice therapy:** The speech language pathologist will improve voice production and its quality using various vocal exercise such as pushing-pulling approach, inhalation phonation, masking, laryngeal massage, relaxation, respiration training and digital manipulation of larynx.
- **Fluency therapy:** This involves improving the proficiency of speaking by facilitating forward flow of speech using fluency reinforcement and fluency modification techniques. These include use of traditional approaches such as voluntary stuttering, cancellation, pullouts, relaxation, airflow therapy, corrective feedback, reinforcement, shadowing and pacing. Cognitive restructuring, behaviour therapy approach and emotional support therapy have also proved to be effective in gaining fluency. Techniques that combine teaching patients a strategy for modifying their speech production with psychological intervention and therapy aimed at improving attitudes seem to be most effective.

When is therapy needed?

Children might need speech-language therapy for a variety of reasons including:

- Hearing impairment.
- Cognitive (intellectual, thinking) or other developmental delays.
- Weak oral muscles.
- Excessive drooling.
- Hoarseness.
- Birth defects such as cleft lip or cleft palate.
- Autism.
- Motor planning problems (Apraxia).
- Respiratory disorders.
- Feeding and swallowing disorders.
- Traumatic brain injury.

Therapy should begin as soon as possible. Children enrolled in therapy early (before they are 5 years old) tend to have better outcomes than those who begin therapy later. This does not mean that older kids can't make progress in therapy; they may progress at a slower rate because they often have learned patterns that need to be changed.

Adults might need speech therapy in cases of:

- Stroke.
- Traumatic brain injury.
- Hyperfunctional voice disorder.
- Dementia.
- Swallowing disorder.
- Alzheimer's and other neurological diseases.
- Voice restoration after total laryngectomy.
- Professional voice users.

CONCLUSION

There are several technical and instrumental advancements in the field of otorhinolaryngology. Speech therapy is a promising tool in the field of rehabilitative otorhinolaryngology. It is enlightening prospect in lives of several families suffering from various forms of speech and language disorders. Otorhinolaryngologists should be aware of the various disorders where speech therapy can be utilised clinically. However, speech therapy is known to be a slow process in treatment of a disorder as it is behavioural in nature, still it is proved to mark effective changes in lives of patients attending regular speech therapy. As suggested by various reviews on speech therapy, for effective results it should be regular, intensive, systematic and evidence based.

SUGGESTED READING

1. Andrews G, Guitar B, Howie P. Meta-Analysis of the effects of stuttering treatment. *J Speech Hear Dis*, 1980; 45: 287–307.
2. Boone D R. Human communication and its disorders. Englewood Cliffs, NJ: Prentice- Hall, 1987.
3. Boone DR, McFarlane SC. The Voice and Voice Therapy (4th ed.). Englewood Cliffs, NJ: Prentice-Hall, 1998.
4. Bowen C. Children's speech sound disorders: Questions and answers. Retrieved from http://www.speech-language-therapy.com.
5. Enderby P. Outcome measures in speech therapy: impairment, disability, handicap and distress. *Health Trends*, 1992; 24: 61–4.
6. Enderby P, Emerson J. Does speech and language therapy work? Whurr publications, *British Med J*, 1996; 312: 1655–8.
7. Hegde MN. Introduction to communicative disorders. Austin, TX; PRO-ED: 1991.
8. http://www.spiritlakeconsulting. com/COPT/intro/communicationdisorder.
9. http://www.aetna.com.
10. Jayaram M, Savithri S R. Fluency disorders: Assessment and management. *ISHA*, 1993; I: 27–34.
11. Olswang LB, Bain BA. Clinical forum: treatment efficacy; when to recommend intervention. *Language Speech and Hearing Services in Schools*, 1991; 22: 253–65.
12. Scarborough HS, Dobrich W. Development of children with early language delay. *J Speech Hear Res*, 1990; 33: 70–83.
13. Shewan CM, Kertesz A. Effects of speech and language treatment on recovery from aphasia. *Brain Language*, 1984; 23: 272–99
14. Singh S, Kent R D. Pocket dictionary of speech language and pathology. Singular Publishing Group, 2000; 279.
15. Van Demark DR, Hardin MA. Effectiveness of intensive articulation therapy for children with cleft palate. *Cleft Palate J*, 1986; 23: 215.
16. Van -Riper C, Erickson R L. Speech correction: An introduction to speech pathology and audiology 1996; Allyn & Bacon Publishing: 110–33.
17. Weiss D A. Cluttering. Englewood Cliffs, NJ: Prentice-Hall, 1964.
18. Wingate M E. Evaluation and stuttering, part III: Identification of stuttering and the use of a label. *J Speech Hear Dis*, 1962; 27, 368–77.

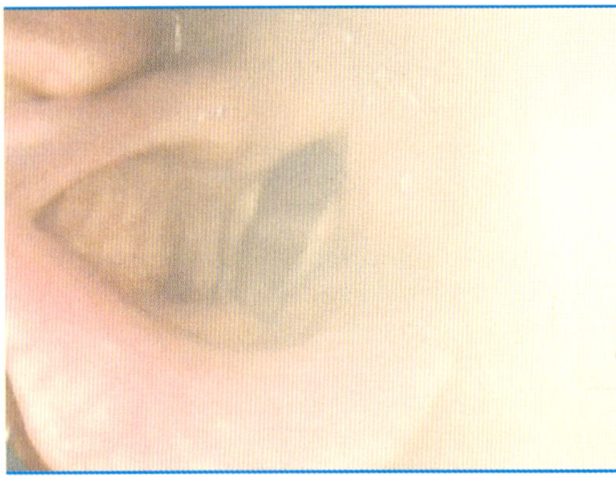

CHAPTER 36

Laryngopharyngeal Reflux

S.P.S. Yadav, J.S. Gulia, Arpit Agrawal

Laryngopharyngeal reflux (LPR) refers to the backflow of stomach contents into the throat that is into hypopharynx. There are numerous synonymous for LPR in medical literature – reflux laryngitis, laryngeal reflux, gastropharyngeal reflux, pharyngoesophageal reflux, extraesophageal reflux and atypical reflux. Although LPR and GERD are both caused by abnormal reflux of gastric contents, yet they are distinct clinical entities.

Gastroesophageal reflux (GER) is defined as the retrograde movement of material from the stomach into the esophagus, in the absence of belching or vomiting. GERD occurs when GER is associated with symptoms. LPR is a gastrointestinal and otolaryngologic condition related to, but distinct from, gastroesophageal reflux disease (GERD). It is estimated that 4% to 10% of patients presenting to an otolaryngology practice have symptoms or findings related to LPR.

LPR is the term which was coined by Koufman et al. and is accepted by the American Academy of Otolaryngology, Head and Neck Surgery. The authors in a landmark article emphasized the otolaryngological importance of reflux and described reflux as an underlying etiology in 40–60% of patients with various voice disorders. Wiener et al. were the first to use concurrent oesophageal and pharyngeal pH monitoring (double probe) for diagnosing and evaluation of patients with LPR symptoms and demonstrated that there are separate episodes of reflux that go up to the laryngopharynx, which are distinct.

PATHOPHYSIOLOGY

There are four main barriers to reflux in a normal individual:

1. Lower esophageal sphincter (LES).
2. Upper esophageal sphincter (UES).
3. Esophageal acid clearance.
4. Epithelial resistance.

Antireflux barriers are the first line of defence against the reflux of gastric contents. They are designed to limit the frequency and volume of refluxates. Once these barriers are breached, a second line of defence, esophageal clearance and esophageal epithelial resistance, protects the esophagus. The reflux of gastric contents into the esophagus is prevented by two mechanisms at the gastroesophageal junction, the LES and the crural diaphragm.

Contraction of lower esophageal sphincter results in circular closure that prevents reflux of gastric contents into oesophagus. Isolated LES dysfunction leads to GERD; however, LES along with UES dysfunction leads to the symptoms of LPR. LES's low resting pressure is associated with CREST (calcinosis, Raynaud's phenomenon, esophageal dysmotility, sclerodactyly and telangiectasia) syndrome, scleroderma and isolated Raynaud's phenomenon.

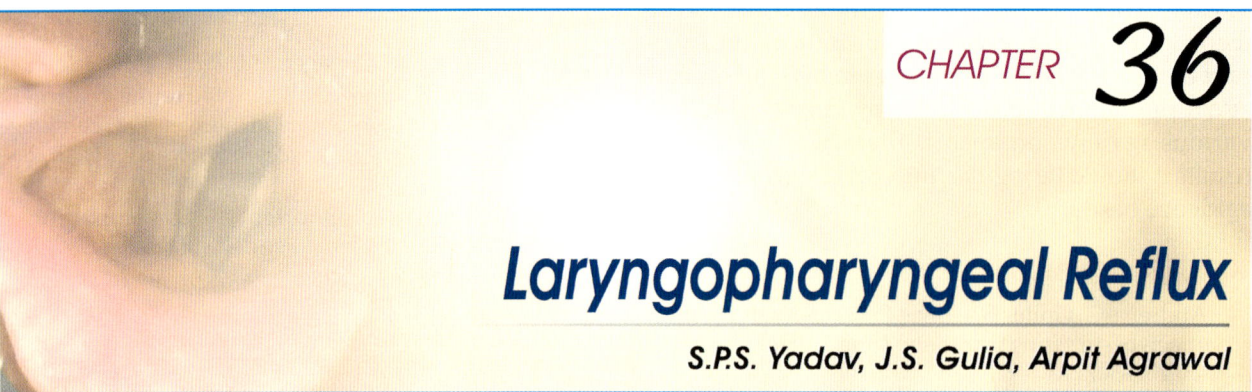

Functionally upper esophageal sphincter is defined as an area of proximal esophagus and distal pharynx, which usually remains closed, but opens for specific physiological demands (swallowing). Unlike other muscular sphincters, UES is not a complete muscular circle but rather a C-shaped sling attached to the cricoid cartilage. UES comprises of thyropharyngeus, cricopharyngeus and proximal cervical oesophagus. UES receives innervations from pharyngeal plexus, a contribution of vagus nerve, glossopharyngeal nerve and sympathetic branches from superior cervical ganglion. Normally UES remains close via tonic contraction of cricopharyngeus. Vagal stimulation causes UES relaxation, while other two nerves are meant for sensory information from UES. Increased UES pressure is seen with laryngeal stimulation (laryngo-upper esophageal sphincter contractile reflex), acidification of distal esophagus and slow balloon dilatation of distal esophagus. Decreased UES pressure is associated with cigarette smoking, peppermint intake and sleep state. The most critical defence mechanism for LPR is UES dysfunction.

Esophageal acid clearance works to clear and neutralize the gastric contents as they pass into oesophagus. Esophageal peristaltic waves, along with the effect of gravity, helps to mechanically clear the esophagus. On the other hand, acidic refluxate left in the esophagus can be neutralized by gastric glandular secretions and buffering agents in the saliva. Radiotherapy, certain drugs and Sjogren's disease causing xerostomia, can abolish this important barrier.

The epithelial resistance factors also prevent the severity of damage. There are pre-epithelial, epithelial and intracellular protective mechanisms. The pre-epithelial layer consists of mucus layer and an aqueous layer with high bicarbonate ions; mucus layer resists penetration by pepsin while aqueous layer buffers acid material. At the epithelial level, cell membrane and the intracellular junctions resist acid and pepsin. The esophageal epithelium constitutes a structural barrier to the diffusion of acid and pepsin because of tight junctions and an intracellular glycoprotein matrix that together result in high epithelial resistance, which limits the entry of acid into the tissues.

In laryngopharyngeal reflux, upper esophageal sphincter dysfunction, along with impaired acid clearance mechanism, allows refluxate to come in contact with laryngopharyngeal segment, especially posterior glottis (Fig. 36.1). The gastric acid and pepsin causes direct damage to larynx mucosa resulting in impaired mucociliary clearance and mucus stasis resulting in decreased resistance to infection. Some studies have revealed the depletion of carbonic anhydrase isoenzyme-III (CA-III) in LPR. The direct stimulation of sensory receptors in the larynx by refluxate can result in reflexive vocal fold adduction or laryngospasm.

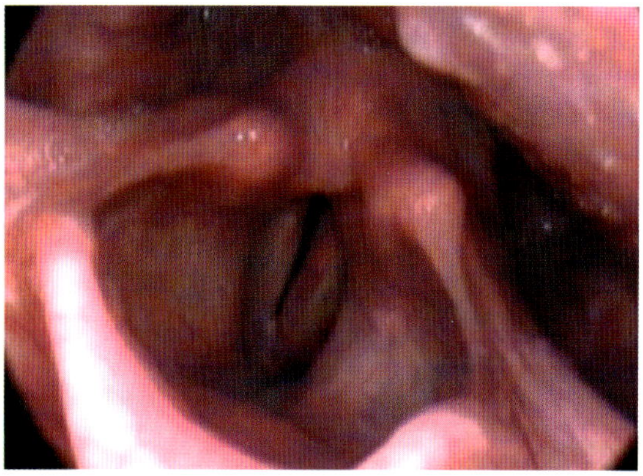

Fig. 36.1. Endoscopic view of laryngopharyngeal segment.

Different tissues have variable epithelial resistance, with esophageal epithelium being more resistant than respiratory epithelium. For the oesophagus up to 50 reflux episodes a day is considered normal, while for the larynx, even 3 episodes a week has been shown to be associated with development of significant disease.

CLINICAL PRESENTATION IN LPR

Symptoms of LPR are diverse, and even not exclusive to LPR, as can also be caused by allergy, degenerative changes, neurological disease, infection, behavioral disorders, medications and neoplasia. The symptoms include intermittent dysphonia, chronic throat clearing of excessive mucus, sialorrhea, cough, sensation of postnasal drainage, cervical dysphagia, dysgeusia, halitosis, globus and throat pain.

Excessive throat mucus and chronic throat clearing are the most common symptoms of LPR. Acid instilled into the oesophagus can result in rapid increase in salivation; this sudden filling of the mouth with saliva is termed 'water brash'. Excessive salivation causes a sense of fullness in the pharynx that typically results in repeated throat clearing. Excessive throat clearing causes hypopharyngeal edema and more secretions to pool in throat, thus stimulating more throat clearing resulting in a self-perpetuating cycle.

Patients with LPR-related postnasal drip (PND) often lack other symptoms suggestive of allergic rhinitis such as rhinorrhea, nasal congestion, sneezing and itchy or running eyes. Patients with rhinitis are usually aware of the colour and odour of PND, whereas inability to characterize PND suggests LPR.

LPR can cause the sensation of a foreign body in the throat (globus). Reflux may be a causative factor in up to two thirds of individuals with globus. The majority of patients with reflux-related globus will improve with antireflux treatment.

Dysphonia caused by LPR is intermittent. Patients with chronic, unremitting and progressive hoarseness are less likely to have reflux as the primary cause of their voice disorder. Similarly progressive dysphonia is not likely to be caused by reflux.

Because these symptoms are nonspecific, the clinician must rely on a combination of the symptoms, laryngoscopic findings and diagnostic tools. In some cases an empirical trial of proton pump inhibitors (PPI) may help to make an accurate diagnosis.

Reflux symptom index

Belafsky et al. (2002) developed a useful 9-item self-administered tool, the Reflux Symptom Index that can help clinicians assess the relative degree of LPR symptoms during initial evaluation and after treatment. The Reflux Symptom Index is based on a careful study of pH probe – confirmed LPR cases. Reflux Symptom Index score greater than 13 is considered abnormal.

Patients are asked to use a 0- to 5-point scale to grade the following symptoms:

1. Hoarseness or voice problem.
2. Throat clearing.
3. Excess throat mucus or postnasal drip.
4. Difficulty in swallowing.
5. Coughing after eating or lying down.
6. Breathing difficulties or choking spells.
7. Troublesome or annoying cough.
8. Sensation of something sticking or a lump in the throat.
9. Heartburn, chest pain, indigestion, or stomach acid coming up.

The authors reported that the Reflux Symptom Index score in untreated LPR patients was significantly higher than in controls (21.2 vs 11.6; $p \geq 0.001$).

The Reflux Finding Score

Since there is no pathognomonic LPR finding, Belafsky et al. (2001) developed an 8-item clinical severity scale for judging laryngoscopic findings, the Reflux Finding Score, which appears to be useful for assessment and follow-up of LPR patients. They rated 8 LPR-associated findings on a variably weighted scale from 0 to 4: subglottic edema, ventricular obliteration, erythema/hyperemia, vocal fold edema, diffuse laryngeal edema, posterior commissure hypertrophy, granuloma, and thick endolaryngeal mucus.

The various possible scores are:

- Pseudosulcus (0 absent, 2 present).
- Ventricular obliteration (0 none, 2 partial, 4 complete).
- Erythema/hyperaemia (0 none, 2 arytenoid only, 4 diffuse).
- Vocal cord edema (0 none, 1 mild, 2 moderate, 3 severe, 4 obstructing [polypoidal]).
- Diffuse laryngeal edema (0 none, 1 mild, 2 moderate, 3 severe, 4 obstructing).
- Posterior commissure hypertrophy (0 none, 1 mild, 2 moderate, 3 severe, 4 obstructing).
- Granuloma/granulation (0 absent, 2 present).
- Thick endolaryngeal mucus (0 absent, 2 present).

The results could range from 0 (normal) to 26 (worst possible score). Based on their analysis, one can be 95% certain that a patient with a Reflux Finding Score of 7 or more will have LPR.

The larynx of patient with LPR can be visualized through indirect laryngoscopy, rigid/flexible direct laryngoscopy. Videoendoscopy and stroboscopy are useful for documenting treatment effects and for visualizing subtle signs associated with acid reflux.

The commonest laryngeal findings in LPR-associated laryngitis include edematous changes as opposed to erythematous, predominantly involving the posterior larynx. As the true and false vocal cords swell in response to reflux, it leads to 'ventricular obliteration'. Chronic irritation can result in thickening of the posterior laryngeal mucosa with hyperkeratosis (pachydermia laryngeus). The posterior mucosal thickening with increased granularity and rough cobblestone appearance is known as 'granular laryngitis'. Increased and thick mucus formation leads to mucus stranding and pooling. 'Pseudosulcus' is a common endoscopy finding in LPR. The term pseudosulcus refers to the edematous changes that are seen at the undersurface of the vocal folds from anterior to posterior commissure, in contrast to true sulcus vocalis which involves the free edge of the fold and terminates at the vocal process. Contact ulcers, granuloma, scarring and stenosis indicate more severe LPR.

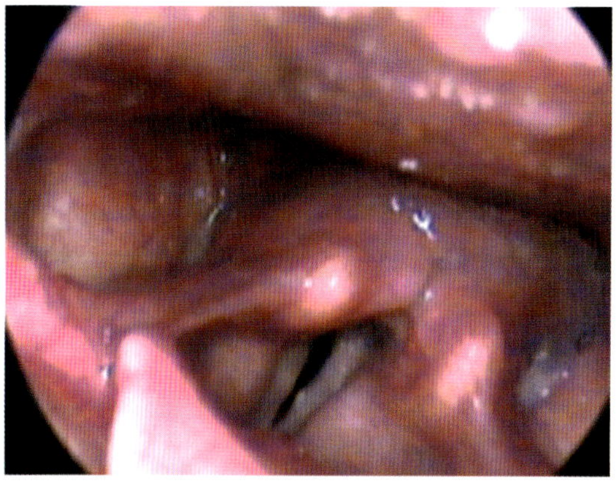

Fig. 36.2. Endoscopic view – pooling of secretions and irregular laryngeal mucosa.

DIAGNOSIS

There is often lack of correlation between symptoms and signs to the extent that laryngeal signs need not to be present in order to diagnose LPR. A normal laryngeal appearance cannot rule out the presence of LPR. The laryngeal findings and the presence of suggestive symptoms gives important information for the diagnosis. Dual probe pH monitoring remains the most specific and sensitive test available to diagnose LPR. The establishment of diagnosis by pH monitoring for LPR is reserved by American Gastroenterological Association for patients who do not respond to initial acid suppression and the use of pH monitoring as the initial diagnostic study is also recommended in patients with more severe conditions possibly related to LPR such as subglottic stenosis and severe laryngospasm.

A. Empiric medical trial

Many clinicians consider an empiric trial with PPIs a reasonable approach to diagnose LPR. The current recommendation for an empiric trial is a PPI taken twice daily for up to 3 months. If there is no response to twice daily PPI therapy after 3 months, treatment failure or more likely an alternative cause for the patient's symptoms should be suspected.

B. 24-hours ambulatory pH monitoring

Currently, 24-hours ambulatory pH monitoring is gold standard to diagnose LPR. For GERD, probe is kept about 5 cm above the manometrically determined site of LES. However, for LPR, additional probe is kept 1 cm above UES in the pharynx. The various types of electrodes available are unipolar glass electrodes, antimony electrodes and combined glass electrodes. They are inserted under local anaesthesia in outpatient setting. The electrodes can be put by endoscopy, fluoroscopy or manometric (most commonly) control. Patient also carries a portable data logger tied with a waist belt. Data from the electrodes are recorded at 6–8 seconds intervals. The parameters studied are as follows:

- Percent upright time pH less than 4.
- Percent total time pH less than 4.
- Percent recumbent time pH less than 4.
- Number of reflux episodes with pH less than 4.
- Number of reflux episodes with pH less than 4, for 5 or more minutes.
- Period of longest single acid exposure.

These values are compared with previously determined normal values.

C. Esophagoscopy

It is essential to endoscopically examine the oesophagus in patients with suspected acid reflux disease because of the proven relationship between acid reflux esophagitis and esophageal adeno-carcinoma.

D. Esophagogram

It is useful method to diagnose structural and functional abnormalities of the oesophagus, including hiatal hernia, strictures, esophageal rings, extrinsic compression, motility disorders, diverticula, possible malignancy, esophageal shortening. It also has a significant use for planning of antireflux surgery.

E. Manometry

Oesophageal manometry may be useful to diagnose motility disorders presenting with atypical GERD-like symptoms such as achalasia or diffuse oesophageal spasm.

F. Laryngeal sensory testing

It is to quantify posterior laryngeal edema that results from acid reflux. With laryngeal sensory testing, a pressure and duration controlled pulse of air is administered to the arytenoids epithelium in order to induce the laryngeal adductor reflux, a brain stem mediated, airway protective reflex. The practical way to regard laryngeal sensory testing is that edematous arytenoids would require a stronger air pulse pressure to cause indentation of the arytenoids epithelium than the air pressure required to indent arytenoids epithelium that is not edematous.

G. Pepsin immunoassay

A recent study has demonstrated that detection of pepsin in throat sputum by immunoassay appears as a sensitive test to detect LPR. The pepsin immunoassay was 100% sensitive and 89% specific.

H. Mucosal biopsies

In the esophageal biopsies basal cell hyperplasia, increased papillary length of squamous epithelium and infiltration by polymorphonuclear leukocytes or eosinophils are some of the findings. However, the esophageal biopsies are positive in only about 30–35% of GERD patients.

Biopsy of posterior laryngeal mucosa

Pepsin is often found on laryngeal epithelial biopsy and in sputum of patients with pH test-proven GERD and symptoms of LPR. Detection of pepsin improves diagnostic accuracy in patients with LPR.

In spite of various tests, the diagnosis of reflux in LPR can be challenging, because they might have a heartburn and negative esophageal mucosal injury during endoscopy. Patients with these symptoms are a heterogeneous subgroup of GERD, either combined with or without typical esophagitis.

TREATMENT

The treatment of these individuals is based on decrease in volume and potency of gastroesophageal reflux and protection of the mucosa from acid-induced injury.

Intermittent and mild symptoms

Initial approach for patients with mild and intermittent symptoms is with dietary and lifestyle modifications including weight loss, exercise and smoking cessation. Reducing the intake of alcohol, beverage, chocolate, peppermint and caffeine is helpful. Eating more frequent, smaller meals may help to reduce reflux. Patients are also instructed to avoid tight-fitting clothing. Patients should avoid food and drink within 3 hours before sleep. During the sleep patients are encouraged to lie on their left side as in left lateral decubitus position the diaphragmatic crura cause a natural kink at the gastroesophageal junction.

Various studies have indicated the efficacy of elevation of the head end of the bed, preferably with six inch blocks (not pillows) to reduce reflux and increase acid clearance. Activities that require lifting, bending, stooping and inversions should be minimized, especially during acute symptoms and after meals. Increased water intake is important for vocal hygiene.

For patients with LPR who fail to respond to dietary and behavioral modifications, antacids or H2 receptor blockers (ranitidine, cimetidine, famotidine and nigatidine) may be used. Sodium alginate, which forms a physical barrier on the top of the stomach, may be used as adjuvant therapy for any type of LPR or as a sole therapy in minor LPR.

Troublesome symptoms

Patients with troublesome symptoms or with complications of GERD in addition to lifestyle changes should be treated with proton pump inhibitors. The AAO-HNS currently recommends treatment for LPR with twice daily PPI (Omeprazole, Rabeprazole, Pantoprazole, etc.) therapy. PPI should be taken 30–40 minutes prior to meals. Its effect on reducing stomach acid production is lost if taken more than two hours before eating. Twice daily PPI therapy for at least 3 months is a reasonable treatment for troublesome LPR. Symptoms usually improve by 2 months. Laryngeal inflammation may continue to resolve after more than 6 months. Twice daily PPI therapy should be continued until laryngeal examination appears normal. Maintenance dose of PPI may be required if symptoms or laryngeal findings recur.

Ambulatory pH monitoring is warranted for patients who do not respond to twice daily PPI therapy. If the second ambulatory pH study is normal, alternative causes of patient's symptoms should be sought for. Combined esophageal pH monitoring with impedance monitoring may be considered to look for nonacid reflux events in patients with persistent reflux symptoms who are receiving prolonged PPI therapy.

Surgery, most commonly Nissen fundoplication, in which the proximal stomach is wrapped around the distal esophagus to create an antireflux barrier, is an alternative management approach to chronic gastroesophageal reflux disease. It can be offered to selected patients with extraesophageal manifestations of reflux, as these cases often require high doses of PPI and may more effectively be controlled with antireflux surgery.

CONCLUSION

The increasing importance of LPR is being recognized in otolaryngology practice. LPR has a significant negative impact in the quality of lives of the patients especially patient's social functioning and vitality. All otolaryngologists need to be sensitized to the presence of LPR and the need for starting treatment whenever required.

SUGGESTED READING

1. Koufman JA, Aviv JE, Casiano RR, Shaw GY. Larynogopharyngeal reflux: position statement of the committee on speech, voice and swallowing disorders of the American Academy of Otolaryngology – Head and Neck Surgery. *Otolaryngol Head Neck Surg*, 2002; 127: 32–5.
2. Wiener GJ, Cooper JB, Wu WC, Koufman JA, Richter JE. Is hoarseness an atypical manifestation of gastroesophageal reflux (GER)? An ambulatory 24 hour pH study. *Gastroenterology*, 1986; 90: 1691.
3. Chevalier JM, Brossard E, Monnier P. Globus sensation and gastroesophageal reflux. *Eur Arch Otorhinolaryngol*, 2003; 260: 273–6.
4. Park W, Hicks DM, Khandwala F, et al. Laryngopharyngeal reflux: propective cohort study evaluating optimal dose of proton-pump inhibitor therapy and pretherapy predictors of response: *Laryngoscope*, 2005; 115: 1230–8.
5. Postma GN, Johnson LF, Koufman JA, Treatment of laryngopharyngeal reflux. *Ear Nose Throat J*, 2002; 81 (9 Suppl 2): 24–6.
6. Belafsky PC, Postma GN, Koufman JA. Laryngopharyngeal reflux symptoms improve before changes in physical findings. *Laryngoscope*, 2001; 111: 979–81.
7. Lindstrom DR, Wallace J, Loehrl TA, et al. Nissen fundoplication surgery for extraesophageal manifestation of gastroesophageal reflux (EER). *Laryngoscope*, 2002; 112: 1762–5.
8. Hunter JG, Trus TL, Branum GD. A physiologic approach to laparoscopic fundoplication for gastroesophageal reflux disease. *Ann Surg*, 1996; 223: 673–87.
9. Jamieson JR, Stein HJ, Demesster TR, et al. Ambulatory 24-H esophageal pH monitoring: normal values, optimal thresholds, specificity sensitivity and reproducibility. *Am J Gastroenterol*, 1992; 87: 1102–11.
10. Kahrilas PJ, Quigley EM. Clinical esophageal pH recording: a technical review for practice guidelines development. *Gastroenterology*, 1996; 110: 1982–6.
11. Hill J, Stuart RC, Fung HK, et al. Gastroesophageal reflux, motility disorders and psychological profiles in the etiology of globus pharynges. *Laryngoscope*, 1997; 107: 1373–7.
12. Knight J, Lively MO, Johnston N, Dettmar PW, Koufman JA. Sensitive pepsin immunoassay for detection of laryngopharyngeal reflux. *Laryngoscope*, 2005; 115: 1473–8.
13. Sen P, Georgalas C. A systematic review of the role of the proton pump inhibitors for symptoms of laryngopharyngeal reflux. *Clin Otolaryngol*, 2005; 31: 20–4.
14. Belfasky PC, Postma GN. The validity and reliability of reflux finding score. *Laryngoscope*, 2001; 111: 1313–7.
15. Belafsky PC, Postma GN, Koufman JA. Validity and reliability of the reflux symptom index. *J Voice*, 2002; 16: 274–7.
16. Jecker P, Orloff LA. Extraesophageal reflux and upper aerodigestive tract diseases. *ORL*, 2005; 67: 185–91.

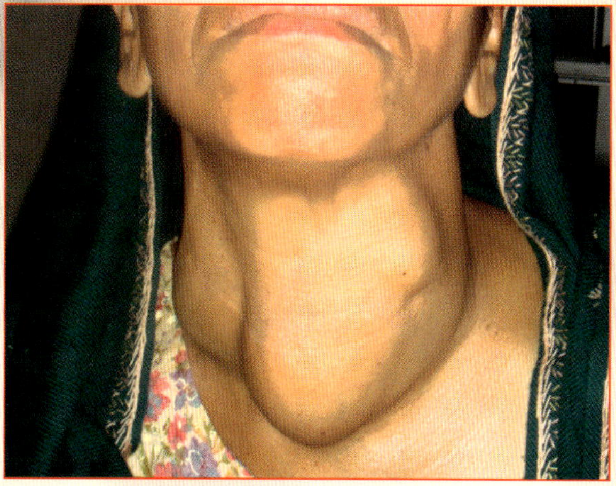

SECTION 6

Head & Neck Surgery

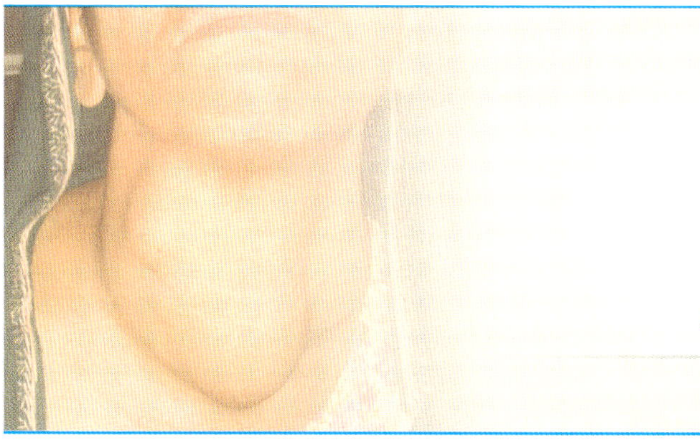

CHAPTER 37

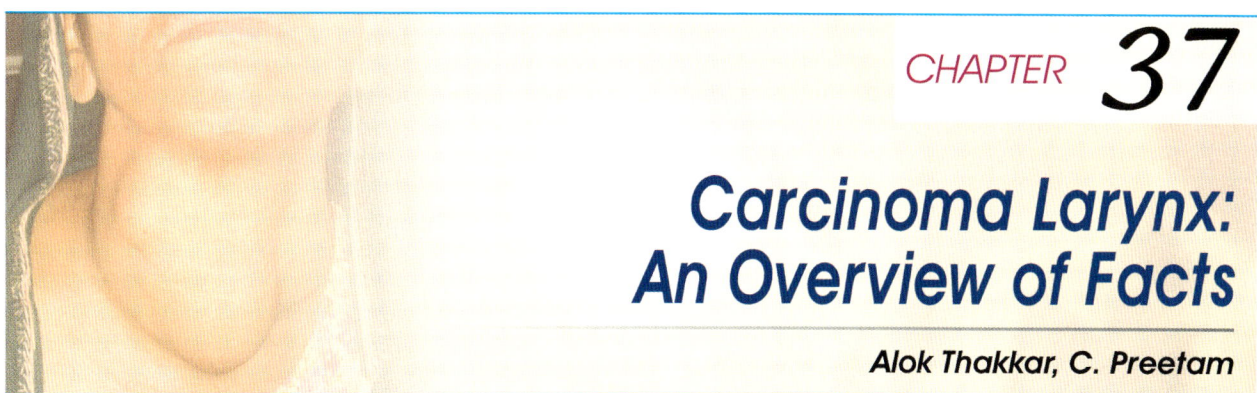

Carcinoma Larynx: An Overview of Facts

Alok Thakkar, C. Preetam

The incidence of laryngeal cancer is relatively low compared with that of carcinomas of all sites, comprising about 2 to 5% of all cancers worldwide. In India, Silchar town (10.7) had the highest incidence followed by Kamrup Urban District (8.2). Most importantly, because of the early presentation and lack of rich lymphatic drainage of larynx, tumours confined to larynx have substantially better prognosis. There is an increasing trend towards radiation therapy with concomitant chemotherapy as a first line management for laryngeal and hypopharyngeal carcinomas. Conservative treatment when not effective still permits reasonable salvage with a more radical surgery. Thus enhancing the importance of need for early detection and proper management of cases of carcinoma larynx.

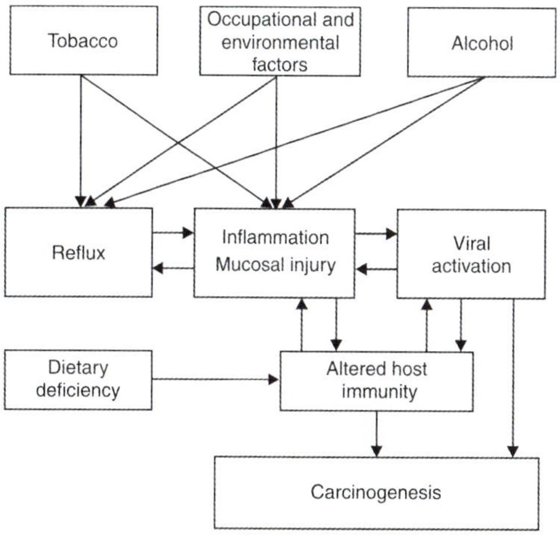

Fig. 37.1. Schematic model of multifactorial development of squamous cell carcinoma of the larynx.

ETIOLOGY (Fig. 37.1)

By far, smoking tobacco has been implicated as the prime factor in causing laryngeal cancer. Persons with various types of immunodeficiency states are also thought to be at higher risk for developing laryngeal cancer. An underlying genetic susceptibility to this type of cancer may also exist and has been theorized as a potential cofactor in oncogenesis. The strain HPV 16 has been most frequently demonstrated in laryngeal squamous carcinomas by using probes for HPV and deoxyribonucleic acid (DNA). Other etiologic factors include gastroesophageal reflux and exposure to wood dust, asbestos, volatile chemicals, nitrogen mustard, and ionizing radiation. Genetic alteration of chromosomal region 9p21 seem to occur frequently and early in progression of paraneoplastic abnormal mucosa to invasive cancer.

INCIDENCE

Over the years, there has been a male predominance noted (about 5 : 1 in the United States). As more women have taken up smoking in recent decades, a shift in this ratio can be expected. The incidence of carcinoma of the larynx was recently reported to be 12% of all tumours diagnosed. The greatest incidence of laryngeal cancer occurs in the fifth, sixth, and seventh decades (more than 80%). For laryngeal cancer in males the highest incidence is noted by Delhi registry (8.5) followed by Mumbai (7.0), Chennai (4.5), Bhopal (4.5), Bangalore (3.8), and Barshi registry (1.9).

PATHOLOGY

Over 95% of all malignant laryngeal tumours are squamous cell carcinomas. The premalignant lesions have clinical relevance since 3% of hyperkeratoses without dysplasia, 7% of mild dysplasias, 18% of moderate dysplasias, and 24% of severe dysplasias of the vocal folds have been shown to ultimately develop invasive carcinoma. Some other rare malignancies are:

- Sarcomas
- Lymphoma
- Adenocarcinoma
- Neuroendocrine carcinoma
- Extramedullary plasmacytoma

Second primary tumours occur synchronously in about 1% of laryngeal cancers and metachronously in 5 to 10%. This occurrence seems to be greater with supraglottic compared with glottic primaries. The most common second primary tumour is bronchogenic carcinoma.

SURGICAL ANATOMY AND PATHWAYS OF SPREAD (Figs. 37.2–37.6)

LARYNX

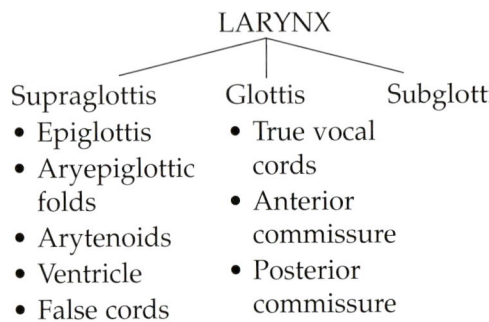

- Supraglottis
  - Epiglottis
  - Aryepiglottic folds
  - Arytenoids
  - Ventricle
  - False cords
- Glottis
  - True vocal cords
  - Anterior commissure
  - Posterior commissure
- Subglottis

The inferior boundry of supraglottis as defined by AJCC is a horizontal plane passing through apex of the ventricle. The anatomic division is located at the arcuate line, which marks the change from the respiratory to squamous epithelium and is reliably located at apex. The marginal zone of the supraglottis is recognized for its aggressive clinical behavior, composing of suprahyoid epiglottis and aryepiglottic folds.

According to UICC the inferior border of glottis is a horizontal plane 1 cm inferior to the level of the upper surface of vocal cord (Fig. 37.2).

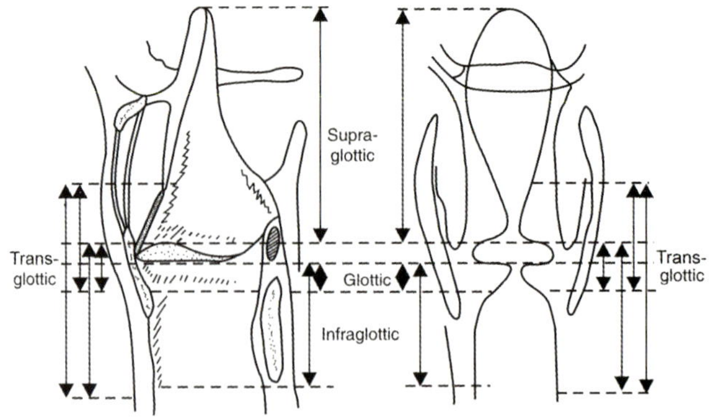

Fig. 37.2. Boundaries of supraglottis, glottis and subglottis.

5 layers of vocal cord (Fig. 37.3):

- Squamous epithelium
- Superficial layer of lamina propria (Reinkes space) } Cover
- Intermediate layer
- Deep layer } Transition
- Vocalis muscle — Body

Lower lymphatics → cricothyroid membrane → prelaryngeal/pretracheal

Superior → thyrohyoid memb

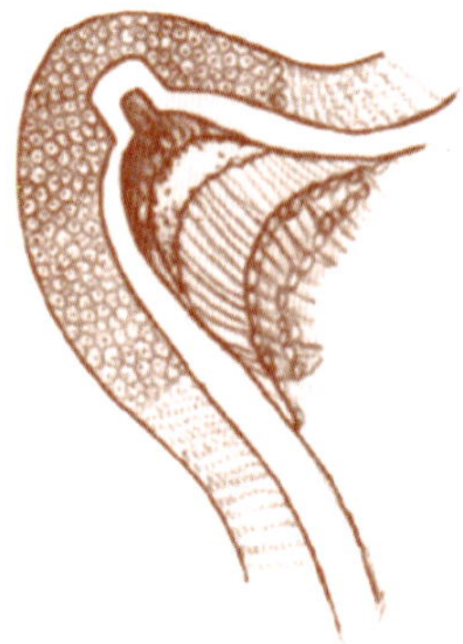

Fig. 37.3. Histology of vocal cord.

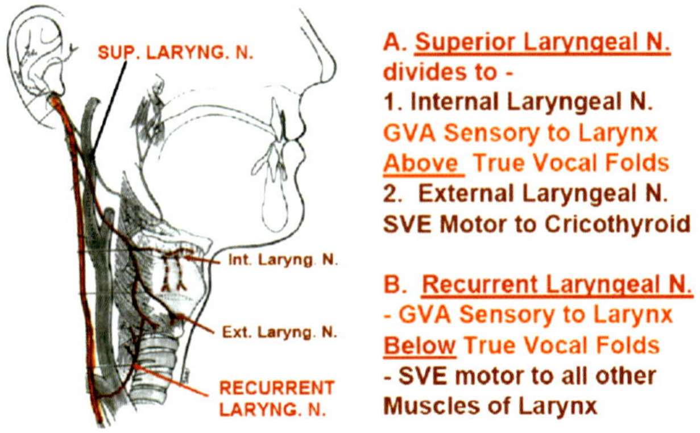

Fig. 37.4. Nerves of the larynx (branches of vagus nerve).

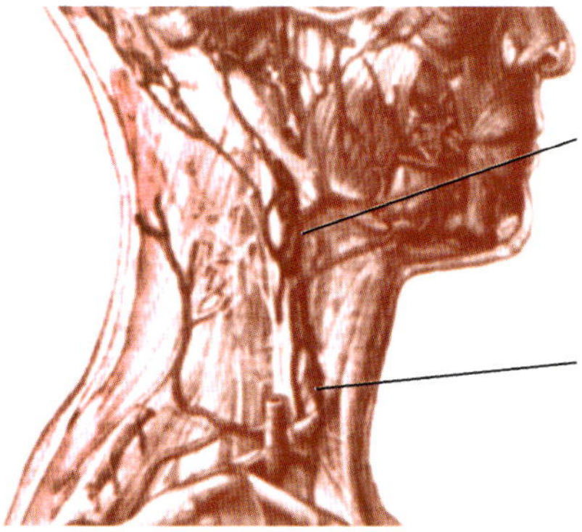

Fig. 37.5. Major lymphatics of larynx.

SPREAD OF TUMOUR (Fig. 37.6)

The endolarynx contains fibroelastic membranes which compartmentalize the endolarynx and act as barriers for spread of tumour and also form the basis for partial laryngectomies. Spread can occur either by mucosal, submucosal, lymphatic, vascular, perineural or direct spread.

Spaces of significance

1. Reinke's space
2. Paraglottic space
3. Pre-epiglottic space
4. Anterior subglottic wedge

Supraglottis

Propensity for bilateral spread and high chance for lymphatic metastasis.

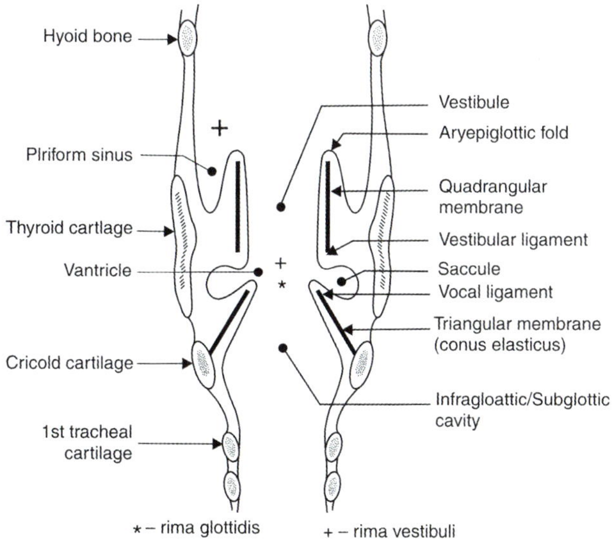

Fig. 37.6. Vertical section of larynx.

Suprahyoid epiglottis – usually exophytic, locoregional spread.

Infrahyoid epiglottis – usually infiltrative

Pores of epiglottic cartilage → pre-epiglottic space → paraglottic space ↓

Extra laryngeal spread ← Thyrohyoid membrane

False vocal cords – quadrangular membrane limits the inferior extension of the tumour. Usually spread superiorly.

Aryepiglottic folds and Arytenoids – marginal zone lesions and usually involve adjacent hypopharynx. They are considered aggressive and carry a poor prognosis.

Glottic tumours: The anterior commissure ligament or Broyle's ligament limits the spread of tumour, but once it is involved the tumour can spread both upward and downward, due to its fibre distribution. The inner perichondrium is dehiscent at anterior commissure, facilitating the spread of tumour. Once the conus elasticus is breached, the tumour extends to subglottis. There can also be lateral extension with involvement of paraglottic space, identified clinically by fixation of vocal cord, due to involvement of thyroarytenoid muscle.

Subglottis: Usually circumferential growth is seen, with early cartilage involvement due to lack of absence of intervening muscle layer. Tumour can breach cricothyroid membrane and can spread to extralaryngeal tissues.

EVALUATION

In current times, a complete oncologic evaluation includes all of the following:

- History and physical exam
- Fiberoptic laryngoscopy – v.c. mobility/site of fixation
- Labs and CXR to rule out metastasis
- USG for evaluation of lymph nodes
- CT or MRI
- Staging panendoscopy – arytenoid mobility
- +/- Pulmonary function tests, Videostroboscopy

Imaging is useful for assessment of :

1. Extent of disease
2. Cartilage invasion
3. Extralaryngeal spread
4. Pre-epiglottic and paraglottic space involvement
5. Tumour volume
6. Nodal disease

STAGING

Supraglottis

- T1: Tumour limited to one subsite of supraglottis with normal vocal cord mobility.
- T2: Tumour invades mucosa of more than one adjacent subsite of supraglottis or glottis or region outside the supraglottis (e.g., mucosa of base of tongue, vallecula, medial wall of pyriform sinus) without fixation of the larynx.
- T3: Tumour limited to larynx with vocal cord fixation and/or invades any of the following: postcricoid area, pre-epiglottic tissues, paraglottic space, and/or minor thyroid cartilage erosion (e.g., inner cortex).
- T4a: Tumour invades through the thyroid cartilage, and/or invades tissues beyond the larynx (e.g., trachea, soft tissues of the neck including deep extrinsic muscle of the tongue, strap muscles, thyroid, or esophagus).
- T4b: Tumour invades prevertebral space, encases carotid artery, or invades mediastinal structures Subsites include the following: ventricular bands (false cords), arytenoids, suprahyoid epiglottis, infrahyoid epiglottis, aryepiglottic folds (laryngeal aspect).

Glottis

- T1: Tumour limited to the vocal cord(s) (may involve anterior or posterior commissure) with normal mobility.
- T2: Tumour extends to supraglottis and/or subglottis, and/or with impaired vocal cord mobility.
- T3: Tumour limited to the larynx with vocal cord fixation and/or invades paraglottic space, and/or minor thyroid cartilage erosion (e.g., inner cortex).
- T4a: Tumour invades through the thyroid cartilage and/or invades tissues beyond the larynx (e.g., trachea, soft tissues of neck, including deep extrinsic muscle of the tongue, strap muscles, thyroid, or esophagus).
- T4b: Tumour invades prevertebral space, encases carotid artery, or invades mediastinal structures.

37

Subglottis

- T1: Tumour limited to the subglottis.
- T2: Tumour extends to vocal cord(s) with normal or impaired mobility.
- T3: Tumour limited to larynx with vocal cord fixation.
- T4a: Tumour invades cricoid or thyroid cartilage and/or invades tissues beyond the larynx (e.g., trachea, soft tissues of neck, including deep extrinsic muscles of the tongue, strap muscles, thyroid, or esophagus).
- T4b: Tumour invades prevertebral space, encases carotid artery, or invades mediastinal structures.

Stage 0	Tis	N0	M0
Stage I	T1	N0	M0
Stage II	T2	N0	M0
Stage III	T3	N0	M0
	T1	N1	M0
	T2	N1	M0
	T3	N1	M0
Stage IVa	T4	N0	M0
	T4	N1	M0
	Any T	N2	M0
Stage IVb	Any T	N3	M0
Stage IVc	Any T	Any N	M1

MANAGEMENT

The first decision with regard to management in any patient with Head-Neck Cancer is essentially with regard to the intent of treatment which is appropriate for a given patient, i.e., whether treatment is to be with curative intent, palliative intent or supportive intent. Cases that may initially be planned for palliative treatment may sometimes be subsequently considered for curative treatment in case of good response to therapy.

Fortunately, with cancer larynx it is almost always possible to consider treatment with curative intent and it is unusual to have situations wherein palliative or supportive treatment has to be resorted to.

The modalities of treatment vary between the following:

- Radiotherapy
- Chemotherapy
- Surgery

The variety of surgical options have increased markedly over the last two decades. The current concept is not only to aim for an oncologic resection but to also look at function preservation. The current surgical options are as below:

- Transoral laser excision
- Laryngofissure
- Vertical laryngectomy
- Supraglottic laryngectomy
- Supracricoid laryngectomy
- Near total laryngectomy
- Total laryngectomy

The following criteria should be met for patients to be candidates for partial laryngectomy of any type:

1. The patient should be in good general health. Elderly, debilitated, or mentally impaired patients who would not be able to tolerate a temporary tracheostomy and/or temporary aspiration with eating should not be candidates for conservation procedures.
2. The patient should have a good understanding of the procedure and the possibility that prolonged rehabilitation of speech and swallowing may be required.
3. Adequate pulmonary function is most critical for supraglottic laryngectomy. Poor exercise tolerance, either by history or demonstrated on pulmonary function tests, excludes most patients from open partial laryngeal surgery, particularly supraglottic laryngectomy. If doubt exists, a formal consultation with a pulmonary specialist should be obtained. (Inadequate pulmonary reserve/FEV1<50%)

Early lesion (T1–T2)

Options include radiation therapy/endoscopic surgery/open conservation laryngectomy

Invasive glottis carcinomas are generally less biologically aggressive and surgery offers 90–95% cure rate, with radiotherapy providing cure rates of about 92%. Conservation procedures run the risk of aspiration and voice problems, though equally effective in managing the cancer.

Subglottic lesions rules out any conservation surgery and requires total laryngectomy/±CT/RT.

Supraglottic lesions can be well managed by conservation surgery like supraglottic laryngectomy, but most important is that one needs to address both sides of neck in view of high chance of bilateral nodal metastasis.

Advanced lesions (T3–T4)

Usually require multimodality treatment with surgery / CT/± RT. Supraglottic and transglottic T3 and selective T4 lesions might be amendable for conservation surgery like supracricoid laryngectomy or near total laryngectomy. Postoperative radiation is recommended for cartilage invasion, subglottic extension, thyroid gland involvement, positive paratracheal nodes or in patients with margins positive for tumour.

VOICE REHABILITATION

Electronic pneumatic, Electrolarynx, Non-pulmonary air, Pulmonary air, Esophageal speech, Stoma to mouth appliances and Trachea-esophageal prosthesis.

CONCLUSION

Carcinoma larynx is more common in men, although more women are developing it today due to increase in smoking in female population. Exact cause is not known, however, tobacco smoking, alcohol, GERD, poor nutrition, human papilloma virus and toxic exposure have been blamed. Change of voice, airway obstruction, neck nodes and difficulty in eating are the chief presenting features. Indirect laryngoscopy, direct laryngoscopy, microlaryngoscopy, biopsy, CT and MRI are important diagnostic tools. The treatment modalities are radiotherapy, chemotherapy and surgery.

SUGGESTED READING

1. American Cancer Society. Cancer fact and figure – 2000. Atlanta: American Cancer society; 2000.
2. Consolidated Report of PBCRs: 2001–2004.
3. Tishler RB et al. An initial experience using concurrent paclitaxel and radiation in treatment of head and neck malignancies. *Int J Radiat Oncol Phys*, 1999; 43: 1001–8.
4. Koufman JA, Buke AG. The etiology and pathogenesis of laryngeal carcinoma. *Otolaryngol Clin North Am*, 1997; 30: 1–17.
5. Brandsma JL, Steinberg BM, Abramson AL, Winker B. Presence of human papilloma virus type-16 related sequences in verrucous carcinoma of larynx. *Cancer Res*, 1986; 46: 2185–88.
6. El-Serag HB, Hepworth EJ, Lee P, Sonnenberg A. Gastroesophageal reflux disease is a risk factor for laryngeal and pharyngeal cancer. *Am J Gastroentrol*, 2001; 96: 2013–18.
7. Yalmaz T, Gedikoglu G, Gursel B. The relationship between tumour thickness and clinical and histopathologic parameters in cancer of larynx. *Otolaryngol Head Neck Surg*, 2003; 129(3): 192–98.
8. Shah J. Larynx and trachea. *In:* Shah J and Patel SG editor. Head and Neck Surgery and Oncology. Philadelphia: Mosby 2002; 267–352.

9. Sliamniku B, Bauer W, Painter C, Session D. The transformation of laryngeal keratosis in to invasive carcinoma. *Am J Otolaryngol*, 1989; 10: 42–54.
10. Hong WK, Lipman SM, Itri LM, et al. Prevention of second primary tumours with isoretintion in squmous cell carcinoma of head and neck. *N Engl J Med*, 1990; 323 (12): 795–801.
11. Geisler SA, Olshan AF. GSTMI, GSTTI and the risk of squamous cell carcinoma of head and neck: a mini-HUGS review. *Am J Epidemol*, 2001; 154: 95–105.
12. Armstrong WB, Vokes DE and Maisel RH. Malignant tumours of the larynx. *In:* Flint PW, Haghey BH, Lund VJ, Niparko JK, Richardson MA, Robins KT and Thomas JR editors. Cumming Otolaryngol Head Neck Surg, Vol-2. Philadelphia: Mosby Elesvier, 2010; 1482–1511.

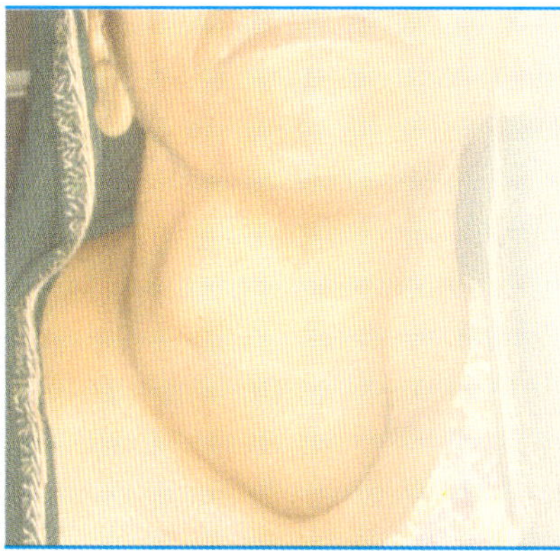

CHAPTER 38

Carcinoma Hypopharynx

Ishwar Singh

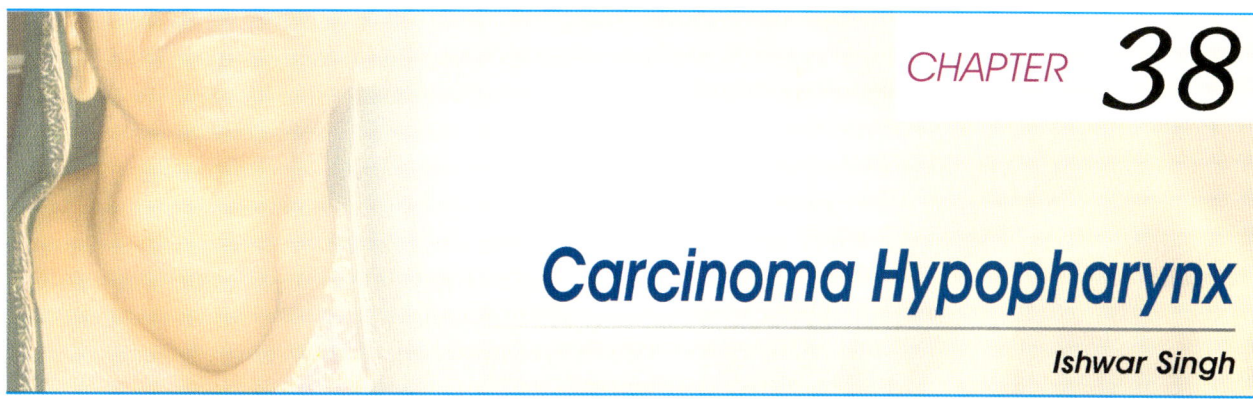

Surgical anatomy of the hypopharynx

Embryologically pharynx develops from the foregut. It is divided into three parts namely: Nasopharynx, Oropharynx and Hypopharynx. The latter is further subdivided in to three parts namely pyriform fossae on either side of larynx, the posterior pharyngeal wall and postcricoid area (Fig. 38.1). The line of demarcation between oropharynx and hypopharynx is an imaginary horizontal line at the tip of epiglottis or at the level of hyoid bone. The inferior limit of hyphopharynx is the lower border of the cricoid cartilage.

Pyriform fossae

These are inverted pyramid-like structures with base upward which is open and the apex at lower end of cricoid cartilage. Apex is located at the crico-arytenoid joint. It has a deep and a shallow part. Medial wall is aryepiglottic fold, lateral wall thyrohyoid membrane in upper part and thyroid cartilage in the lower part. Two pyriform fossae open into postcricoid area. Postcricoid area is just behind the cricoid cartilage and posterior wall is limited by the upper and lower border of cricoid cartilage. Lateral extent is by backward extension of the imaginary line in the long axis of fully abducted vocal cords (Fig. 38.2).

Posterior pharyngeal wall

It extends from the hyoid bone to the inferior border of the cricoid cartilage.

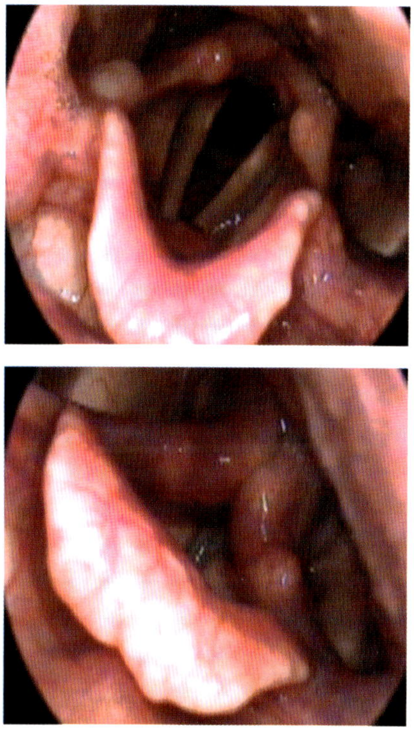

Fig. 38.1. Endoscopic vew of hypopharynx.

It has a good lymphatic supply as compared to the larynx, therefore, its carcinoma has poor prognosis as compared to the larynx. Carcinoma of the hypopharynx is 10% of the total upper aero-digestive tract while it constitutes far less than 1% of the total body cancer. Squamous cell carcinoma is usually seen on histopathology.

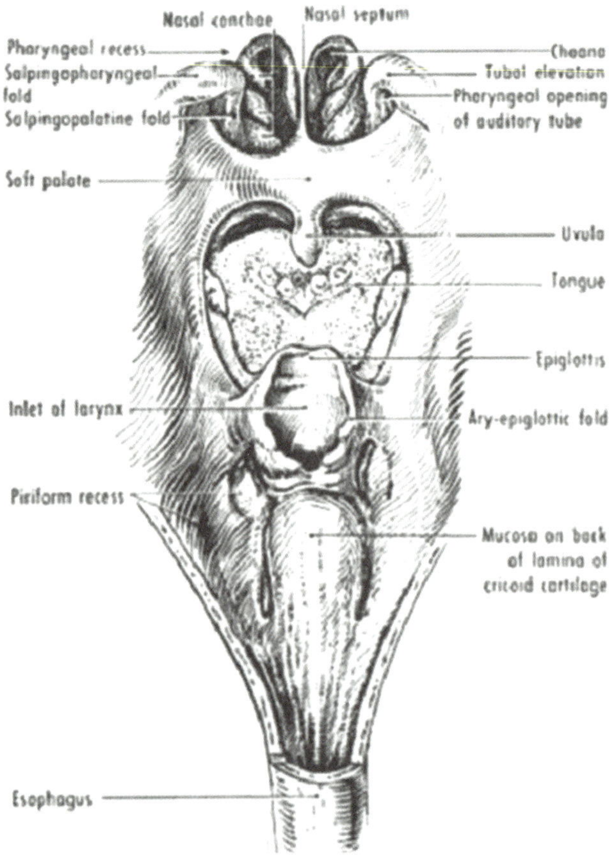

Fig. 38.2. Various parts of hypopharynx piriform fossa postcricoid area seen from back.

Age

Individuals over 50 years with peak incidence in sixth and seventh decades. Postcricoid is the only area in head neck region with slight female preponderance especially in Scandinavia.

Site of involvement

Medial wall of pyriform fossae is commonest site (66–75% cases), posterior pharyngeal wall and postcricoid area is involved in 20–25% cases.

Etiology

- SCC of hypopharynx is also associated with tobacco and alcohol. Tobacco is more strongly causative yet these two substances act synergistically when consumed together.
- **Human papilloma virus** has been found in the SCC. It may play a part in the carcinogenesis in this site.
- **Laryngopharyngeal reflex** is also thought to play a carcinogenic role.
- Patients with **Plummer-Vinson syndrome** have a high risk of developing hypopharyngeal SCC. SCC occurs just proximal to the web because of chronic irritation in Paterson-Kelly syndrome. Iron-deficiency anemia has been treated with supplementation of vitamins A and B, and lead to decreased incidence of postcricoid carcinoma.
- Mutations in tumour suppressor p53 gene occurs in 40–70% in head neck cancers.

Symptoms

Most symptoms are related to the loco-regional spread of the disease.

Early symptoms may be

- Foreign body sensation.
- Progressive dysphagia initially for the solids later on with liquids.
- Repeated clearing of the throat.

Later on

- Sore throat.
- Dysphagia/odynophagia with weight loss.
- Hoarseness.
- A neck mass is seen in 25 % of the cases (Fig. 38.3).
- Referred otalgia is more common with the carcinoma of pyriform sinus innervated by the internal branch of the superior laryngeal nerve, a branch of vagus.

Clinical examination

Clinical examination may show following features. Neck needs to be thoroughly examined for any secondary.

1. Pooling of secretions will obscure the apex of the piriform sinus called Jackson sign. It is one of the sites for the occult primary (Fig. 38.3).
2. Postcricoid may be difficult to visualize (Fig. 38.4).
3. Arytenoid edema.
4. Laryngeal crepitus may be absent.

In advanced cases laryngeal functions may be impaired

5. Vocal cord mobility is impaired.
6. Fiberoptic laryngoscopy with Valsalva manoeuvre helps in the delineation of the superficial tumour extension.

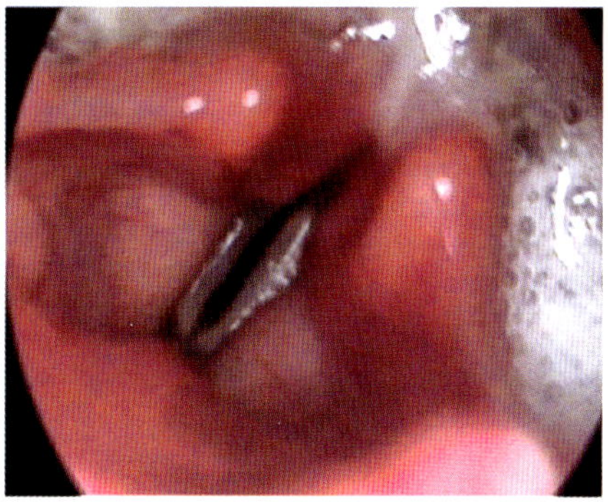

Fig. 38.3. Endoscopic view showing pooling of secretion into piriform fossae.

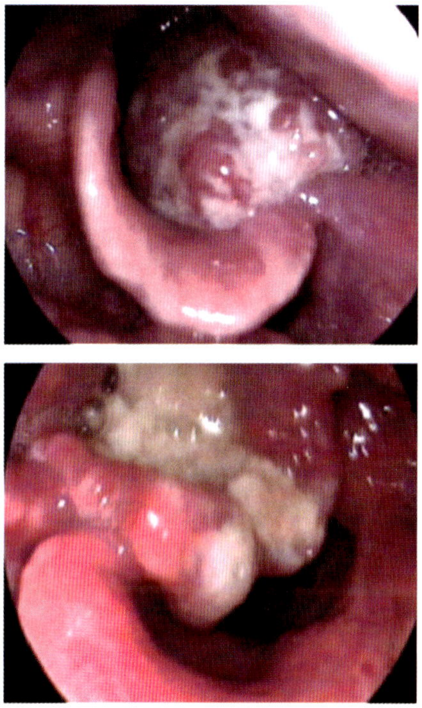

Fig. 38.4. Endscopic view showing hypopharyngeal growth.

7. Panendoscopy under general anesthesia will allow better define the macroscopic limits of the disease and rule out second primary.

Spread of the tumour

If the medial wall of pyriform sinus is involved, i.e., lateral surface of aryepiglottic fold than laryngeal involment, false vocal cord, true vocal cord, arytenoid, is more common. Vocal cord infiltration, cricoarytenoid joint invasion by tumour or the recurrent laryngeal nerve inovolment leads to vocal cord paralysis. Later on pre-epiglottic space and paraglottic space may be infiltrated. If the tumour origin is located in the lateral wall of pyriform sinus then it may extend to posterior pharyngeal wall or the thyroid cartilage may be involved. If on posterior pharyngeal wall, it may extend superiorly in the oropharynx or inferiorly in to the postcricoid area (Fig. 38.5).

Investigations

Radiological

CT or MRI may be done depending on the availability of the facility. MRI defines the soft tissue more accurately as compared to CT. In carcinoma hypopharynx retropharyngeal lymph nodes are involved first. It is essential for the staging of the disease (Figs. 38.6, 38.7). FDG-PET may also be used for the diagnosis if the primary is occult.

Staging of the primary tumours

Tis	Carcinoma in situ
T1	Tumour limited to one subsite of hypopharynx and ≤ 2 cm in the greatest dimension
T2	Tumour invades more than one subsite of hypopharynx or an adjacent site or measure > 2 cm but ≤ 4 cm without fixation of hemilarynx
T3	Tumours > 4 cm or with fixation of hemilarynx
T4	Tumour invades thyroid/cricoid cartilage, hyoid bone, thyroid gland, esophagus or central compartment soft tissue
T4b	Tumour invades prevertebral fascia, encases carotid artery or involves mediastinal structures.

Nodal staging for tumours of the hypopharynx

Nx	Regional lymph nodes cannot be assessed
No	No regional lymph node metastasis
N1	Single ipsilateral lymph node metastasis ≤ 3 cm in the greatest dimension
N2a	Single ipsilateral lymph node metastasis > 3 cm but ≤ 6 cm
N2b	Multiple ipsilateral lymph node metastasis none > 6 cm
N2c	Bilateral or contralateral lymph node metastasis none > 6 cm
N3	Lymph node metastasis > 6 cm in greatest dimension

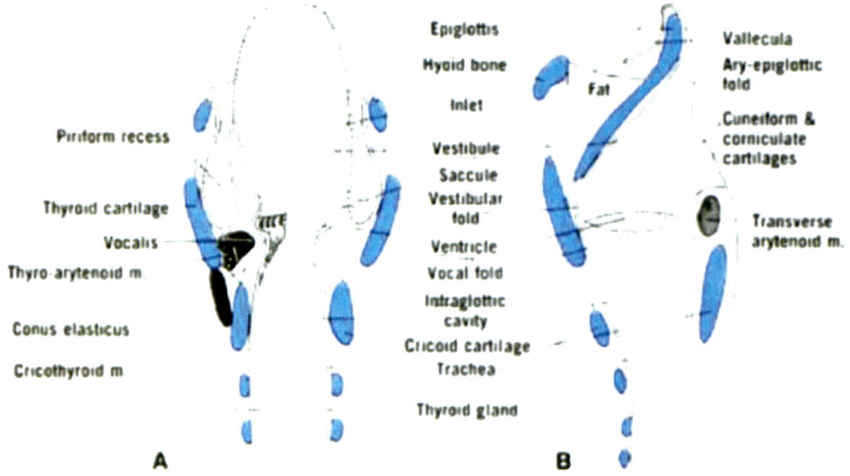

Fig. 38.5. Different barriers for spread of tumour.

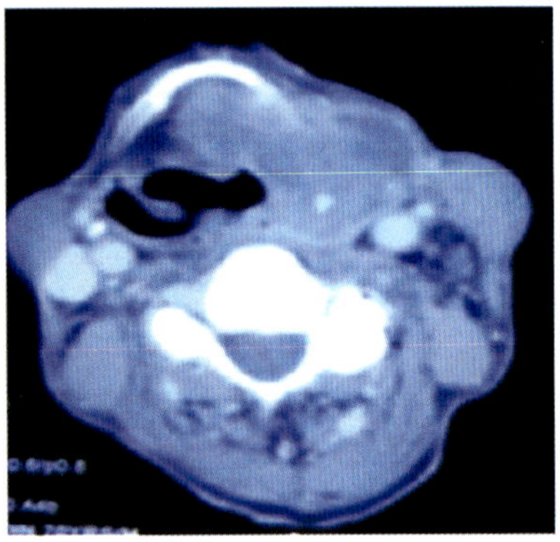

Fig. 38.6. CT scan showing growth in lateral pharyngeal wall.

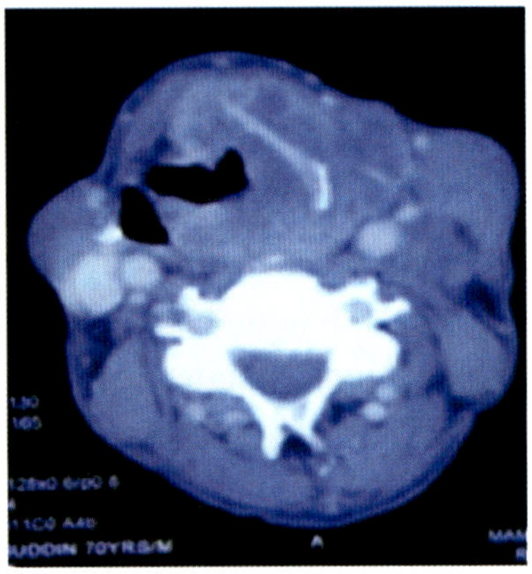

Fig. 38.7. CT showing growth and secondaries in neck.

Treatment policy

Hyphopharyngeal SCC is treated with organ preservation protocols. Chemotherapy and radiotherapy are the initial treatments. If there is any residual or recurrent disease after the initial treatment then radical resection is carried out. Reconstruction is done with free tissue transfer. European Organization for Research and Treatment for Cancer (EORTC) showed favorable results comparing induction chemotherapy followed by radiation in treatment of hypopharyngeal SCC. In cases of early T category tumours (T1, T2) without nodes, these are treated with radiotherapy.

Radical radiotherpy

It is indicated for the following cases:

1. Pyriform fossa T1 or T2 stage.
2. Postcricoid < 5 cm long and not bulky.
3. Low volume posterior pharyngeal wall.

Laryngectomy and partial pharyngectomy (± flap)

1. Pyriform fossa with opposite side clear and not extending to the midline posteriorly.
2. Posterior pharyngeal wall not invading larynx.

Total pharyngolaryngectomy (usually jejunal loop repair)

1. Large postcricoid.
2. Cervical oesophagus.
3. Second tumour in oesophagus.
4. Tumour and perforation.
5. Thyroid cancer invading pharynx.
6. Heavy irradiation damage.
7. Peristomal recurrence.
8. Failed previous methods.

FLOW DIAGRAM FOR MANAGEMENT OF CARCINOMA HYPOPHARYNX

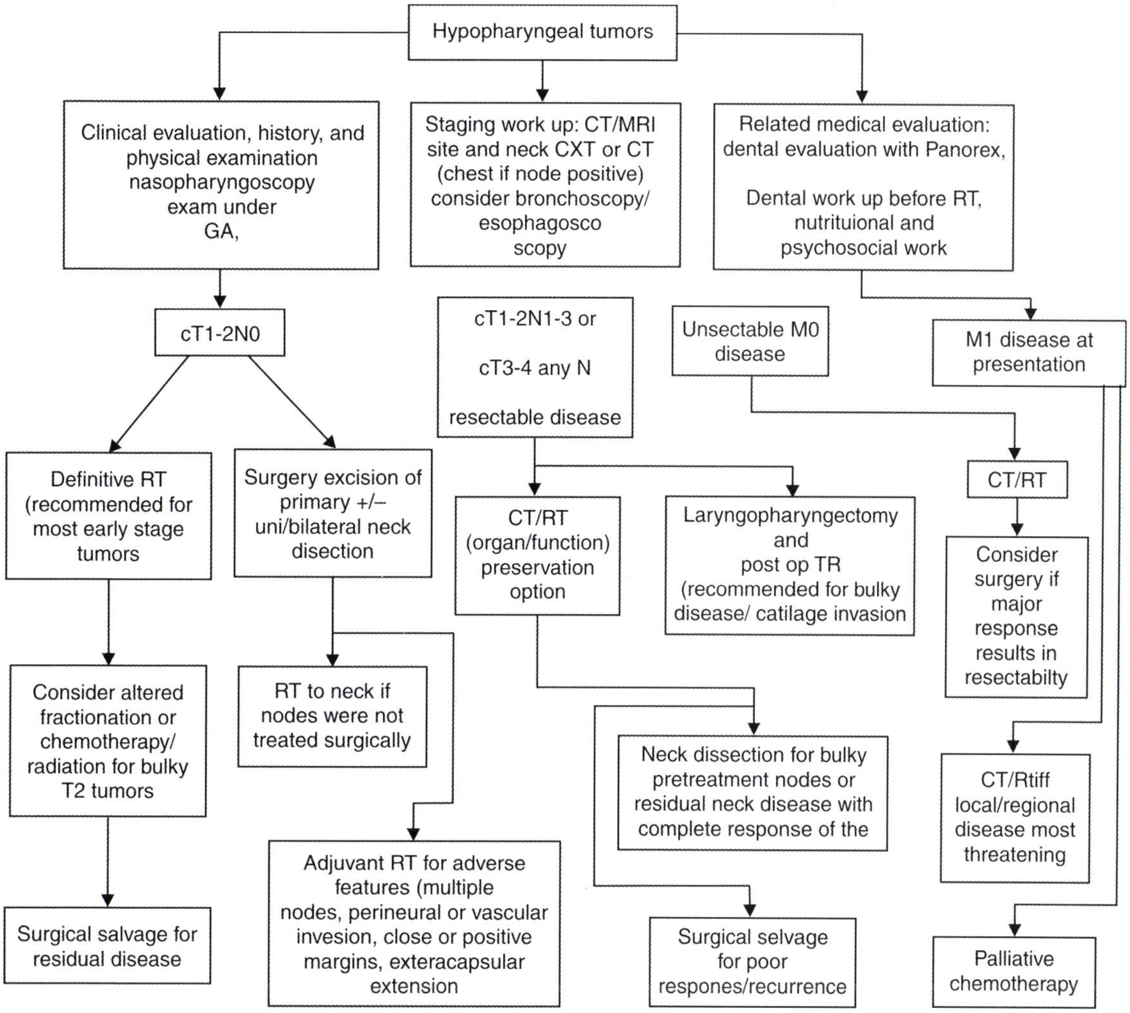

CONCLUSION

Carcinoma hypopharynx is common in elderly males who are chronic smokers. It may present as simple sore throat, dysphagia, odyniophasia, with pain in ear or as mass in the neck. Clinical examination may show uleroprolifarative growth in hypopharynx or level II, III or IV level lymph nodes enlargement. Biopsy, CT or MRI are the main investigations for the extent of the tumors. Chemoradiation or surgery may be carried out with a flap repair.

SUGGESTED READING

1. David G Pfister, Kenneth S Hau, Jean-Louis Lefebvre. Cancer of the Hypopharynx and Cervical Esophagus, *In:* Head and Neck Cancer: A Multidisciplinary Approach Third edition. Ed Louis B Harrison, Roy B Sesssion, Waun Ki Hong. Lippincott Williams & Wilkins Philadelphia 2004; pp. 397–450.
2. Lin DT, Seth M, Cohen, George L, Coppit, Burkey BB. Squamous cell carcinoma of the Oropharynx and Hypopharynx. *Otolaryngol Clin North Am*, 2005; 3891: 59–74.
3. Thawley SE, Session DG, Genden EM. Surgical Therapy of Pharyngeal Tumours. *In:* Comprehensive Management of Head and Neck Tumours, Thawley SE, Panje WR, Batsakis JG, Lindberg RD. WB Saunders Company Philadelphia, 1999, Vol. 2, pp. 1039–68.
4. Uppaluri R, Sunwoo JB. Neoplasm of the Hypopharynx and Cervical Esophagus. *In:* Otolaryngology Head Neck Surgery, 4th edition by Charles W Cummings, Paul W Flint, Lee A Harker, Bruce H haughey, Mark A Richardson et al. Elsevier Mosby Philadelphia, pp. 1899–1931.
5. Andrew S Jones. Tumours of the hypopharynx and Oesophagus. *In:* Scott-brown's Otolaryngology Head Neck Surgery Ed Gleeson M, Browning GG, Burton MJ, et al. Hodder Arnold 7th ed, 2008, Vol. 2, pp. 2633–60.

38

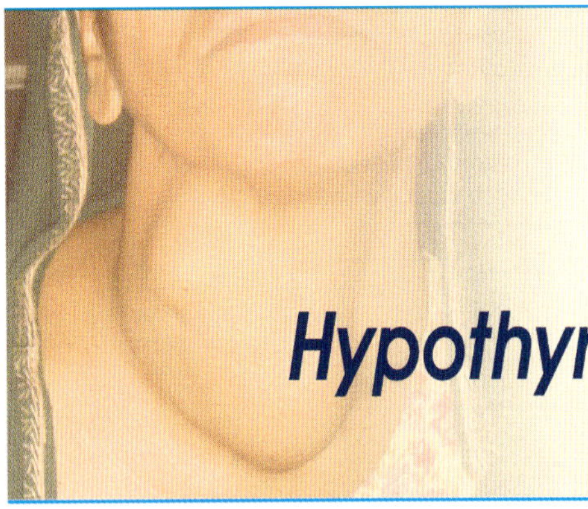

CHAPTER 39

Diseases of Thyroid Gland: Hypothyroidism and Hyperthyroidism

Rajesh Rajput

The thyroid gland is the biggest gland in the neck. It is situated in the anterior neck below the skin and muscle layers. The thyroid gland takes the shape of a butterfly with the two wings being represented by the left and right thyroid lobes which wrap around the trachea. The sole function of the thyroid is to make thyroid hormone. This hormone has an effect on nearly all tissues of the body where it increases cellular activity. The function of the thyroid, therefore, is to regulate the body's metabolism. The thyroid gland is prone to several very distinct problems, out of which two extremely common conditions, i.e., hypothyroidism and hyperthyroidism are described in this chapter.

HYPOTHYROIDISM

Hypothyroidism is a common endocrine disorder resulting from deficiency of thyroid hormone. It is called as primary hypothyroidism if thyroid gland produces insufficient amounts of thyroid hormone and secondary if lack of thyroid hormone secretion is due to inadequate secretion of thyroid-stimulating hormone (TSH) from the pituitary gland. The patient's presentation may vary from asymptomatic to, rarely, coma with multisystem organ failure (myxedema coma). Worldwide iodine deficiency is the most common cause of hypothyroidism followed by autoimmune thyroiditis (i.e., Hashimoto's thyroiditis) and postablative (surgical, radiation exposure) hypothyroidism. Other causes include postpartum thyroiditis, subacute granulomatous thyroiditis, drug induced (amiodarone, interferon alpha, thalidomide, lithium, stavudine) hypothyroidism. It is more common in females and its prevalence increases with age with as many as 10% of elderly females having some degree of hypothyroidism.

Pathophysiology

Because all metabolically active cells require thyroid hormone, deficiency of the hormone has a wide range of systemic effects. Clinical manifestations are due to either derangements in metabolic processes or direct effects by myxedematous infiltration (i.e., accumulation of glucosaminoglycans in the tissues). The myxedematous changes in the heart result in decreased contractility, cardiac enlargement, pericardial effusion, decreased pulse, and decreased cardiac output. In the GI tract, achlorhydria and decreased intestinal transit with gastric stasis can occur. Delayed puberty, anovulation, menstrual irregularities, and infertility are common. Decreased thyroid hormone effect can cause increased levels of total cholesterol and low-density lipoprotein (LDL) cholesterol and a possible change in high-density lipoprotein (HDL) cholesterol due to a change in metabolic clearance. In addition, hypothyroidism may result in an increase in insulin resistance.

Clinical features

Symptoms and signs of this disease are often subtle and neither sensitive nor specific. Classic signs and symptoms, such as cold intolerance, puffiness, decreased sweating, and coarse skin, previously reported in 90–97% of patients, may actually occur in only 50–64% of younger patients. Many of the more common symptoms are nonspecific and difficult to attribute to a specific cause. Individuals can also present with obstructive sleep apnea (secondary to macroglossia) or carpal tunnel syndrome, muscle cramps and frequent muscle aches. Women can present with galactorrhea and menstrual disturbances. Consequently, the diagnosis of hypothyroidism is based on clinical suspicion and confirmed by laboratory testing. Physical signs of hypothyroidism include hypothermia, weight gain, slowed speech and movements, dry skin, jaundice, pallor, coarse, brittle, strawlike hair, loss of scalp, axillary and pubic hair, dull and coarse facial features, periorbital puffiness, macroglossia, goiter, hoarseness, decreased systolic blood pressure and increased diastolic blood pressure, bradycardia, pericardial effusion, abdominal distension, ascites (uncommon), nonpitting edema (myxedema), hyporeflexia with delayed relaxation, ataxia, or both (Fig. 39.1A & B). Metabolic abnormalities associated with hypothyroidism include anemia, dilutional hyponatremia, hyperlipidemia, and reversible increase in creatinine.

A scoring system based on 12 symptoms and signs with score ≥6 has a positive predictive value of 96.9% for diagnosing hypothyroidism and a score of ≤3 has a negative predictive value to rule out hypothyroidism (Table 39.1).

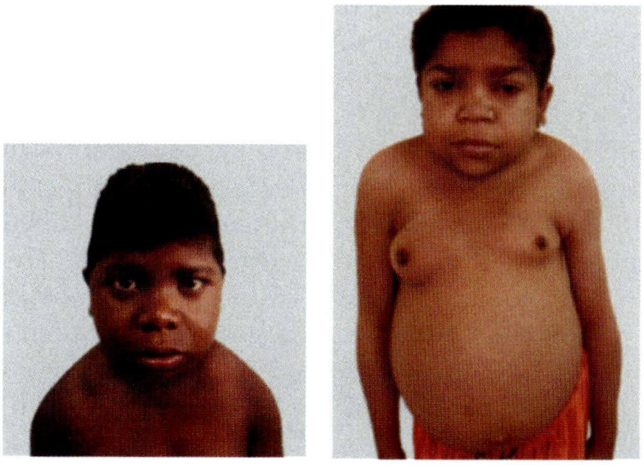

Fig. 39.1A. Typical facial features of a hypothyroid patient. **B.** Hypothyroid girl with short stature and thelarche.

Table 39.1. Scoring system for evaluation of a patient suspected to have hypothyroidism

Symptoms	*Score if present*
Hearing impairment	1
Diminished sweating	1
Constipation	1
Paraesthesia	1
Hoarseness of voice	1
Weight increase	1
Dry skin	1
Physical signs	1
Slow movements	1
Periorbital puffiness	1
Delayed ankle reflex	1
Coarse skin	1
Cold skin	1
Sum of all symptoms and signs	12

1. Add 1 point for women younger than 55 years
2. Hypothyroid ≥6 points, Intermediate 3–5 points, Euthyroid ≤2 points

Investigations

Third-generation TSH assays are readily available and are generally the most sensitive screening tool for primary hypothyroidism. The generally accepted reference range for normal serum TSH is 0.17–4.05 mIU/L. Patients with primary hypothyroidism have elevated TSH levels and decreased T4 and T3 levels. As the TSH level increases early in the disease, an increased conversion of T4 to T3 occur, this maintains T3 levels within normal limits in early hypothyroidism. Patients with elevated TSH levels but normal free hormone levels are considered to have subclinical hypothyroidism. Evaluation of the presence of thyroid autoantibodies (antimicrosomal or anti-TPO antibodies) is helpful in determining the etiology of hypothyroidism and in predicting future hypothyroidism. In addition, anti-TPO antibodies have been associated with a higher risk of infertility and miscarriage.

In patients with nonthyroid disease who are severely ill, TSH secretion is normal or decreased, total T4 levels are decreased, and total T3 levels are markedly decreased. This can be confused with secondary hypothyroidism. In these patients, the primary abnormality is the decreased peripheral production of T3 from T4. They have an increased reverse T3, which can be measured. Other abnormalities seen in patients who are critically ill include decreased TBG levels and abnormalities in the hypothalamic-pituitary axis. During recovery, some patients have transient elevations in serum

39

TSH concentrations (up to 20 mIU/L). Hence, thyroid function should not be evaluated in a critically ill person unless thyroid dysfunction is strongly suspected, and, if so, screening with TSH alone is insufficient.

In patients with hypothalamic or pituitary dysfunction, TSH levels do not increase in appropriate relation to the low free T4 levels. The absolute levels may be in the normal or even slightly elevated range but inappropriately low for the severity of the hypothyroid state. Hence, when secondary or tertiary hypothyroidism is suspected, T4 should be measured and should be used for future monitoring of such patients.

Imaging studies has little use in hypothyroidism per se unless a secondary anatomic lesion in the gland is of clinical concern. Radioactive iodine uptake (RAIU) and thyroid scanning are not useful in hypothyroidism because these tests require some level of endogenous function in the hypofunctioning gland to provide information. Patients with Hashimoto thyroiditis may have relatively high early uptake (after 4 h) but do not have the usual doubling of uptake at 24 hours consistent with an organification defect.

Treatment

The treatment goals for hypothyroidism are the reversal of clinical progression and the corrections of metabolic derangements as evidenced by normal blood levels of TSH and T4. No specific diets are required for hypothyroidism. There is no role of iodine supplementation as treatment of hypothyroidism. Infact in post iodination era there is increase in subclinical hypothyroidism with greater iodine intake. The World Health Organization recommends a daily dietary iodine intake of 150 mcg for adults, 200 mcg for pregnant and lactating women, and 50–120 mcg for children. Thyroid hormone is administered to supplement or replace decreased endogenous production. In general, hypothyroidism is adequately treated with a daily dose of levothyroxine (LT4). Clinical benefits begin in 3–5 days and level off after 4–6 weeks. Anticipated full replacement doses may be initiated in individuals who are otherwise young and healthy. In elderly patients or those with known ischemic heart disease, treatment should begin with one fourth to one half the expected dose, and the dose should be adjusted in small increments no sooner than 4–6 weeks. Achieving a TSH level within the reference range may be slowed because of delay of hypothalamic-pituitary axis readaptation and may take several months. Patients should take thyroid hormone fasting as a single dose in the morning. Thyroid hormone is better absorbed in fasting state from the small bowel; therefore, absorption can be affected by malabsorptive states, small bowel disease. Many drugs (e.g., iron, calcium carbonate, aluminum hydroxide, sucralfate) can interfere with absorption. After dose stabilization, patients can be monitored with annual clinical evaluations and TSH monitoring. Patients should be monitored for symptoms and signs of overtreatment, which include tachycardia, palpitations, nervousness, tiredness, headache, increased excitability, sleeplessness, tremors, and possible angina.

Pregnancy and hypothyroidism

Hypothyroidism in pregnancy is associated with preeclampsia, anemia, postpartum hemorrhage, cardiac ventricular dysfunction, spontaneous abortion, low birth weight, impaired cognitive development, and fetal mortality. Even mild disease may be associated with adverse effects for offspring. Thyroid hormone replacement dosage should be increased during pregnancy, especially in the first and second trimesters. Studies have suggested that patients with hypothyroidism should augment the LT4 dose by 30% at the confirmation of pregnancy, followed by adjustments according to TSH levels. For previously diagnosed women, serum TSH should be measured every 3–4 weeks during the first half of pregnancy and every 6 weeks thereafter. LT4 dose should be adjusted to maintain a serum TSH less than 2.5 mIU/L. TSH and free T4 levels should be measured every 3–4 weeks after every dosage adjustment. Autoimmune thyroid disease without overt hypothyroidism has been associated with a higher miscarriage rate. Negro et al showed that euthyroid Caucasian women with positive anti-TPO antibodies treated with levothyroxine during the first trimester had lower miscarriage rates when compared with those who were not treated. They also had lower incidence of premature delivery, comparable to women without thyroid antibodies. This will need to be confirmed by other studies, and, if confirmed, there will be an indication to treat euthyroid pregnant women who have thyroid antibodies. LT4 should not be taken with vitamin preparations containing iron and calcium. After delivery, the LT4 dose can be reduced to the prepregnancy level and TSH should be checked in 6 weeks.

Postpartum thyroiditis

Up to 10% of postpartum women may develop lymphocytic thyroiditis in the 2–10 months after delivery. The frequency may be as high as 25% in women with type 1 diabetes mellitus. The condition is usually transient (2–4 mo) and can require a short course of treatment with levothyroxine (LT4), but postpartum patients with lymphocytic thyroiditis are at increased risk of permanent hypothyroidism. The hypothyroid state can be preceded by a short thyrotoxic state. High titers of anti-TPO antibodies during pregnancy have been reported to be 97% sensitive and 91% specific for postpartum autoimmune thyroid disease.

Subclinical hypothyroidism

Significant controversy persists regarding the treatment of patients with mild hypothyroidism. Some have argued that treatment of these patients improves symptoms, prevents progression to overt hypothyroidism, and may have cardioprotective benefits. The American Association of Clinical Endocrinologists (AACE) guidelines state that treatment is indicated in patients with TSH levels above 10 mIU/mL or in patients with TSH levels between 5 and 10 mIU/mL in conjunction with goiter and/or positive antithyroid peroxidase antibodies, as these patients have the highest rates of progression to overt hypothyroidism. An initial dose of 25–50 mcg/d of LT4 can be used and can be titrated every 6–8 weeks, to achieve a target TSH of between 0.3 and 3 mIU/mL.

Myxedema coma

Myxedema coma is a severe form of hypothyroidism that results in an altered mental status, hypothermia, bradycardia, hypercarbia, and hyponatremia. Cardiomegaly, pericardial effusion, cardiogenic shock, and ascites may be present. Myxedema coma most commonly occurs in individuals with undiagnosed or untreated hypothyroidisms who are subjected to an external stress, such as low temperature, infection, or medical emergencies like myocardial infarction, CVA, surgical stress or hypnotic drugs. An effective approach is to use intravenous LT4 at a dose of 4 mcg/kg of lean body weight, or approximately 200–250 mcg as a bolus followed by 100 mcg 24 hours later and then 50 mcg daily IV or PO along with stress doses of intravenous glucocorticoids. Adjustment of the dose can then be made based on clinical and laboratory parameters along with stress doses of intravenous glucocorticoids. Use of intravenous triiodothyronine is controversial as it has a higher frequency of adverse cardiac events and is generally reserved for patients who are not improving clinically on LT4. LT3 can be given initially as a 10 mcg IV bolus and repeated every 8–12 hours until the patient can take maintenance oral doses of T4. Advanced age, high dose T4 therapy, and cardiac complications had the highest associations with mortality.

HYPERTHYROIDISM

Background

Thyrotoxicosis is the hypermetabolic condition associated with elevated levels of thyroid hormones. Thyrotoxicosis needs to be differentiated from hyperthyroidism which is a subset of thyrotoxicosis characterized by excess synthesis and secretion of thyroid hormone by the thyroid itself. The most common forms of hyperthyroidism include diffuse toxic goiter (Graves' disease), toxic multinodular goiter (Plummer's disease), and toxic adenoma. Together with subacute thyroiditis, these conditions constitute 85–90% of all causes of thyrotoxicosis. Hyperthyroidism occurs more frequently in women than in men. Graves' disease occurs in a male-to-female ratio of 1 : 5–10. The male-to-female ratio for toxic multinodular goiter and toxic adenomas is 1 : 2–4. Table 39.2 summarizes the causes of thyrotoxicosis and hyperthyroidism.

Graves' disease

The most common cause of thyrotoxicosis is Graves' disease (50–60%). Graves' disease is an organ-specific autoimmune disorder characterized by a variety of circulating antibodies, including anti-thyroid peroxidase (anti-TPO), antithyroglobulin (anti-TG) antibodies and thyroid-stimulating immunoglobulin (TSI). TSI is directed toward epitopes of the thyroid-stimulating hormone (TSH) receptor and acts as a TSH-receptor agonist. Similar to TSH, TSI binds to the TSH receptor on the thyroid follicular cells to activate thyroid hormone synthesis and release and thyroid growth (hypertrophy). This results in the characteristic picture of Graves' thyro-

Table 39.2. Various causes of thyrotoxicosis and hyperthyroidism

	Radioactive iodine uptake over neck
Common forms (85–90% of cases)	
Diffuse toxic goitre (Graves' disease)	Increased
Toxic multinodular goiter (Plummer's disease)	Increased
Toxic adenoma	Increased
Thyrotoxic phase of subacute thyroiditis	Decreased
Less common forms	
Iodide-induced thyrotoxicosis	Variable
Thyrotoxicosis factitia	Decreased
Uncommon forms	
Pituitary tumours producing thyroid-stimulating hormone	Increased
Excess human chorionic gonadotropin (molar pregnancy/choriocarcinoma)	Increased
Pituitary resistance to thyroid hormone	Increased
Metastatic thyroid carcinoma	Decreased
Struma ovarii with thyrotoxicosis	Decreased

toxicosis, with a diffusely enlarged thyroid, very high radioactive iodine uptake, and excessive thyroid hormone levels compared with a healthy thyroid. Clinical findings specific to Graves' disease include thyroid ophthalmopathy and, rarely, dermopathy over the lower extremities (Fig. 39.2). Graves' disease is usually associated with other autoimmune diseases, such as pernicious anemia, myasthenia gravis, vitiligo, adrenal insufficiency, and type 1 diabetes mellitus.

Toxic multinodular goitre

Toxic multinodular goiter also known as Plummer's disease occurs in 15–20% of patients with thyrotoxicosis. It occurs more commonly in elderly individuals, especially in patients with a long-standing goiter. Thyroid hormone excess develops very slowly over time and often is only mildly elevated at the time of diagnosis. Symptoms of thyrotoxicosis are mild, often because only a slight elevation of thyroid hormone levels is present, and the signs and symptoms of thyrotoxicosis often are blunted (apathetic hyperthyroidism) in older patients. A typical nuclear scintigraphy scan of a toxic multinodular goiter demonstrates an enlarged thyroid gland with areas of increased and decreased activity. Sometimes very high thyroid hormone levels may occur in this condition after high iodine intake, ie, with contrast or amiodarone exposure

Toxic adenoma

Toxic adenoma is caused by a single hyperfunctioning follicular thyroid adenoma. Patients with a toxic thyroid adenoma comprise approximately 3–5% of patients who are thyrotoxic. The excess secretion of thyroid hormone occurs from a benign monoclonal tumour that usually is larger than 2.5 cm in diameter. The excess thyroid hormone suppresses TSH levels. Radioactive iodine uptake usually is normal, and the radioactive iodine scan shows only the hot nodule, with the remainder of the normal thyroid gland suppressed because the TSH level is low.

Other causes of thyrotoxicosis

Several rare causes of thyrotoxicosis exist that are described below:

Subacute thyroiditis: Seen in approximately 15–20% of patients, is a destructive release of preformed thyroid hormone. A typical nuclear scintigraphy scan shows no radioactive iodine uptake in the thyrotoxic phase of the disease.

Iodide-induced thyrotoxicosis: Also known as Jod-Basedow syndrome occurs in patients with

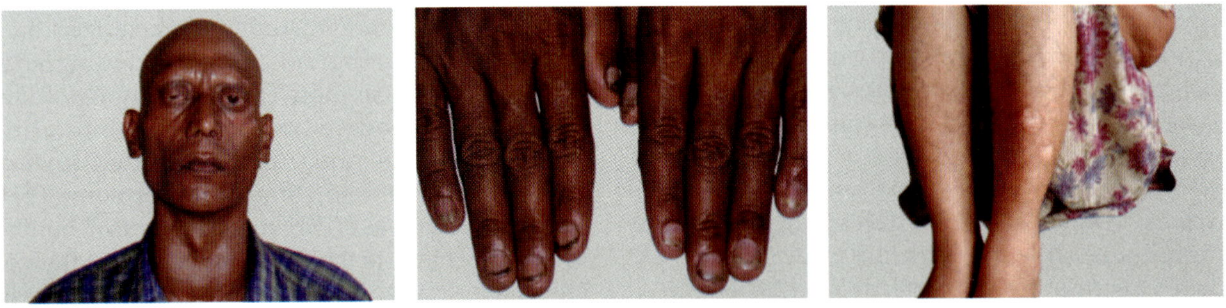

Fig. 39.2A. Typical facial features of a hyperthyroid patient. **B.** Onycholysis in Graves disease patient. **C.** Infiltrative dermopathy in Graves disease patient.

excessive iodine intake, such as after an iodinated radio-contrast study. It occurs in patients with areas of thyroid autonomy, such as a multinodular goiter or autonomous nodule. The thyrotoxicosis appears to be a result of loss of the normal adaptation of the thyroid to iodide excess. It is treated by cessation of the excess iodine intake and administration of antithyroid medication. Usually, after depletion of the excess iodine, thyroid functions return to preexposure levels.

Struma ovarii: It is ectopic thyroid tissue associated with dermoid tumours or ovarian teratomas that can secrete excessive amounts of thyroid hormone and produce thyrotoxicosis.

Metastatic follicular thyroid carcinoma: It maintains the ability to make thyroid hormone and can cause thyrotoxicosis in patients with bulky tumours.

Molar hydatidiform or choriocarcinoma: It is characterized by extremely high levels of beta human chorionic gonadotropin (βHCG) that can weakly activate the TSH receptor. At very high levels of βHCG, activation of the TSH receptor occurs that is sufficient to cause thyrotoxicosis. Physiologic maximum elevation of βHCG at the end of the first trimester of pregnancy is associated with a mirror-image temporary reduction in TSH. Despite the reduction in TSH, the FT_4 levels usually remain normal or only slightly above the reference range. As the pregnancy progresses and the βHCG plateaus at a lower level, TSH level reverts back to normal levels.

Clinical features

The presentation of thyrotoxicosis is variable among patients. Younger patients tend to exhibit symptoms of more sympathetic activation, such as anxiety, hyperactivity, and tremor, while older patients have more cardiovascular symptoms, including dyspnea and atrial fibrillation with unexplained weight loss. Common symptoms of thyrotoxicosis include nervousness, anxiety, increased perspiration, heat intolerance, tremor, hyperactivity, palpitations, weight loss despite increased appetite, reduction in menstrual flow or oligomenorrhea. Common signs of thyrotoxicosis include hyperactivity, tachycardia or atrial arrhythmia, systolic hypertension, warm, moist, and smooth skin, lid lag, stare, tremor, hyperkinesis, large-muscle weakness, and soft, smooth skin.

Physical examination often can help the clinician determine the etiology of thyrotoxicosis. Thyrotoxicosis due to Graves' disease is associated with a diffusely enlarged and slightly firm thyroid gland. Sometimes, a thyroid bruit is audible using the bell of the stethoscope. Toxic multinodular goiters occur when goiters generally are enlarged to at least 2 to 3 times normal size. The gland often is soft, but individual nodules occasionally can be palpated. A toxic adenoma generally does not cause thyrotoxicosis in a patient until it is at least 2.5 cm in diameter. If the thyroid is enlarged and painful, the diagnosis is likely to be subacute painful or granulomatous thyroiditis, but consider degeneration or hemorrhage into a nodule or suppurative thyroiditis.

Graves' thyrotoxicosis can be associated with mild thyroid ophthalmopathy in 50% of patients (Fig. 39.3). Evidence of thyroid eye disease and high thyroid hormone levels confirms the diagnosis of autoimmune Graves' disease. Graves' disease rarely can affect the skin by deposition of glycosaminoglycans in the dermis of the lower leg. This causes nonpitting edema, usually associated with erythema and thickening of the skin, without pain or pruritus.

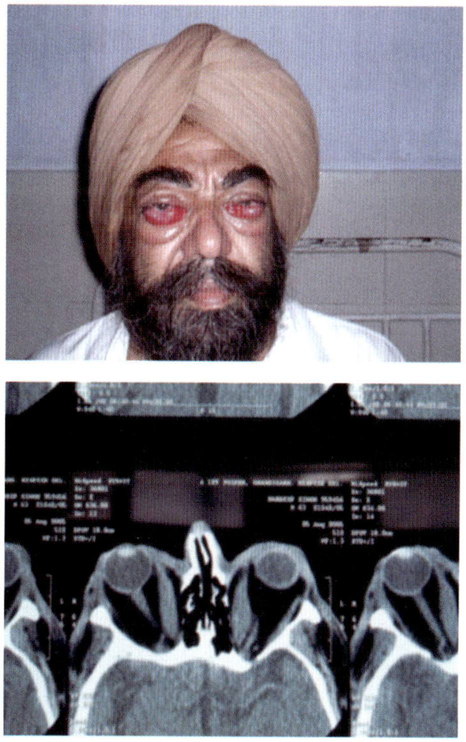

Fig. 39.3A. Active Graves' ophthalmopathy. **B.** CT scan orbit showing extraocular muscle thickening in a patient with active Graves' ophthalmopathy.

39

Investigations

The most reliable screening measure of thyroid function is a TSH level. TSH levels usually are suppressed to immeasurable levels (< 0.05 μIU/mL) in thyrotoxicosis. Of patients with thyrotoxicosis, 5% have only elevated T_3 levels. Therefore, measuring T_4 and T_3 if T_4 levels are normal is recommended in patients with suspected thyrotoxicosis when TSH is low. The most specific autoantibody for autoimmune thyroiditis is ELISA for anti-TPO antibody. The titers usually are significantly elevated in the most common type of hyperthyroidism, Graves' thyrotoxicosis, and usually are low or absent in toxic multinodular goiter and toxic adenoma. TSI, if elevated, helps establish the diagnosis of Graves' disease.

Imaging studies

If the etiology of thyrotoxicosis is not clear after physical examination and other laboratory tests, it can be confirmed by an ^{123}I or technetium-99m (^{99m}Tc) thyroid scanning, which provides anatomic information on the type of goiter (e.g., diffuse vs nodular). Values are elevated in patients with Graves' disease and toxic multinodular goiters. Graves' disease is associated with diffuse enlargement of both thyroid lobes, with an elevated uptake. A toxic multinodular goiter demonstrates an enlarged thyroid with multiple nodules and areas of increased and decreased isotope uptake. A toxic adenoma demonstrates a solitary hot nodule with suppression of function in the surrounding normal thyroid tissue (Fig. 39.4). Subacute thyroiditis usually demonstrates very low ^{123}I isotope uptake.

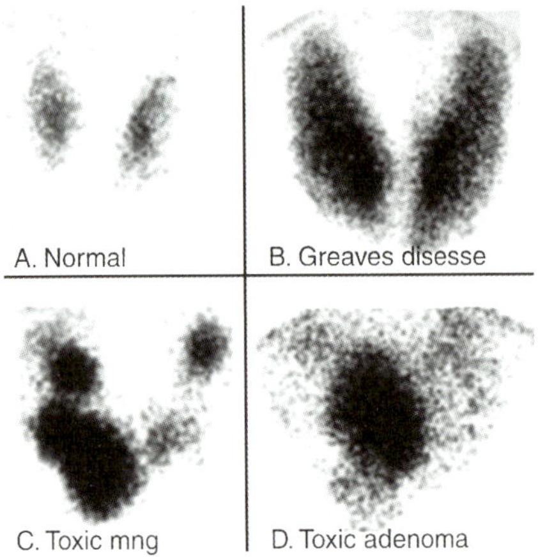

Fig. 39.4. Iodine^{123} nuclear scintigraphy: ^{123}I scans of a normal thyroid gland (A); Graves' disease (B); toxic multinodular goitre (C); and toxic adenoma (D).

39

If a dominant nodule is found upon examination of a patient with thyrotoxicosis, obtain an ^{123}I thyroid scan to assure that the dominant nodule is functioning. If the nodule is cold, perform a biopsy on the nodule by fine-needle aspiration to exclude concomitant malignancy.

Treatment

With the exception of low ^{123}I uptake hyperthyroidism e.g., subacute thyroiditis treatment options for hyperthyroidism includes antithyroid medications, radioactive iodine ^{131}I, or thyroidectomy. No special diet is recommended for patients with hyperthyroidism. However it is important to note that excess amounts of iodide found in some expectorants, radiographic contrast dyes, seaweed tablets, and health food supplements should be avoided, because the iodide interferes with and complicates the management with antithyroid and radioactive iodine therapies. Routine administration of beta-blocker to the patients should be avoided except in those with marked sympathetic overactivity. Calcium-channel blockers can be used for the same purposes when beta blockers are contraindicated or poorly tolerated.

Antithyroid drugs

Antithyroid drugs e.g., methimazole, propylthiouracil have been used for hyperthyroidism since their introduction in the 1940s. These drugs inhibit multiple steps in the synthesis of T_4 and T_3, leading to a gradual reduction in thyroid hormone levels over 2–8 weeks or longer. Antithyroid drug dosage should be titrated every 4 weeks until thyroid functions normalize. Perform follow-up tests of thyroid function at least every 3 months for the first year. Some patients with Graves' disease go into a remission after treatment for 12–18 months, and the drug can be discontinued. But half of the patients who go into remission have a recurrence of hyperthyroidism within the following year. Nodular forms of hyperthyroidism (toxic multinodular goiter and toxic adenoma) are permanent conditions and will not go into remission. The antithyroid medications are used for the long-term control of hyperthyroidism in children, adolescents, and pregnant women (propylthiouracil only for pregnancy). The choice between propylthiouracil and methimazole is somewhat arbitrary. Methimazole is a more potent and longer-acting drug. Often, patient compliance is better with methimazole taken once or twice daily than with propylthiouracil given 3 or 4 times daily. Propylthiouracil often is the drug of choice in severe thyrotoxicosis because of the additional benefit of inhibition of T_4 to T_3 conversion. The reduction in T_3, which is 20–100 times more potent than T_4, theoretically helps to reduce the thyrotoxic symptoms more quickly than does methimazole. The most common adverse effects of antithyroid medications are allergic reactions of fever, rash, urticaria, and arthralgia, which occur in 1–5% of patients, usually within the first few weeks of treatment. Serious adverse effects include agranulocytosis, aplastic anemia, hepatitis, polyarthritis, and a lupus like vasculitis. All of these adverse effects, except agranulocytosis, occur more frequently with propylthiouracil. Agranulocytosis occurs in 0. 2–0.5% of patients, with an equal frequency for both drugs. Patients with agranulocytosis usually present with fever and pharyngitis. After the drug is stopped, granulocyte counts usually start to rise within several days but may not normalize for 10–14 days. Granulocyte colony-stimulating factor (G-CSF) appears to accelerate recovery in patients with a bone marrow aspiration showing a granulocyte-to-erythrocyte (G : E) ratio of 1 : 2 or greater than 0.5. The US Food and Drug Administration (FDA) added a boxed warning, the strongest warning issued by the FDA, to the prescribing information for propylthiouracil. The FDA recommends the following criteria be considered for prescribing propylthiouracil:

- Reserve propylthiouracil use during first trimester of pregnancy or in patients who are allergic to or intolerant of methimazole
- Closely monitor propylthiouracil therapy for signs and symptoms of liver injury, especially during the first 6 months after initiation of therapy
- For suspected liver injury, promptly discontinue propylthiouracil therapy, evaluate the patient for evidence of liver injury, and provide supportive care
- Propylthiouracil should not be used in pediatric patients unless the patient is allergic to or intolerant of methimazole and no other treatment options are available
- Counsel patients to promptly contact their health care provider for the following signs or symptoms: fatigue, weakness, vague abdominal pain, loss of appetite, itching, easy bruising, or yellowing of the eyes or skin.

Radioactive iodine therapy

It is the most common treatment for hyperthyroidism in adults in the United States. Although the effect is less rapid than it is in antithyroid medication or thyroidectomy, it is effective and safe and does not require hospitalization. It is administered orally as a single dose, in capsule or liquid form. The radioactive iodine is quickly absorbed and taken up by the thyroid. No other tissue or organ in the body is capable of retaining the radioactive iodine and, therefore, very few adverse effects are associated with this therapy. The treatment results in a thyroid-specific inflammatory response, causing fibrosis and destruction of the thyroid over weeks to many months. Generally, the dose of ^{131}I administered is 75–200 µCi/g of estimated thyroid tissue divided by the percent of ^{123}I uptake in 24 hours. This dose is intended to render the patient hypothyroid as hypothyroidism is considered by many experts to be the expected goal of radioactive iodine therapy. In several large epidemiologic studies of radioactive iodine therapy in patients with Graves' disease, no evidence indicated that radioactive iodine therapy caused the development of thyroid carcinoma. No evidence of increased mortality exists for any other form of cancer, including leukemia, with radioactive iodine therapy of hyperthyroidism. Long-term follow-up data of children and adolescents treated with radioactive iodine are lacking. Consequently, long-term antithyroid medications, rather than radioiodine therapy, usually are recommended in children less than 10 years of age. Radioactive iodine is never administered to pregnant or lactating women; as it can cross the placenta and can be excreted into milk, which can ablate the infant's thyroid and result in hypothyroidism. Checking for pregnancy prior to radioactive iodine therapy and suggesting that the patient not become pregnant for at least 3–6 months after the treatment and until thyroid functions are normal are standard practice. Retrospective reviews have demonstrated no excess in fetal malformations or miscarriage rates in women previously treated with radioactive iodine for hyperthyroidism. Radioactive iodine usually is not administered to patients with severe ophthalmopathy, because clinical evidence suggests that usually mild, but occasionally severe, worsening of thyroid eye disease occurs after radioactive iodine therapy. The risk of ophthalmopathy is worse in patients who smoke cigarettes, but apparently it can be reduced by glucocorticoid therapy (prednisone 0.5 mg/kg for 1 mo with subsequent taper) after the radioactive iodine therapy.

Surgery

Because of excellent effectiveness in regulating thyroid function with antithyroid medications and radioactive iodine, thyroidectomy is reserved for special circumstances, including the following:

- Severe hyperthyroidism in children.
- Pregnant women who are noncompliant or intolerant of antithyroid medication.
- Patients with very large goiters or severe ophthalmopathy.
- Patients who refuse radioactive iodine therapy.
- Refractory amiodarone-induced hyperthyroidism.
- Patients who require normalization of thyroid functions quickly, such as pregnant women, women who desire pregnancy in the next 6 months.

With current operative techniques, bilateral subtotal thyroidectomy should have a mortality rate approaching zero in patients who are properly prepared. Preoperative preparation includes antithyroid medication, stable (cold) iodine treatment (to decrease gland vascularity), and beta-blocker therapy. Generally, antithyroid drug therapy should be administered until thyroid functions normalize (4–8 wk). Propranolol should be titrated until the resting pulse rate is less than 80 bpm. Finally, administer iodide as SSKI (1–2 drops bid for 7–10 d) before surgery. An additional benefit from stable iodide therapy, besides the reduction in thyroid hormone excretion, is a demonstrated decrease in thyroid blood flow and possible reduction in blood loss during surgery. Adverse effects of surgery include recurrent laryngeal nerve damage and hypoparathyroidism due to damage of parathyroid glands during surgery.

Special problems

Subclinical hyperthyroidism

Subclinical hyperthyroidism is defined as a suppressed TSH level (< 0.17 μU/mL in many laboratories) in combination with normal serum concentrations of T_3 and T_4. It is associated with no clinical symptoms of thyrotoxicosis. However, certain conditions, such as atrial fibrillation, osteoporosis, or hypercalcemia, may suggest the possibility of thyrotoxicosis. In fact, subclinical hyperthyroidism may be associated with a 3-fold increase in the risk of atrial fibrillation. The prevalence of subclinical hyperthyroidism may be as high as 12% in the general population.

Graves' ophthalmopathy

The eye disease usually occurs within 1 year before or after the diagnosis of hyperthyroidism, but sometimes precede or follow thyrotoxicosis by several years accounting for some cases of euthyroid opthalmopathy. Cigarette smoking is a significant risk factor, increasing the odds of ophthalmopathy approximately 7-fold. It is manifested by periorbital edema, conjunctival edema (chemosis), injection, poor lid closure, extraocular muscle dysfunction (diplopia), and proptosis (Fig. 39.3). It is more common in women than in men. Although 50% of patients with Graves' disease have clinical evidence of thyroid eye disease, only 5% develop severe ophthalmopathy. The unilateral signs are found in up to 10% of patients. The earliest manifestations of opthalmopathy are sensation of grittiness, eye discomfort and excess tearing. About one third have proptosis, best detected by visualisation of the sclera between the lower border of iris and the lower eyelid, with eye in primary position. The other clinical signs include Von Graefe's sign (lid lag on infraduction), Kocher's sign (eye globe lag on supraduction), Dalrymple's sign (a widened palpebral fissure during fixation) and lagophthalmos (incapacity of closing the eyelids completely). Many scoring systems have been used to gauge the extent and activity of the orbital changes in Graves' disease. The NO SPECS is an acronym derived from the following classes of eye changes:

Class 0	No signs or symptoms
Class 1	Only signs (limited to upper lid retraction and stare, with or without lid lag)
Class 2	Soft tissue involvement (oedema of conjunctivae and lids, conjunctival injection, etc.)
Class 3	Proptosis
Class 4	Extraocular muscle involvement (usually with diplopia)
Class 5	Corneal involvement (primarily due to lagophthalmos)
Class 6	Sight loss (due to optic nerve involvement)

When eye disease is active referral to ophthalmologist for objective measurement such as lid fissure width, corneal staining with fluorescein, extraocular muscle function evaluation (Hess chart), intraocular pressure, visual fields, acuity and color vision and referral to endocrinologist for treatment of active eye disease is indicated. The clinical course of ophthalmopathy does not follow that of thyroid disease. Ophthalmopathy typically worsens over the initial 3–6 months, followed by a plateau over next 12–18 months, with spontaneous improvement, particularly in the soft tissue changes. However, the course is fulminant in 5% of patients and immediate intervention in form of immunosuppressive therapy is required.

Dermopathy

This is an infiltrative dermopathy, usually over the lower extremity that is characterized by an accumulation of glycosaminoglycans and inflammatory cells in the dermis. The skin changes usually include a nonpitting erythematous edema of the anterior shins. Dermopathy can occur at other sites of repeat trauma. The dermopathy usually only occurs in the presence of significant ophthalmopathy. No effective treatment exists. Nightly occlusive wraps of the affected site are recommended with plastic wrap after application of a high-potency topical steroid cream.

SUGGESTED READING

1. Baskin HJ, Cobin RH, Duick DS, et al. American Association of Clinical Endocrinologists medical guidelines for clinical practice for the evaluation and treatment of hyperthyroidism and hypothyroidism. *Endocr Pract*, 2002; 8(6): 457–469.
2. Brent P GA, Larsen PR, Davies TF. Hypothyroidism & Thyroiditis. *In:* Kronenberg HM, Melmed S, Polonsky KS, Larsen PR, eds. Williams Textbook of Endocrinology. 11th ed. Philadelphia, Pa: Saunders Elsevier; 2008: Chap 12.
3. Davies TF, Larsen PR. Thyrotoxicosis. In: Kronenberg HM, Melmed S, Polonsky KS, Larsen PR, eds. Williams Textbook of Endocrinology. 11th ed. Philadelphia, Pa: Saunders Elsevier; 2008: Chap 11.

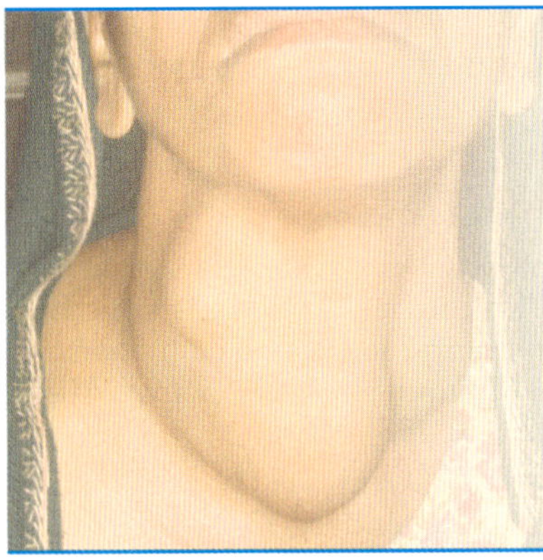

CHAPTER 40

Carcinoma Thyroid

Ishwar Singh

The normal thyroid gland is responsive to both the internal and external environment. It weighs about 20 gm and has smooth and homogenous structure. The Himalayan region and sub-Himalayan plains show a marked prevalence of goitre on an average of 29% with areas as high as 60% (Figs. 40.1, 40.2). Thyroid cancer includes a spectrum of disease with relatively very indolent variety of differentiated cancers to highly aggressive anaplastic neoplasms. Epidemiologic studies have reported palpable thyroid nodules to be 5% in females while 1% in males residing in iodine-sufficient parts of the world. Thyroid cancer occurs in 5–10% of thyroid nodules with high risk factors – age, male gender, radiation exposure history, but only in 0.1% of nodules in general population. Thyroid nodule is the most common presentation of thyroid cancer. A complete history and physical examination focusing on thyroid gland and adjoining lymph nodes should be performed. Any history of head neck irradiation, family history of carcinoma in a first-degree relative and rapid growth and hoarseness are some features of thyroid carcinoma. Clinical examination may reveal vocal cord paralysis, ipsilateral lymphadenopathy and fixation of the nodules to surrounding tissue.

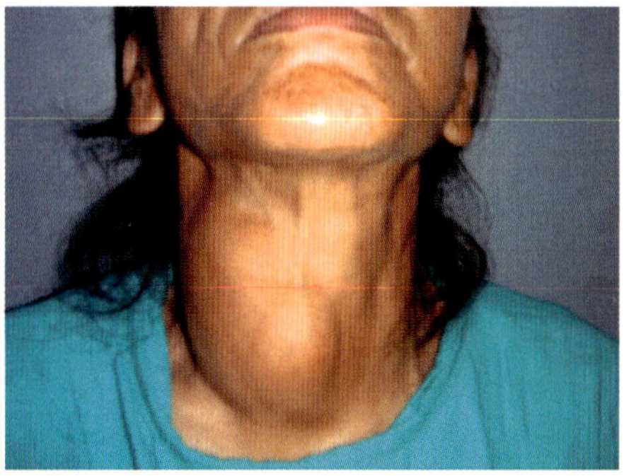

Fig. 40.1. Thyroid enlargement.

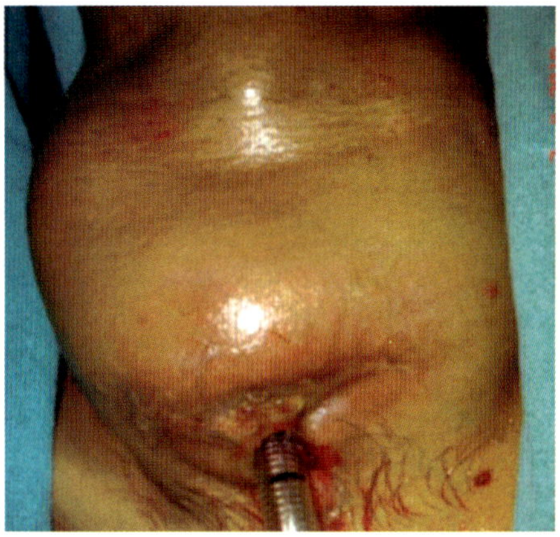

Fig. 40.2. Preoperative trachestomy in a case of thyroid carcinoma.

Investigations

Clinical assessment

- Thyroid function test
- Serum anti-thyroid antibodies
- Serum thyroglobulin antibodies
- Scintiscannings

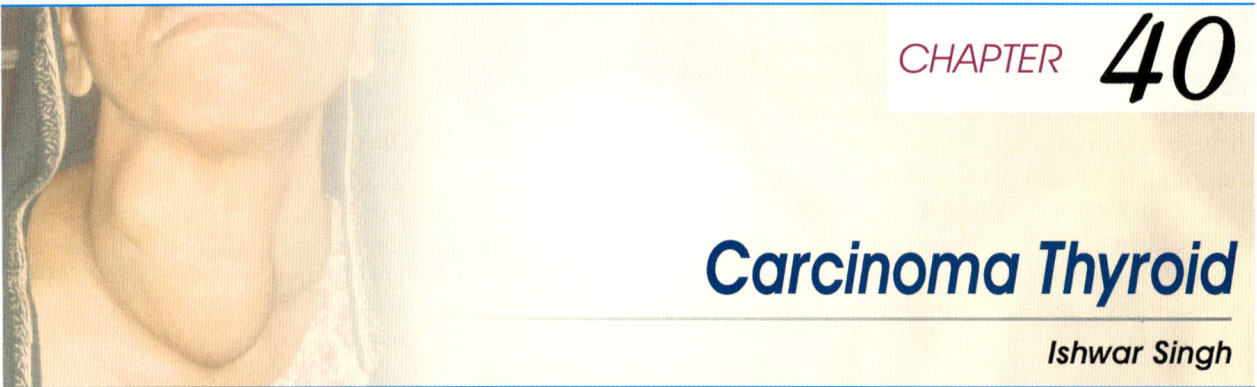

Ultrasonography

Ultrasound can classify nodules as solid and cystic in 90% cases. A solid nodule is most often benign but one out of three is most likely to be malignant. On the other hand cystic nodules are not always benign since carcinoma of more than 3 cm can undergo cystic changes.

Ultrasound features suggestive of malignancy are as follows:

1. Absent "Halo" sign.
2. Solid or hypoechogenicity.
3. Heterogeneous echo structure.
4. Irregular margin.
5. Fine calcification.
6. Extraglandular extension.

FNAC

FNAC has emerged as a very valuable tool in the diagnosis and management of thyroid lesions as it is safe, inexpensive, quick and has a good diagnostic accuracy in experienced hands. There may be some complications following this simple procedure.

Complications of FNAC

1. Pain
2. Hematoma
3. Entry into trachea
4. Transient thyroid swelling
5. Cystic degeneration
6. Transient bradycardia
7. Transient vocal cord paralysis
8. Formation of calcification
9. Necrosis of nodule
10. Capsular pseudoinvasion
11. Fibrosis
12. Transient thyrotoxicosis
13. Elevation of thyroglobulin

WHO CLASSIFICATION-2004

Thyroid carcinoma

1. Pappilary carcinoma
2. Follicular carcinoma
3. Poorly differentiated carcinoma
4. Undifferentiated (anaplastic) carcinoma
5. Squamous cell carcinoma
6. Mucoepidermoid carcinoma
7. Sclerosing mucoepidermoid carcinoma with eosinophilia
8. Mucinous carcinoma
9. Medullary thyroid carcinoma
10. Spindle cell tumour with thymus-like differentiation (SETTLE)
11. Carcinoma showing thymus-like differentiation (CASTLE)
12. Hurthle cell tumour.

Thyroid adenomas

1. Follicular adenoma
2. Hyalinizing trabecular tumours

Other thyroid tumours

1. Teratoma
2. Primary lymphaoma
3. Ectopic thymoma
4. Angiosarcoma
5. Smooth muscle tumours
6. Peripheral nerve sheath tumours
7. Paraganglioma
8. Solitary fibrous tumours
9. Follicular dendritic cell tumours
10. Langerhans cell histocytosis

PROGNOSTIC CLASSIFICATION OF MALIGNANT THYROID TUMOURS

1. Low grade malignancy

(a) Papillary carcinoma
(b) Minimally invasive follicular carcinoma
(c) Mucoepidermoid carcinoma with eosinophilia
(d) Sclerosing mucoepidermoid carcinoma with eosinophilia
(e) Tumours with thymic or related branchial pouch differentiation

2. Intermediate grade malignancy

(a) Tall cell and columnar variant of papillary carcinoma
(b) Widely invasive follicular carcinoma
(c) Medullary carcinoma
(d) Poorly differentiated including insular carcinoma
(e) Mixed medullary-follicular carcinoma
(f) Malignant lymphoma

3. High grade malignancy

(a) Undifferentiated (anaplastic) carcinoma
(b) Squamous cell carcinoma
(c) Angiosarcoma
(d) Other sarcoma

Thyroid nodule is the most common presentation of thyroid malignancy. A detailed history and examination, that of gland as well as of cervical lymph nodes is done. Find out if patient had any exposure to radiation in the past or any other member of the family is having similar complaints or history of thyroid carcinoma. If there is hoarseness of voice or difficulty in swallowing or respiratory distress, these are indicators that the thyroid swelling may be carcinoma. If clinical examination reveals vocal cord fixation or ipsilateral cervical lymphadenopathy and fixation of the nodule to the surrounding structures, it is again suggestive of thyroid carcinoma.

However, even in the absence of all these, any thyroid nodule more than 1 cm need to be evaluated for the possibility of malignancy. Ultrasonography and FNAC are the main investigations for the diagnosis of thyroid cancer.

CT scan may be necessary to find out if surrounding structures are involved or not. Trachea may be compressed by thyroid lobe giving rise to scabbard trachea (Fig. 40.3). Fig. 40.4 shows invasion of trachea by follicular carcinoma of thyroid.

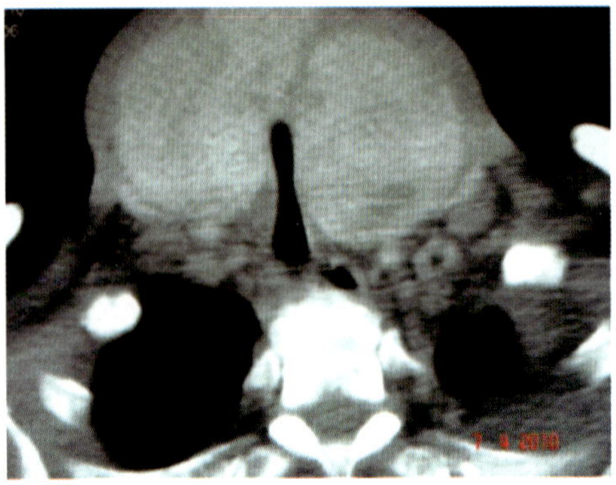

Fig. 40.3. Scabbard trachea due to pressure on it by thyroid.

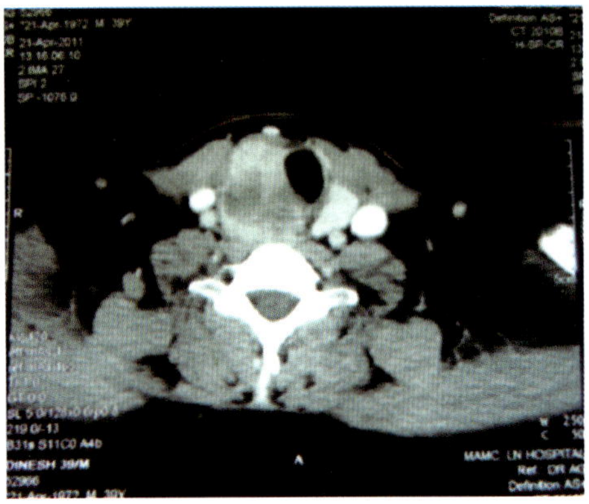

Fig. 40.4. Carcinoma thyroid infiltrating the trachea.

The flowchart will guide how to investigate a thyroid nodule.

AJCC STAGING OF DIFFERENTIATED THYROID CANCER

Primary tumour (T)

- TX Primary tumour cannot be assessed
- T0 No evidence of primary tumour
- T1 Tumour 2 cm or less in greatest dimension limited to thyroid
- T2 Tumour more than 2 cm but not more than 4 cm in greatest dimension limited to the thyroid
- T3 Tumour more than 4 cm in greatest dimension limited to the thyroid or any tumour with minimal extrathyroid extension (e.g., extension to sternothyroid muscle or perithyroid soft tissue)
- T4a Tumour of any size extending beyond the thyroid capsule to invade the subcutaneous soft tissue, larynx, trachea, esophagus or recurrent laryngeal nerve
- T4b Tumour invades prevertebral fascia or encases carotid artery or mediastinal vessels

All anaplastic carcinomas are considered T4 tumours

- T4a Intrathyroid anaplastic carcinoma – surgically resectable
- T4b Extrathyroidal anplastic carcinoma – surgically unresectable

Regional lymph nodes (N)

Regional lymph nodes are the central compartment, lateral cervical and upper mediastinal lymph nodes.

- NX Regional lymph nodes cannot be assessed
- N0 No regional lymph node metastasis
- N1 Regional lymph node metastasis
- N1a Metastasis to level VI (pretracheal, paratracheal and prelaryngeal also known as Delphian lymph node)
- N1b Metastasis to unilateral, bilateral, or contra-cervical or superior or mediastinal lymph nodes

Distant metastasis (M)

- MX Distant metastasis cannot be assessed
- M0 No distant metastasis
- M1 Distant metastasis

Algorithm outlining evaluation and management of nodular thyroid disease practised by Mayo Clinics

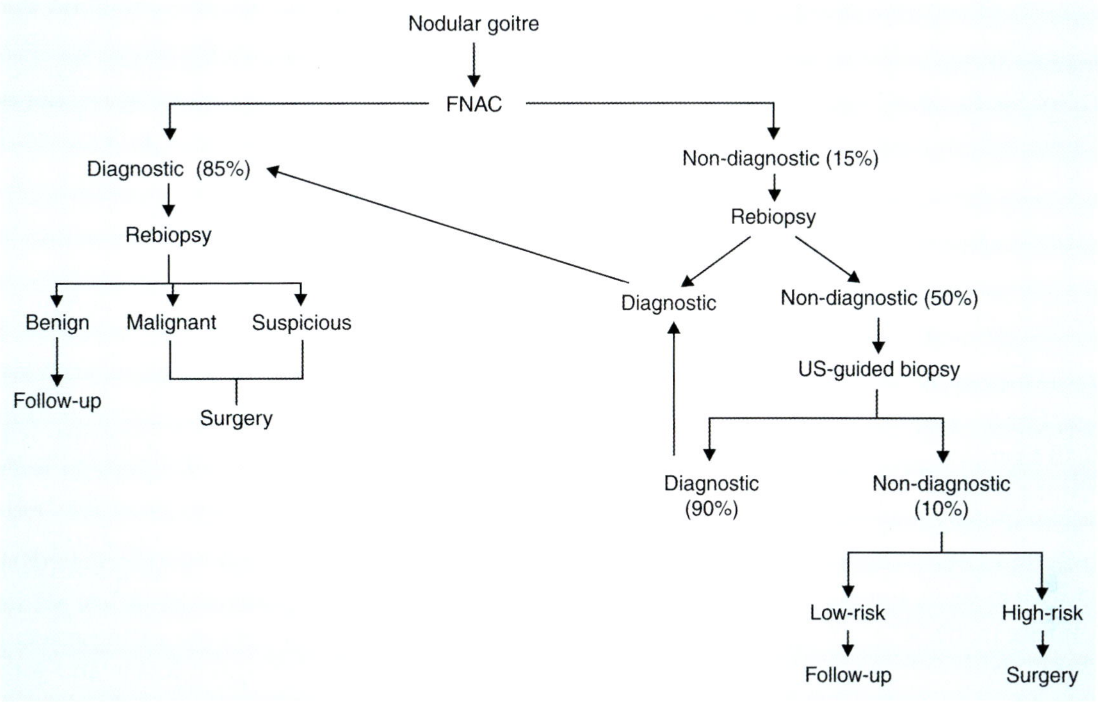

An algorithm for the rational approach to the evaluation and management of a thyroid nodule

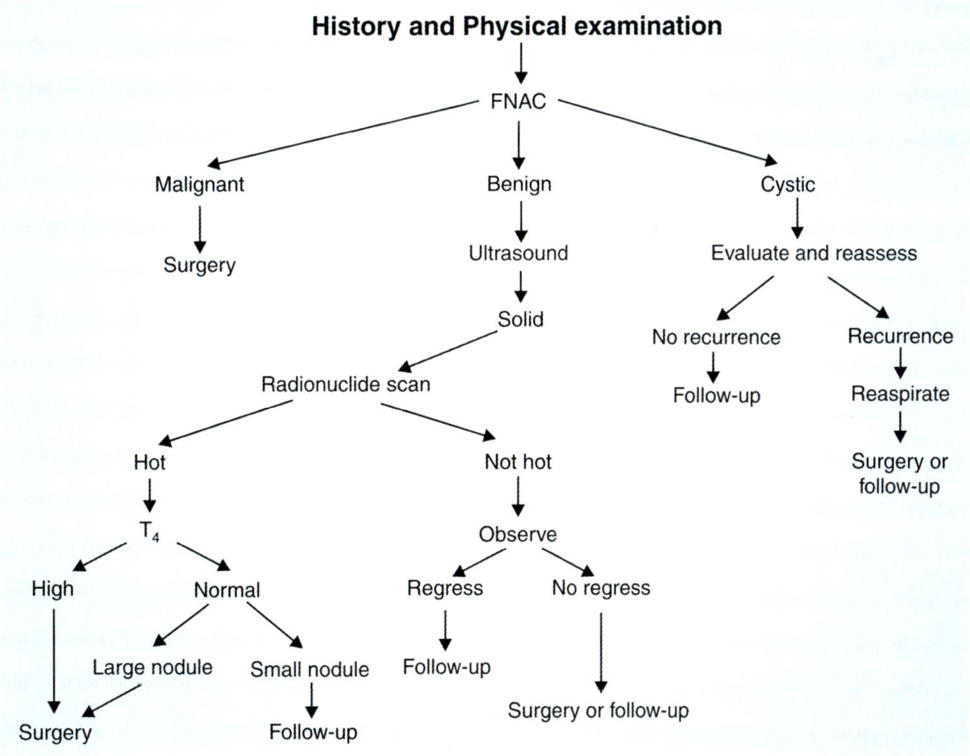

40

Patient-related and tumour-related risk stratification is therefore the management of well-differentiated thyroid tumours. Various risk factors are:

- Age of patient
- Size of the tumour
- Distant metastasis
- Extent of tumour
- Completeness of resection
- Local invasion and grade of tumour

GAMES from Memorial Hospital (MSCC)
- **G**rade, **A**ge, **M**etastasis, **E**xtension, **S**ize

AGES from Mayo Clinic, 1987
- **A**ge, **G**rade, **E**xtension, **S**ize

MACIS from Mayo Clinic, 1993
- Distant **M**etastasis, **A**ge, **C**ompleteness of resection, **I**nvasion, **S**ize

AMES from Lahey Clinic
- **A**ge, **M**etastasis, **E**xtension, **S**ize

Karolinska Institute
DAMES
- **D**NA, **A**ge, **M**etastasis, **E**xtension, **S**ize

Extent of surgery

Completeness of resection is one of the most important prognostic factors. Lobectomy with satisfactory margins is adequate for low risk category patients. Total thyroidectomy in low risk patients may lead to more of complications than any benefits. Total thyroidectomy is advised in cases with intermediate and higher risk cases. It should be followed by radioiodine scan.

Role of lymph node dissection

Central compartment node's elective clearance may be done with explained risk of hypoparathyroidism.

Follow-up

40

A diagnostic radioactive scan should be done at 4–6 weeks to rule out any remnant disease. Any remnant or metastatic node may be treated by radioactive iodine. Thyroglobulin and anti-Tg antibodies to be done periodically at six months interval.

Role of adjuvant external RT

It is reserved for cases above 45 years of age. Those that had extra nodal spread of disease or had microscopic residual of disease.

Special consideration

Thyroid cancer in children

It has same psychological and emotional effect like any other childhood cancer on the family and patient. Cases of well-differentiated thyroid cancer present in well advanced stage. Fifty percent of the cases present with enlarged lymph nodes. The 20-years survival rate is 95% while 10-year survival is almost 100%. An aggressive surgical therapy like total or near total thyroidectomy and central compartment neck dissection which includes paratracheal, pretracheal, and prelaryngeal lymph nodes clearance bilaterally. In cases where secondary lymph nodes are present then level II to VI clearance should be done. Use of ^{131}I remains controversial in paediatric age-group. Although these patient have advanced disease at the time of presentation, the long-term risk of the radioactive iodine exposure must be considered. Despite excellent response initially a long-term follow-up is required. These patients have late widespread recurrence. Early recognition of these recurrences with periodic thyroglobulin levels and total body scans is essential in maximizing long-term survival.

Steps of thyroid surgery

- It can be done under local or general anesthesia depending on the situation. In case of local anesthesia cervical block to be given. One would prefer to operate under general anaesthesia.
- **Position.** Patient is kept in supine position with extension of neck.
- **Incision.** A collar incision is made two fingers above the clavicle (Fig. 40.5). It may be modified if neck dissection is required. Local infiltration with 1 : 1,00,000 adrenaline saline is done. Incision is made upto the platysema and flaps are elevated upto the thyroid notch superiorly and clavicle inferiorly (Fig. 40.6).
- The strap muscles are separated in midline in avascular plane. Muscles are retracted and middle thyroid vein is ligated.
- Recurrent laryngeal nerve is identified in relation to inferior thyroid artery. Left side is more vertical and seen in tracheoesophageal groove. It comes up in the neck from the thorax while the right turns around the subclavian artery.

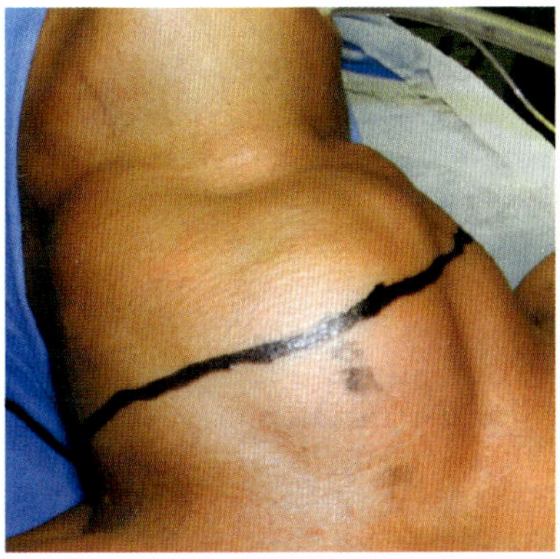

Fig. 40.5. Collar incision marked for thyroid surgery.

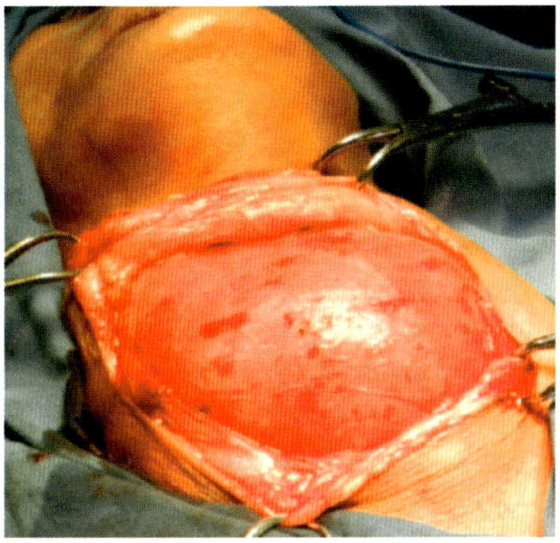

Fig. 40.6. Skin flaps raised.

- External branch of superior laryngeal nerve supplies the cricothyroid muscle of the larynx. This nerve is to be preserved by tying the vascular pedicle close to the upper pole of thyroid.
- Parathyroid glands are to be preserved. These appear as amber-coloured. Upper glands are lower than the lower one. Lower ones are more constant in position just at the point of entry of recurrent laryngeal nerve. Its blood supply needs to be preserved by subcapsular dissection.
- Berry's ligament needs to be dissected from the trachea and thyroid gland mobilised (Figs. 40.7 and 40.8).
- If there are any lymph nodes in the neck then modified neck dissection should be carried out. Middle compartment clearance should be done, i.e., level VI nodes should be cleared.
- Wound should be sutured in two layers after inserting a drain.
- The excised specimen (Fig. 40.9) should be sent for histopathology.

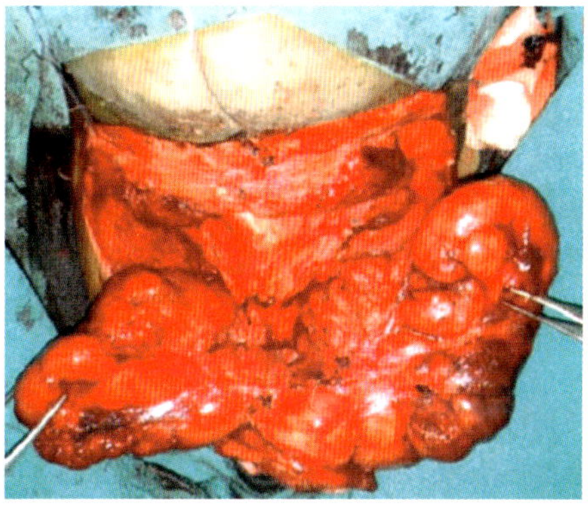

Fig. 40.7. Thyroid gland mobilised.

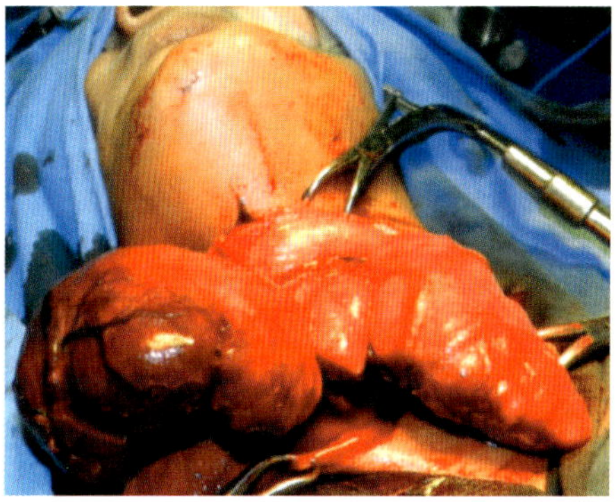

Fig. 40.8. Thyroid gland excised.

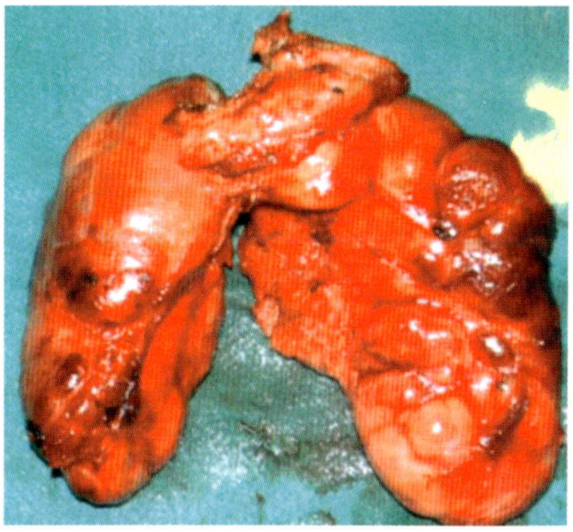

Fig. 40.9. Excised specimen of the thyroid.

Complications

1. Injury to recurrent laryngeal nerve.
2. Hypocalcemia.
3. Injury to the superior laryngeal nerve.

CONCLUSION

Goitre or thyroid enlargement is very common in Terai region of Himalayas. It is more common in females as compared to males. A detailed history and physical examination and movement of vocal cords should be examined. Fine needle aspiration and ultrasound are the main stay of investigations. CT scan or MRI may also be done to see the extent of thyroid enlargement. There is long list of risk factors such as age, sex, etc. Follicular and papillary cell carcinoma are two well differentiated types. Treatment for the carcinoma is either hemi- or total thyroidectomy with or without central compartment clearence. Postoperative radioactive iodine may be given. External beam radiotherapy may be given depending on the extent of tumor.

SUGGESTED READING

1. PK Pellitteri, Steven Ing. Disorders of the thyroid gland. *In:* Otolaryngology Head Neck Surgery, 4th ed. by Charles W Cummings, Paul W Flint, Lee A Harker, Bruce H Haughey, Mark A Richardson et al. Elsevier Mosby, Philadelphia, pp. 2661–2723.
2. Frank R Miller, Randal A Otto. Disorders of thyroid. *Otolaryngol Clin of North Am*, 2003; 3(1): 17–35.
3. Stefan KG Grebe, Ian D Hay. Clinical Evaluation of thyroid tumours. *In:* Comprehensive Management of Head and Neck Tumours, Vol 2, 2nd ed. Eds. Stanley E Thawley, William R Panje, John G Batsakis, Robert D Lindberg. WB Saunders Company, Philadelphia, pp. 1694–1700.
4. Shilpa Chatni, Anil D'Cruz. Management of thyroid cancer. *In:* Current Concepts in Head & Neck Oncology by Head Neck Institute, Amrita Institute of Medical Sciences & FHNO. Teaching Manual, 2009 pp. 25–32.

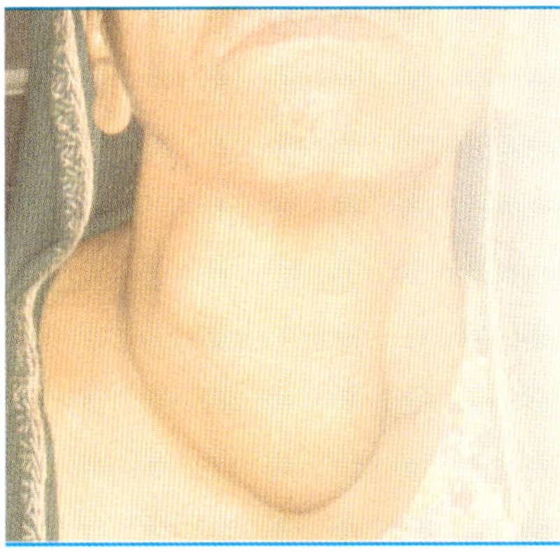

CHAPTER **41**

Lasers in ENT

Sonal Modi, K.P. Morwani

The word laser is an acronym derived from "Light Amplification by Stimulated Emission of Radiation". A laser-equipped device can generate a high-intensity light that makes the laser useful for commercial as well as medical applications. An understanding of the general properties of lasers allows the physician as well as the patient to appreciate the technology and its capabilities and also its limitations.

Laser has certainly proved to be a boon to medical fraternity and for patients as well as surgeons. Laser certainly has an added advantage over conventional techniques in fair number of cases. Laser has not replaced the conventional technique but has definitely contributed tremendously due to extreme precision and minimal penetration.

HISTORICAL BACKGROUND

The first gas laser, which was developed in 1961, used a mixture of helium and neon. Although its beam was not powerful enough to trigger a thermal reaction, its red colour allowed it to be used as an aiming beam for invisible lasers such as the carbon dioxide (CO_2) laser.

In 1964, Patel at Bell Laboratories developed the CO_2 laser. It emitted spectral energy in the far IR portion of the electromagnetic spectrum at 10,600 nm. At this wavelength, energy is heavily absorbed by water, which is the primary constituent and chromophore of cells in living tissue. Thus, the energy generated by this laser can be used for cutting or volume ablation by means of tissue vaporization. This unique characteristic makes the CO_2 laser the most widely used medical laser today.

TYPES OF LASERS

Till date there are various types of lasers and these have been differentiated depending upon the specific tissue reaction each produces depending upon their wavelengths. CO_2 laser, diode, KTP and Nd:Yag lasers are more frequently used in medical applications.

- CO_2 (Laryngeal, Nasal, Oral)
- Diode (Tracheal and Nasal)
- Argon (Opthalmology and Dermatology)
- KTP (Stapedectomy)
- Nd:Yag (Neodymium yttrium aluminium garnet) (Gastric, Urology and Dermatology)

CO_2 LASER

Properties of laser

The CO_2 beam has special properties:

- **Coherent:** Laser light shows coherent light waves. All waves are in same phase.
- **Monochromatic:** Laser light consists of just one wavelength, and cannot be split.
- **Unidirectionality:** Laser light is unidirectional.

Physics

LASER is the energy used to excite atoms and produce photons that resonate in a laser chamber. These photons excite other atoms in the laser chamber until a highly concentrated beam of light is produced. Laser light is produced by energizing the molecules of a crystal or gaseous compound causing them to give off light at a specific wavelength.

The basic laser device consists of 3 components:

1. An active medium, or lasing medium.
2. An optical cavity, or resonator.
3. An energizing source, or pump.

The active medium in lasers may be a solid, liquid, or gas. Different active media emit different energies or wavelengths of light. However, they all operate with the same basic principles.

The resonator contains an active medium. At each end of the resonator, parallel reflectors or mirrors are placed facing each other. The front of the output mirror is designed to be partially reflective. It reflects only a portion of the light impinging on it, allowing some portion of the total energy or light to escape. The rear mirror is a total reflector that reflects 100% of the energy impinging on it. The pump source provides the energy (thermal, electric, or optical, e.g., a flash lamp) for absorption by the active medium.

When the active medium is pumped with sufficient energy, a population inversion occurs, causing the spontaneous emission of photons. Some of these photons are reflected back and forth between the 2 mirrors (others are dissipated as heat) and then collide with atoms in the excited state; these collisions subsequently stimulate the emission of radiation. As other photons collide with excited atoms, energy within the resonator builds and is amplified by reflections between the parallel mirrors. At the front output mirror, a portion of the energy is permitted to escape. This energy is in the form of an intense beam of monochromatic (same wavelength), collimated (parallel, nondiverging), and coherent (same direction) light.

Power density

When the laser beam exits the resonator, its diameter is often too large and diffuse, and the beam itself may have inadequate power to be useful. Therefore, the laser beam is passed through a focusing lens to reduce its diameter, which increases its intensity and energy so that it is of more suitable size for manipulation and practicality. Its intensity is the power density (Pd) and is defined as the energy delivered per unit area of incident tissue. It is measured in terms of wattage of laser per diameter of the beam.

For a given wattage, a wide or unfocused beam has less penetration ability and is more useful for procedures such as skin resurfacing, vaporization of tissue, and coagulation of blood vessels. A focused beam penetrates to a greater depth and is more useful in procedures involving delicate cutting and volume ablation.

Duration of exposure

To accurately determine the total amount of energy delivered to the tissue by the laser, the duration of exposure is vital. Prolonged exposures result in tissue destruction, and too short an exposure results in an inadequate effect. The dose is a measure of the total energy. It is expressed in terms of energy per unit area of incident tissue.

Wavelength

The effect of light on skin depends on the wavelength of the light. In general, the effects of light in the mid-to-far IR region of the spectrum are limited to the superficial layers. The degree of absorption and its thermal effect on skin vary with the amount and type of chromophores that are present in the recipient. As stated earlier, hemoglobin and melanin are natural endogenous chromophores. An example of an exogenous chromophore is tattoo ink. Different chromophores have different absorption coefficients. The absorption coefficient is a measure of the degree of absorption by the chromophores at a particular wavelength. Because the laser is monochromatic and a very narrow bandwidth, it permits selective targeting of chromophores in the tissue for treatment.

Interaction with tissues

When the laser beam is focused on target tissue, not all the energy aimed at the tissue is effective. A portion of this energy is lost either by reflection at the surface or by transmission through the target tissue. The part of the beam which is neither reflected nor absorbed will ultimately give up its energy to the tissue concerned.

Thermal effects

Vapourization

- 650°C – Protein denaturation
- 1000°C – Intracellular water boils
- 400–5000°C – Cellular debris burns

Application technique

Contact technique

Fibre tip touches the tissue surface.

Non-contact technique

Laser probe directed to target tissue from some distance. With increase in distance from the tip of the laser the power density decreases.

The pathologies which are easily accessible to the naked eye can be dealt with using the hand-held probe (Fig. 41.1) like a pen and the lesions in the depth can be addressed using the micromanipulator attached to the microscope (Fig. 41.2). With the help of micromanipulator one can reflect and direct the beam to the desired target area.

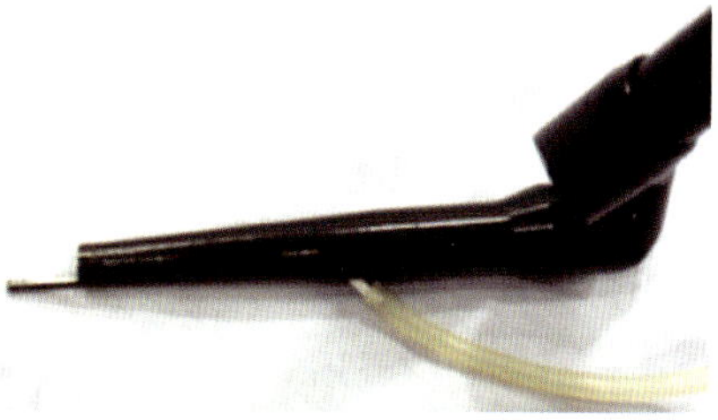

Fig. 41.1. Handpiece.

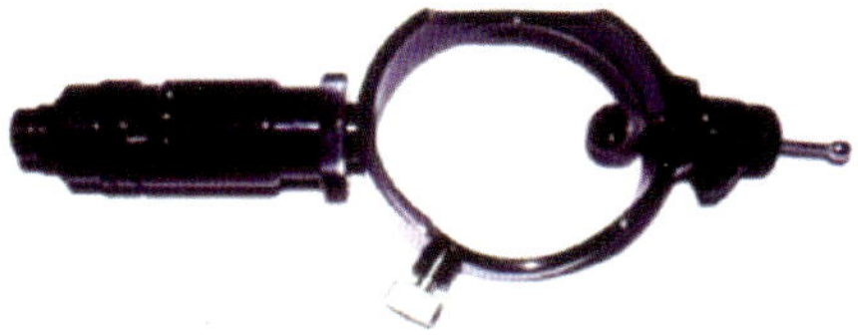

Fig. 41.2. Micromanipulator.

The laser can be successfully used in ENT practice, but the surgeon should be well aware of the benefits as well as the drawbacks of the facilities of the equipment and for this the surgeon should have more than adequate training before indulging in this sophisticated surgery.

Understanding the equipment (Fig. 41.3)

To understand the equipment better one needs to understand the control panel of the equipment. On this panel there are settings for:

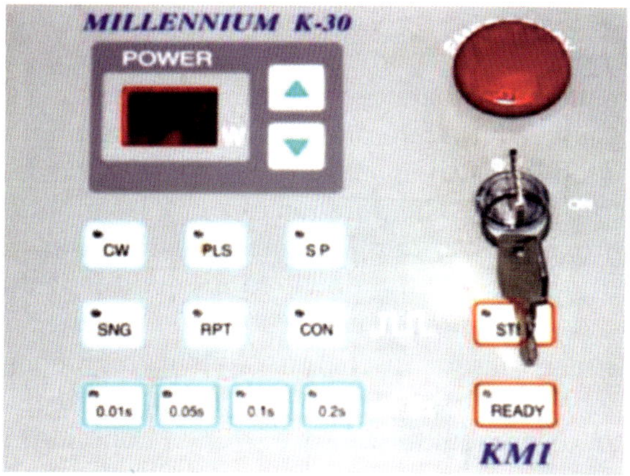

Fig. 41.3. Control panel of laser.

- Power control 1 to 30 watts depending upon the current required
- Red Knob Emergency button to put off the equipment in times of crisis or fire hazard
- CW – Continuous Mode
- PLS – Pulse Mode
- SP – Super Pulse Mode
- SNG – Single Shot
- RPT – Repeat Shots
- CNT – Continuous Shots
- 0.01 to 0.2 s – Time duration between two pulses
- ON – Key to start the equipment
- STANDBY – The equipment is on but not functional
- READY – The laser is functional

The depth and width of excision depends on the type of mode.

- Continuous Mode – CW is the continued emission of laser with constant power
- Pulse Mode – Pulse beam is the form of emission for adjustable short time
- Super Pulse Mode – Super pulse is the form of emission for very short time with very high peak power.

The light generated with a laser, in general, can be delivered in 2 ways:

- a constant flow of energy (continuous wave), or
- multiple discrete pulses (pulsed laser).

The 2 types of lasers are fundamentally different in design, light delivery, and operation.

A CW laser is generated by continuously pumping energy into the active medium to achieve an equilibrium between the number of atoms raised to the excited state and the number of photons emitted. At such an equilibrium, continuous laser output results. The duration of a CW laser pulse is approximately 0.25 s. With this duration and with relatively constant power delivery to tissues, significant thermal damage occurs.

Pulsed lasers, in contrast, deliver high-energy beams in very short pulses in the range of milliseconds without the use of a shutter. Emissions are produced when the pump is modulated to create discrete laser pulses, which usually are broad and randomly shaped.

Pulse and super pulse beams are available with single emission (SNG) or repetitive emission (RPT) for set time (for example, 0.01/0.05/0.1/0.2 sec) or continuously repetitive emission (CON) in 80 Hz. Choice of continuous, pulse or super pulse mode is made for each individual case, based on depth of incision required, size of necrosis area, surrounding damage, size of incision opening, haemostasis and healing time. These modes are to be utilized individually or simultaneously depending upon the type of lesion. At times all three modes or any two can be used alternatively for same pathology. The duration of the pulse delivered can be controlled using this equipment which has duration control of 0.01 s, 0.05 s, 0.1 s and 0.2 s thus avoiding excessive thermal damage.

- **Focused beam:** Highly focused laser beam generates heat causing tissue vaporization resulting in incision.
- **Defocused beam:** With the defocused mode, there is a wider zone of removal but a shallower depth of penetration as compared to the focused mode. CO_2 laser in laser beam coagulates and seals blood vessels upto 1 mm, providing bloodless surgical site.

41

CONTINUOUS MODE (Fig. 41.4)

Continuous mode is used on lesions where deeper penetration is required and in lesions of solid consistency.

- Excision of bulky lesions
- Excision of benign as well as malignant lesions
- Supraglottic, glottis and subglottic stenosis
- Excision of T1, T2 carcinoma of vocal cord
- Base of tongue lesions
- Partial glossectomy

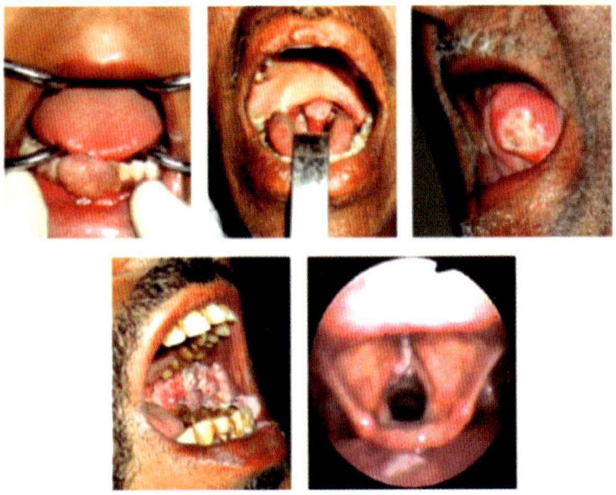

Fig. 41.4. Lesions fit to be dealt with continuous mode.

- Vaporisation of arytenoid cartilage in cases of laser partial arytenoidectomy for bilateral vocal cord palsy

PULSE MODE (Fig. 41.5)

When penetration with laser has to be reduced, one can use pulse mode and one can give continuous pulse or intermittent pulses.

- Benign lesions
- Multiple papillomas of vocal cord
- Vocal cord polyp, and nodule
- Nasal septal mass
- Pedunculated mass in oropharynx
- Residual adenoid tissue
- Superficial lesions
- Deeper part of malignant lesions
- Ca in situ

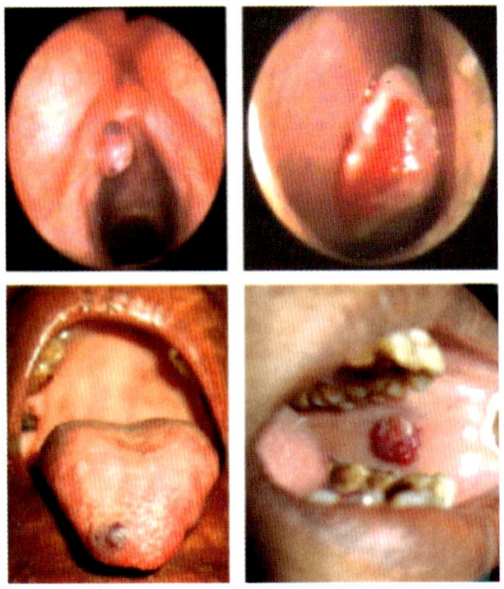

Fig. 41.5. Lesions where pulse mode should be used.

SUPER PULSE MODE (Fig. 41.6)

Super pulse mode is used when the penetration required is least and beam can be given in single pulse, repeatedly or continuously. Besides the duration of each pulse can be controlled.

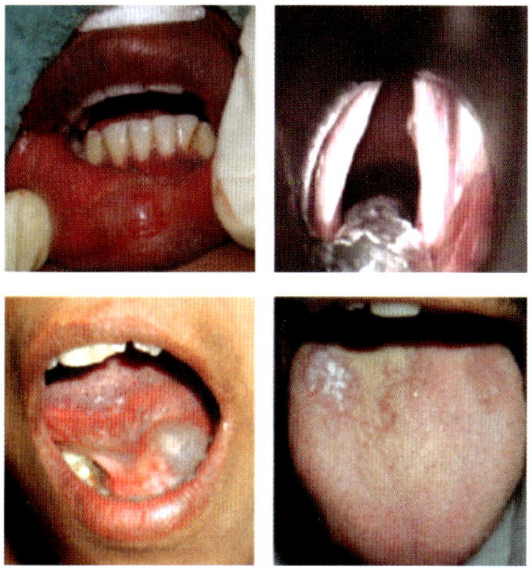

Fig. 41.6. Lesion to be dealt with super pulse mode.

- Vocal cord cyst
- Leukoplakia of vocal cord
- Premalignant lesions of oral cavity or oro-pharynx
- Epistaxis secondary to bleeding from little area
- Deeper part of benign lesions of VC
- Deeper part of multiple papilloma

At times in a certain case one can keep on changing the type of mode as required for a particular situation, e.g., in a case of carcinoma in situ of vocal cord initially one will require pulse mode on main tumour mass and super pulse mode on periphery and the safe margins of the lesion. In short the surgeon must be very well versed with the laser equipment and the various modes.

The major drawback of laser is thermal damage which is minimized by upgradation of the equipment. So, it is of utmost importance to have good quality equipment.

Laser safety precautions (Fig. 41.7)

The only dreaded complication of laser is the fire hazard but with utmost care one can certainly avoid these complications.

The precautions to be strictly followed are:

- Laser control area
- Area limited to specific personnel

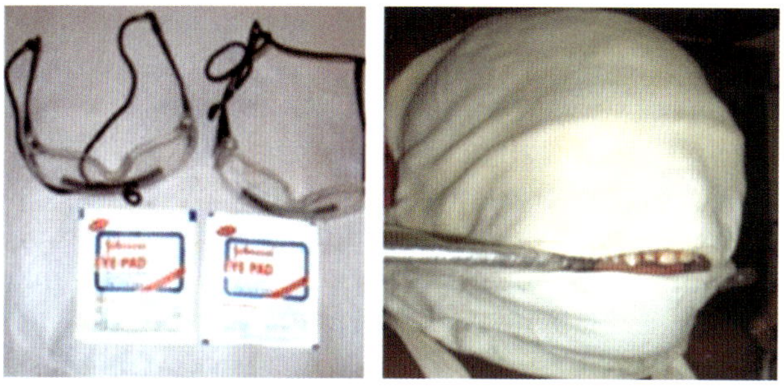

Fig. 41.7. Laser safety precautions.

- Observers not allowed without permission
- Appropriate protective and safety device (safety goggles)
- Protection of body tissues (draping the non-target area with wet mops)
- Heavy duty smoke evacuatous – for vaporization of large plumes.
- Laser ON
- Laser STANDBY

Anaesthesia (Fig. 41.8)

Anaesthesia for laser surgery is somewhat similar to conventional surgery except for a few advances which can avoid complications of laser surgery.

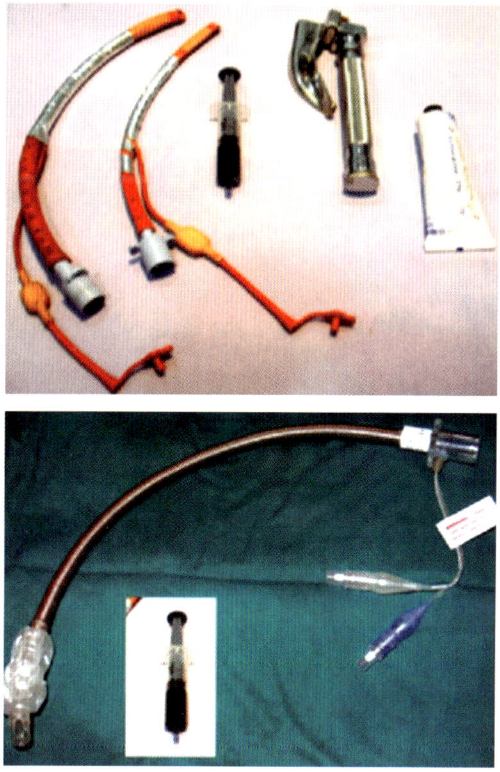

Fig. 41.8. Anaesthesia equipment for laser.

The focus of concern is mainly centred on the endotracheal tube. With the rapid advancement in ENT laser surgery the anesthetist and laser surgeons are presented with new challenges. Carbon dioxide laser surgery in the airway presents the anesthetist with new problems. The mode of action of carbon dioxide lasers and its effects on anesthetic agents and equipment must be anticipated. Complications, especially of fire hazards in the airway, and methods of avoiding them are most important.

- Possible intubation problems due to narrow upper airway.
- The team should be familiar with the problems of lasers in the airway.
- Have good cooperation and communication with each other.
- Maintain constant vigilance during surgery.
- Because of the intense heat generated, lasers must not be used with flammable agents.
- Nitrous oxide, although not flammable, does support combustion at high temperatures and should be avoided with open anesthetic systems.
- The oxygen concentration should be as low as possible with adequate oxygenation.

The original method of protecting tracheal tubes involved the use of self-adhesive, nonreflective aluminium tape. The tube is carefully wrapped with the tape in a spiral fashion with overlapping edges, commencing just above the cuff or at the distal tip of endotracheal tubes. Tape edges are then smoothed to decrease injury to pharyngeal and laryngeal tissue. This significantly retards ignition of both red rubber and PVC tubes. Although adequate, it is not without danger.

Narrow tubes can become occluded as a result of compression by the foil as it accommodates to the curvature of the pharynx The tape does not always adhere adequately to the tube and may loosen or break off, resulting in acute airway obstruction. The outer wall of the tube is protected, but the cuff and the distal end of the tube can be ignited by direct or indirect contact with the laser beam.

The cuff, when ruptured, allows a massive leak of anesthetic gases, leading to hypoventilation as well as providing a richer environment for ignition of the tube. The cuff can be protected by filling it with saline and placing saline-soaked cottonoids around it and these are kept moist throughout the procedure.

Laser resistant cuffed endotracheal tube made from silicone and having an outer coating of metallic oxide are more resistant to lasers than red rubber and PVC tubes. However, the cuffs of these tubes do present a hazard when inflated with air. Multiple impacts from a laser will penetrate the cuff, which could ignite. Hence, the cuff is inflated with saline which is diluted in methylene blue so as to identify immediately the leak from the cuff due to bluish seepage of saline. The high volume, low pressure floppy cuff may present difficulty during its passage through a narrow larynx.

The development of a flexible metal tube provides a partial solution to the problem. All the fleximetallic tubes in use are non-combustible, easily sterilized, gas-tight and non-reactive with human tissue. Wet cottonoids can be placed around the tube to act as a pack, as well as a protective shield for normal tissue distal to the lesion. The walls of these tubes are relatively thick, with a large external diameter which precludes their use in the younger patient. They can be reused many times and provide long-term economy.

Indications of CO_2 laser

CO_2 laser can practically be used in each and every field of ENT, be it a benign oral lesion which is accessible, to lesions in the depth, i.e., subglottis and trachea. Laser can be used in:

- Benign lesions like papillomas, fibromas, polyps, cyst, haemangiomas.
- Premalignant lesions like keratosis, leukoplakia, melanoplakia and carcinoma in situ.
- Malignant lesions depending on the stage of lesion.

1. Oral cavity and oropharynx (Fig. 41.9)

- Gums
- Lip lesions
- Angle of mouth
- Buccal mucosa
- Floor of mouth
- Tongue
- Tonsil
- Palate
- Uvula

2. Laryngopharynx and larynx (Fig. 41.10)

- Posterior pharyngeal wall
- Epiglottis

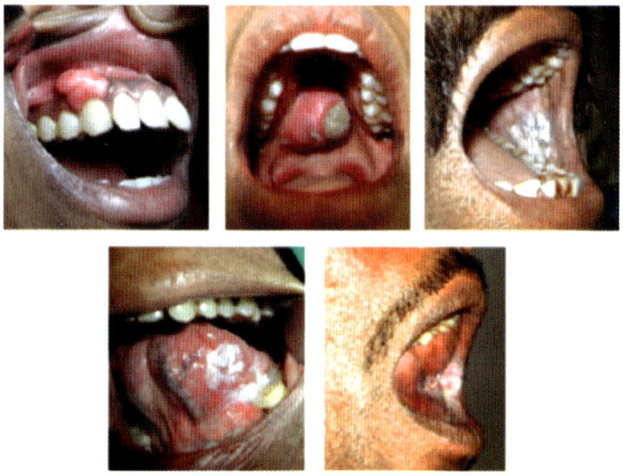

Fig. 41.9. Oral cavity lesions fit for laser surgery.

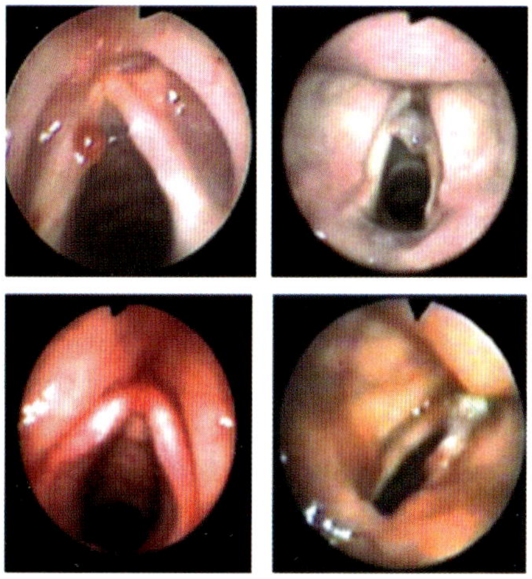

Fig. 41.10. Laryngeal and laryngopharyngeal disease fit for laser excision.

- Pyriform fossa
- Arytenoids
- Vocal cords
- Laser partial arytenoidectomy
- Ca larynx
- Subglottic lesions
- Tracheal lesions

3. Nose and nasopharynx (Fig. 41.11)

- Epistaxis
- Septal mass, polyp, haemangioma
- Synechiae
- Residual polyps
- Adenoids
- Choanal atresia

4. Ear

- Stapedectomy

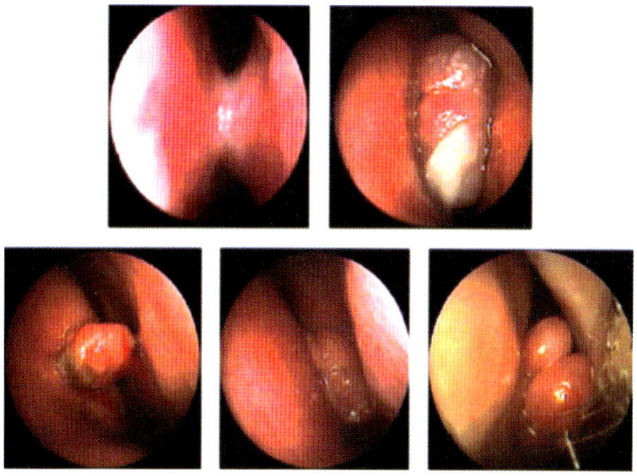

Fig. 41.11. Nasal cavity disease fit for laser surgery.

Advantages

Minimal pain

The CO_2 laser beam automatically seals nerve endings when incising through tissue. So, patient feels less pain during and after surgery. Patient needs no or less anesthesia during surgery.

Excellent haemostasis

The laser beam can cauterise and seal small blood vessels up to 1 mm in diameter, resulting in haemostasis and providing the surgeon with a virtually bloodless surgical field during surgery.

Minimal post-op oedema

There is no physical contact between the laser and the surgical region, thus the crushing, tearing and bruising of tissue associated with traditional surgical methods is reduced and thereby causing less of inflammation and quickens the healing. Similarly the lymphatic vessels are also sealed.

Minimal post-op care

Laser seals lymphatic, sterilizing surgical site with high temperature, thus reducing much of the post-op care.

Minimal or no chances of post-op infection

The laser sterilizes surgical region by producing high temperature as it removes diseased tissue, thereby causing sterilization and reducing chances of infection.

Excellent precision

The laser beam is accurately delivered to a point of focus that can remove unhealthy tissue with minimal damage to surrounding healthy tissue.

Super pulse beam vaporizes target tissue with no or least effect on adjacent tissue.

Early mobilisation

Combination of the above attributes including minimal pain, practically no postoperative bleeding and minimal post-op oedema certainly helps the patient to return to normal activity sooner.

Advantages in laryngeal lesions

- Fewer tracheotomies.
- No fistulae.
- Less disfigurement.
- Less pain.
- Earlier swallowing.
- Lower risk of over-treatment.
- Shorter length of stay.
- Repeatable treatment.
- Second primaries – all treatment options remain open.

Limitations

- Cost factor.
- Though the cost is a bit on higher side eventually one realizes that it is very much cost effective.
- Special training.
- Every sophisticated equipment requires special training, be it a microscope, endoscope or laser.
- Fire hazard – direct or indirect.
- Anesthetic complications.

Fire hazard is one particular aspect which has to be taken very seriously but it is something which is certainly an avoidable complication.

Two types of burn injury are produced by laser explosions. The thermal effect from dry heat dissipated by vaporization of cellular and surface water gives rise to a mummified appearance of the tissue. The second type of injury arises from the chemical response of tissues to toxic PVC fumes.

- First, stop ventilation.
- Disconnect oxygen.
- Remove endotracheal tube.
- Place oral airway and ventilate with anesthesia mask.
- Perform rigid bronchoscopy to remove large foreign bodies (if any), and lavage the trachea.
- Fibreoptic bronchoscopy to visualize small airways, remove small foreign bodies and lavage to distal airways.
- Evaluate injury to laryngotracheobronchial tree.
- Remove fragmented mucosa and debris.
- If necessary, perform a low tracheostomy.
- Administer antibiotics and short-term steroids.
- Provide a high humidity environment and positive end expiratory pressure ventilation.
- Culture tracheal aspirate daily.
- Perform endoscopy 3–5 days post-burn to evaluate extent of injury.

Just because a debrider can cause injury to vital structures or an ear surgery can cause facial nerve palsy we don't stop operating. These complications occur once in a lifetime and once you know how to take care of these situations the fear of these complications is certainly negligible.

CONCLUSION

Laser can be used in practically each and every area of not only oral cavity and oropharynx but also in nose, larynx and laryngopharynx, either through direct or endoscopic vision. Today laser has changed the complete scenario of surgery with added advantage of minimal blood loss, excellent haemostasis, improved healing process, less morbidity and hospitalization and better post-operative results. The CO_2 laser is considered as state of art equipment in every field of surgical specialty more so for managing pathologies in oral cavity, oropharynx, larynx, laryngopharynx, nose and nasopharynx. Laser has an added advantage over conventional surgeries in certain lesions like cysts, fibromas, papillomas and haemangiomas.

However, in malignant cases laser can work as a miracle. Imagine a patient coming for your consultation on day one for hoarseness of voice. You diagnosis him as a case of malignancy of vocal cord. The next day you operate him and laserise the malignant lesion and within twenty four hours your patient is free of malignancy. In such a case patient need not go for radiotherapy nor any mutilating surgery which is certainly a benefit not only for the surgeon but also for the patient.

The advantages of laser are tremendous. At times one can avoid antibiotics, IV fluids and Ryle's tube feeding. As bleeding is minimized, major lesions can be operated without the need of transfusion in most of the cases. The duration of surgery and anaesthesia is reduced. Though the surgical principle remains the same, the added advantage of bloodless field and pinpoint precision is certainly exceptional. This magic wand requires fair amount of training and is not free of complications unless treated very delicately.

SUGGESTED READING

1. Satar B, Shah AR. Laser in head and neck surgery. *In:* Lalwani AK, editor. Current Diagnosis and Treatment in Otolaryngology – Head & Neck Surgery, 2nd edition. McGraw Hill Medical, New York, 2008; 177–91.
2. Remacle M. Laser assisted microphonosurgery. *In:* Remacle M, Eckel HE, editors. Surgery of Larynx and Trachea. Springer- Verlag, Heidelberg, New York, 2010; 51–56.
3. Jakobowicz M. Nd:YAG laser and the treatment of nasal and sinus pathology. *In:* Levine HL, Clemente MP, editors. Sinus Surgery: Endoscopic and Microscopic Approaches. Thieme, New York, 2009; 245–55.
4. Hiittenbrink KB. Current topics in otolaryngology – head & neck surgery. Laser in otorhinolaryngology. Thieme, New York, 2005.
5. McGill TJI, Friedman EM, Healy GB. Laser surgery in pediatric airway. *Otolaryngol Clin North Am*, 1983; 16: 865–72.
6. Oswal V, Remacle M. Principles and practice of laser in otorhinolaryngology and head & neck surgery. Kugler Publication, The Hague, Netherland, 2002.
7. Steiner W, Ambrosch P. Endoscopic laser surgery of the upper aerodigestive tract, with special emphasis on cancer surgery. Thieme, New York, 2000.

The Magic Is In the Magician,
Not in the Wand.

CHAPTER 42

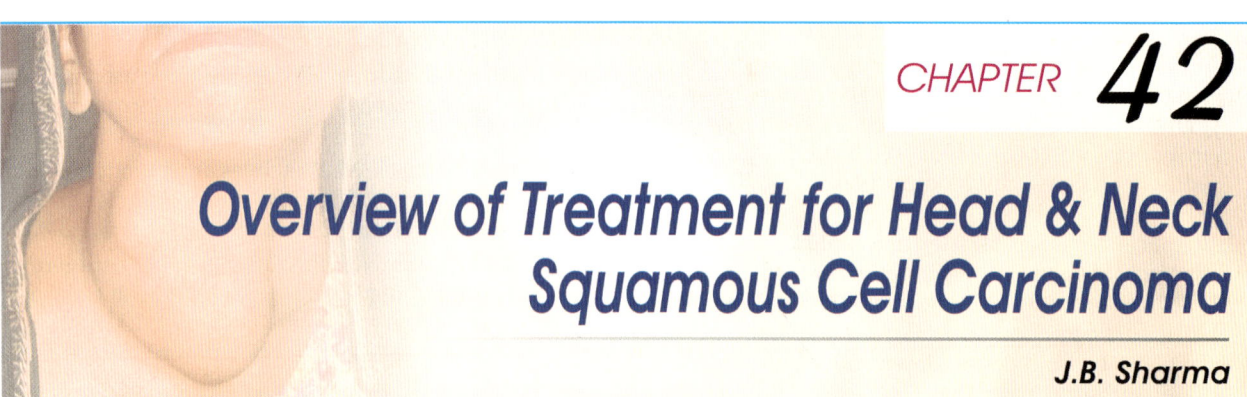

Overview of Treatment for Head & Neck Squamous Cell Carcinoma

J.B. Sharma

Head & neck cancers arise from a variety of sites within the head and neck region, which is divided into five basic areas (Fig. 42.1).

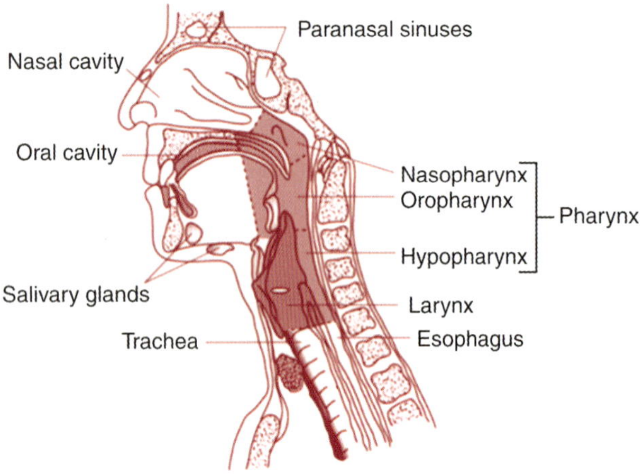

Fig. 42.1. Anatomical landmarks of head & neck.

- The oral cavity includes the lips, buccal mucosa, anterior tongue, floor of the mouth, hard palate, upper gingiva, lower gingiva, and retromolar trigone (Fig. 42.2).
- The pharynx is divided into the oropharynx, the nasopharynx, and the hypopharynx.
  - Nasopharynx, the narrow tubular passage behind the nasal cavity, is the upper part of the pharynx.
  - Oropharynx, the middle part of the pharynx, includes the tonsillar area, the tongue base, the soft palate, and the posterior pharyngeal wall.

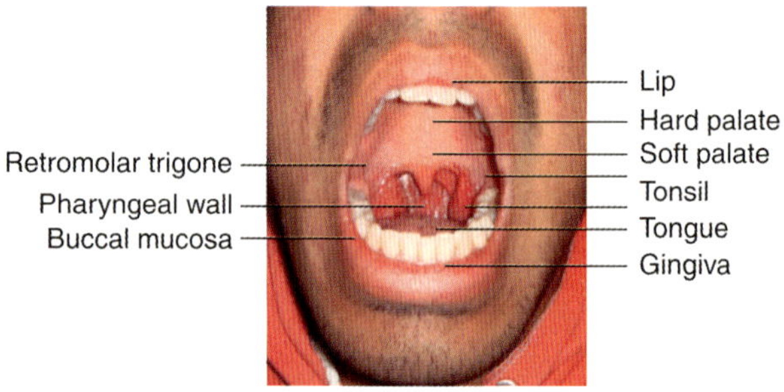

Fig. 42.2. Anatomy of oral cavity.

  - Hypopharynx, which is the lower part of the pharynx, includes the pyriform sinuses, the posterior surface of the larynx (postcricoid area) and the inferoposterior, and inferolateral pharyngeal walls.
- The larynx (voice box) contains the vocal cords and epiglottis. It is divided into three anatomic regions: the supraglottic larynx, the glottic larynx (true vocal cords and the anterior and posterior commissures) and the subglottic larynx.
- The nasal cavity and the paranasal sinuses, which include the maxillary, ethmoid, sphenoid, and frontal sinuses.
- The major salivary glands (parotid, submandibular, and sublingual) and the minor salivary glands, which are located throughout the submucosa of the mouth and upper aerodigestive tract, including the oral cavity (especially the palate), paranasal sinuses, larynx, and pharynx.

Most head and neck cancers begin in the mucosal surfaces of the head and neck region (upper aero-digestive tract) and are predominantly squamous cell carcinomas.

STAGING

The tumour node metastases (TNM) staging system of the American Joint Committee on Cancer (AJCC) and the International Union for Cancer Control (UICC) is used to classify cancers of the head & neck. The T classifications indicate the extent of the primary tumour and are site specific; there is considerable overlap in the cervical node (N) classifications.

TNM staging tables are separated according to head & neck site.

- Oral cavity
- Nasopharynx
- Oropharynx
- Hypopharynx
- Larynx
- Nasal cavity and paranasal sinuses
- Salivary glands

For example, Tumour node metastases (TNM) staging system for cancer of the **lip and oral cavity primary tumour (T)**

TX	Primary tumour cannot be assessed
T0	No evidence of primary tumour
Tis	Carcinoma in situ
T1	Tumour 2 cm or less in greatest dimension
T2	Tumour more than 2 cm but not more than 4 cm in greatest dimension
T3	Tumour more than 4 cm in greatest dimension
T4a	Moderately advanced local disease*

Lip: Tumour invades through cortical bone, inferior alveolar nerve, floor of mouth, or skin of face, i.e., chin or nose.

Oral cavity: Tumour invades adjacent structures only, e.g., through cortical bone (mandible or maxilla), into deep (extrinsic) muscle of tongue (genioglossus, hyoglossus, palatoglossus, and styloglossus), maxillary sinus, skin of face.

T4b Very advanced local disease

Tumour invades masticator space, pterygoid plates, or skull base and/or encases internal carotid artery.

* Superficial erosion alone of bone/tooth socket by gingival primary is not sufficient to classify a tumour as T4.

Regional lymph nodes (N)

NX	Regional lymph nodes cannot be assessed
N0	No regional lymph node metastasis
N1	Metastasis in a single ipsilateral lymph node, 3 cm or less in greatest dimension
N2	Metastasis in a single ipsilateral lymph node, more than 3 cm but not more than 6 cm in greatest dimension; or in multiple ipsilateral lymph nodes, none more than 6 cm in greatest dimension; or in bilateral or contralateral lymph nodes, none more than 6 cm in greatest dimension
N2a	Metastasis in single ipsilateral lymph node more than 3 cm but not more than 6 cm in greatest dimension
N2b	Metastasis in multiple ipsilateral lymph nodes, none more than 6 cm in greatest dimension
N2c	Metastasis in bilateral or contralateral lymph nodes, none more than 6 cm in greatest dimension
N3	Metastasis in a lymph node more than 6 cm in greatest dimension

Distant metastasis (M)

M0	No distant metastasis
M1	Distant metastasis

Anatomic stage/prognostic groups

Stage 0	Tis	N0	M0
Stage I	T1	N0	M0
Stage II	T2	N0	M0
Stage III	T3	N0	M0
	T1	N1	M0
	T2	N1	M0
	T3	N1	M0
Stage IVA	T4a	N0	M0
	T4a	N1	M0
	T1	N2	M0
	T2	N2	M0
	T3	N2	M0
	T4a	N2	M0
Stage IVB	Any T	N3	M0
	T4b	Any N	M0
Stage IVC	Any T	Any N	M1

Note: cTNM is the clinical classification, pTNM is the pathologic classification.

42

SPECIAL CIRCUMSTANCES

Head and neck cancers occurring at certain sites, including the nasopharynx, nasal vestibule and cavity, paranasal sinuses, and salivary glands, and/or in certain circumstances, i.e., cancer of unknown primary and human papilloma-virus associated head and neck squamous cell carcinomas (HNSCCs), have different histology and biology than typical HNSCCs and have particular treatment considerations.

Nasopharyngeal cancer

Nasopharyngeal cancer differs from other head and neck cancers in its epidemiology, pathology, natural history, and treatment. Radiation therapy (RT) is the mainstay of treatment for nasopharyngeal cancer, but the integration of chemotherapy has been instrumental in improving survival for advanced stage disease. Surgery is not typically used because of the deep anatomical location of the nasopharynx and its close proximity to critical neurovascular structures.

Nasal vestibule and nasal cavity cancers

Tumours of the nasal vestibule are essentially skin cancers and are treated with surgery and/or RT, depending on size and location within the nasal vestibule. Cancers of the nasal cavity are similar to those that occur in the paranasal sinuses, and have a wide variety of histologies. Both early and moderately advanced tumours of the nasal cavity are treated with surgical resection and postoperative radiation.

Paranasal sinus cancer

Paranasal sinus cancers encompass multiple histologies, with adenocarcinoma and squamous cell carcinoma being predominant. Aggressive surgical resection remains the mainstay of treatment, but multimodality approaches with surgery, RT, and chemotherapy may be appropriate for certain histologies and for advanced stage cancers.

Salivary gland cancers

Salivary gland tumours represent a wide array of benign and malignant histologies that occur in salivary gland tissue throughout the head and neck. Surgical extirpation of the salivary gland is important in diagnosis and treatment. Patients with benign and low-grade tumours are typically treated with surgery alone, whereas patients with high-grade carcinomas and other high-risk features are usually treated with surgery and postoperative RT.

Cancer of unknown primary

Squamous cell carcinoma of occult (unknown) primary that involves the upper cervical lymph nodes most likely originated from a head and neck primary, while squamous cell carcinomas involving the lower neck may represent metastases from a head and neck, esophagus, lung, gastrointestinal, or genitourinary tract primary. Patients without other obvious sites of metastatic disease (e.g., lung, liver, or bone) should be treated with definitive therapy for locoregional disease.

Human papillomavirus-associated oropharynx cancer

Human papillomavirus (HPV) infection has been established as a causative agent for HNSCC. HPV-associated HNSCCs occur primarily in the oropharynx (tonsils and base of tongue), account for the changing epidemiology of oropharyngeal squamous cell carcinoma, and define a subset of patients with improved clinical behavior and treatment outcome. However, the use of HPV status in clinical decision-making remains investigational at this time.

EARLY STAGE

Approximately 30 to 40 percent of patients with head and neck squamous cell carcinomas (HNSCCs) present with early (stages I and II) disease. In general, these patients are treated with either primary surgery or definitive radiation therapy (RT). Because both modalities result in similar rates of local control and survival, the choice is typically based upon surgical accessibility of the tumour and the functional outcomes and morbidity associated with each modality. In general, surgery is used as the main modality of treatment in the oral cavity, whereas RT is more commonly used in the other mucosal sites.

When surgery is used, traditional surgical approaches, i.e., wide local excision, are usually used for oral cavity cancers, which are easily accessible. Minimally invasive surgery techniques, such as transoral laser resection and robotic surgery, have demonstrated improvements in access, functional outcomes, and morbidity for cancers at other sites, such as the oropharynx and larynx, which are not easily approached with standard instruments.

Definitive radiation therapy (RT) approaches incorporate external beam therapy and brachytherapy. As with surgery, advances in RT techniques and delivery, such as three-dimensional conformal treatment planning (3D-CRT, with intensity modulated RT [IMRT] and image-guided RT [IGRT]), have demonstrated improved efficacy and reduced morbidity.

For patients treated with primary surgery, postoperative RT with or without concurrent chemoradiation is indicated for close or positive margins and other risk factors including perineural invasion and lymphovascular invasion.

ADVANCED STAGE

Historically, local therapy alone, i.e., primary surgery or definitive radiation therapy (RT), for locoregionally advanced (stages III, IVA, and IVB) head and neck squamous cell carcinomas (HNSCCs) resulted in high rates of locoregional recurrence and considerable morbidity, including loss of tongue and larynx function (speech and swallowing). The risk for distant metastasis after local therapy is also high. The integration of chemotherapy into standard surgery and/or RT has improved survival and permitted organ function preservation for many patients with locoregionally advanced HNSCC.

Effective approaches for locoregionally advanced HNSCC include primary surgery followed by either postoperative RT or concurrent chemoradiation (CRT), induction chemotherapy (the addition of chemotherapy prior to surgery and/or RT), concurrent CRT, and sequential therapy (induction chemotherapy followed by concurrent CRT). Decisions about the sequencing and selection of surgery, RT, and/or chemotherapy should be made with multidisciplinary input; tailored to the individual patient, disease sites, and the likely functional consequences and morbidity of each treatment approach; and take into account the experience and technology available at the medical institution.

RADIATION SCHEDULE

A standard approach for patients treated with concurrent CRT is to use conventional fractionation external beam RT often with three-dimensional conformal treatment planning (3D-CRT), including intensity-modulated RT (IMRT) and image-guided RT (IGRT). Conventional RT typically delivers 70 Gray (Gy) in 2 Gy daily fractions, over seven weeks. Most common chemotherapy regimen used with concurrent radiotherapy is cisplatin 30 to 40 mg/m^2 weekly. Other agents which are used with RT include Carboplatin, Paclitaxel, Hydroxyurea and recently approved molecularly targeted therapy against EGFR receptor-Cetuximab.

INDUCTION CHEMOTHERAPY REGIMEN

Early clinical trials established cisplatin and 5-fluorouracil (PF, cisplatin, 100 mg/m^2, and 5-fluorouracil, 1000 mg/m^2 continuous 24-hour infusion for five days) as the standard regimen for induction chemotherapy; it is associated with higher rates of complete response and survival relative to other cisplatin and bleomycin-based regimens and regimens with shorter infusions of 5-fluorouracil. However, the addition of a taxane, paclitaxel or docetaxel to PF induction chemotherapy has enhanced the effectiveness of contemporary induction chemotherapy.

For organ preservation in hypopharynx and larynx cancer, the addition of docetaxel to the standard cisplatin and 5-fluorouracil induction regimen (TPF, docetaxel 75 mg/m^2 day 1, cisplatin 75 mg/m^2 day 1, and 5-fluorouracil 750 mg/m^2 continuous infusion days 1 to 5) for 3 cycles q3 weekly resulted in improved larynx preservation. The three-year actuarial larynx preservation rate was 70 percent following TPF versus 58 percent with PF.

Surgery is generally preferred for oral cavity squamous cell carcinomas (OCSCCs) since most cases are easily accessible, and simultaneous resection and reconstruction can be accomplished with acceptable functional outcomes. However, since OCSCCs are aggressive cancers with high rates of locoregional recurrence, postoperative RT with or without chemotherapy should be strongly considered. Definitive radiation therapy (RT), concurrent chemoradiation (CRT), and sequential therapy are typically reserved for patients who are medically inoperable, who have unresectable disease, or who have resectable disease where surgical resection cannot be accomplished with acceptable long-term functional consequences (e.g., total glossectomy).

In contrast, organ sparing approaches rather than primary surgery are preferred for most patients with resectable cancers of the oropharynx, hypopharynx, and larynx. Concurrent CRT is a standard option for organ function preservation, but sequential therapy may be preferable in certain circumstances, in particular, for patients with advanced primary tumours (T4b) and/or advanced nodal disease. Unresectable cancers of the oropharynx, hypopharynx, and larynx are treated with concurrent CRT or sequential therapy. Definitive RT remains a treatment option for elderly patients and those with a poor performance status.

LOCALLY RECURRENT AND METASTATIC DISEASE

Most patients with recurrent disease have a poor prognosis, with a median survival of six to nine months. Treatment options are limited by previous treatment received. All patients with locoregionally recurrent disease should be evaluated for distant metastases prior to initiating retreatment. Those with a good performance status and whose disease is confined to the head and neck may benefit from surgical salvage and/or reirradiation. However, many patients with locally recurrent and metastatic disease are most appropriate for palliative chemotherapy and/or supportive care. Many chemotherapy agents, both conventional and molecularly targeted, have activity in metastatic and recurrent HNSCC, i.e., Cetuximab, Cisplatin and Carboplatin, Docetaxel, Erlotinib, Etoposide, Fluorouracil and Capecitabine, Gefitinib, Gemcitabine, Irinotecan, Liposomal doxorubicin, Methotrexate, Paclitaxel and Pemetrexed.

MANAGEMENT OF THE NECK

Head and neck squamous cell carcinomas (HNSCCs) frequently metastasize to the cervical lymph nodes, an occurrence that has a markedly negative impact on prognosis. Consequently, treatment of the cervical neck nodes, even if involvement is clinically occult, is often part of the treatment strategy for HNSCC.

The risk of developing nodal metastases varies by primary tumour site and factors such as size, histology, tumour thickness, and perineural invasion. Most agree that when the probability of occult metastases exceeds 20 percent, the risk of neck recurrence without elective (prophylactic) treatment is sufficiently high to outweigh the morbidity of neck dissection and/or irradiation.

RECONSTRUCTION AND REHABILITATION FOR SURGICAL DEFECTS

Surgical resection of the mandible, palate, and the larynx can lead to problems in airway management, mastication, deglutition, speech, and cosmesis. Function is also impaired by radiation therapy and chemotherapy.

Prosthetic rehabilitation of patients with hard palate defects (the result of tumour resections involving the maxilla) consists of placement of an obturator prosthesis, which serves to restore orofacial functions, including deglutition, control of secretions, mastication, phonetics, and to aesthetically replace the missing orofacial structures. Surgical reconstruction alone or combined with an obturator prosthesis can be used to remedy palatal defects. In addition, a variety of reconstruction options, including free flaps and autogenous bone grafts, are available to restore mandibular defects. (Speech and swallowing rehabilitation are critical to restoring function and quality of life.)

COMPLICATIONS

Treatment-related toxicity associated with treatment, whether surgery, radiation therapy, and/or chemotherapy, for head and neck cancer is substantial and negatively impacts upon patient quality of life.

Throughout the course of therapy, including surgery, radiation, and chemotherapy, complications can arise which also have the potential to be severe, and sometimes fatal. Due to the anatomic location of the vital organs of speech, swallowing, and respiration, the side effects of treatment for HNC are more common than similar treatments for cancers at other sites. It is critical that these side effects be discussed with patients prior to therapy. This is particularly important when multiple therapeutic options exist for their HNC, and considerations of toxicities might have an impact on treatment choice.

The specific complications include:

- Airway compromise
- Swallowing dysfunction (including dysphagia, odynophagia, stricture, and tongue complications)
- Speech complications (including hoarseness and loss of normal speech)
- Soft tissue and bone complications (including soft tissue edema, fibrosis, necrosis, and osteoradionecrosis)

- Vascular complications ("carotid blowout", carotid artery stenosis, and ischemic stroke)
- Pain
- Xerostomia and change in sputum consistency
- Cosmetic deformities
- Alteration of taste
- Mucositis
- Aspiration pneumonia, oral infections, and soft tissue infections
- Hypothyroidism
- Scarring, fibrosis and esophageal stenosis
- Psychosocial distress.

DISEASE RELATED DYSFUNCTION AT PRESENTATION

Many presenting symptoms and potential complications are dependent upon the primary tumour site. In general, however, patients with HNC most commonly come to medical attention because of site nonspecific symptoms such as pain (oral pain, odynophagia, or otalgia), hoarseness, dysphagia, or after noticing an asymptomatic mass in the neck. Loose teeth may be a manifestation of tumours of the mandible, maxilla, hard palate or maxillary sinus.

Beyond the uncomfortable symptoms described above, patients may have other complications at presentation that can lead to severe morbidity and, rarely, mortality.

Weight loss and malnutrition are common, generally as a result of direct interference with oral intake or pharyngeal function. Weight loss due to the tumour itself (cancer-related cachexia) is less common.

The magnitude or the importance of weight loss may be multiplied by the frequent comorbidities in this patient population (e.g., complications of smoking or alcohol abuse).

Cranial nerve abnormalities, most frequently seen with large tumours of the nasopharynx, most commonly involve the fifth and sixth nerves, followed by the twelfth, third, and fourth cranial nerves. Parotid cancers may present with facial nerve dysfunction.

Respiratory or airway compromise is another frequent complication found on presentation with HNC. In particular, patients with laryngeal tumours or bulky pharyngeal tumours may present with progressive or acute shortness of breath or stridor. Some of these patients will require an emergency tracheotomy, which may need to be performed with the patient awake, as a result of airway compromise.

Aspiration pneumonia, due to loss of normal pharyngeal motility, epiglottic distortion, cranial nerve abnormalities, or decreased level of awareness, is common and can be severe.

COMPLICATIONS OF SURGERY

Most surgical complications are subsite specific. Common to any of the surgical procedures is the possibility for cosmetic deformities. With the advent of soft tissue transfers, advances in surgical techniques, and organ preservation approaches, these are somewhat less common than they were in the past. Nonetheless, major or even minor surgical defects in these areas may be very evident because of their location on the face and neck, resulting in emotional and psychological distress (Fig. 42.3).

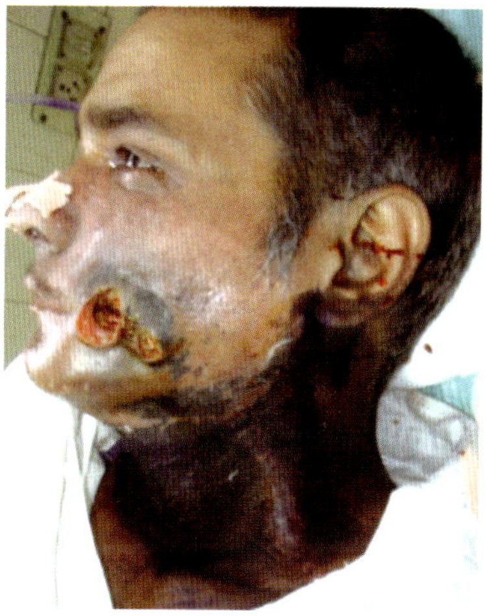

Fig. 42.3. Cosmetic deformity of surgery and chemoradiation.

Oral cavity

Patients who undergo partial glossectomy for T1 or T2 anterior or lateral tumours usually have reasonably good function postoperatively. Some have mild speech impairment or swallowing dysfunction that may lead to altered diet and/or aspiration.

Total or near-total glossectomy leads to severe deficits in speech and swallowing. Surgical procedures for tumours involving the gingiva, mandible, maxilla and retromolar trigone may lead to malocclusion or temporomandibular joint (TMJ) dysfunction. In addition, flap failure or revision may complicate microvascular free flaps used in oral

42

cavity reconstruction to improve cosmesis and function. The use of preoperative radiotherapy does not appear to predispose to flap failure.

Oropharynx

Oropharyngeal surgery, including tonsillar resection for tumours requiring more than just simple tonsillectomy, soft palate procedures, base of tongue resection, or pharyngeal wall resection, frequently causes swallowing dysfunction. Altered diet and limitation of oral intake may occur, and aspiration pneumonitis is common in this setting. In addition, a pharyngeal stricture may develop following therapy, limiting oral intake or requiring a change in diet, and airway edema may lead to airway compromise and the need for tracheostomy.

Larynx

Partial laryngectomy may be associated with significant hoarseness or preservation of some or all of the normal voice features, and may lead to swallowing dysfunction and an increased risk of aspiration. Approximately 20 percent of patients require prolonged tracheostomy due to edema induced by surgery or subsequent radiation therapy.

Total laryngectomy imparts less of a risk of aspiration since the larynx no longer communicates with the upper airway. There are some exceptions to this general rule. On occasion, a tracheo-esophageal fistula develops either naturally or as a result of a tracheoesophageal puncture (TEP) surgically placed for voice restoration. The main adverse effect of total laryngectomy is the loss of natural voice. Additional complications include pharyngocutaneous fistulae and stomal stenosis.

Neck dissection

Patients who undergo surgery for HNC frequently undergo neck dissection for management of occult or clinically evident malignant lymphadenopathy. Complications of neck dissection are dependent upon the extent and type of dissection.

Patients having a classic radical neck dissection (RND) undergo resection of the spinal accessory nerve with resulting denervation of the trapezius muscle and destabilization of the scapula. A shoulder syndrome results, with pain and weakness of the shoulder and a shoulder girdle deformity. In addition, the cervical plexus may be injured, resulting in neuropathic pain and sensory loss in the anterolateral neck extending to the shoulder.

Modified and selective neck dissections lead to less morbidity than an RND. However, shoulder pain, disability, and weakness may still occur after these nerve-sparing procedures.

Early diagnosis of shoulder syndrome and prompt initiation of physical therapy are encouraged to reduce pain and disability. A program of progressive resistance exercise training as compared to a standard therapeutic exercise protocol has been shown to improve shoulder pain and disability in patients presenting with shoulder dysfunction.

Other potential complications include hardening of the tissues of the neck or face, and facial, submental, or less commonly, cerebral edema. This is generally worse with bilateral neck dissection, or when neck dissection follows or precedes radiation, and is caused by venous and lymphatic compromise. Postoperative bleeding, infection, chylous fistula, and, rarely, blindness due to posterior ischemic optic neuropathy, can also occur. Contractures or loss of normal range of motion of the neck can occur, especially if neck dissection is combined with radiotherapy.

Carotid artery rupture

In some cases, especially when surgery is coupled with radiation, vascular compromise leads to devastating complications. Rupture of the carotid artery (sometimes called "carotid blowout syndrome") is most common in the setting of a surgically exposed carotid artery with limited residual normal tissue to cover it, recurrent tumour, infection, or severe radiation damage. Although this devastating complication can sometimes be managed with endovascular therapy, it recurs in up to 25 percent of patients often as a manifestation of recurrent tumour or of multifocal iatrogenic arteriopathy and occasional wound complications.

Hard palate and sinuses

Surgical procedures on the hard and soft palate or sinuses may lead to major defects in speech or swallowing[3]. As an example, nasal regurgitation of food and altered voice may occur after hard palate surgery. Resection of the hard palate, and in some instances, the soft palate requires reconstruction with soft tissue flaps or prostheses to restore or maximize speech, swallowing and mastication.

COMPLICATIONS OF RADIATION AND CHEMORADIATION

Complications of these therapies are included together since, in general, the complications of concurrent chemotherapy plus radiation are similar qualitatively, although the acute complications of concurrent therapy are often more severe than those of radiation alone.

Radiotherapy complications are somewhat site-specific, and radiation fields, particularly for advanced disease, may encompass tissue beyond the primary site. The neck and oral and pharyngeal mucosa may be included in the field to encompass gross disease and suspected microscopic disease. This increases the potential for complications beyond the involved HNC subsite.

Acute complications include mucositis, dysphagia, pain, hoarseness, dermatitis, weight loss, xerostomia, loss of taste, and thick sputum and secretions

Acute complications

The acute side effects and complications of radiation with or without chemotherapy are more predictable than the chronic toxicities, and are dependent upon the dose and schedule of radiation used and the accompanying chemotherapy drugs.

Mucositis is a predictable complication. When aggressive regimens are used, mucositis is sufficiently severe that gastrostomy feeding tubes are required in 50 percent or more patients. Weight loss, even with full gastrostomy support, generally accompanies mucositis. With aggressive regimens, weight loss of 8 to 10 percent of body weight is common even with early gastrostomy support.

Dermatitis occurs commonly in the radiation field. The spectrum of effects ranges from hyper-pigmentation and dry desquamation of the epithelial layers to moist desquamation and skin necrosis.

The most common long-term complication of treatment within the oral cavity is xerostomia, which occurs to some degree in up to 100 percent of patients undergoing radiotherapy for the oral cavity or oropharynx. Although xerostomia begins during treatment, it often manifests fully only after healing of mucositis. Xerostomia is dose dependent and severe xerostomia nearly always occurs with doses exceeding 50 Gy to the bilateral parotid glands. Improvement in xerostomia over time has been demonstrated to result from parotid-sparing radiation therapy.

Pilocarpine may improve or prevent xerostomia when given before or after completing radiotherapy. Improvement in symptoms may occur only after many weeks of treatment, and cholinergic side effects, in particular sweating, may stop a significant number of patients from continuing the drug.

The other important adjunctive drug that has been used in an attempt to diminish xerostomia is amifostine. In three randomized trials in patients with HNC receiving radiation therapy, concurrent daily intravenous amifostine reduced the incidence, severity, and duration of mucositis, and/or diminished post-treatment dry mouth and eating difficulties, compared to placebo. Other studies have been less positive.

Cost, the inconvenience of daily intravenous infusion, and side effects have limited the widespread use of amifostine. A possible alternative route of administration is subcutaneous which, during radiation therapy, appears to provide similar toxicity protection as the intravenous route, and is more convenient, less expensive, and may be better tolerated. Even with subcutaneous administration, as many as 25 percent of patients will not complete a full course of this drug in conjunction with their radiation. The benefit of amifostine when given in conjunction with concurrent chemoradiation and/ or with parotid sparing IMRT is not well defined.

Dental caries are very common after radio-therapy. The treatment of dental caries becomes more difficult after radiotherapy; in particular, tooth extraction is made difficult because of the tendency toward non-healing and osteoradionecrosis following radiotherapy. Thus, patients should have pre-treatment dental evaluation to include necessary tooth extractions, and to initiate fluoride treatments, and other preventative dental and oral hygiene. Long-term follow-up by an experienced dentist should also be provided. Preliminary data suggest a possible benefit of amifostine on the prevention of dental caries following radiation therapy of HNC.

Late effects

A number of late sequelae can occur at various sites within the head and neck. These include sub-cutaneous fibrosis, skin ulceration and necrosis, thyroid dysfunction, pharyngeal and esophageal stenosis, swallowing dysfunction, xerostomia, hoarseness, dysphonia, cartilage necrosis, osteoradionecrosis (particularly of the mandible), delayed wound healing, fistulae, dental decay, damage to the middle or inner ear, myelopathy, ischemic stroke, carotid stenosis, and neck contractures.

Osteoradionecrosis

Osteoradionecrosis of the jaw (ORN) is a severe complication of RT for HNC. The presentation of post-RT ORN ranges from small asymptomatic bone exposures that remain stable for months to years and heal with conservative management, to severe necrosis necessitating surgical intervention and reconstruction. Depending on the location and extent of the lesion, symptoms can include pain, bad breath, dysgeusia, dysesthesia or anesthesia, trismus, difficulty with mastication, deglutition, and/or speech, fistula formation, pathologic fracture, and local, spreading, or systemic infection.

The mandible is the most frequently affected bone, because in the majority of patients treated for HNC, a large part is inevitably exposed to high RT doses. Possibly because of the collateral circulation it receives, maxillary ORN is reported infrequently. It is most often seen in the setting of irradiation for nasopharyngeal cancer (in which both jaws are at risk).

Mandibular ORN occurs in 5 to 10 percent of patients treated with conventional RT or high dose rate brachytherapy, and is severe in about 2 percent. The incidence of this complication appears to be higher with hyperfractionated regimens, especially with a short interfraction interval.

Tooth extraction and dental disease in irradiated regions are major factors in the development of both mandibular and maxillary ORN. Although opinion differs as to pre-irradiation versus post-irradiation, many authors report that post-irradiation extraction of diseased and nonrestorable teeth produces a higher rate of mandibular ORN. Furthermore, at least some data suggest that mandibular ORN associated with post-irradiation extraction more often requires radical resection than cases of ORN that develop after pre-irradiation extraction. Repair of nonrestorable and diseased teeth prior to RT may reduce the risk of this complication. However, most authorities do not recommend the pre-irradiation extraction of healthy or restorable teeth.

Treatment

For mild osteoradionecrosis, treatment with conservative debridement, antibiotics, and occasionally ultrasound is usually successful. Some authors advocate pentoxifylline and vitamin E. However, when bone and soft tissue necrosis are extensive, radical resection of the mandible with immediate microvascular reconstruction may provide better results. Persistent ORN, despite aggressive treatment, should raise the suspicion of recurrent cancer.

Hyperbaric oxygen therapy (HBO) has been suggested as a beneficial therapeutic manoeuvre in patients developing ORN of the jaw after RT. ORN may be triggered by a predominantly fibro-atrophic mechanism. At least in theory, HBO simulates the function of monocytes and fibroblasts, increasing collagen synthesis and vascular density.

RT-induced fibrosis

A serious complication of RT in the treatment of cancer patients is the late onset of fibrosis in normal tissues including the neck, pharynx and/or esophagus (leading to a pharyngoesophageal stricture), and temporomandibular joint. At least some data suggest benefit from pentoxifylline, with or without alpha-tocopherol (vitamin E).

Thyroid dysfunction

Irradiation of the low neck is associated with hypothyroidism, detectable by an elevation in serum TSH, but clinically significant in only a limited number of patients. The incidence varies widely and is dose-dependent as well as time-dependent, increasing with time elapsed since treatment.

Most of these cases reflect primary hypothyroidism (i.e., caused by damage to the thyroid gland itself), but some are centrally mediated (i.e., caused by damage to the hypothalamus or pituitary region).

RT-induced hypothyroidism develops at a median of 1.4 to 1.8 years (range 0.3 to 7.2 years). It is more common in patients undergoing both neck surgery and RT and possibly intensity-modulated RT (IMRT), but is not higher in patients who undergo chemotherapy in addition to radiation compared to radiation alone. Although some studies suggest that this complication is more frequent in women than in men, this is not a universal finding.

For patients treated with neck RT, expert groups recommend that serum TSH should be checked within 12 months of completing therapy and repeated every 6 to 12 months.

COMPLICATIONS SPECIFIC TO CHEMOTHERAPY

In general, the complications of chemotherapy given for HNC are not unique to these patients. The most common drugs used in the treatment of HNC include cisplatin and carboplatin, 5-fluorouracil, and the taxanes, paclitaxel and docetaxel.

The main unique side effects of cisplatin and carboplatin are neurotoxicity, nephrotoxicity, and ototoxicity. These can be severe and irreversible and are all more common with cisplatin than carboplatin.

Fluorouracil commonly causes mucositis (independent of radiation), diarrhea, and acral erythema (also called hand-foot syndrome or palmar-plantar erythrodysesthesia). Mucositis and acral erythema are more common when fluorouracil is given by prolonged infusion, as it is frequently administered in patients with HNC. Fluorouracil is also the second most common chemotherapy drug causing cardiotoxicity, after the anthracyclines. Infusional regimens are more likely to cause this complication than are bolus regimens. The most common symptom is chest pain associated with electrocardiographic changes. The taxanes can cause an acute allergic reaction during infusion or shortly after the infusion of the drug is stopped. This can usually be prevented by pretreatment with steroids

Peripheral neuropathies (generally cumulative) and myalgias (not as cumulative) are also common with the taxanes. Fluid retention often occurs with docetaxel, and its onset can be delayed with concomitant treatment with corticosteroids. High dose therapy may also be associated with pulmonary toxicity.

As with most chemotherapy drugs, these drugs may all cause myelosuppression, which may predispose to sepsis, and nausea and vomiting, which is especially common with cisplatin.

POSTTREATMENT EVALUATION AND SURVEILLANCE

Upon completion of therapy, post-treatment imaging is important to evaluate for residual disease and establish a baseline. However, imaging should not be performed too soon. Obtaining imaging studies, in particular positron emission tomography-computed tomography (PET-CT) scans, prior to 12 weeks following treatment can lead to false positive results. We recommend waiting at least four to six weeks following radiation or chemoradiation therapy for CT scans or magnetic resonance imaging (MRI) and 8 to 12 weeks for PET scans.

Regular post-treatment follow-up has become an essential part of the care of patients after potentially curative treatment of head and neck cancer. Patients should be educated about possible signs and symptoms of tumour recurrence, including hoarseness, pain, dysphagia, bleeding, and enlarged lymph nodes.

In general, the intensity of follow-up is greatest in the first two to four years, since approximately 80 to 90 percent of all recurrences after curative intent treatment will occur within this timeframe, while the risk of second primary malignancy is higher than recurrence risk for most patients beyond three years. However, continued follow-up is generally suggested since the risk of recurrence (and second primary malignancy) remains elevated beyond the first five years, especially for cancers of the hypopharynx, larynx, nasopharynx, and salivary glands. Because of the higher risk of recurrence and second primary malignancy in those who continue tobacco use, many schedule more frequent surveillance visits for these patients and continue for longer duration (i.e., beyond five years).

CONCLUSION

Selection of treatment for head and neck squamous cell carcinoma (HNSCC) depends upon tumour site and stage, the functional outcomes and morbidity associated with various treatment approaches, and patient-related factors, such as performance status, comorbidities, and preference. A multidisciplinary approach, including surgeons, medical oncologists, and radiation oncologists, as well as dentists, dieticians, and rehabilitation therapists, is generally required for treatment planning and managing patients with head and neck cancer.

Patients with early (stages I and II) HNSCC are generally managed with single modality treatment, either surgery or radiation therapy (RT).

Patients with advanced (stages III, IVA, and IVB) HNSCC are typically managed with multimodality treatment; organ function sparing approaches are preferred.

Effective approaches for locoregionally advanced HNSCC include:

1. Primary surgery followed by either postoperative RT or concurrent chemoradiation (CRT).

2. Induction chemotherapy (the addition of chemotherapy prior to surgery and/or RT).
3. Concurrent CRT.
4. Sequential therapy (induction chemotherapy followed by concurrent CRT).

Most patients with locally recurrent and metastatic disease are most appropriate for palliative chemotherapy and/or supportive care, but select patients with disease confined to the head and neck may benefit from surgical salvage and/or reirradiation. Treatment of the cervical neck nodes, even if involvement is clinically occult, is often part of the treatment strategy for HNSCC. Regular posttreatment follow-up is an essential part of the care of patients after potentially curative treatment of head and neck cancer.

SUGGESTED READING

1. Cancer – Principles and Practice of Oncology by DeVita, Hellman, Rosenberg, DePinho and Weinberg, 8th Edition, 2008.
2. Vokes EE, Weichselbaum RR, Lippman SM, Hong WK. Head and neck cancer. *N Engl J Med*, 1993; 328: 184–194.
3. Herrmann, T, Baumann, M, Dörr, W. Clinical Radiation Biology. Munich, Germany: Elsevier; 2006.
4. Dörr W, Hendry JH. Consequential late effects in normal tissues. *Radiother Oncol*, 2001; 61: 223–31.
5. Pointreau Y, Garaud P, Chapet S, et al. Randomized trial of induction chemotherapy with cisplatin and 5-fluorouracil with or without docetaxel for larynx preservation. *J Natl Cancer Inst*, 2009; 101: 498–506.
6. Edge, SB, Byrd, DR, Compton, CC, et al (Eds). AJCC (American Joint Committee on Cancer) Cancer Staging Manual, 7th ed, Springer, New York, 2010.
7. Furness S, Glenny AM, Worthington HV, et al. Interventions for the treatment of oral cavity and oropharyngeal cancer: chemotherapy. *Cochrane Database Syst Rev*, 2010; CD006386.
8. Pignon JP, le Maître A, Maillard E, et al. Meta-analysis of chemotherapy in head and neck cancer (MACH-NC): an update on 93 randomised trials and 17, 346 patients. *Radiother Oncol*, 2009; 92: 4–14.

CHAPTER 43

Hair Transplant and the ENT Surgeon

Brajendra Baser

Hair transplantation is a surgical technique that involves moving skin containing hair follicles from one part of the body (the donor site) to bald or balding parts (the recipient site). It is primarily used to treat male pattern baldness, whereby grafts containing hair follicles that are genetically resistant to balding are transplanted to bald scalp. Since hair naturally grows in follicles that contain groupings of 1 to 4 hairs, most advanced techniques transplant these naturally occurring 1–4 hair "follicular units" in their natural groupings. Thus modern hair transplantation can achieve a natural appearance by mimicking nature hair for hair. This recent hair transplant procedure is called "Follicular Unit Transplantation".

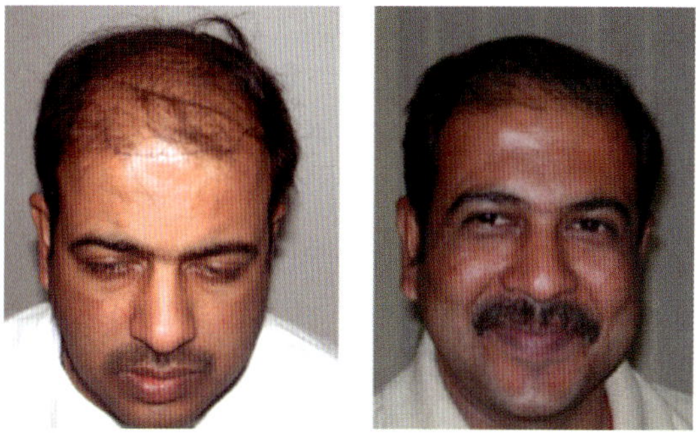

Fig. 43.1. Preoperative and postoperative of hair implant.

The Role of ENT Surgeon

Hair transplant surgery is new to India and most of it is performed by plastic surgeons, dermatologists and maxillofacial surgeons. For some reasons ENT surgeons are little shy to accept new developments. ENT surgeons are familiar with head and neck anatomy, can easily harvest a strip and many have a daycare surgery unit and they can develop and start practising this technically not so difficult procedure. It is definitely rewarding and now with the increasing prosperity in the society many customers are available.

History of Hair Transplant

The origins of hair transplant surgery stem from Japanese dermatologist, Dr. Okuda, who in 1939 published a revolutionary method in a Japanese medical journal of using small grafts that were similar to the way hair transplantation is performed today. This method involved using hair transplant grafts to correct lost hair from various body areas, including the scalp, eyebrow, and moustache areas.

In the late 50s one physician in particular, Dr. Norman Orentreich, began to experiment with the idea of relocating or transplanting the hair from the back and sides of the head to the balding areas. Dr. Orentreich's experiments showed that when bald-resistant hairs from the back and sides of the head were relocated, they maintained their bald-resistant genetic characteristic regardless of where they were transplanted.

This principle, known as Donor Dominance, established that hair could be transplanted from the

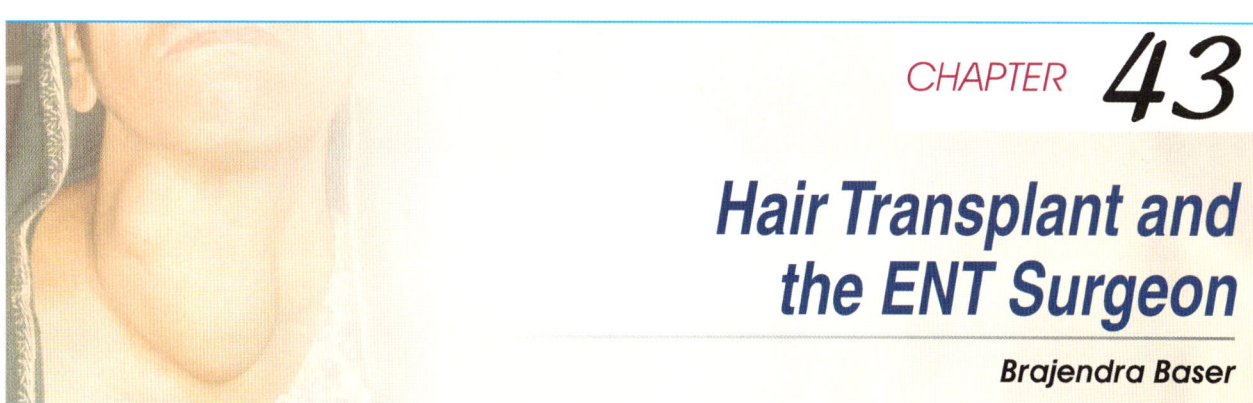

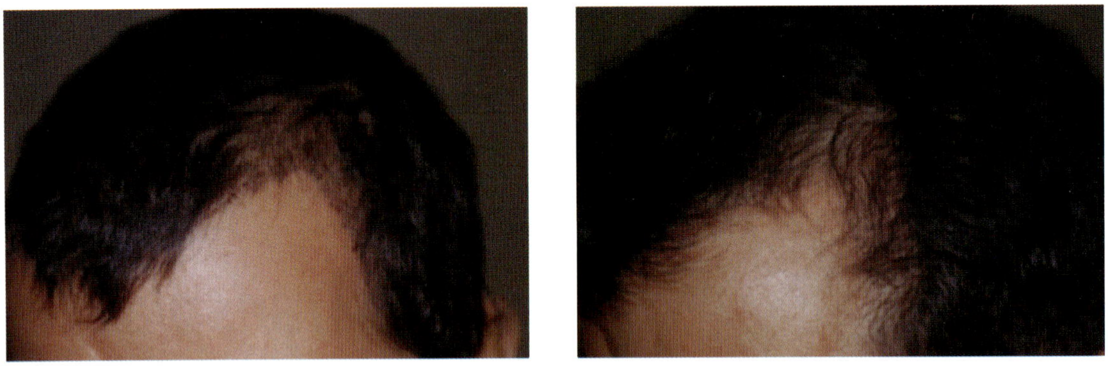

Fig. 43.2.

bald-resistant donor areas to the balding areas and continue to grow for a life time. This laid the foundation for modern hair transplantation. During the 60s and 70s hair transplants grew in popularity. However, the standard of care involved the use of larger grafts that were removed by round punches and often contained many hairs.

In the 80s hair restoration surgery evolved dramatically, as the large punch grafts were gradually replaced with a more refined combination of mini- and micrografts. This combination mini-micrografting hair transplantation procedure no longer used the punch to extract the bald-resistant grafts. Rather a strip of bald-resistant hair was surgically removed from the back of the head and then trimmed into mini- and micrografts.

Types of Hair Transplant

There are two main methods of follicular unit hair transplant surgery. Follicular unit transplant commonly known as FUT or strip surgery and follicular unit extraction, commonly known as FUE. The main difference is the method of extracting the transplanted hair. FUT and FUE are really complimentary forms of HT, not competing methods of which one must make a choice.

FOLLICULAR UNIT TRANSPLANT

43

Technique

Transplant operations are performed on an outpatient basis, with mild sedation (optional) and injected topical anesthesia, and typically last about four hours. The scalp is shampooed and then treated with an antibacterial chemical prior to the donor scalp being harvested.

Donor site

Several methods are used to provide anesthesia to the donor site. Some surgeons prefer to infiltrate the donor site locally or use a ring block using 1% or 2% xylocaine with 1 : 100,000 adrenaline. A 26 No. needle is used to infiltrate the solution.

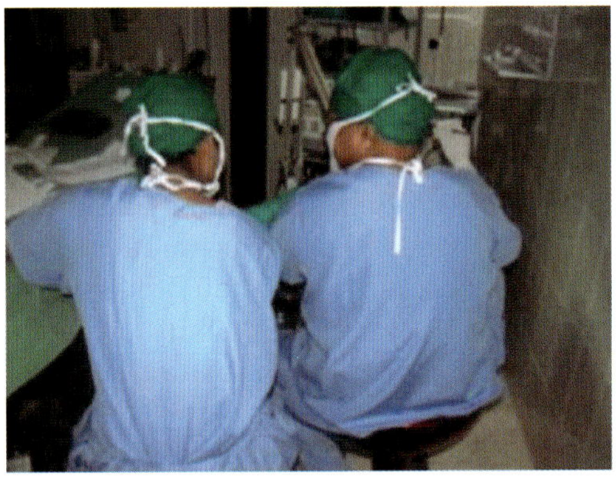

Fig. 43.3. Implant hair unit.

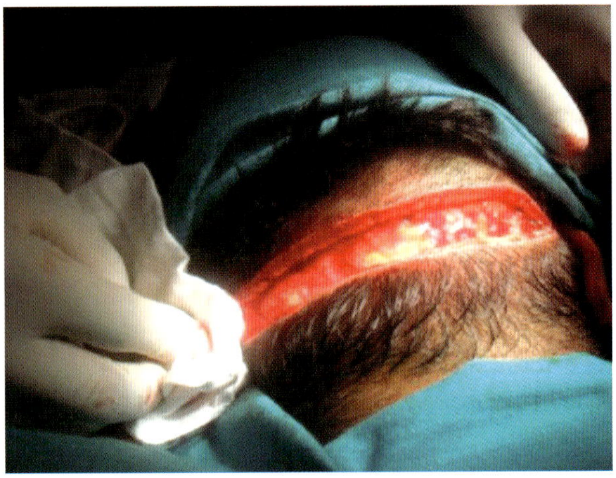

Fig. 43.4. Donor site incision.

Harvesting the strip

The donor site is excised as an elongated fusiform ellipse of full-thickness scalp using a scalpel blade size 10 or 15. Take care when excising not to damage hair follicles at the edge of the donor tissue. The resultant defect is closed using suture or skin staples, and the scar is minimal. Then, donor tissue is dissected carefully into the desired number of grafts, which can vary in size.

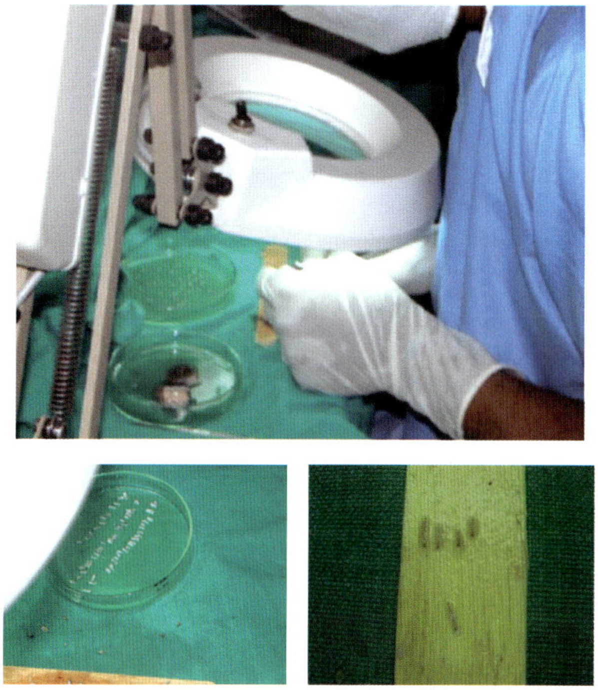

Fig. 43.4. Harvesting graft follicle.

Dissecting follicular units

Grafts harvested by excision or strip harvesting can be cut to single grafts, minigrafts, or micrografts by using a size 15 blade or razor blade. This is done under magnification and a team of technicians can be trained to do this. Each follicular unit may have 1–4 follicles. Care is taken to avoid trauma to the bulb of the hair follicle.

Recipient sites

Local anesthesia is given with ready 2% xylocaine and adrenaline. Sensorocaine can be mixed in the solution for longer duration of anesthesia.

Pain relief can be given with intramuscular diclofenac or pentazocine.

Placing the Graft

Single hair and slit grafting: Using an 18-gauge needle, multiple 0.5 to 3 mm slits are made in the scalp in which the grafts are placed. Single hair or micrografting is most often used to recreate the frontal hairline. The graft is holed with the fat below the follicle and is gently slid in the hole with the help of a microvascular forceps. Closer the graft placement, denser will be the hair growth. A magnifying loupe is of great help in placing the graft.

Postoperative care

Medicated paraffin gauze dressing is kept for 24 hours and removed after that. There is no need for dressing after 24 hours. A short course of antibiotics is generally given for 7 to 10 days.

If non-absorbable sutures are used at the donor site the stitches are removed after 7 days.

Complications

As with any surgical procedure, a risk exists of the following infrequent complications:

- Bleeding
- Infection
- Scarring at donor site
- Scarring at recipient sites
- Dyspigmentation at recipient sites
- Cobblestone appearance at recipient sites
- Failure of graft
- Cyst formation

Postoperative edema is expected; therefore, it is not a complication, although it can be severe.

The FUE transplantation procedure itself involves a different approach to extraction that pinpoints individual follicular grafts from the donor area as opposed to more traditional linear strip extraction. Each follicular unit graft, or compact bundle of 1 to 4 hair follicles, replete with oil glands, muscle and connecting tissue is removed individually and transplanted to the affected hair loss area.

An excellent procedure for selected patients. The transplantation procedure does not result in a linear scar which may be a serious consideration for those who wear their hair short and wish to avoid a linear excision. Patients with very tight scalps or that have existing donor scarring that cannot be excised may also be good candidates.

The most significant drawback to follicular unit extraction (FUE) transplantation is the limit of donor supply and because each follicular unit is removed individually, the procedure takes a considerably larger amount of time. As such, each procedure is limited usually to 500 grafts per session though some skilled surgeons can do more.

CONCLUSION

Hair transplant is a new concept to otorhinolaryngologist, previously it was practised by plastic surgeons, dermatologists and faciomaxillary surgeons. In this technique transfer of hair follicle graft from one part to bald area is done. This procedure is performed in local anesthesia. Hair unit graft is placed using 18-gauge needle with multiple slit in scalp; closer the graft placement better will be the hair growth. Negligible post-op morbidity is seen in this procedure.

SUGGESTED READING

1. Headington JT. Transverse microscopic anatomy of the human scalp. A basis for a morphometric approach to disorders of the hair follicle. *Arch Dermatol*, 1984; 120: 449–56.
2. Orentreich N. Autografts in alopecias and other selected dermatological conditions. *Ann NY Acad Sci*, Nov 20 1959; 83: 463–79. Vogel JE. Hair restoration complications: An approach to the unnatural-appearing hair transplant. *Facial Plast Surg*, 2008; 24: 453–61.
3. Beehner M. Hairline design in hair replacement surgery. *Facial Plast Surg*, 2008; 24: 389–403.
4. Rousso DE, Presti PM. Follicular unit transplantation. *Facial Plast Surg*, 2008; 24: 381–8.
5. Limmer BL. Elliptical donor stereoscopically assisted micrografting as an approach to further refinement in hair transplantation. *J Dermatol Surg Oncol*, 1994; 20: 789–93.
6. Hamilton JB. Patterned loss of hair in man; types and incidence. *Ann NY Acad Sci*, 1951; 53: 708–28.
7. Seager D. Binocular stereoscopic dissecting microscoping – should we use them? *Hair Transplant Forum Int*, 1996; 6: 2–5.
8. Bernstein RM, Rassman WR, Szaniawski W. Follicular transplantation. *Int J Aesthetic Restor Surg*, 1995; 3: 119–32.
9. Bradshaw W, Unger WP, Nordstrom REA, eds. Quarter-grafts: a technique for minigrafts. *In:* Hair Transplantation. 2nd ed. New York, NY: Marcel Dekker; 1988: 333–51.
10. Fujita K. Reconstruction of eyebrow. *La Lepro*, 1943; 22: 364.

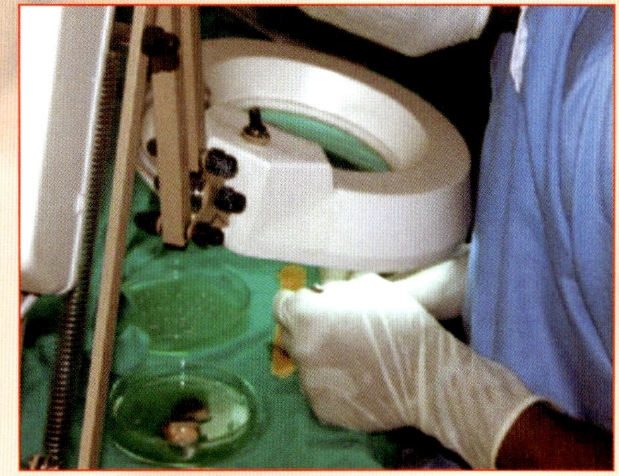

SECTION 7

Miscellaneous

CHAPTER 44

Anaesthesia in Otorhinolaryngology

Susheela Taxak, Rohtas Singh Sehrawat, Ravi Sehrawat

Anaesthesia for ear, nose and throat surgery encompasses a range of operations varying in duration, severity and complexity from high volume cases such as myringotomy, tonsillectomy and simple nasal procedures to complex procedures in head and neck cancer patients. Probably in no other branch of surgery is the requirement for understanding between the surgeon and anaesthesiologist greater than in otorhinolaryngology because of the 'shared airway' procedures. Hence careful planning, preoperative evaluation and close cooperation are essential.

PRE-OPERATIVE ASSESSMENT

The goals of preoperative evaluation are to reduce patient risk and morbidity of surgery, as well as to reduce the costs. The American Society of Anesthesiologists (ASA) has approved basic standards for preanaesthetic care, which outline the minimum requirements for preoperative evaluation (Table 44.1).

A recent history of an upper respiratory infection especially in children can predispose patients to pulmonary complications including broncho- and laryngospasm during induction of, and emergence from, general anaesthesia.

Preexisting medical conditions should be controlled or stabilized before surgery.

Table 44.1. American Society of Anaesthesiologists Physical Status classification

Status	*Disease state*
ASA Class 1	No organic, physiological, biochemical or psychiatric disturbance
ASA Class 2	Mild to moderate systemic disturbance that may not be related to the reason for surgery
ASA Class 3	Severe systemic disturbance that may or may not be related to the reason for surgery
ASA Class 4	Severe systemic disturbance that is life threatening with or without surgery
ASA Class 5	Moribund patient who has little chance of survival but is submitted to surgery as a last resort (resuscitation effort)
Emergency Operation (E)	Any patient in whom an emergency operation is required

PREOPERATIVE PREPARATION AND PREOPERATIVE MEDICATION

Anaesthetic management for patients begins with preoperative psychological preparation and if necessary, preoperative medication. Because it is part of beginning of the anaesthetic, choice of preoperative medication is based on the same consideration as the choice of anaesthesia, including the patient's medical problems, requirements of the surgery, and the anaesthesiologist's skills.

Satisfactory preoperative preparation and medication facilitates an uneventful perioperative course. Informing the patients of the events of the perioperative period includes the following:

1. The time after which the patient must have nothing to eat or drink [NPO] (Table 44.2).
2. The estimated time of surgery
3. The medications to be continued on the day of surgery. In general, antihypertensives (beta blockers, calcium channel blockers, clonidine), anticonvulsants, antiarrhythmic agents, inhaled bronchodilators, antireflux medications, steroids and hormonal supplements should be continued. Angiotensin converting enzyme inhibitors and angiotension receptor blocking agents are sometimes discontinued because they can cause refractory hypotension intraoperatively.

Table 44.2. Guideline for NPO status preoperatively

Age	*Clear liquids*	*Breast milk*	*Nonhuman milk, light shakes*	*Fried fatty foods*
Infant	2 hours	4 hours	6 hours	8 hours
Child	2 hours	4 hours	6 hours	8 hours
Adult	2 hours	NTA	6 hours	8 hours

The doses of various drugs which need to be altered in different group of patients:

1. Doses of sedatives and analgesics should be reduced in elderly, debilitated, intoxicated and in those with upper airway obstruction or trauma, central apnoea, and severe pulmonary or valvular heart disease.
2. Patients addicted to opioids and barbiturates and patients on chronic pain therapy should receive sufficient premedication to overcome tolerance and to prevent withdrawal during or shortly after surgery.
3. Diabetes mellitus patients may be hyperglycemic or hypoglycemic preoperatively and intraoperatively. The signs and symptoms of hypoglycemia in patients who have taken insulin or hypoglycemic agents is masked by general anaesthesia.
4. Untreated hypertension (HTN) can cause end organ damage in the perioperative period. Acute treatment of chronic HTN may be indicated in patients with systolic blood pressure greater than 20% of their baseline.
5. Patients with moderate to severe asthma require pre-treatment with bronchodilators to reduce the incidence of bronchospasm intraoperatively.

Drugs commonly given in premedication are:

1. **Benzodiazepines:** These are highly effective for the treatment of anxiety.
   (a) Midazolam 0.3 mg – 0.5 mg/oral or 0.3 mg/kg intravenously on induction is a short acting benzodiazepine that provides excellent amnesia and sedation.
   (b) Lorazepam 1 to 2 mg orally or intravenously but it can cause prolonged amnesia and postoperative sedation.
2. **Anticholinergics:** Glycopyrrolate (0.2–0.4 mg intravenously for adults and 10–20 $\mu g.kg^{-1}$ for paediatric patients) or atropine (0.4 to 0.6 mg for adults and 20 $\mu g.kg^{-1}$ for paediatric patients) is given during induction as antisialagogue specifically for bronchoscopy.
3. **Antiemetic agents:** These can be given before induction or intraoperatively to prevent postoperative nausea and vomiting (PONV). Prophylactic antiemetics should be given to patients who are high risk for PONV.

Guidelines for prophylaxis of pulmonary aspiration have been recommended for patients with high risk for aspiration pneumonitis e.g. patients with difficult airway, obesity.

Some important antiemetic agents are shown in Table 44.3.

PRE-OPERATIVE AIRWAY ASSESSMENT AND MANAGEMENT

Induction and maintenance of anaesthesia for ENT surgery requires interdisciplinary cooperation. Communication between surgeon and anaesthesiologist is crucial to assure success due to either sharing of airway or head movement.

Airway obstruction and may make intubation extremely difficult and in some cases, impossible requiring tracheostomy. Airway obstruction upon induction of anaesthesia can occur even with seemingly simple procedures such as tonsillectomy.

There should be a low threshold for awake fiberoptic intubation if the airway is questionable. If the anaesthesiologist decides to proceed with conventional means of securing the airway, the patient's head position should be optimized

Table 44.3. Antiemetic agents

Agent	*Mechanism of action*	*Side effects*	*Dose*
Ondansetron	5HT3 receptor antagonist	Dizziness, headache QTc prolongation	4 mg iv
Droperidiol	Dopamine (D2) receptor antagonist	Dystonia, prolongs QT, decreases seizure threshold	0.5 to 2.5 mg iv
Dexamethasone	Unknown	Hyperglycemia	4 mg iv
Metoclopramide	Dopamine receptor antagonist	GI upset with abdominal cramping, dystonia	10 mg iv
Promethazine	Antihistamine	Sedation, decreases seizure threshold	25 mg iv
Scopolamine	Anticholinergic	Dry mouth, blurred vision, confusion, urinary retention	1.5 mg transdermal

carefully and intubating aids (stylets, gum elastic bougies) as well as endotracheal tubes (ETT) of different sizes should be available.

Tools for intubation of a difficult airway are:

- Fiberoptic scope – for nasal or oral intubation in an awake or anaesthetized patient;
- Eschmann stylet;
- Laryngeal mask airways (LMA);
- Intubating LMA;
- Bullard intubating scope;
- Light wand/Trachlight; and
- C-Mac laryngoscope.

For certain procedures (e.g. excision of tongue base, tongue suspension for obstructive sleep apnoea (OSA) etc., nasal intubation may be desirable to facilitate surgical access.

General Principles of Anaesthetic Management for ENT

The essential anaesthetic requirements for ENT surgery are:

1. Assurance of good intraoperative and post-operative analgesia.
2. Quiet surgical field (the operated areas are highly vascular): Controlled hypotension (SBP <100 mmHg and MAP = 60 mmHg) is widely employed. Deliberate hypotension is usually accompanied easily by a potent inhalational anaesthetic and/or intermittent boluses of agents like esmolol 0.3–1 µg.kg,$^{-1}$ labetalol 0.1–0.3 mgkg^{-1} or hydralazine 0.05–0.15 mgkg^{-1}), infusion of nitroglycerine or sodium nitroprusside as necessary.
3. Patient immobility: For certain procedures profound muscle relaxation may be required, while for others administration of neuro-muscular blocking drugs is avoided.
4. Smooth emergence from anaesthesia: Straining, bucking and coughing will cause an increase in venous pressure that may promote postoperative bleeding, disruption of delicate suture lines and graft dislodgement following tympanoplasty.

Given below is a brief description of various drugs used during general anaesthesia.

Intravenous induction agents

All intravenous induction agents are administered in aqueous solution ,or as an oil or an emulsion that is readily miscible with plasma. In addition they must be partially or entirely non toxic and lipid soluble at pH 7.4, in order to cross the blood brain barrier and produce rapid loss of consciousness.

The intravenous induction agents in current use in our country are sodium thiopental, propofol, ketamine and midazolam.

Inhalational anaesthetic agents

The inhalational anaesthetic agents in current practice are nitrous oxide, halothane, isoflurane, sevoflurane and desflurane. The safe administration of inhalational anaesthetic agents requires a good understanding of their pharmacokinetics. The depth of anaesthesia is directly proportional to the tension (or partial pressure) of the agent in the brain or arterial blood.

Similarly speed of induction and recovery are related to rate of rise and fall of arterial/brain tensions. The factors that affect the tension of anaesthetic vapour in brain and in arterial blood are:

- alveolar ventilation;
- Concentration or tension of the agent in the inspired gas mixture;
- transfer of vapour from alveoli to blood in the lungs; and

- transfer of vapour from arterial blood to body tissues.

Neuromuscular blocking agents (muscle relaxants)

Muscle relaxants belong to two groups – the depolarizers and non-depolarizers.

Depolarizing muscle relaxants mimic the effect of acetylcholine at the neuromuscular junction, first causing muscle contractions (fasciculations) and then paralysis. Suxamethonium is the only depolariser in use.

Non-depolarizers have slower onset (2–3 minutes) and are therefore unsuitable for rapid control of airway. They work by competitive blockade of the neuromuscular junction and are reversed with anticholinesterases such as neostigmine. There is no initial muscle fasciculation. The non-depolarizers are benzylisoquinolinium diesters (such as atracurium, mivacurium, doxacurium and cisatracurium) and aminosteroids (vecuronium, pancuronium, rocuronium and pipecuronium).

Cholinesterase inhibitors

These drugs, also known as anticholinesterases, are used to reverse the neuromuscular blockade of non-depolarizing relaxants, e.g., neostigmine. Non-depolarizing relaxants compete with acetylcholine to bind to nicotinic cholinergic receptors. The anticholinesterases indirectly increase the amount of acetylcholine available to compete with the non-depolarizing agent thereby re-establishing neuromuscular transmission.

Suggammadex

Suggammadex is a modified γ-cyclodextrin, a novel, selective muscle relaxant binding agent, that is currently approved for clinical use. Following IV administration, it forms tight water-soluble complexes at a 1 : 1 ratio with steroidal NMBDs (rocuronium > vecuronium >> pancuronium) thereby reducing the amount of neuromuscular blocking agent available to bind to AChRs in the NMJ.

44

Opioid analgesics

These include all naturally-occurring or synthetic drugs which have stereospecific actions at μ-opioid receptors, whose effects can be antagonized by naloxone. Opioid analgesics are either pure agonists, e.g., morphine, fentanyl, etc. or agonist-antagonists, e.g., pentazocine. Morphine is the gold standard analgesic. The choice of an opioid depends on the degree of surgical stimulation, anticipated post-operative pain and duration of surgery. Highly potent opioids (fentanyl loading dose of 2–4 $\mu g.kg^{-1}$, alfentanil loading dose of 0.5–1 $\mu g.kg^{-1}$ followed by other intermittent boluses or continuous infusion) is one of the protocols for major ENT surgery. For procedures that are characterized by minimal postoperative discomfort, e.g., laser surgery, short-acting opioids may be preferred.

Adjuvant drugs

1. Benzodiazepines

- Diazepam
- Midazolam

(a) Diazepam

- Long-acting sedative – metabolites are also active
- Causes anterograde amnesia and hypnosis

Dose: Given in the increments of 2–2.5 mg till the desired effect is achieved.

Side effects:

- Painful on injection – given in a running drip
- May cause respiratory depression
- Hypotension
- In hypovolemic patients

(b) Midazolam

- Three times more potent than diazepam
- Short-acting

Dose: Given in the increments of 1 mg

2. Antacids/Antiemetics/Prokinetics

These are the drugs given for reducing the acidity of gastric contents and prevention or suppression of vomiting

LOCAL ANAESTHESIA

Local anaesthesia results from the blockade of voltage – gated sodium channels and interruption of initiation and propagation of nerve impulses. Local anaesthetic agents can be defined as drugs that are used clinically to produce reversible inhibition of excitation and conduction in peripheral nerve fibers and nerve endings, and thus produce the loss of sensation in circumscribed area of the body.

During conduction blockade, different modalities may be affected to an unequal extent by local anaesthetics. The sensation of pain usually disappears before touch and pressure, while motor fibers may remain functional although sensory pathways are blocked. Currently available local anaesthetics are of two chemical classes: aminoesters and aminoamides.

Local anaesthetic preparations

Most local anaesthetics are bases that are almost insoluble in water. Consequently, their hydrochloride salts which are extremely water soluble, are usually dissolved in saline to form acidic solution (pH 4.0–6.5). Preparations with added adrenaline often contain a reducing agent (e.g. sodium metabisulphite) to prevent oxidation. Some local anaesthetic preparations (particularly multidose vials) also incorporate a preservative / fungicide e.g. (methyl p-hydroxybenzoate). Most local anaesthetic solutions are extremely stable and usually have an effective shelf life of more than 2 years.

Vasoconstriction

Many local anaesthetics have a vasodilator effect and are rapidly absorbed after local injection. Consequently they are often used with added vasoconstrictors, which enhance their potency and prolong their duration of action. Vasoconstrictors also decrease the systemic toxicity and increase the safety margin of local anaesthetics by reducing their rate of absorption.

Adrenaline is the most commonly used vasoconstrictor and is added to local anaesthetic solutions in concentrations ranging from 1 in 500,000 (2 $\mu g.ml^{-1}$) to 1 in 200,000 (5 $\mu g.ml^{-1}$). Higher dose may have toxic effects on the cardiovascular system and peripheral nerves. Felypressin is an exon catecholamine vasoconstrictor (0.03 $\mu g.ml^{-1}$) that is chemically related to vasopressin, the posterior pituitary hormone. It is a synthetic octapeptide that only affects peripheral vessels and has no effect on heart. Although it produces less marked vasoconstriction it may be useful for patients with ischaemic heart disease when the use of catecholamines is undesirable.

Local anaesthetics in clinical practice

Lidocaine

Lidocaine is extremely versatile amide local anaesthetic. It remains a popular and widely used agent due to its potency, rapid onset and intermediate duration of action. The maximum safe dose is 3 $mg.kg^{-1}$ (or 200 mg) in plain solutions and 7 $mg.kg^{-1}$ (500 mg) with adrenaline.

Lidocaine is a widely used topical agent and numerous preparations are available as aqueous solutions (2–4%) or in water miscible bases as gels, ointments, creams and sprays (2–10%). Preparation may be applied to the mouth, the nose or the ear, as well as other mucous membranes. Lidocaine spray is frequently used to produce anaesthesia of the bronchial tract prior to endotracheal intubation and bronchoscopic examination. In these conditions, lidocaine has rapid onset of action (3–5 minutes) and a moderate duration of action (30–60 minutes).

Local anaesthetic toxicity

A. Allergic reactions

True allergic reactions to local anaesthetics are uncommon. It is important to differentiate them from common nonallergic responses such as vasovagal episodes and responses to intravascular injection of local anaesthetics.

B. Systemic toxicity

Usually occurs from intravascular injection or overdose. Intravascular injection most commonly occurs during nerve blockade in areas with large blood vessels. This can be minimized by the following:

(a) Aspiration before injection
(b) Use of epinephrine – containing solutions for test doses
(c) Use of small incremental volumes in establishing the blocks.

Central nervous system toxicity

(a) Clinical features of CNS toxicity include metallic taste, light headedness, tinnitus, visual disturbances and numbness of tongue and lips. These may progress to muscle twitching, loss of consciousness, grandmal seizures and coma.
(b) Treatment: At the first sign of toxicity; injection must be discontinued and oxygen administered. If seizure activity interferes with ventilation or is prolonged, anticonvulsant treatment is indicated with midazolam (1 to 2 mg) or thiopentone (50 to

200 mg in adults). If required airway is secured by an endotracheal tube.

Cardiovascular toxicity

(a) Clinical features – Cardiovascular toxicity produces decreased ventricular contractility, refractory cardiac arrhythmias, and loss of peripheral vasomotor tone; which may lead to cardiovascular collapse.

(b) The intravascular injection of bupivacaine or etidocaine may cause cardiovascular collapse, which is often refractory to therapy because of high degree of tissue binding by these agents.

(c) Treatment:

1. Oxygen must be administered and circulation supported by volume replacement and vasopressor including inotropes as necessary. Advanced cardiac support may be necessary.
2. Ventricular tachycardia should be treated by electrical cardioversion, local anaesthetic-induced cardiac arrhythmias are difficult to treat but usually subside over time if the haemodynamics can be maintained.
3. Amiodarone may be more effective than lidocaine for ventricular arrhythmias associated with intravenous injections of bupivacaine.

Anaesthesia Equipment

In each anaesthetising location where general anaesthesia is to be performed, there must be an anaesthesia delivery system which is capable of delivering an accurately measured flow of oxygen and preferably medical air. The anaesthesia machine must have calibrated vaporisers or other systems designed for the accurate delivery of inhalational anaesthetic agents and equipment for automatic ventilation of the lungs incorporating alarms.

Monitoring equipment for ECG, blood pressure (both non invasive and invasive), oxygen saturation, end tidal CO_2, temperature, etc is required.

44

An appropriate range of face masks; oro-pharyngeal, nasopharyngeal and laryngeal masks and other artificial airways, two laryngoscopes with a range of suitable blades, an appropriate range of endotracheal tubes and connectors, a range of endotracheal tube introducers and bougies, Magill's forceps and throat packs must be at hand. Equipments for managing difficult intubations in all locations where endotracheal intubation is electively performed are essential.

SOME SPECIFIC ANAESTHETIC CONSIDERATIONS

Tonsillectomy and Adenoidectomy

Most patients for tonsillectomy and or adenoidectomy are young and otherwise healthy; a subset of both paediatric and adult patients may present with signs of obstructive sleep apnoea(OSA) and upper repiratory infection(URI). The presence of chipped, loose and missing teeth should be documented preoperatively.

Specific considerations are:

- Mask ventilation prior to intubation may be difficult due to large tonsils and adenoids.

- Nasal intubation with large adenoids predisposes to excess bleeding.

- Sharing of operative field.

- Compression of ETT by mouth gag

- Aspiration and/or ingestion of blood

- Adequate muscle relaxation to allow mouth gag and to prevent any bucking,coughing and straining

- Rapid and smooth recovery with adequate airway reflexes is desired to prevent reactionary haemorrhage, laryngospasm and aspiration. This also limits the use of sedatives in premedication.

Induction of anaesthesia can be done with inhalational agent (sevoflurane, preferred in small children especially when iv line is not in place and in OSA patients). An intravenous induction with propofol (2 $mg.kg^{-1}$) and fentanyl (1 to 2 $\mu g.kg^{-1}$) is suitable for majority of patients (consider avoiding thiopentone sodium for outpatient surgery).

Flexible LMA may be used for adenotonsillectomy surgeries and is routinely used in some centres. Advantages are that it requires light plane of anaesthesia and no need for muscle relaxants with resultant rapid induction and smooth recovery. The LMA is not removed until full return of reflexes. Its use for this purpose has not become very popular, the main disadvantage is if airway is lost during surgery it can be difficult to rectify the situation.

Maintenance with inhaled anaesthetics and short acting opioids like fentanyl or remifentanil using spontaneous ventilation and/or muscle relaxants with controlled ventilation is acceptable however adequate depth should be maintained to prevent any reflex stimulation during surgery. The mouth gag may be repositioned several times during the procedure and is removed only at the end of the case.

Prevention of PONV is of major importance. The stomach should be suctioned at the end of the case and further emptying will be facilitated by metoclopromide. Administration of 5HT3, blocker with or without steroids, will constitute adequate antemetic prophylaxis.

Local anaesthetic plus adrenaline in the tonsillar fossa gives the advantages of bloodless dissection, and reduced postoperative pain. If large volumes are injected can give rise to respiratory obstruction once the patients is extubated because of bilateral glossopharyngeal nerve block. Blood loss during tonsillectomy may be difficult to estimate. Intravenous fluids like RL may be used to maintain adequate volumes status.

Patient should be transported in recovery room in tonsillar position with oxygen supplementation. Tonsillar position is left lateral position with one knee flexed and the hand under the face along with slight head low position. This allows the blood and secretion to drain out rather than flow back onto the vocal cords.

Post-tonsillectomy pain is usually mild to moderate and can be taken care of with inj. paracetamol, fentanyl, etc. The NSAIDs are usually avoided, especially aspirin, because of their tendency to increase bleeding and cause bronchospasm. The role of steroids with single intravenous doses of dexamethasone, 0.05–0.15 $mg.kg^{-1}$, to improve recovery after tonsillectomy has been investigated. Steroids decreased postoperative emesis, increased tolerance to regular diet, and reduced pain.

It is recommended that patients be observed for early hemorrhage for a minimum of 6 hours and be free from significant nausea, vomiting, and pain. Excessive somnolence and severe vomiting are indications for hospital admission.

LOCAL ANAESTHESIA FOR TONSILLECTOMY

Following topical anaesthesia of the mucous membrane, three separate injections of local anaesthetic solutions are made, one each in the region of the upper pole, anterior pillar and the lower pole. In each instance attempt is to deposit the solution between the capsule and the pharyngeal wall. This is a very vascular area and special care must be taken not to inject intravascular. The protective laryngeal reflexes don't guarantee laryngeal obstruction and aspiration of blood and debris. Tonsillectomy under these circumstances is however unpleasant for the patients and surgeons alike is rarely performed under local anaesthesia.

Complications

Potential complications after extubation include laryngospasm, airway obstruction, pulmonary edema, aspiration and vomiting (often due to blood in the airway or stomach). Delayed complications include bleeding, sore throat, pharyngeal edema, pain and emesis.

ANAESTHESIA FOR BRONCHOSCOPY

The planned technique for bronchoscopy should be discussed with the surgeon before the operation, and all equipment and connectors should be checked for compatibility, monitoring during bronchoscopy include an electrocardiogram, a blood pressure cuff, a precordial stethoscope, a pulse oximeter and a capnometry. Many anaesthetic techniques are useful for bronchoscopy.

General Anaesthesia

This permits effective suctioning of the trachea and bronchi and the patient recovers gradually from general anaesthesia.

General anaesthesia for bronchoscopy is often combined with topical laryngeal anaesthesia. A balanced technique uses N_2O/O_2, incremental doses of propofol or thiopental, an opioid and a neuromuscular drug. A potent inhaled anaesthetic is also satisfactory. In most cases trachea is intubated with an endotracheal tube after bronchoscopy under general anaesthesia.

Rigid Bronchoscopy

A modern rigid ventilating bronchoscope have a side arm for anaesthesia. A number of techniques have been described for maintenance of ventilation and oxygenation during rigid bronchoscope examination.

- Apnoeic oxygenation
- Apnoea and intermittent ventilation.
- Sanders injection system that applies venturi principle to provide ventilation.
- Mechanical ventilation
- High frequency positive pressure ventilation
- Complications of bronchoscopy like mechanical trauma to the teeth, haemorrhage, bronchospasm,

bronchial or tracheal perforation, subglottic oedema and barotrauma have all to be kept in mind.

Foreign body bronchus

Types of foreign body: Commonly inhaled objects are organic food-seeds, nuts, bones coins, beetlenut, pins and needles.

Goals of anaesthesia in this case are control of airway, suppression of airway reflexes, amnesia, unobstructed surgical field, no time restriction for the surgeon, decreased secretions,prevention of aspiration and smooth and safe extubation.

To achieve these goals we must rush for surgery (bronchoscopic removal of FB) if there is acute stridor with air hunger and cyanosis, severe respiratory obstruction. Administer 100% oxygen by face mask. Choice of induction of anaesthesia can be inhalational or intravenous depending on patient's condition and situation.

ANAESTHESIA FOR LASER SURGERY

Anaesthesia for laser surgery depends on the expected length of procedure and the location of the target. While all endotracheal tubes are flammable, special endotracheal tubes have been developed that may be more resistant to ignition e.g. stainless steel endotracheal tube, foil wrapped polyvinyl chloride (PVC) tube, red rubber endotracheal tube, silicon tube with laser resistant coating. To further prevent combustion, it is recommended that the cuff be filled with saline instead of air. The saline may be colored (e.g. methylene blue) to allow faster identification of cuff rupture. Some have a double cuff to ensure protection of the airway in the event of a cuff rupture, whereas others have a special matte finish that is effective in deflecting the laser beam throughout the entire length.

The lowest acceptable inspired oxygen level should be used and nitrous oxide should be avoided. Air or helium can be used to lower the inspired oxygen concentration. Inhaled anaesthetics or intravenous agents such as propofol can be used. Neuromuscular blockade is often helpful to limit motion of airway structures.

Postoperatively laryngospasm is a potential complication due to swelling or debris in the airway. Other hazards include potential laser injury to blood vessels or other structures as well as to operating room personnel.

Options that avoid endotracheal intubation include mask ventilation with intermittent apnea during laser use jet ventilation through a bronchoscope, or hyperventilation followed by intermittent extubation and reintubation. All these techniques require close monitoring of pulse oximetry and inspired oxygen levels.

Management of airway fire

1. Turn off all gas flow, especially nitrous oxide, disconnect endotracheal tube from circuit.
2. Remove the endotracheal tube and extinguish any fusing material
3. Ventilate patient by mask with 100% oxygen
4. Perform bronchoscopy and oesophagoscopy to assess damage and remove any debris
5. Reintubate patient or perform tracheostomy if necessary.
6. Patient may require prolonged ventilation in case of extensive damage.
7. Bronchial lavage and intravenous steroids may be helpful.

ANAESTHESIA FOR EAR SURGERY

Local Anesthesia

Simple external ear and some middle ear procedures involving the tympanic membrane and stapes are suitable for local anaesthesia (LA) with or without sedation. Preoperative assessment and intra-operative monitoring should be the same as for general anaesthesia. The choice of local anaesthesia or general anaesthesia depends on numerous factors, including patient cooperation, duration of procedure, patient's and surgeon's preference. Patient's understanding and cooperation are vital to prevent sudden movements at critical stages of the surgery, children and uncooperative adults require a general anaesthetic.

Light sedation during these procedures can be achieved by careful bolus doses of midazolam, titrated infusion of propofol, and, more recently, careful titration with an infusion of remifentanil. Local anesthetic can be administered by infiltration with lidocaine and epinephrine, topical instillation of lidocaine on the tympanic membrane and topical application of LA cream on the tympanic membrane.

Nerve Block

The sensory nerve supply of the ear comes from the auriculotemporal, greater auricular nerve, auricular branch of the vagus, and tympanic nerves. Local anaesthesia involves infiltration of the anterior and posterior external meatal wall blocking the auriculotemporal and greater auricular nerve. Infiltration through an aural speculum blocks the auricular branch of the vagus, and topical infiltration of local anesthetic on the tympanic membrane blocks the tympanic nerve.

General anaesthesia

The essential surgical requirements are a clear surgical field, absence of patient movement, smooth emergence from anesthesia to avoid straining and rapid awakening to assess facial nerve function. The incidence of PONV can be as high as 80% after tympanomastoid surgery if no antiemetic prophylaxis is given.

Opioid-based technique is preferred for induction of anaesthesia and the induction and maintenance doses of opioids can be reduced safely if one of the LMAs is used. Propofol is preferred because of its intrinsic antiemetic effect. Both TIVA and inhalational agents can be used for maintenance. Nitrous oxide if used, should not exceed 50% concentration and must be discontinued at least 15 min before tympanic membrane graft placement to avoid pressure-related displacement.

Ear surgery often involves surgical identification and preservation of the facial nerve, which requires isolation of the nerve by the surgeon and verification of its function by means of electrical stimulation. This is accomplished by brainstem auditory-evoked potential and electrocochleogram monitoring, which requires that muscle relaxation be avoided and a volatile drug is the primary anaesthetic. If an opioid-relaxant technique is chosen, however, at least 30% of the muscle response, as determined by a twitch monitor, should be preserved.

ANESTHETIC CONSIDERATIONS FOR NASAL SURGERY

Surgery on the nose includes procedures on the external aspect of the nose, nasal cavity, nasal sinuses and bony structures. Most sinus surgeries are undertaken using endoscopes and is called functional endoscopic sinus surgery.

Some nasal procedures are done under local anaesthesia with or without sedation and others may require general anaesthesia. This choice depends on patient factors, type of procedure contemplated, duration and site of surgery etc. Generally, local anaesthesia is suitable for procedures on the anterior septum, septoplasty, turbinectomy, cauterization, simple polypectomy and simple nasal fractures. For bigger and complex surgeries like septorhinoplasty, nasolacrimal surgery, craniofacial resections,general anaesthesia may be required.

Nasal vasoconstrictors

In order to reduce bleeding from vascular nasal mucosa, many nasal vasoconstrictor agents alone or in combination are commonly used. Cocaine, epinephrine, phenylephrine are some of these. Lignocaine has only local anaesthetic properties.

Cocaine has a rapid onset of action and excellent vasoconstrictor properties. Small doses are vagotonic producing a reduction in heart rate, whereas increasing blood concentration cause tachycardia, hypertension, ventricular tachycardia, and direct cardiac muscle depression leading to increased morbidity and mortality. So, use of cocaine should be avoided in patients with a history of myocardial infarction, coronary artery disease, congestive heart failure, irregular heart rhythm and hypertension, and in patients taking monoamine oxidase inhibitors. It has been used as a nasal vasoconstriction in a topical solution, paste or gel and spray. The safe recommended maximum dose of cocaine is 1.5–3 $mg.kg^{-1}$ with a maximum dose of 200 mg.

Phenylephrine is a potent alpha – adrenergic agonist and is used as a topical vasoconstrictor alone or in combination with lidocaine. Initial phenylephrine dose should not exceed 0.5 mg, and in children weighing 25 kg or less, it should not exceed 20 $\mu g.kg^{-1}$. Blood pressure and pulse rate should be closely monitored. Severe hypertension should be treated immediately with direct vasodilators or alpha receptor antagonists.

General anaesthesia

The essential surgical requirements are: patient's immobility, clear surgical field and smooth emergence from anesthesia to avoid postoperative haemorrhage. General anaesthesia with an endotracheal tube or a flexible LMA and spontaneous or controlled ventilation can be used. Significant nasal blockage can make facemask ventilation difficult, and an oral airway may be needed. Airway maintenance can be a particular problem in obese patients with obstructed supraglottic airway (OSA) and nasal blockade.

Propofol (1–2 mg.kg^{-1}) is an ideal induction agent. Fentanyl can be used for analgesia. For maintenance a balanced inhalational or TIVA technique can be used safely. A moderate degree of hypotension without compensatory increase in HR is desirable.

Emergence from anaesthesia after nasal surgery presents significant challenges to the anaesthesiologist. Nearly all nasal surgeries have the potential to contaminate the lower airway with blood or secretions, and it is essential to prevent it.

SUGGESTED READING

1. Soreide E, Eriksoson LI, Hirilekar G, Eriksson H,

ARMAMENTARIUM USED IN ANESTHESIA

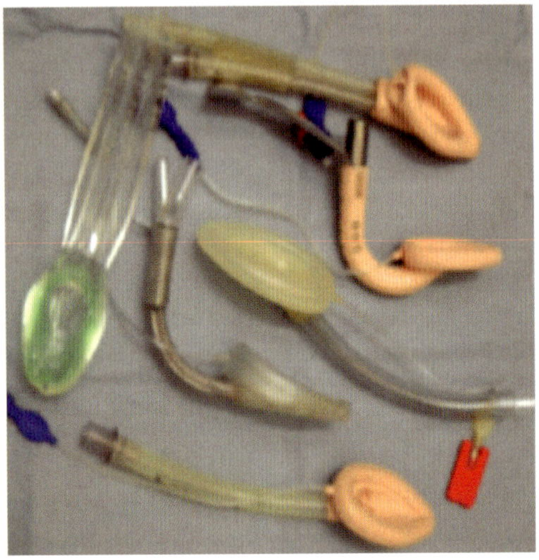

Fig. 44.1. Different sizes of laryngeal mask airway (LMA).

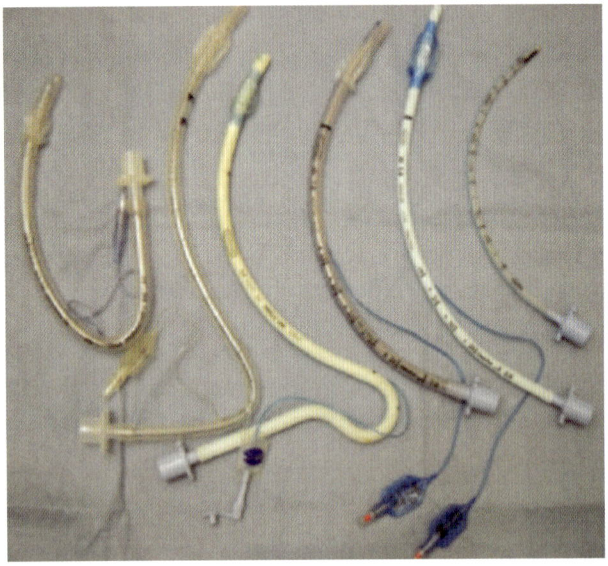

Fig. 44.2. Different sizes and shapes of cuffed endotracheal tube pattern.

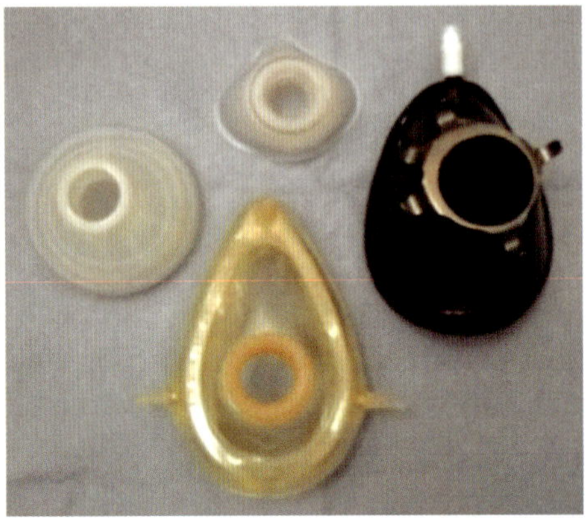

Fig. 44.3. Different sizes and shapes of facial mask.

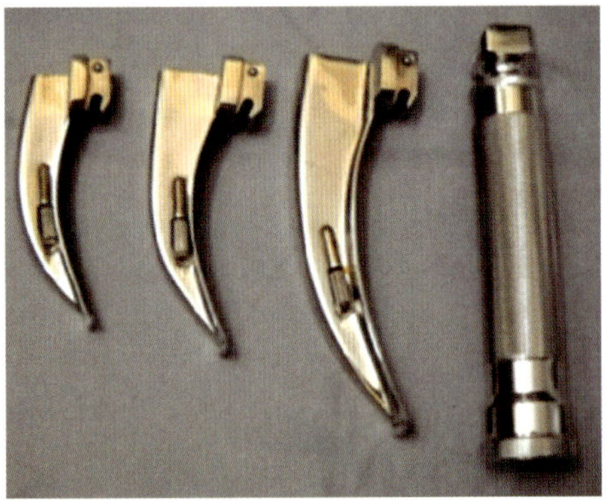

Fig. 44.4. Laryngoscope handle with an assortment of Macintosh blade (Large for adult and small for pediatrics).

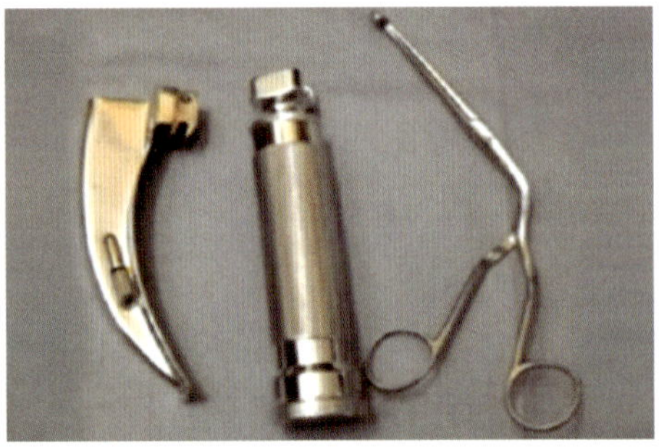

Fig. 44.5. Laryngoscope with Magill forceps.

44

ARMAMENTARIUM USED IN ANESTHESIA (contd.)

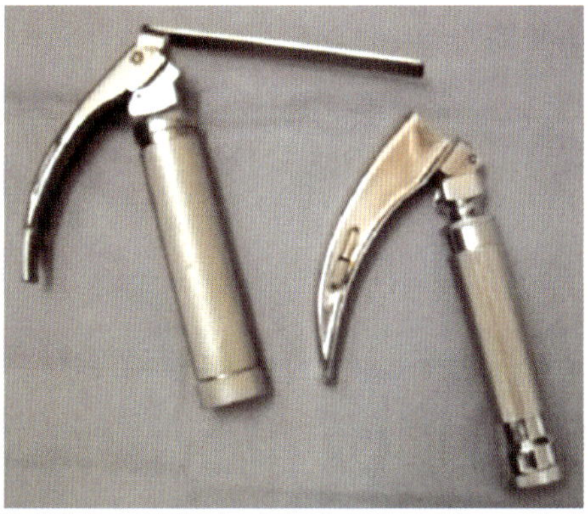

Fig. 44.6. McCoy blade with a hinged tip.

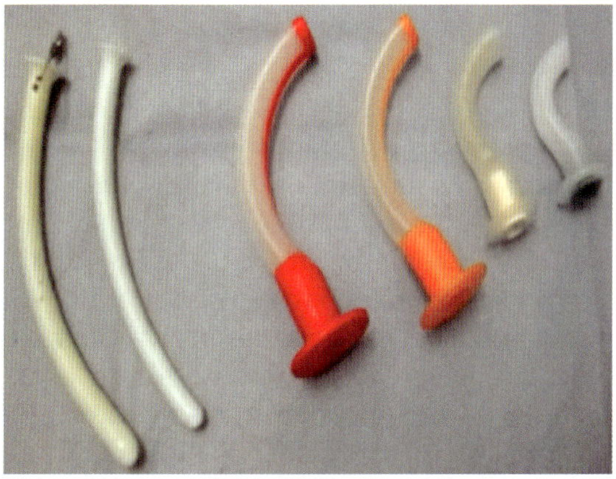

Fig. 44.7. Nasopharyngeal and oropharyngeal airways.

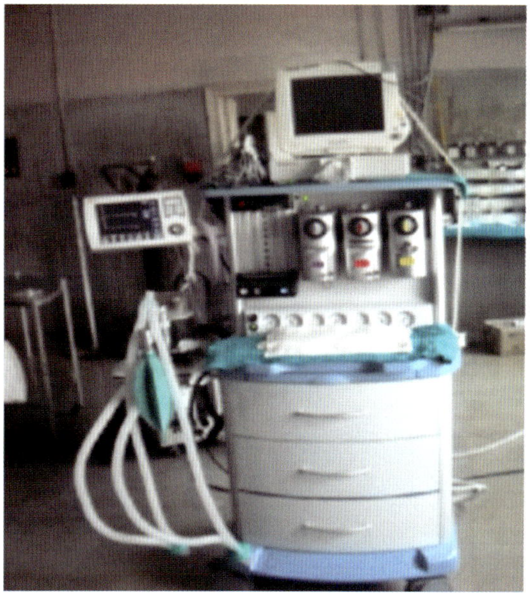

Fig. 44.8. Anaesthesia machine.

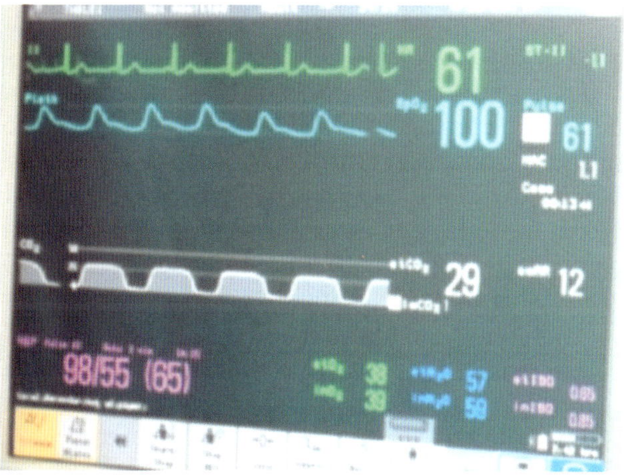

Fig. 44.9. Multi Parameter Monitor.

Henneberg SW, Sandir R et al. Preoperative fasting guidelines: an update. *Acta Anaesthesiol Scand*, 2005; 49: 1041–7.
2. Pearce A. Recognition and management of difficult airway. In: Gleeson M, Browning GG, Burton MJ, Clarke R, Hibbert J, Lund VJ, Luxon LM, Watkinson JC editors. Scott-Brown's Otorhinolaryngology, Head and Neck Surgery Vol-1. Edward Arnold (Publisher) Ltd. London, 2008; 467–87.
3. Mayers D, Hildebrandt MM. Anaesthesia for sinus surgery. In: Levine HL, Clemente MP editors. Sinus surgery: endoscopic and microscopic approaches. Thieme New York 2005; 316–21.
4. Peterson LJ, Indresano AT, Marciani RD, Roser SM. Principles of oral and maxillofacial surgery. JB Lippincott Philadelphia, 1992; 1539–46.
5. Smith G. Inhalational anaesthetic agents. In: Aitkenhead AR, Rowbotham DJ, Smith G editors. Textbook of Anaesthesia 4th edition. Churchill Livingstone 2001.
6. White PF, Waddle JP. Anaesthesia for plastic surgery. In: Mathes SJ editor. Plastic surgery 2nd edition. Saunders Elsevier Philadelphia 2006.
7. Lobo E, Pellegrini F. Anaesthesia for head and neck surgery. In: Lalwani AK editor. Current Diagnosis and Treatment in Otolaryngology – Head & Neck Surgery. McGraw Hill New York, 2008; 160–76.
8. Lee KJ. Anesthesia for head and neck surgery. In: Essential of Otolaryngology Head & Neck Surgery. McGraw Hill Professional, 2003; 897–926.

CHAPTER 45

National Programme for Prevention and Control of Deafness*

R.G. Aiyer

Hearing loss is the most common sensory deficit in humans today. World over, it is the second leading cause for 'Years Lived with Disability (YLD)' the first being depression. It is responsible for 24.9 million YLD globally and gives it a larger non-fatal burden than alcohol use disorders, osteoarthritis and schizophrenia. As per WHO estimates in India, there are approximately 63 million people, who are suffering from 'Significant Auditory Impairment' i.e. hearing threshold >40 dB in better ear in adults and 30 dB in better ear in children. Of these, a large percentage is children between the ages of 0 to 14 years. This segment forms 40% of our population.

The common causes leading to all degrees of hearing loss are:

S. No.	Disease	% of population suffering
1.	Ear wax	15.9%
2.	Chronic suppurative otitis media	5.2%
3.	Serous otitis media	3%
4.	Dry perforation	0.5%
5.	Congenital deafness	0.2%
6.	Non-infectious and other unknown causes (presbyacusis, NIHL, ototoxicity)	10.3%

Overall ear care in terms of primary, secondary prevention and rehabilitation have not been paid due attention. The studies have also shown that it is feasible to focus attention to primary, secondary prevention and rehabilitation of hearing impairment and deafness through the existing health infrastructure with some inputs. An urgent need of a nationwide program to pay focused attention to the primary and secondary prevention of hearing impairment and deafness in addition to rehabilitation of those already affected was felt.

Justification for the National Programme

1. As per WHO, the overall prevalence of significant auditory impairment is 6.3% in Indian population (WHO, 2003). The burden of deafness was disproportionately high in Indian context and required immediate action.
2. Of the 420 million children in India, it is estimated that about 26.4 million suffer from hearing loss, which is of a magnitude and nature that it hinders their acquisition of communication skills and academic capabilities leading to severe loss of productivity (physical and economical) on account of the functional loss.
3. Over 50% of the causes of hearing impairment are preventable including hearing loss caused by infections of the ear (ASOM, CSOM),

* Compiled from programme guidelines issued by Govt. of India

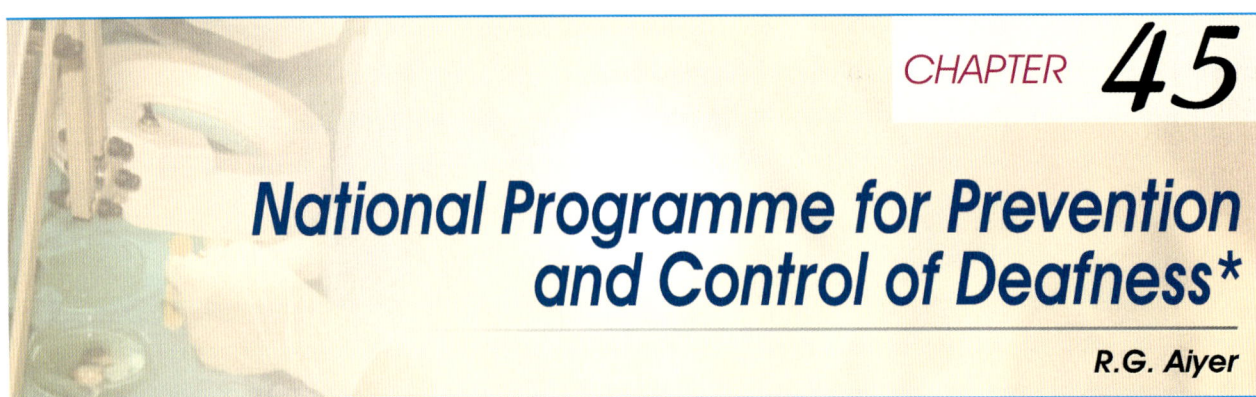

secretory otitis media, traumatic, rubella, noise-induced hearing loss and ototoxicity. 30% of deafness, though not preventable, is treatable.

Thus, a total of 80% of all deafness is avoidable by medical or surgical methods while other patients can be rehabilitated with the use of hearing aid, speech and hearing therapy. This strongly indicated the need to strengthen ear and hearing care services.

OBJECTIVES OF THE PROGRAMME

1. To prevent the avoidable hearing loss on account of disease or injury.
2. Early identification, diagnosis and treatment of ear problems responsible for hearing loss.
3. To medically rehabilitate persons of all age groups, suffering with deafness.
4. To strengthen the existing inter-sectoral linkages for continuity of the rehabilitation programme, for persons with deafness.
5. To develop institutional capacity for ear care services by providing support for equipment and material and training personnel.

STRATEGIES

1. To strengthen the service delivery including rehabilitation.
2. To develop human resource for ear care.
3. To promote outreach activities and public awareness through innovative and effective IEC strategies with special emphasis on prevention of deafness.
4. To develop institutional capacity.

COMPONENTS

1. Manpower training and development.
2. Capacity building.
3. Service provision including rehabilitation.
4. Awareness generation through Information, Education and Communication (IEC) activities.

Organisational Structure of National Programme for Prevention and Control of Deafness (NPPCD)

The NPPCD is governed by a central core committee which guides the state level committees and in turn the state committee directs the functioning of the programme through district health society. The finances are drawn from national rural health mission (NRHM).

Service Delivery and Referral System

I. Primary level

CHCs/PHCs/SCs/Primary School teachers/Health Workers/Panchayats

Functions

- Early identification of cases of hearing impairment and their management.
- Primary ear care.
- Promoting public awareness in respect of prevention of deafness.
- Sensitization training of health workers.
- Support to school ear care programme

II. Secondary level

District Hospital

Functions

- Management of cases referred from PHCs/CHCs.
- Organization of ear care screening camps.
- Organization of school ear care programme.
- Training of manpower – PHC doctors, nurses, audiometric assistants, health workers and school teachers.

III. Tertiary level

State Medical College

In each state, medical colleges have been identified to act as the centres of excellence and referral centre for the districts covered under the programme in that area. Two ENT surgeons and one audiologist will be trained under the programme for skill up-gradation in ENT/audiology procedures.

Functions

- Training of manpower i.e. sensitization programmes and surgical training workshops.
- Management of referral cases, especially the difficult cases for diagnosis and management.

MANPOWER TRAINING & DEVELOPMENT

Objectives

1. To orient all the health care personnel from the district to grass root level about prevention, promotion, early identification and rehabilitation of all types of ear diseases leading to deafness.
2. To make these personnel aware of the existing facilities available for deafness in order to facilitate appropriate referral.

3. To sensitize the health care personnel regarding their specific roles in the programme.
4. To enable the health providers to provide a leadership role in creating awareness about hearing impairment.
5. To facilitate development of suitable manpower, in order to be able to implement this programme in the entire nation.

TRAINING SCHEME

I. Sensitization and awareness of the doctors and audiologists at the medical college level.
II. Training of district hospital ENT doctors and audiologists.
III. Sensitization training of pediatricians and obstetricians.
IV. Training of the doctors at the PHC and CHC.
V. Training of public health nurses, multipurpose health workers male and female, ANMs, anganwadi supervisors (AWW supervisor) and child development project officers (CDPO).
VI. Training of health workers at grass root level: anganwadi workers (AWW), ASHAs and TBAs.
VII. Training of the primary school teachers at the village level.

SERVICE PROVISION INCLUDING REHABILITATION

Service components will include:

- Early detection
- Ear screening camps
- Treatment: medical and surgical
- Appropriate referral
- Rehabilitation of hearing and speech disorders and hearing aid provision.
- Awareness creation in the community.

Early Detection

45

- The detection would be by sensitized personnel at grass root level including family members/ parents, selected school teachers, MPWs at subcentre level, public health nurses and medical officers in PHCs and CHCs and district level personnel. Personnel at all levels would be assigned a specific task in order to ensure that the right guidance is provided at the appropriate time to the affected persons.
- House to house surveys will be conducted by the AWWs and ASHAs, under the supervision of the male and female MPWs for detection of cases of hearing impairment and deafness. The deafness cases will be noted in the disability column of ANM's village register.
- The MPWs will maintain records of each family based on a family proforma provided to them.
- The district level paediatricians and gynaecologists will be responsible for referring any child born of a high risk pregnancy or delivery, as well as other children who are exposed to a high risk factor in infancy and who show features suggestive of hearing impairment. These children will be screened by the district level ENT doctor/ audiologist with OAE and then subjected to diagnostic tests.

Ear Screening Camps

Functions

- Screening camps will be organized at the PHC/ CHC and district level for screening the general population in respect of ear problems, hearing impairment and deafness.
- Detection and treatment of common ear problems.
- Spreading awareness regarding ear problems, early detection of deafness, available treatment and health care facilities for referral of such cases.
- Education of community, especially the parents of young children regarding importance of right feeding practices, various common ear problems, early detection of deafness in young children and available treatment for hearing impairment/ deafness.
- Education of panchayat members, members of mahila mandals and youth leaders.

Conduction of Screening Camps

- Ear screening camps will be conducted by the PHC/CHC doctors and district level ENT specialists, trained under the programme.
- The screening camps will be facilitated by the NGOs, identified by the District Health Society. These NGOs will require to have adequate infrastructure to carry out screening camps and experience of work at the community level.
- One screening camp will be organized per month at any PHC or CHC or district hospital by rotation. Total 24 camps will be organized in each district over a period of 2 years.

Treatment

Treatment of all affected persons would be undertaken at the following levels:

- Public Health Nurses and MPWs would provide treatment of common ear ailments such as wax, acute suppurative otitis media, etc. under the guidance of the PHC doctor. The Public Health Nurses & MPWs will have the capacity to distribute relevant ear drops and medicines under the guidance of the PHC doctor.
- Trained PHC/CHC doctors will provide early diagnosis of ear diseases and treatment of all common ear ailments. All persons requiring special diagnostic facilities, complicated cases and those needing surgical intervention will be referred to the District hospital.
- District hospital: The district level ENT doctors, audiologists will provide comprehensive preventive, promotive, curative and medical rehabilitative services. Wherever feasible, suitable linkages would be developed with the comprehensive rehabilitation centres (CRC) and DDRC in coordination with the Ministry of Social Justice & Empowerment, for provision of rehabilitative services.
- The district level paediatricians will also be responsible for treating ear diseases such as acute otitis media, so that progress to deafness can be prevented.

Referral services

Effective linkages would be developed from peripheral level to district level with the help of functionaries and personnel from grass root level (AWW, ASHA and sensitized parents and PRIs), subcentre level (Male and female MPWs), PHC level medical officers, public health nurses, school teachers and school health doctors, private practitioners and district level officers.

Rehabilitation and Hearing Aid provision

- All patients who are identified as having an ear problem that either requires surgery, hearing aid fitting or rehabilitative therapy will be referred to the ENT doctor and audiologist at the district level.
- Those who need surgery will be given the appropriate treatment at the district hospital.
- Complicated cases that cannot be adequately handled at the district hospital will be further referred to the state medical college for expert treatment.
- Patients who suffer with sensorineural hearing loss that is not amenable to medical or surgical correction and which requires hearing aid will be fitted with the same at the district level. This will include children who are suffering with bilateral sensorineural hearing loss.
- The hearing aids will be issued as per existing rules. It is proposed that collaboration with the Ministry of Social Justice & Empowerment will be established for this purpose.
- The requirement for speech therapy and hearing therapy will be met with by the audiologist at the district level.

Awareness Creation among Parents/community

- Community level health workers and doctors will undertake this activity on a continuous basis. This will also form a part of the IEC activities at various levels.
- Sensitization will be done regarding various aspects relating to early detection of hearing loss. They will be educated about the various ill effects of hearing loss on the speech, mental and social development of the child.
- Information regarding various treatment modalities as well as techniques of rehabilitation.
- Sensitization to ill effects of hearing loss in the elderly so that they may refer the aged hearing impaired persons for suitable management/ rehabilitation.

Activities envisaged at different levels

Grassroots: Anganwadi workers, ASHA, Trained dais, Health workers

1. IEC for hearing and speech problems through
   (a) Sensitization of community
   (b) House to house visits
2. Early detection and primary prevention
3. Referral to appropriate facility

- **Sensitization of Community:** All grass root level workers in collaboration with MPWs would be having regular meetings with community-based organizations such as Gram panchayat, village health committee, Mahila mandal to create awareness for hearing and speech problems. This component would be reinforced in regular meetings of mahila mandals. The screening camps would also serve as useful platform for awareness creation and motivation of individuals for early diagnosis and check up.

- **House to house visits:** The ASHA under NRHM/AWW under ICDS scheme would be instructed to enquire about any ear and hearing problems in the family during their home visits. They would serve as link workers between the community and mahila mandals, village health committee and health care facilities. Any problem identified would need to be referred for further treatment. ASHA/AWW would be trained to diagnose and ensure treatment of acute suppurative otitis media as untreated ASOM is an important aetiological factor for development of CSOM.
- **AWW & ANM** would be trained about the correct posture for feeding the baby which she must convey to the mother at the time of the birth of the baby or during postnatal visits. This too will bring down the incidence of ASOM and CSOM as poor feeding practices are rampant and an important cause of CSOM.
- She would also be told to refer all patients who had a difficult labour or where the child suffered birth asphyxia to the nearest health care facility. Any child who fails these criteria may be reassessed at the next visit and then sent for testing to the District hospital.

Health Workers at Subcentre level

At the time of immunization by the female MPW at the subcentre at the age of 3 months and 6 months, the worker will screen the child for hearing loss. This can be done simply by building into the already existing immunization card, the assessment of the child's hearing by pertinent questions such as:

- Does the mother feel that the child can hear normally?
- Does he turn his head towards a loud noise/bang?
- Does he smile when hearing his mother's voice?
- Is startle reflex (sudden startle response on hearing a loud noise) present?
- **Sensitization and education of the parents** is an important part of this programme. This would occur at all levels (primary, secondary and tertiary) and would also involve the grass root level workers, panchayat, mahila mandals and village health committees.
- MPW (male) would maintain a family-based proforma in order to keep a record of all hearing-impaired members in the community and the actions taken in that respect.
- The MPWs and PHNs will be able to provide basic treatment for common ear diseases such as ASOM, otitis externa, wax, etc, under the guidance of the PHC doctor.
- The male MPW will be involved in the IEC activities. They will be responsible for creation of awareness and encouraging the involvement of male family members which would facilitate detection and referral of the hearing impaired child.
- Local, culture sensitive innovative strategies would be used for awareness creation and sensitization of the community.

Primary School Teachers

- Education of children regarding hearing loss and speech problems: Towards this aim, the teacher will talk to children regarding the common unhealthy and healthy ear practices. A document in simple language containing the dos and don'ts regarding ear care will be circulated to the children and discussed with them by the teacher.
- Identification of children with hearing loss/ear disease: As schools are the place where children can be easily accessed, this would be an essential part of the programme. At school level the screening would be carried out through the use of a questionnaire. The children with any suspicion of hearing loss will be identified for further diagnosis.
- Referral to the school health doctor/PHC doctor/district level ENT doctor.

Doctors at PHC level

Integration of primary ear care with general health services is likely to yield most cost effective solutions by:

- Early diagnosis and management of common hearing ailments. The management of patients referred to the PHC from the village or the subcentre level. The medical treatment would be provided by the PHC doctor.
- Referral of patients requiring special investigations, surgical management or an expert's opinion will be referred to the district hospital.
- IEC and awareness creation regarding deafness including hereditary disorders.

District Hospital

- Capacity of district health systems would be enhanced by providing facilities for diagnosis and management of hearing problems.
- Cases reporting to the district hospital or referred from the primary level will be dealt with through medical and surgical means. Provision for care of specialized ear problems and audiological diagnosis will be done here.
- Microsurgeries of the ear will be performed by the doctors at the district level.
- Facilitate the training of doctors at primary care level, school health doctors, doctors in the industry.
- Rehabilitation of the cases with hearing impairment would also be undertaken at the district level with provision of hearing aids along with hearing therapy and speech therapy.
- Educational and therapeutic aspects of the pre-school going children suffering with hearing impairment will be looked after at the district level by the audiologist. This would help in early language development of these children and in mainstreaming them into the regular schools.
- Screening Camp: The District level ENT specialist along with audiologists will be responsible for monitoring and supervising the organization of camps by NGOs in their respective districts.

State Medical College

- Training of manpower
- Management of referral cases
- Programme monitoring and evaluation

INFORMATION, EDUCATION & COMMUNICATION ACTIVITIES (IEC)

Innovative IEC strategies would be devised for the purpose of creating awareness regarding hearing impairment, its causes, ill effects and treatment and to dispel the commonly held beliefs and myths in this regard.

The strategies would focus on :

- IEC activities by workers and doctors at all levels of health care delivery during home visits or patient care in the health care facility.
- Through Electronic Media: By advertisements/messages over the radio or TV.
- Through print media such as:
  - Posters
  - Advertisements in newspapers, magazines, etc.
  - Leaflets on hearing loss and its causes, treatment and ill effects.

EXPECTED BENEFITS OF THE PROGRAMME

The programme is expected to generate the following benefits in the short as well as in the long run.

1. Large scale direct benefit of various services like prevention, early identification, treatment, referral, rehabilitation, etc. for hearing impairment and deafness as the district hospitals largely cater to their need.
2. Decrease in the magnitude of hearing impaired persons.
3. Decrease in the severity/extent of ear morbidity or hearing impairment in large number of cases.
4. Improved service network for the persons with ear morbidity/hearing impairment in the states and districts covered under the project.
5. Awareness creation among the health workers/grassroot level workers through the medical officers and district officers which will percolate to the lowest level as the lower level health workers function within the community.
6. Larger community participation to prevent hearing loss through PRIs, mahila mandals, village bodies and also creation of a collective responsibility framework in the broad spectrum of the society.
7. Leadership building in the medical officers to help create better sensitization at the grass root level which will ultimately ensure better implementation of the Programme.
8. Capacity building at the district hospitals to ensure better care.
9. State of the art department of ENT at the medical colleges in the state/union territory under the project.

CHAPTER 46

ENT – Internet Review

R.K. Ranga, Saroj Bala, Rahul Jeet Singh, Shubhrica

The use of computer and information technology is on escalation over the past two decades. The internet, one of the key developments in otorhinolaryngology, provides instant information regarding recent advances and management. Therefore, World Federation for Medical Education (WFME) recommends integration of worldwide web (www) into the medical curriculum with a view to improve quality of patient care and keep medical knowledge updated.

ENT images and information at otolaryngology Houston
http://www.ghorayeb.com/pictures.html

Wikipedia
http://www.wikipedia.com
Wikipedia is a free web-based encyclopedia that is developed, researched and edited by users.

The Hearing Centre
http://www.hearingcentreonline.com

The European Academy of facial plastic Surgery
http://www.eafps.org

The Chelsea Physics Garden at:
http://www.chelseaphysicgarden.co.uk/garden

The House Ear Institute at:
http://www.hei.org

National Temporal Bone, Hearing and Balance Pathology Resource Registry
http://www.tbregistry.org

American Tinnitus Association
http://www.ata.org

Facial Surgery
http://www.aafprs.org

Live Surgical broadcasts at:
http://www.or-live.com

Smell and Taste and Anosmia
http://www.cf.ac.uk/biosi/staffinfo/jacob/

Video fluoroscopy Tutorial
http://www.d.umm.edu/csd/current/courses/swallowing/index.html

ENT Charities
http://www.brinos.org.uk
http://www.geoutreac.org

Deafness Research Foundation
http://www.drf.org

Your guide to pressure equalization surgery
http://www.petube.org

American Academy of paediatrics
http://www.aap.org/otitismedia/www/vc/ear/ruw/pre.cfm

Medical education at:
http://www.123doc.com/

Audiology Interviews at:
http://audiologyonline.com/interview/archives.asp.

Dog for the deaf
http://dogsforthedeaf.org/

Hearing Exchange
http://www.hearingexchange.com

Patient-Centered Video at:
http://www.entman.com

National Institute on Deafness and other Communication Disorders
http://www.nidcd.nih.gov

American Academy of Sleep Medicine
http://www.aasmnet.org

Flexible Endoscopic Evolution of Swallowing with sensory testing at:
http://www.feesst.com/index.html

Dysphagia
http://www.dysphagia.com

Sjogren's Information at:
http://www.dry.org/welcome.html

Head & Neck clinical teaching presentation at:
http://www.ecancermedicalscience.com/

Patient thyroid cancer at:
http://butterfly.org.uk

Extensive medical resources at:
http://www.univadis.co.uk

Baylor College of Medicine: Otolaryngology – Head & Neck Surgery
http://www.bcm.edu/oto/

New York Eye and Ear Infirmary at:
http://www.nyee.edu/

ENT resource page for medical students at:
http://www.entformedstudents.co.uk

Otolaryngology images at:
http://www.ghorayeb.com/pictures.html

Mouth Cancer Foundation (awareness)
http://www.rdoc.org.uk

New Zealand Audiological Society at:
http://www.audiolog.org.nz
http://www.bshaa.com

Audiology Online at:
http://www.healthyhearing.com
http://www.audiology.online.com

Hearing website at:
http://www.cubex.co.uk

Union for International Cancer Control
http://www.uicc.org

Benign positional paroxysml vertigo at:
http://www.tchain.com/otoneurology/disorders/bppv/bvvp.html

Jean Causse Ear Clinic at:
http://www.clinic-causse.com

Starkey Hearing and Hearing Aid Website at:
http://www.starkeydirect.co.uk

Facial Surgery – a one stop website
http://www.facialsurgery.com

NHS connecting for health at:
http://www.connectingforhealth.nhs.uk

ENT patient information at:
http://www.tonsil.org
http://www.petube.org
http://www.entinformation.com

ENT nursing at:
http://www.entnursing.com

Otoacoustic emissions portal at:
http://www.otoemission.org

American Academy of Otolaryngology Head & Neck Surgery
http://www.entnet.org

British Association of Head & Neck Oncologists
http://www.bahno.org.uk

British Tinnitus Association
http://www.anausa.org

Cochlear at:
http://www.cochlear.com

Dizzy page at:
http://www.vertigo-dizziness.com

Bell's Information at:
http://www.bellsplasy.ws
http://www.bellsplasy.org.uk

Voice and Swallowing Centre at:
http://www.voiceandswallowing.com

Surgical Planning Laboratory at:
http://splweb.bwh.harvard.edu:8001/index.html

What hearing loss sounds like at:
http://facstaff.uww.edu/bradleys/radio/hlsimulation/

Laryngeal disorders at:
http://www.texasvoicecenter.com/diseases.html

Otohns at:
http://www.otohns.net/default.asp?id=15102

Recurrent respiratory papillomatosis at:
http://www.rrpwebsite.org
http://www.rrpf.org/index.html

Trigeminal nerve anatomy at:
http://www.medinfo.ulf.edu/year1/trigen/home.html

British thyroid association at:
http://www.british-thyroid-assocation.org/info-for-patients

Vesalius clinical folios and image archive
http://www.vesalius.com

Information at clinicians & other healthcare
http://www.medscape.com

Digital anatomy at:
http://www.anatomy.com

Grand rounds archive at UTMB
http://www.utmb.edu/otoref/grnds/grndsindex.html

Patient and cancer information at:
http://www.mdanderson.org/patient-and-cancer-information/index.html

Online free cancer books at:
http://www.ncbi.nlm.nih.gov/books?term=cancer

Sense of smell institute at:
http://www.senseofsmell.org

Quit smoking website at:
http://www.quit.org.uk

ENT Linx
http://www.entlinx.com

Cosmetic Surgery at:
http://www.PersonalSurgeon.com

ENT history, facts and artefacts at:
http://www.entnet.org/museum/index.cfm

Chat forum for anyone affected by cancer at:
http://www.oncochat.org

Oral Cancer Foundation at:
http://www.oralcancerfoundation.org

Abbreviations and acronyms for oncdogg at:
http://www.staff.ncl.ac.uk/s.j.cottorill/medim15a.html

And who named it at:
http://www.whonamedit.com

Epistaxis Pearls at:
http://www.utmb.edu/otoref/Grnds/epi-pearls.html

Educational Programs for Eye & ENT at:
http://www.nyee.edu/page-deli.html?page_no=312#requirements

Functional Endoscopic Sinus Surgery Tutorial at:
http://www.otohns.net/library/ess.asp

ENT Consent home page at:
http://www.entconsent.co.uk/

Dream anatomy exhibition at:
http://www.nlm.nih.gov/exhibition/dreamanatomy/index.html

Otic anatomy at:
http://www.iurc.montp.inserm.fr/cric/audition/english/start.html

Discharge information online at:
http://www.entdischargeinfo.org.uk

PET scanning information at:
http://www.petscaninfo.com

Audiology resources at:
http://www.aud.org.uk

Compendium of medical humor at
http://www.doctorspage.net/humor.asp

Free microsurgery textbook at:-
http://www.buncke.org/book/contents.html

British academy of audiology at:-
http://www.baaudiology.org

Fractured nose at:
http://www.aboutrhinoplasty.com
http://www.abroken/nose.com

Lies, Damned Lies and Statistics at:
http://cancerguide.org/median_not_msg.html

Otoscopy tutorial online at:

http://www.uwcm.ac.uk:9080/otoscopy/index.html

Medline Plus Interactive health tutorials at:
http://www.nlm.nih.gov/medlineplus/tutorial.html

Deaf Library at:
http://www.deaflibrary.org

Oral Pathology images at:
http://www.usc.edu/hsc.dental/opts/
http://www.uiowa.edu/woprm/atlasHome.html
http://www.usc.edu/hsc/denta/opfs

ENT Surgical Videos and Images at:
http://www.entusa.com
http://www.handstable.com/ear_surgery.html

Deafening sound at:
http://net.unl.edu/artsfeat/deafening_sound/ds_splash.html

Children and hearing website at:
http://www.widex.com/children

Pathology reporting guideline at:
http://www.rcpath.org/activities/publications/headnek.html

Hearing Loss Video Clips at:
http://www.vastvideo.com/i/2.1/navigate.asp?cid=289

Otolaryngology and Facial Plastic Surgery at:
http://www.emedicine.com/ent/contents.html

Health humour at:
http://www.thebestmedicalcare.com/numour/index.html

LINKS OF JOURNALS

JARO-Journal of the association for Research in Otolaryngology
http://www.springerlink.com/content/1525-3961

Head and Neck – Journal for the Sciences and Specialties of the Head and Neck
http://www3.interscience.wiley.com/journal/117934747/grouphome/home.html

Audiology and Neurotology
http://content.karger.com/produkte.asp?Aktion=journalhome&produktnr=224213

Ear and Hearing
http://journals.lww.com/ear-hearing/pages/default.aspx

Laryngoscope
http://www3.interscience.wiley.com/journal/12460873

Archives of Otolaryngology-Head and neck Surgery
http://archotol.ama-assn.org/

Otology and Neurotology
http://journals.elsevierhealth.com/periodical/ymhn

American Journal of Rhinology
http://www.ingentaconnect.com/content/ocean/ajra

Clinical Otolaryngology
http://www3.interscience.wiley.com/journal/119877277/grouphome/home.html

Annals of Otology, Rhinology and Laryngology
http://www.annals.com/index.php

Rhinology
http://www.rhinologyjournal.com/

British medical journal at:
http://www.springerlink.com/content/100357

Otolaryngologic clinics in North America
http://www.oto.theclinics.com

Journal of Rhinology & Otology
http://www.jlo.co.uk

HNO
http://www.springerlink.metapress.com/content/1433-0458

B-ENT
http://www.b-ent.be/

Skull Base - an interdisciplinary approach
http://www.thieme-connect.com/ejournals/toc/sbs

CHAPTER 47

Doctor and Law

P.K. Anand

Nobility of medical profession is undoubted, but there had been instances of malpractices where doctors have indulged in making a quick buck and also the situations where the medical men had been negligent or have failed to deliver hundred percent. Doctor is not a God but expectations are no less. Before embarking on the issues of medical ethics, malpractices, or violation of legal provisions, it would be pertinent to have quick review of what is obligatory on the part of the medical practitioner.

From the dawn of civilization every system of medicine has brought out a set of regulations to maintain the professional conduct and etiquette among its members. The earliest known such code is Hippocratic Oath. The modern version of the Hippocratic Oath is the International Code of Medical Ethics, 1948.

Medical Council of India brought out the new code of medical ethics in 2002 replacing the older one introduced in 1972 and updated on 18 July 2000.

Code of Medical Ethics

Declaration

Each applicant, at the time of making an application for registration under the provisions of the Act, shall be provided a copy of the declaration and shall submit a duly signed Declaration as provided and the applicant shall read and agree to abide by the same.

1. I solemnly pledge myself to consecrate my life to service of humanity.
2. Even under threat, I will not use my medical knowledge contrary to the laws of humanity.
3. I will maintain the utmost respect for human life from the time of conception.
4. I will not permit considerations of religion, nationality, race, party politics or social standing to intervene between my duty and my patient.
5. I will practice my profession with conscience and dignity.

- The health of my patient will be my first consideration.
- I will respect the secrets which are confined in me.
- I will give to my teachers the respect and gratitude which is their due.
- I will maintain by all means, in my power, the honours and noble traditions of medical profession.
- I will treat my colleagues with all respect and dignity.
- I shall abide by the code of medical ethics as enunciated in the Indian Medical Council (Professional Conduct, Etiquette and Ethics) Regulations, 2002.

1. Duties and responsibilities of the physician in general

1.1. A physician shall uphold the dignity and honours of his profession.

The prime object of the medical profession is to render service to humanity; reward or financial gain is a subordinate consideration.

No person other than a doctor having qualification recognized by Medical Council of India and registered with Medical Council of India/State Medical Council(s) is allowed to practice modern system of medicine or surgery. A person obtaining qualification in any other system of medicine is not allowed to practice modern system of medicine in any form.

1.2. **Maintaining good medical practice:**

1.2.1. The principal objective of the medical profession is to render service to humanity with full respect for the dignity of profession and man. Physicians should try continuously to improve medical knowledge and skills and should make available to their patients and colleagues the benefits of their professional attainments.

1.2.2. Membership in medical society for the advancement of his profession: A physician should affiliate with associations and societies of allopathic medical professions and involve actively in the functioning of such bodies.

1.2.3. A physician should participate in professional meetings as part of continuing medical education programmes for at least 30 hours every five years, organized by reputed professional academic bodies or any other authorized organizations. The compliance of this requirement shall be informed regularly to Medical Council of India or the State Medical Councils as the case may be.

1.3. Maintenance of medical records:

1.3.1. Every physician shall maintain the medical records pertaining to his/her indoor patients for a period of 3 years from the date of commencement of the treatment in a standard proforma laid down by the Medical Council of India and attached as Appendix 3.

1.3.2. If any request is made for medical records either by the patients/authorized relatives or legal authorities the same may be duly acknowledged and documents shall be issued within the period of 72 hours.

1.3.3. A registered medical practitioner shall maintain a register of Medical Certificates giving full details of certificates issued. When issuing a medical certificate he/she shall always enter the identification marks of the patient and keep a copy of the certificate. He/she shall not omit to record the signature and/or thumb mark, address and at least one identification mark of the patient on the medical certificate or report.

1.4. Display of registration numbers:

1.4.1. Every physician shall display the registration number accorded to him by the State Medical Council/Medical Council of India in his clinic and in all his prescriptions, certificates, money receipts given to his patients.

1.4.2. Physicians shall display as suffix to their names only recognized medical degrees or such certificates/diplomas and memberships/honours which confer professional knowledge or recognizes any exemplary qualification achievements.

1.5. **Use of generic names of drugs** – Every physician should, as far as possible, prescribe drugs with generic names and he/she shall ensure that there is a rational prescription and use of drugs.

1.6. **Highest quality assurance in patient care** – Every physician should aid in safeguarding the profession against admission to it of those who are deficient in moral character or education.

1.7. **Exposure of unethical conduct** – A physician should expose, without fear or favour, incompetent or corrupt, dishonest or unethical conduct on the part of members of the profession.

1.8. **Payment of professional services** – The physician, engaged in the practice of medicine, shall give priority to the interests of patients. A physician should announce his fees before rendering service and not after the operation or treatment is under way.

1.9. **Evasion of legal restrictions** – The physician shall observe the laws of the country in regulating the practice of medicine and shall also not assist others to evade such laws. He should be cooperative in observance and enforcement of sanitary laws and regulations in the interest of public health. A physician should observe the provisions of the interest of public health. A physician should observe the provisions of the State acts like Drugs and Cosmetics Act, 1940; Pharmacy Act, 1948; Narcotic Drugs and Psychotropic Substances Act, 1985; Medical Termination of Pregnancy Act, 1971;

Transplantation of Human Organ Act, 1994; Mental Health Act, 1987; Environmental Protection Act, 1986; Prenatal Sex Determination Test Act, 1994; Drugs and Magic Remedies (Objectionable Advertisement) Act, 1954; Persons with Disabilities (Equal Opportunities and Full Participation) Act, 1995; and Bio-Medical Waste (Management and Handling) Rules, 1998 and such other acts, rules, regulations made by the central/state governments or local administrative bodies or any other relevant act relating to the protection and promotion of public health.

2. Duties of physicians to their patients

2.1. **Obligations to the sick:**

2.1.1. Though a physician is not bound to treat each and every person asking his service he should not only be ever ready to respond to the calls of the sick and the injured, but should be mindful of the high character of his mission and the responsibility he discharges in the course of his professional duties. No physician shall arbitrarily refuse treatment to a patient. However, for good reason, when a patient is suffering from an ailment which is not within the range of experience of the treating physician, the physician may refuse treatment and refer the patient to another physician.

2.1.2. Medical practitioner having any incapacity detrimental to the patient or which can affect his performance vis-à-vis the patient is not permitted to practice his profession.

2.2. **Patience, delicacy and secrecy:** Patience and delicacy should characterize the physician. Confidences concerning individual or domestic life entrusted by patients to a physician and defects in the disposition or character of patients observed during medical attendance should never be revealed unless their revelation is required by the laws of the state.

2.3. **Prognosis:** The physician should neither exaggerate nor minimize the gravity of a patient's condition.

47

2.4. **The patient must not be neglected:** A physician is free to choose whom he will serve. He should, however, respond to any request for his assistance in an emergency. Once having undertaken a case, the physician should not neglect the patient, nor should he withdraw from the case without giving adequate notice to the patient and his family. Provisionally or fully registered medical practitioner shall not wilfully commit an act of negligence that may deprive his patient or patients from necessary medical care.

2.5. **Engagement for an obstetric:** When a physician who has been engaged to attend an obstetric case is absent and another is sent for and delivery accomplished, the acting physician is entitled to his professional fees, but should secure the patient's consent to resign on the arrival of the physician engaged.

3. Duties of physician in consultation

3.1. **Unnecessary consultations should be avoided**.

3.1.1. However, in case of serious illness and in doubtful or difficult conditions, the physician should request consultation, but under any circumstances such consultation should be justifiable and in the interest of the patient only and not for any other consideration.

3.1.2. Consulting pathologists/radiologists or asking for any other diagnostic lab investigation should be done judiciously and not in a routine manner.

3.2. Consultation for patient's benefit: In every consultation, the benefit to the patient is of foremost importance.

3.3. **Punctuality in consultation:** Utmost punctuality should be observed by a physician in making themselves available for consultations.

3.4. Statement to patient after consultation.

3.4.1. All statement to the patient or his representatives should take place in the presence of the consulting physicians, except as otherwise agreed.

3.4.2. Differences of opinion should not be divulged unnecessarily but when there is irreconcilable difference of opinion the circumstances should be frankly and impartially explained to the patient or his relatives or friends. It would be opened to them to seek further advice as they so desire.

3.5. **Treatment after consultation:** No decision should restrain the attending physician from making such subsequent variations in the treatment, if any unexpected change occurs, but at the next consultation, reasons for the variations should be discussed/explained.

3.6. **Patients referred to specialists:** When a patient is referred to a specialist by the attending physician, a case summary of the patient should be given to the specialist, who should communicate his opinion in writing to the attending physician.

3.7. Fees and other charges:

3.7.1. A physician shall clearly display his fees and other charges on the board of his chamber and/or the hospitals he is visiting.

3.7.2. A physician shall write his name and designation in full along with registration particulars in his prescription letter head.

4. Responsiblities of physicians to each other

4.1. Dependence of physicians on each other: A physician should consider it as a pleasure and privilege to render gratuitous service to all physicians and their immediate family dependants.

4.2. Conduct in consultation: In consultation no insincerity, rivalry or envy should be indulged in.

4.3. Consultant not to take charge of the case: When a physician has been called for consultation, the consultant should normally not take charge of the case, especially on the solicitation of the patient or friends. The consultant shall not criticize the referring physician. He/she shall discuss the diagnosis treatment plan with referring physician.

4.4. Appointment of substitute: Whenever a physician requests another physician to attend his patients during his temporary absence from his practice, professional courtesy requires the acceptance of such appointment only when he has the capacity to discharge the additional responsibility along with his/her other duties. The physician acting under such an appointment should give the utmost consideration to the interests and reputation of the absent physician and all such patients should be restored to the care of the latter upon his/her return.

4.5. Visiting another physician's case: When it becomes the duty of a physician occupying an official position to see and report upon an illness or injury, he should communicate to the physician in attendance so as to give him an option of being present. The medical officer/physician occupying an official position should avoid remarks upon the diagnosis or the treatment that has been adopted.

5. Duties of physician to the public and to the paramedical profession

5.1. Physician as citizens: Physicians, as good citizens, possessed of special training should disseminate advice on public health issues.

5.2. Public and community health physician, especially those engaged in public health work, should enlighten the public concerning quarantine regulations/measures for the prevention of epidemic and communicable diseases.

5.3. Pharmacists/nurses: Physicians should recognize and promote the practice of different paramedical services such as pharmacy and nursing as professions and should seek their cooperation wherever required.

6. Unethical acts

A physician shall not aid or abet or commit any of the following acts which shall be construed as unethical:

6.1. Advertising:

6.1.1. Soliciting of patients, directly or indirectly, by a physician, by a group of physicians, or by institutions or organisations is unethical. A medical practitioner is, however, permitted to make a formal announcement in press regarding the following:

- on starting practice;
- on change of type of practice;
- on changing address;
- on temporary absence of duty;
- on resumption of another practice;
- on succeeding to another practice; and
- public declaration of charges.

6.1.2. Printing of self photograph, or any material of publicity in the letter head or on sign board of the consulting room or any such clinical establishment shall be regarded as acts of self-advertisement and unethical conduct on the part of the physician.

6.2. **Patent and copyrights:** A physician may patent surgical instruments, appliances and medicine or copyright application methods and procedures.

6.3. Running an open shop (dispensing of drugs and appliances by physicians): A physician should not run an open shop for sale of medicine for dispensing prescriptions prescribed by doctor other than himself or for sale of medical or surgical appliances. It is not unethical for a physician to prescribe or supply drugs, remedies or appliances as long as there is no exploitation of the patient. Drugs prescribed by a physician or brought from the market for a patient should explicitly state the proprietary formulae as well as generic name of the drug.

6.4. Rcbatcs and commission

6.4.1. A physician shall not give, solicit, or receive nor shall he offer to solicit or receive, any gift, gratuity, commission or bonus in consideration of or return for the referring, recommending or procuring of any patient for medical, surgical or other treatment. A physician shall not, directly or indirectly, participate in or be a party to act of division, transference, assignment, subordination, rebating, splitting or refunding of any fee for medical, surgical or other treatment.

6.4.2. Provisions of para 6.4.1 shall apply with equal force to the referring, recommending or treating physician.

6.5. **Secret remedies:** The prescribing or dispensing by a physician of secret remedial agents of which he does not know the composition, or the manufacture or promotion of their use is unethical and as such prohibited. All the drugs prescribed by a physician should always carry a proprietary formula and clear name.

6.6. **Human rights:** The physician shall not aid or abet torture nor shall he be a party to either infliction of mental or physical trauma or concealment of torture inflicted by some other person or agency in clear violation of human rights.

6.7. **Euthanasia:** Practising euthanasia shall constitute unethical conduct. However, on specific occasion, the question of withdrawing supporting devices to sustain cardiopulmonary function, even after brain death, shall be decided only by a team of doctors.

7. Misconduct

The following acts of commission or omission on the part of physician shall constitute professional misconduct rendering him/her liable for disciplinary action:

7.1. Violation of the regulations: If he/she commits any violation of these regulations.

7.2. If he/she does not maintain the medical records of his/her indoor patients for a period of three years as per regulation 1.3 and refuses to provide the same within 72 hours when the patient or his/her authorized representative makes a request for it as per regulation 1.3.2.

7.3. If he/she does not display the registration number accorded to him/her by the State Medical Council or the Medical Council of India in his clinic, prescriptions and certificates etc. issued by him or violates the provisions of regulation 1.4.2.

7.4. Adultery or improper conduct: Abuse of professional position by committing adultery or improper conduct with a patient or by maintaining an improper association with a patient will render a physician liable for disciplinary action as provided under the Indian Medical Council Act, 1956 or the concerned State Medical Council Act.

7.5. Conviction by court of law: Conviction by a court of law for offences involving moral turpitude/criminal acts.

7.6. Sex determination tests: On no account sex determination test shall be undertaken with the intent to terminate the life of a female foetus developing in her mother's womb, unless there are other absolute indications for termination of pregnancy as specified in the Medical Termination of Pregnancy Act, 1971. Any act of termination of pregnancy of normal female foetus amounting to female foeticide shall be regarded as professional misconduct on the part of the physician leading to penal censure, besides rendering him liable to criminal proceedings as per the provisions of this Act.

7.7. Signing professional certificates, reports and other documents: Registered medical practitioners are, in certain cases, bound by law to give, or may from time to time be called upon or requested to give, certificates, notification, reports and other documents of similar character signed by them in their professional capacity for subsequent use in the courts or for administrative purposes, etc.

7.8. A registered medical practitioner shall not contravene the provisions of the Drugs and Cosmetics Act, and regulations made thereunder. Accordingly, prescribing steroids/psychotropic drugs, when there is no absolute medical indication, selling schedule 'H' & 'L' drugs and poisons to the public, except to his patient.

7.9. Performing or enabling unqualified person to perform an abortion or any illegal operation for which there is no medical, surgical or psychological indication.

7.10. A registered medical practitioner shall not issue certificates of efficiency in modern medicine to unqualified or non-medical person.

7.11. A physician should not contribute to the lay press articles and give interviews regarding diseases and treatments which may have the effect of advertising himself or soliciting practices; but is open to write to the lay press under his own name on matters of public health, hygienic, living or to deliver public lectures, give talks on the radio/TV/internet chat for the same purpose and send announcement of the same to lay press.

7.12. An institution run by a physician for a particular purpose such as a maternity home, nursing home, private hospital, rehabilitation centre or any type of training institution, etc. may be advertised in the lay press, but such advertisements should not contain anything more than the name of the institution, type of patients admitted, type of training and other facilities offered and the fees.

7.13. It is improper for a physician to use an unusually large signboard and write on it anything other than his name, qualifications obtained from a university or a statutory body, titles and name of his speciality, registration number including the name of the State Medical Council under which registered.

7.14. The registered medical practitioner shall not disclose the secrets of a patient that have been learnt in the exercise of his/her profession except:

(1) in a court of law under orders of the presiding judge;

(2) in circumstances where there is a serious and identified risk to a specific person and/or community; and

(3) notifiable diseases.

In case of communicable/notifiable diseases, concerned public health authorities should be informed immediately.

7.15. The registered medical practitioner shall not refuse on religious grounds alone to give assistance in or conduct of sterility, birth control, circumcision and medical termination of pregnancy when there is medical indication, unless the medical practitioner feels himself/herself incompetent to do so.

7.16. Before performing an operation, the physician should obtain in writing the consent from the husband or wife, parent or guardian in the case of minor, or the patient himself as the case may be. In an operation which may result in sterility, the consent of both husband and wife is needed.

7.17. A registered medical practitioner shall not publish photographs or case reports of his/her patients without their permission, in any medical or other journal in a manner by which their identity could be made out. If the identity is not to be disclosed, the consent is not needed.

7.18. In the case of running of a nursing home by a physician and employing assistants to help him/her, the ultimate responsibility rests on the physician.

7.19. A physician shall not use touts or agents for procuring patients.

7.20. A physician shall not claim to be specialist unless he has a special qualification in that branch.

7.21. No act of in vitro fertilization or artificial insemination shall be undertaken without the informed consent of the female patient and her spouse as well as the donor.

7.22. **Research:** Clinical drug trials or other research involving patients or volunteers as per the guidelines of ICMR can be undertaken, provided ethical considerations are borne in mind. Violation of existing ICMR guidelines in this regard shall constitute misconduct.

7.23. If a physician posted in rural area is found absent on more than two occasions during inspection by the head of the district health authority or the chairman, Zilla Parishad, the same shall be construed as a misconduct if it is recommended to the Medical Council of India/State Medical Council by the State Government for action under these regulations.

7.24. A physician posted in a medical college/institution both as teaching faculty or otherwise shall remain in hospital/college during the assigned duty hours. If they are found absent on more than two occasions during this period, the same shall be construed as a misconduct if it is certified by the principal/medical superintendent and forwarded through the State government to Medical Council of India/State Medical Council for action under these regulations.

8. Punishment and disciplinary action

8.1. It must be clearly understood that the instances of offences and of professional misconduct which are given above do not constitute and are not intended to constitute a complete list of the infamous acts which calls for disciplinary action, and that by issuing this notice the Medical Council of India and/or State Medical Council are in no way precluded from considering and dealing with any other form of professional misconduct on the part of a registered practitioner. Circumstances may and do arise from time to time in relation to which there may occur questions of professional misconduct which do not come within any of these categories. Every care should be taken that the code is not violated in letter or spirit. In such instances, as in all others, the Medical Council of India and/or State Medical Council have to consider and decide upon the facts brought before the Medical Council of India and/or State Medical Councils.

8.2. It is made clear that any complaint with regard to professional misconduct can be brought before the appropriate Medical Council for disciplinary action. Upon receipt of any complaint of professional misconduct, the appropriate Medical Council would hold an enquiry and give opportunity to the registered medical practitioner to be heard in person or by pleader. If the medical practitioner is found to be guilty of committing professional misconduct, the appropriate Medical Council may award such punishment as deemed necessary or may direct the removal altogether or for a specified period, from the register of the name of the delinquent registered practitioner and publications of different Medical Associations/ Societies/Bodies.

8.3. In case the punishment of removal from the register is for a limited period, the appropriate council may also direct that the name so removed shall be restored in the register after the expiry of the period for which the name was ordered to be removed.

8.4. Decision on complaint against delinquent physician shall be taken within a time limit of 6 months.

8.5. During the pendency of the complain the appropriate council may restrain the physician from performing the procedure or practice which is under scrutiny.

8.6. Professional incompetence shall be judged by peer groups as per guidelines prescribed by the Medical Council of India.

Since it has been made clear what is expected out of an upright, honest, straightforward physician, we shall be deliberating on a practice which is deviant from normal or optimal. In today's era there is rapid development and growth in every area coupled with increased awareness among people. Patients often confront negative medical outcomes, occasionally due to negligence or complications of illness or combination of circumstances, and in turn they become legally injured. Over 500,000 practising doctors see millions of patients every day in India, 20% patients have sued their physicians. Medical errors each year in India are estimated to be between 34000 and 79000. The overall picture which emerges out of these studies is disheartening.

Once there is a legal injury its redressal is obligatory. Under the following fora and courts the complaint against the doctor shall lie:

- **Indian Medical Council or State Medical Council**
  - Warning, Deletion – temporarily or permanent your name from the medical register
- **Consumer Court**
  - Usually compensation
- **Civil Court**
  - Usually compensation, occasionally imprisonment
- **Criminal Court**
  - Usually imprisonment and/or fine

Why the complaint arises

It arises because of

(1) Negligence

(2) Professional Misconduct.

Negligence

Negligence is the breach of a duty to take care which results in damage to the person receiving service. Legally defined "Negligence as Tort is the breach of a duty caused by omission to do something which a reasonable man would do or doing something which a prudent and reasonable man would not do".

Constituents of negligence

(a) A legal duty to exercise due care

(b) Breach of duty

(c) Consequential damage

(a) **Legal duty:** This duty arises when there is a doctor patient relationship which can be contractual or gratuitous and also when patient is a consumer and service rendered to the patient is "service" under CPA.

(b) **Breach of duty:** Whenever the doctor readies to deliver medical advice and treatment he owes to the patient following duties:

- Duty of care in deciding whether to undertake the case.
- Duty of deciding what treatment to give.
- Duty of care in administering such treatment.

A breach of any of the above gives a right of action for negligence to the patient.

(c) **Consequential damage:** When as a result of breach of duty the patient suffers damage, the doctor becomes liable.

Negligence can be

- CIVIL or
- CRIMINAL.

Civil Negligence: Resultant damage to the patient has to be compensated by claims decided either in civil court under the law of torts or consumer forum. It is a milder form of negligence founded on a mere error of judgment or defect of intelligence or lack of care.

A professional may be held liable for negligence if he was not possessed of the requisite skill which he professed to have possessed or he did not exercise with reasonable competence in the given case the skill which he did possess.

Criminal Negligence: Here the degree of negligence would justify a conviction and must be culpable or of gross nature. It should be something more than a mere omission or neglect of duty. In criminal cases there must be mens rea or guilty mind. Rashness or a guilt of a degree which can be described as criminal negligence, mere carelessness is not enough.

Rea Ipsa loquitor

It means "the thing speaks for itself". The three elements to prove the above are:

1. Nature of injury is such that even a lay man can recognize it.
2. The person (doctor) in command had the exclusive control over the instrument or treatment that caused the injury.
3. The patient did not contribute to the injury, e.g.,

(a) Treatment by quack/unqualified person.

(b) Amputation of wrong limb/finger.

(c) Operating the wrong patient/wrong side/wrong eye.

(d) Leaving sponges/instrument inside the body cavity during operation.

(e) Causing extensive burns during surgery/anesthesia.

But simply because a patient has not responded favourably to a treatment given by the doctor or a surgery has failed, the doctor cannot be held straightaway liable for medical negligence by applying the doctrine of rea ipsa loquitor. No sensible professional would intentionally commit an act or omission which would result in harm or injury to the patient.

Professional misconduct

(a) Violation of regulation (under the mode of medical ethics).

(b) Adultery or improper conduct.

(c) Conviction by court of law for offences involving moral turpitude/criminal acts.

(d) Signing false/improper certificates, reports and other documents.

Criminal offences

These are punishable with various terms of imprisonment following violation of different statutory acts. PNDT Act, Organ Transplant Act, Biomedical Waste Management, M.T.P. Act and others.

How to diffuse the grievance, avoid the complaint or else defend it

(a) Doctor patient relationship

Physicians who carefully listen to patient and comfortably share medical information with them have discovered the cornerstone of the art of medicine.

A healthy doctor patient relationship can make a difficult diagnosis more bearable for the patient. It can help a resistant patient understand the need for a medication or procedure. Evidence shows that a clear two-way conversation is a key element in the prevention of patient dissatisfaction and malpractice claim. In fact, many episodes of patient dissatisfaction triggered by an iatrogenic injury or other adverse outcome can be defused by a reasonable explanation from the physician who has established a good basis for communication. On the other hand, inadequate communication and misunderstanding is often the inciting agent that transforms a poor medical outcome into legal action against a physician even when quality care was delivered.

(b) Do's & Don'ts for doctors

DOs

(1) Mention your qualification/warning/experience/designation on the prescription. Avoid mentioning memberships/scholarships or awards.

(2) Always mention date and time of consultation.

(3) Mention age/sex of patient and also the weight in pediatric patients.
(4) Address your patient appropriately and modify your greeting as your relationship progresses.
(5) Maintain healthy eye contact.
(6) Limit the use of medical jargon.
(7) Provide emotional support to grieving anxious frightened depressed patient.
(8) Maintain the condition of patient in specific/objective terms.
(9) Record history of drug allergy.
(10) Write name of drugs clearly. Use correct dosage.
(11) Give instruction to the patient in comprehensible terms.
(12) Mention likely side effects.
(13) Remember major drug interactions.
(14) Always advise the patient not to stop taking a drug suddenly which required to be tapered before it is stopped.
(15) Prescription with cautions during pregnancy/lactation.
(16) Adjust dose in case of child/elderly patient and in renal/hepatic disorders.
(17) If you are not sure about the disease, get a consultation, develop a list of physicians you trust and respect in the concerned speciality.
(18) Whenever referring a patient, provide him with a referring note.
(19) Always keep with you and refer to the latest edition on standard textbooks of your branch of medicine. Always subscribe to at least one standard journal and participate in at least 2 updates/conferences every year.
(20) Preferably employ qualified assistants. If not, impart proper training and skill at your, or some appropriate, centre.
(21) Always obtain a legally valid consent before undertaking a surgical/diagnostic procedure.
(22) It is important to screen every patient for hepatitis B/HIV infection before every surgery/blood transfusion to avoid false claims.
(23) Routinely advise X-rays in injury to bones and joint-related diseases of bones and joint.
(24) Always read reports carefully and interpret the result of test/X-ray properly and make a note of it.
(25) In case of death of patient occurring while during surgery/diagnostic/procedure, police authorities must be informed without loss of time. In such cases autopsy/post mortem is mandatory.
(26) In case hospital/clinics claiming to provide 24 hours emergency service, availability of necessary equipment in working order and competent staff within reasonable time is mandatory.

DON'Ts

(1) Don't be overconfident or look confident.
(2) Don't prescribe a drug or include a procedure if you can't justify its indication.
(3) Don't prescribe a drug which is banned.
(4) Don't over/under-prescribe or prescribe multiple drugs.
(5) Don't do anything beyond your level of competence.
(6) Don't refuse if the patient/attendant want to leave against medical advice. It is their right, document this properly.
(7) Don't hold the patient back in the hospital even if the dues are not paid. This is wrongful confinement and criminal. You can file a separate civil suit for recovery of the dues.
(8) Never guarantee the outcome of a treatment orally or in writing. Prepare patient for any pain discomfort and disability that they can responsibly expect from diagnostic or therapeutic intervention.
(9) Never criticize another physician's management with words or gestures. Malpractice cases have often been precipitated by criticism of this kind and you may find yourself as an expert witness, based on your comments.
(10) Don't refuse the patients right to know about diagnosis and treatment of his illness.
(11) Don't tell patient/attendant any bad news unless you are very sure.
(12) Don't leave at the moment of death.
(13) Don't divulge secrets you come to know during your professional duties unless there are exceptions as carved out in the code of medical ethics.
(14) Don't inform that the patient is infected with HIV unless confirmatory test result is available.
(15) Don't issue a false medical certificate.

(16) Don't refuse first aid/medical care to accident and emergency cases if it is a medicolegal case. It is a primary duty of every doctor/hospital to provide treatment up to its true level of competence before referring them to a higher center if required.

(17) Don't dump hospital garbage including used disposable in the open. It is criminal. If the facility of treatment of biomedical waste is not available at your end, contact such service providers.

(18) Don't adopt experimental method in treatment.

(19) Don't evade questions regarding hospital charge. Be open and frank concerning the cost of care.

(20) Avoid suddenly terminating the relationship with the patient. You may have to offer to continue treatment for at least 30 days and provide the alternative avenues of treatment.

(c) Defence

(1) Proper documentation and record-keeping: Mention date, time, history, positive physical findings, investigation, treatment and instruction given. History of drug allergies, referrals and second opinions should be mentioned, a note of erring patient should be made, of unreliable history refusing admissions, not following instructions, etc.

The prognosis should be explained in simple language, value of legally valid consent cannot be overemphasized, record of patient should be preserved for three years because:

(a) **Under CPA limitation of filing a complaint is two years.**

(b) **Under law of tort, limitation is three years.**

(2) Professional indemnity insurance: Presently all insurance companies are nationalized and hence term & conditions are almost identical, however, proper discussions are helpful to avoid later complications.

(3) Establishment policy: This will help taking care of your subordinate staff and any untoward incidence occurring on account of any system failure.

Be careful because no liability would arise on the part of company in respect of any criminal act/unlawful act, such as:

- Service rendered under the effect of intoxicants or narcotics.
- Claims arising from any condition directly/indirectly caused by HIV.
- Use of drugs for weight reduction, cosmetic surgery.

Any policy is void if there is misstatement or suppression of fact at your end.

Remember you are consumer for insurance companies. If these companies fail to reimburse, you can also take them to consumer court.

(4) Be a part of any medical defence societies and develop a strong peer support.

(5) Avoid defending a case of gross negligence or glaring deviation from the accepted norms of code of ethics.

Also note a doctor will not be held negligent under the following grounds:

(1) Contributory negligence.

(2) Damage due to consultation to the third party without knowledge of the doctor.

(3) Complaint is time-barred.

(4) Damage was due to some unavoidable risk taken in good faith with the consent of patient.

(5) Therapeutic/diagnostic misadventure – which is not due to carelessness.

(6) Merely because doctor chose one course of action in preference to other one available. He would not be liable if the course of action chosen by him was acceptable to medical profession.

Present day legal scenario

Since the promulgation of Consumer Protection Act in 1986 when service provided by the medical professional was included as 'service' u/s 2, the wheel of medicolegal cart has turned a full circle. As the awareness of a common man grew, he started dragging his doctor, whom he once considered God, into the courtroom. Number of cases were decided against the doctors and equally they were dismissed. Claims ranging from few thousands to crores were slapped against the doctors in district, state consumer forums and national commission.

Average medical man was on the backfoot. He started defensive practice, indulged in costly investigation, refusing emergency and referring serious patient and in turn valuable lives were lost and resources wasted. The patient who once looked happy receiving the redressal for his grievance started becoming the ultimate loser. This was most appropriately observed by the Hon'ble Supreme court when it observed in "Jacob Mathews" case.

"A medical practitioner faced with an emergency ordinarily tries his best to redeem the patient out of his suffering. He does not gain anything by acting with negligence or by omitting to do an act. A surgeon with shaky hands under fear of legal action cannot perform a successful operation and a quivering physician cannot administer the end dose of medicine to his patient."

The Hon'ble Supreme Court in a recently decided case viz. Martin F D'souza v/s Mohd Ishfaq (Civil appeal of No. 3541 of 2002 old 17.02.09 2009 (2) RCR p 64-86) elaborated its observations on the subject of medical negligence.

(1) The professional may be held liable for negligence on the ground that he was not possessed of the requisite skill which he professes to have. Thus a doctor who has a qualification in Ayurvedic or Homeopathy medicine will be liable if he prescribes Allopathic treatment which causes some harm.

(2) Whenever a court or consumer forum receives a complaint against a doctor it should refer the matter to a panel of experts. A notice should be issued to the concerned doctor only after the committee finds that there was a prima facie case of medical negligence.

(3) A private complaint should not be entertained unless the complainant has produced prima facie evidence before the court in the form of credible opinion by another competent doctor to support the charge of rashness on the part of the accused doctor.

(4) The investigating officer, before proceeding against the doctor accused of rash or negligent act or omission, obtain an independent and competent medical opinion preferably from a doctor in government service qualified in that branch of medical practice who can normally be expected to give an impartial opinion applying the BOLAM Test.

(5) A doctor accused of negligence should not be arrested in a routine manner, simply because a charge has been levelled against him unless his arrest is necessary for furthering or collecting evidence and unless the investigating officer feels satisfied that the doctor proceeded against would not make himself available to face the prosecution unless arrested.

(6) The medical practitioner is not liable to be held negligent simply because things went wrong from mischance or misadventure or through an error of judgement in choosing one reasonable course of treatment in preference to another. He would be liable only when his conduct fell below that of a reasonably competent doctor in his field, for instance he would be liable if he leaves a surgical gauge inside the patient after an operation.

(7) To fasten liability in criminal proceedings, e.g., Section 304 A IPC, the degree of negligence has to be higher than the negligence which is enough to hold the doctor liable in civil proceedings.

(8) Basic principle relating to law of medical negligence is the BOLAM rule – The test in fixing negligence is the standard of ordinary skilled doctor exercising and professing to have that skill, but a doctor need not have to possess the highest expert skills.

(9) Doctors who cause death and agony due to negligence should certainly be penalized and it must be remembered that like all professionals doctors too can make errors of judgement and if they are punished left and right, no doctor can practise his vocation with equanimity. Indiscriminate proceedings and decisions against doctors are counterproductive and serve society no good. They inhibit the free exercise of judgement by a professional in a particular situation.

For the benefit of medical fraternity certain observations of the Hon'ble Supreme Court and National Consumer Forum are quoted below from recently decided cases viz. Malay Kumar Ganguly v/s Sukumar Mukherjee & Others (decided on 7/8/09), Postgraduate Institute of Medical Education & Research, Chandigarh v/s Jaipal Singh and others (decided on 29/5/09), V. Krishana Rao v/s Nikhil Superspeciality and Anr (decided on 8/3/2010), Ashok Kumar Upadhaya v/s Dr. D.N. Mishra (National Commission decided on 2/2/2011).

The jurisprudential concept of negligence differs in civil and criminal law. For negligence to amount to an offence the element of mens rea must be shown to exist. To prosecute a medical professional for negligence under criminal law it must be shown that accused did something or failed to do something which in the given facts and circumstances no medical professional in his ordinary senses would have done or have failed to do.

Medical science is a difficult one, the court for the purpose of arriving at a decision on the basis of opinion of experts must take into consideration the difference between an expert witness and ordinary witness. The opinion must be based on a person having special skill or knowledge in medical science. It could be admitted or denied. Whether such evidence could be admitted or how much weight should be given thereto lies within the domain of the court. The evidence of an expert should, however, be interpreted like any other evidence.

If a decision is taken that all cases of medical negligence had to be proven on the basis of expert evidence, in that event efficacy of the remedy provided will be unnecessarily burdened and in many cases such remedy would be illusory fact.

Giving a word of caution to District Consumer Fora the Hon'ble Supreme Court said that there cannot be a mechanical or straitjacket approach that each and every case must be referred to experts for evidence. When the forum finds that expert evidence is required, the forum must keep in mind that an expert witness in a given case normally has to discharge two functions. First duty of the expert is to explain the technical issue as clearly as possible so that it can be understood by a common man. Other function is to assist the forum in deciding whether the act or omission of the medical personnel or hospital constitute negligence. Medical negligence is a mixed question of fact and law and the forum is not bound in every case to accept the opinion of the expert witness.

Regarding the burden of proof, the Hon'ble Supreme Court said the simple law would be that once the initial burden has been discharged by the complainant by making out a case of negligence against the hospital or the doctor concerned, the onus then shifts onto the hospital or to the attending doctor and it is for the hospital to satisfy the court that there was no lack of care or diligence (Savita Garg v/s Director National Heart Institute).

The Hon'ble Supreme Court reemphasized the precautions which a doctor or hospital should take:

(1) Current practices, infrastructure, paramedical and other staff, hygiene and sterility should be observed strictly.
(2) No prescription should ordinarily be given without actual examination. The tendency to give prescription over phone except in acute emergency should be avoided.
(3) A doctor should not merely go by the version of the patient regarding his symptoms, but should also make his own analysis including tests and investigations where necessary.
(4) A doctor should not experiment unless necessary and even then he should ordinarily get the written consent from the patient.
(5) An expert should be consulted in case of any doubt.

VIOLENCE AGAINST DOCTORS

In the recent past it was observed that incidences of violence against medical fraternity are on the rise. Man in the street has become more intolerant. Unsatisfied patients or their relatives are no more hesitant in abusing or else assaulting the doctors or nurses and paramedics. They find gratification in damaging hospitals and smashing medical equipments. Be it a crowded emergency of Hindu Rao Hospital, PGIMS Rohtak, nursing homes of Haryana or the posh hospitals of Mumbai the scenes of violence are not rare. Junior doctors, nurses and paramedics have borne the brunt. Keeping all this in view the government has enacted "The MEDICARE SERVICE PERSONS and MEDICARE INSTITUTIONS (Prevention of Violence and Damage to Property) ACT 2008". Such Act was already in vogue in few other States. Under this Act any individual himself or as a member/leader of a group indulges in or abets or incites any act of violence against Medicare Service Person including doctor, student doctor, nurses, student nurses or any Medicare Service Institutions including any medical equipment shall get a three year term in jail and a fine of Rs 50,000/- and shall be liable to pay twice the amount of the cost of the equipment destroyed. The offence under this Act has been made cognizable and nonbailable.

IT IS HOPED THAT NOW DOCTORS SHALL BE ABLE TO WORK IN MORE CONGENIAL ATMOSPHERE AND GIVE THEIR BEST TO THE AILING COMMUNITY.

"THOUGHTS BECOME ACTIONS, ACTIONS BECOME HABITS, HABITS BECOME CHARACTER". Remember you have chosen the medical profession to serve the ailing humanity.

Index

Q

R

S

T